Leptin

Sam Dagogo-Jack
Editor

Leptin

Regulation and Clinical Applications

Springer

Editor
Sam Dagogo-Jack, MD
Division of Endocrinology, Diabetes and Metabolism
University of Tennessee Health Science Center
Memphis, TN, USA

ISBN 978-3-319-09914-9 ISBN 978-3-319-09915-6 (eBook)
DOI 10.1007/978-3-319-09915-6
Springer Cham Heidelberg New York Dordrecht London

Library of Congress Control Number: 2014952453

Printed on acid-free paper

Springer is part of Springer Science+Business Media (www.springer.com)

This book is dedicated to the memory of Douglas Coleman (1931–2014) for his insightful and prescient contributions to our understanding of the biological and genetic basis of obesity and the regulation of body weight.

Foreword

Jeffrey Friedman, MD, PhD

Background

The American author F. Scott Fitzgerald wrote that "there are no second acts in American lives" meaning that in the USA, life's narrative deviated from the standard framework for a classic story in which things start out well in the first act, fall apart in the second, and are happily resolved in the third. By this criterion, leptin is not an American hormone. Leptin's first act was filled with great excitement about the intrinsic importance of its discovery and the excitement that it might become, if not a panacea for the treatment of obesity, an effective treatment. In its second act, with the realization that its utility for treating obesity was limited, the excitement withered; despite that fact, it and other contemporaneous advances paved the way for a deeper and still evolving understanding of the neural mechanisms that control food intake, body weight, and metabolism. These findings established that body weight and appetite are regulated by a previously undiscovered hormonal system that provides an alternative to the explanation that obesity was simply caused by a lapse in willpower.

This year may mark the beginning of leptin's third act as last February, 20 years after its discovery, leptin is now an FDA-approved human therapeutic for the treatment of severe lipodystrophy with potential for the treatment of other disorders, http://www.fda.gov/newsevents/newsroom/pressannouncements/ucm387060.htm. In addition, though leptin's utility as a monotherapy for obesity appears limited, other evidence suggests that it still has potential as part of a combination therapy for this disorder.

Thus 50 years after the original identification of the ob mutation and 20 after the identification of leptin, we know that food intake and body weight are regulated by a classical endocrine feedback loop [1–3]. That the ob gene encoded a hormonal signal was suggested in the original paper reporting the identification of this ob gene in which it was found that there is marked overexpression of the *ob* gene in C57Bl/6J *ob/ob* adipose tissue. This suggested that the gene was under feedback control, with a secondary increase in the level of ob gene expression in obese animals.

This finding that the *ob* gene was induced in *ob/ob* fat tissue was consistent with data from classic parabiosis experiments of Doug Coleman in a now-iconic set of experiments that involved stitching together the skins of living mice so that animals with different mutations shared a circulatory

Friedman J 2014 20 YEARS OF LEPTIN: Leptin at 20: an overview.
Journal of Endocrinology 223 T1–T8. (doi:10.1530/JOE-14-0405)

system [4]. *ob* mice surgically joined to normal or *db* mice (on the same inbred strain background) ate less and lost weight. In contrast, normal mice paired to *db* mice starved to death. From this, Coleman concluded that *ob* mice normally lacked a circulating factor, provided by the conjoined partner, that suppressed food intake and body weight. He further suggested that *db* mice lacked a receptor to detect the weight-suppressing factor in their blood and so overexpressed it, producing levels so high that conjoined mice sensitive to the factor stopped eating. Implicit in this hypothesis was the prediction that the *ob* gene was under feedback control and that obesity would be associated with increased levels of *ob* RNA. However Coleman's experiments did not predict where the hormone that was missing in *ob* mice was expressed, though prior experiments from Hervey predicted that the receptor would be expressed in the hypothalamus [5]. The aggregate data at the time thus suggested the hypothesis that the *ob* gene encoded a novel adipocyte hormone which functioned as the afferent signal in a negative feedback loop that maintains homeostatic control of adipose tissue mass.

Subsequent studies have confirmed that leptin is an adipose tissue hormone that acts on the hypothalamus as part of a new endocrine system that maintains homeostatic control of fat mass [6–9]. This system regulates food intake and metabolism and also links changes in nutritional state to adaptive changes in most other physiologic systems. While some of the features of this new hormonal system were predicted at the time, others were not. Science seldom proceeds in a straight line, and the field spawned by the identification of leptin and other genes that cause obesity is no exception.

Thus there have been surprises and disappointments and the passage of time now provides an opportunity to chronicle, as this timely volume does, what has been learned, what was surprising, and what some of the key questions are.

Wiring Diagram of a Complex Behavior

One can describe the phenotype of *ob* and *db* mice in several different ways. Historically these animals have been described as obesity mutations but one could also think of these animals as showing a behavioral phenotype. *ob* and *db* mice show abnormalities in numerous behaviors [10]. They show profound hyperphagia, exhibit a dramatic decrease in locomotor activity, are quite gentle and non-aggressive, and are not sexually active. Thus the identification of leptin and later the localization of the leptin receptor [8, 9], encoded by the *db* gene, have provided an entry point for delving into the neural mechanisms that control complex behaviors. Moreover the elucidation of the pathogenesis of the obesity resulting from the Ay (yellow agouti) mutation has identified hypothalamic neurons expressing POMC, the precursor of αMSH, as a key neural target of leptin, and as integrators of numerous metabolic signals [11]. αMSH acts on the MC4 receptor, a GPCR, and MC4R mutations replicate the obese phenotype of Ay mice [12]. The subsequent identification of AGRP as an endogenous inhibitor in a second group of hypothalamic neurons also expressing NPY identified another population of leptin-responsive neurons [13, 14]. We now know that leptin acts in part by activating POMC neurons and inhibiting NPY/AGRP neurons though clearly many other neural populations also play a role either as additional neural targets or downstream of these neurons [15]. Indeed enormous progress has been made in defining a set of overlapping neural circuits that control food intake and body weight. These findings provide entry points for a deeper understanding of how feeding behavior is controlled as well as advancing our understanding of the control of other behaviors.

Thus, leptin's neurobiologic effects are not limited to feeding circuits. Extreme weight loss in human has been shown to induce a set of emotional sequelae including depression. A possible role for a reduction in leptin in mediating some portion of this was suggested by the finding that leptin injection into the hippocampus can improve the performance of animals in a forced swim test [16]. This assay provides a quantitative indication of the level of depression in animals and robustly predicts the efficacy of antidepressant drugs in human. Other studies have shown that leptin has significant effects on reward processing by dopaminergic centers in the midbrain and that it can reduce the value of a sucrose reward [17]. This is important because it shows that the pleasure we derive from eating is not fixed but rather reflects the status of metabolic signals such as leptin. Leptin also has potent effects on many other neural circuits including those controlling hormones that regulate reproduction and reproductive behaviors, activity, thermoregulation, and stress [16, 18, 19].

Obesity Has a Substantial Genetic Component

The identification of mutant genes that cause obesity in mice provided a molecular framework for identifying mutant genes that cause obesity in human. Thus, mutations in leptin, the leptin receptor (LepR), the MC4R as well as PCSK1, and enzymes required for the processing of POMC cause human obesity as do other components of the neural circuit that regulates food intake including BDNF, and Sim1. Indeed it now appears that >10 % of morbid human obesity is a result of Mendelian defects in these and other genes, which in the majority of cases are in MC4R and LepR [20]. This is a level of Mendelian inheritance that exceeds that for any other complex trait that has been studied. The realization that obesity is often the result of genetic mutations in human provides strong evidence that this condition is a result of alterations in a neural circuit that controls the basic drive to eat as well as metabolism (and perhaps other behaviors) and provides an alternative to the widely held view that obesity develops from a failure of willpower or consequent to the modern environment.

Furthermore, it is interesting all of the obesity genes identified thus far are expressed in the brain. This is despite the fact that there is large body of evidence indicating that differences in metabolic rate can predict changes in weight [21] and that an increase in peripheral metabolism such as after treatment with thyroid hormone, or uncouplers of respiration such as dinitrophenol, leads to weight loss [22, 23]. Moreover, while a defect in leptin signaling is associated with hyperphagia and a marked decrease in energy expenditure in mice, the principal effect in human is on appetite with little or no discernible effect on metabolism [24].

The hereditability of obesity has been reported to be between 0.7 and 0.8, which is higher than that for most other traits [25]. That there is a substantial genetic contribution to obesity is also supported by adoption and familial aggregation studies [26, 27]. However, while some fraction of obesity can be attributed to the aforementioned Mendelian defects as well as variation in genes identified in GWAS studies such as FTO, it is clear that many new genes remain to be discovered [28]. It is likely that the use of high-throughput genomic sequencing to look for variation in patients with extreme phenotypes, will lead to the identification of new genes [29]. It will be of particular interest to learn whether these new genes also function in the neural circuit that is modulated by leptin. It is quite likely that future volumes on leptin will need to take into account additional as yet unidentified components of the neural circuit that regulates weight that one can anticipate will be found in genetic analyses of human patients.

Leptin Deficiency

Leptin-deficient *ob* mice show abnormalities in most, perhaps all, physiologic systems [10]. Thus these animals show defects in the entire neuroendocrine axis and are infertile or subfertile and euthyroid sick and have markedly increased plasma corticosterone levels. In addition to these global effects on the neuroendocrine axis, *ob* mice are hypothermic and diabetic, and have profound immune and hematologic dysfunction. Indeed the complex phenotype of these animals initially led some to question whether the identification of the *ob* gene would advance our understanding of how food intake and body weight are regulated. In retrospect, the complex phenotype of these mice can be most easily understood by noting that the abnormalities they manifest are generally associated not with obesity, but rather starvation [30, 31]. This observation is consistent with the findings that plasma leptin falls after fasting and that that leptin administration suppresses the neuroendocrine response to food restriction in mice [32]. These findings and others suggest that a key function of leptin is to communicate information to the brain that there are adequate fat stores and that the organism is not starving. In its absence, a set of physiologic responses in many organ systems are elicited, the aggregate effect of which is to reduce energy expenditure at the same time as appetite is stimulated.

In addition to its intrinsic importance, this aspect of leptin function provides a framework for understanding its efficacy for treating a series of leptin deficient states. In each case, leptin treatment improves one or more abnormalities generally associated with starvation. As outlined in this volume, lipodystrophy, the complete or partial absence of fat, is a heterogeneous disorder associated with leptin deficiency and a severe, sometimes intractable, insulin resistance and diabetes as well as hyperlipidemia and NASH [33]. Similarly, as also discussed in this volume, the leanness of young women who often exercise with great avidity is also associated with leptin deficiency and hypothalamic amenorrhea (HA) [34]. This condition is characterized by a failure to menstruate, infertility, and also osteoporosis [35]. Leptin replacement therapy improves the abnormalities associated with lipodystrophy and HA and also includes a significant improvement of bone mineral density in HA patients. Leptin confers these beneficial effects despite causing weight loss in treated patients. In addition, leptin-deficient patients also show extreme weight loss after leptin therapy with marked improvements in their metabolic profile, a restoration of fertility and improvements in immune function despite losing weight. These data strongly suggest that overall nutritional state, as reflected by fat stores, is conveyed by leptin and not by the actual amount of lipid stored in adipose tissue.

In general the more extreme the abnormalities of patients with low leptin levels, the more significant the clinical response to leptin therapy. This raises the possibility that leptin might have potential as a treatment for other pathologies that develop in the setting of leptin deficiency. For example, some female leptin deficient patients fail to enter puberty in adolescence even though their bone age indicated they should have, and leptin treatment led to the onset of menses. This suggests that leptin might be used to induce puberty in very lean young women with a delayed onset of puberty [24].

Both leptin-deficient and -starved individuals show immune abnormalities with a shift from TH1 to TH 2 immunity and an increased susceptibility to infectious disease and leptin treatment of leptin-deficient humans and -starved animals reverses these changes [31, 32, 36]. Thus it is possible that leptin could be used as an immune adjuvant in settings of extreme cachexia such as starvation, cancer or chronic inflammatory or infectious disease. It has even been proposed that leptin might be useful in patients with end stage anorexia nervosa with the hope that low-dose leptin treatment could ameliorate some of the pathology associated with leptin deficiency without significantly reducing food intake (further) and/or as an adjunct to parenteral nutrition (C. Mantzoros, personal communication).

Leptin might also be of benefit in patients who do not manifest signs or symptoms of pathologic deficiency of leptin (i.e., starvation) but who, nonetheless, are leptin sensitive (in contrast to most obese patients who are leptin resistant, see below). Prior studies in animals have shown that leptin stimulates glucose metabolism in wild-type mice independent of weight loss and that it can improve the diabetes of lipodystropic mice independent of insulin [37, 38]. This raised the possibility that leptin might show efficacy for the treatment of type 1 diabetes. This possibility has now been tested in streptozotocin-treated mice that are either partially or completely insulin deficient. In both cases, leptin markedly lowered blood glucose. Indeed in one study, untreated insulin-deficient animals all died within 1 month while treated animals survived as long as leptin continued to be expressed from an adenoviral vector [39]. Further evidence has suggested that leptin elicits its antidiabetic effects by inhibiting glucagon [39]. This has raised the possibility that leptin might also be of benefit for patients with type 1 diabetes who often present with weight loss and hyperphagia as a consequence of complete or partial insulin deficiency. In this setting leptin could either alleviate the demands on the decreasing number of surviving β cells at the onset of the disease and/or be used to supplement insulin at later stages of the disease as a means for smoothing glucose control with less hyperglycemia. Leptin treatment might also minimize the weight gain that is often associated with insulin therapy. Further studies will be necessary to evaluate these possibilities.

Leptin Resistance

Physiologic increases in plasma leptin level in wild-type mice lead to a dose dependent reduction of food intake and loss of weight [40]. While leptin has potent effects to reduce food intake and body weight in *ob* and wild type animals, its efficacy in obese animals is variable and often reduced [40]. Animals with mutations in the leptin receptor fail to respond to leptin treatment as do Ay mice that, as mentioned, have a defect in melanocortin signaling. Diet-induced obese animals show only a small response to leptin while New Zealand obese mice, a strain that develops a polygenic form of obesity, fail to respond to leptin when delivered peripherally but lose significant amounts of weight when leptin is delivered ICV. Each of these strains has high plasma levels of leptin which in combination with the diminished effect of leptin treatment suggests that they, and by extension hyperleptinemic obese patients, are leptin resistant.

The extreme case of leptin resistance is the *db* mouse which has a mutation in the leptin receptor [8, 9]. In the absence of leptin action, animals become obese and secondarily overproduce the hormone. Thus obesity satisfies the hallmarks of a hormone resistance syndrome, with an attenuated response to exogenously administered hormone and elevated endogenous levels [41]. In addition, mutations in genes in the leptin signal transduction pathway, PTP1B and SOCS3, increase leptin signaling and lead to a resistance to obesity, thus identifying potential biochemical mechanisms [42, 43]. Both PTP1B and SOCS3 act to suppress leptin signaling and knocking these genes out amplified leptin signaling. It is not clear whether these genes contribute to the leptin resistance that develops in animals or humans. Moreover, leptin resistance is complex, and can in principle develop at many points in the neural circuit that regulates feeding. Thus leptin resistance can also develop downstream of leptin target neurons as in Ay and MC4R knockout mice, which abrogates melanocortin signaling from POMC neurons [11]. Similar to other hormones, leptin resistance can also develop in response to chronically elevated hormone levels via tachyphylaxis [44]. Finally, as discussed in this volume, leptin resistance can develop because of impaired leptin transport although little is known about the transcytotic mechanism by which leptin crosses the blood brain barrier [45].

In humans, leptin is highly potent in patients with low endogenous levels but its effects in otherwise normal lean patients have not been studied [24, 33–35]. In contrast, leptin has variable effects as monotherapy for obesity in the general population. Initial studies showed encouraging effects at very high doses (0.3 mg/kg bid) but this dose was too high for general usage and a lower dose (0.1 mg/kg bid) did not show efficacy [46]. However a more recent study treating obese patients with an even lower dose (0.05 mg/kg) led to ~5 % weight loss equivalent with efficacy equivalent to other pharmacotherapies for obesity [47]. It is thus possible that higher doses of leptin led to tachyphylaxis and that larger study of patients treated with leptin at 0.05 mg/kg or lower could replicate the weight loss observed in the earlier study. There is also evidence that some obese patients show a greater response to leptin than others. In light of the potency of leptin in leptin deficient patients with low endogenous leptin levels, it is possible that the one could enrich for the responder subset by selecting obese patients with low leptin levels. Indeed, while leptin level is highly correlated with adipose tissue mass ($r=0.9$), plasma leptin still can vary by tenfold or more among patients of the same BMI [41]. That obese patients with low leptin levels might show a greater response to leptin therapy is suggested by studies in mice with constitutively low levels of leptin gene expression. These animals become obese and remain leptin sensitive [48, 49]. Consistent with this, patients with heterozygous leptin mutations are obese with low leptin levels [48, 49].

The efficacy of leptin for the treatment of obesity increases when it is combined with other agents that cause weight loss, in particular short-term signals including intestinal peptides that modulate meal pattern. For example, both leptin and amylin (pramlintide), a pancreatic peptide that is approved for the treatment of diabetes, caused ~5 % weight loss in a selected group of patients while the two agents appeared were synergistic when co-administered with an average weight loss of 13 % [47]. Studies in animals showed that pretreatment of diet induced obese animals with amylin restored leptin's ability to phosphorylate Stat3 in the hypothalamus suggesting that this gut peptide might reduce the activity of neural circuits that cause leptin resistance [50]. In, animals, leptin's efficacy has also been augmented in combinations with other peptides or hormones, raising the possibility that in time it could emerge as part of a combination therapy for obesity [51]. Bariatric surgery is an alternative means for inducing weight loss and, while invasive, can be extremely effective. Leptin falls after this procedure, in proportion to the amount of the weight loss, and it is possible that leptin treatment in this setting could reduce recidivism and/or mitigate some of the sequelae of the procedure that might be secondary to the relative leptin deficiency that develops [52].

Questions for the Future

While much has been learned, the road ahead is likely to lead to new advances and some surprises. Still some key questions remain unanswered including the aforementioned. How is leptin transported into the CNS?

What regulates leptin gene expression? Leptin gene expression is correlated with the intracellular lipid content of adipocytes, suggesting that its regulation might be coupled to a lipid-sensing mechanism [41, 53]. The nature of this putative lipid-sensing mechanism is unknown.

How does leptin control metabolism? What is the role of leptin signaling in peripheral tissues or, instead, are most or all of its effects mediated by the CNS? What are the physiologic and cellular mechanisms by which leptin reduces adipose deposits in fat and other tissues? What are the physiologic and cellular mechanisms by which leptin improves glucose metabolism?

Finally, how does leptin modulate a complex motivational behavior? Leptin acts directly on a number of CNS sites to reduce food intake and body weight in animals and humans and provides an entry point to study the control of feeding [40]. Feeding is a complex motivational behavior controlled by many inputs including smell, taste, hormonal state, cognitive inputs, etc. Recently it has been shown that leptin acts in part by regulating hedonic circuitry but the anatomic site(s) responsible for initiating feeding behavior have proven elusive [17]. Thus it is not known how or even when the multiple inputs are processed to formulate a "binary" decision. So perhaps the biggest question is how do we decide to eat or don't eat. Perhaps, the answer to this timeless question will be part of leptin's fourth act.

The present volume, *Leptin-Regulation and Clinical Applications*, which is graciously dedicated to the memory of Doug Coleman, is a timely rendition of the journey leptin has taken so far from bench to bedside. The chapters and authors of this volume have been carefully selected to present an authoritative account of the biology and clinical applications of leptin that expands on the themes summarized in this Foreword. This book should prove valuable to clinicians and scholars interested in obesity, energy homeostasis, neuroendocrinology of weight regulation, and intermediary metabolism. Sam Dagogo-Jack and his colleagues are to be commended for crafting this important work.

References

1. Ingalls AM, Dickie MM, Snell GD. Obese, a new mutation in the house mouse. J Hered. 1950;41:317–8.
2. Zhang Y, Proenca R, Maffei M, Barone M, Leopold L, Friedman JM. Positional cloning of the mouse *obese* gene and its human homologue. Nature. 1994;372:425–32.
3. Moon BC, Friedman JM. The molecular basis of the obese mutation in ob^{2J} mice. Genomics. 1997;42:152–6.
4. Coleman DL. Obese and Diabetes: two mutant genes causing diabetes-obesity syndromes in mice. Diabetologia. 1978;14:141–8.
5. Hervey GR. Regulation of energy balance. Nature. 1969;222:629–31.
6. Friedman JM, Halaas JL. Leptin and the regulation of body weight in mammals. Nature. 1998;395:763–70.
7. Halaas JL, Gajiwala KS, Maffei M, et al. Weight-reducing effects of the plasma protein encoded by the *obese* gene. Science. 1995;269:543–6.
8. Lee GH, Proenca R, Montez JM, et al. Abnormal splicing of the leptin receptor in *diabetic* mice. Nature. 1996;379:632–5.
9. Tartaglia LA, Dembski M, Weng X, et al. Identification and expression cloning of a leptin receptor, OB-R. Cell. 1995;83:1263–71.
10. Bray GA. Obesity, a disorder of nutrient partitioning: The MONA LISA hypothesis. J Nutrition. 1991;121:1146–62.
11. Lu D, Willard D, Patel IR, et al. Agouti protein is an antagonist of the melanocyte-stimulating-hormone receptor. Nature. 1994;371:799–802.
12. Huszar D, Lynch CA, Fairchild-Huntress V, et al. Targeted disruption of the melanocortin-4 receptor results in obesity in mice. Cell. 1997;88:131–41.
13. Ollmann MM, Wilson BD, Yang Y, et al. Antagonism of central melanocortin receptors in vitro and in vivo by agouti-related protein. Science. 1997;278:135–8.
14. Stephens TW, Bashinski M, Bristow PK, et al. The role of neuropeptide Y in the anti-obesity action of the obese gene product. Nature. 1995;377:530–4.

15. Friedman JM. The alphabet of weight control. Nature. 1997;385:119–20.
16. Lu X-Y, Kim C, Frazer A, Zhang W. Leptin: A potential novel antidepressant. Proc Natl Acad Sci USA. 2006;103:1593–8.
17. Domingos AI, Vaynshteyn J, Voss HU, et al. Leptin regulates the reward value of nutrient. Nat Neurosci. 2011;14:1562–8.
18. Atasoy D, Betley JN, Su HH, Sternson S. Deconstruction of a neural circuit for hunger. Nature. 2012;488:172–7.
19. Wu Q, Boyle MP, Palmiter RD. Loss of GABAergic signaling by AgRP neurons to the parabrachial nucleus leads to starvation. Cell. 2009;137:1225–34.
20. Barsh GS, Farooqi IS, O'Rahilly S. Genetics of body-weight regulation. Nature. 2000;404:644–51.
21. Ravussin E, Lillioja S, Knowler WC, et al. Reduced rate of energy expenditure as a risk factor for body-weight gain. N Eng J Med. 1988;318:467–72.
22. GrundlinghJ, Dargan PI, El-Zanfaly M, Wood DM. 2,4-Dinitrophenol (DNP): A weight loss agent with significant acute toxicity and risk of death. J Med Toxicol. 2011;7:205–12.
23. Pearce E. Thyroid hormone and obesity. Curr Opin Endocrinol Diabetes Obes. 2012;19:408–13.
24. Farooqi IS, Jebb S, Langmack G, et al. Effects of recombinant leptin therapy in a child with congenital leptin deficiency. N Engl J Med. 1999;341:879–84.
25. Stunkard AJ, Harris JR, Pedersen NL, McClearn GE. The body-mass index of twins who have been reared apart. N Engl J Med. 1990;322:1483–7.
26. Stunkard AJ, Sorensen T, Hanis C. An adoption study of human obesity. N Eng J Med. 1986;314:193–8.
27. Adams T, Hunt S, Mason L, Ramirez M, Fisher A, Williams R. Familial aggregation of morbid obesity. Obes Res. 1993;1:261–70.
28. Fawcett K, Barroso I. The genetics of obesity: FTO leads the way. Trends Genet. 2010;26:266–74.
29. Ku C, Naidoo N, Pawitan Y. Revisiting Mendelian disorders through exome sequencing. Hum Genet. 2011;129:351–70.
30. Frisch R. Female Fertility and the Body Fat Connection. 2002, Chicago: The University of Chicago
31. Lord G. Leptin modulates the T-cell immune response and reverses starvation induced immunosuppression. Nature. 1998;394:897–91.
32. Ahima RS, Prabakaran D, Mantzoros C, et al. Role of leptin in the neuroendocrine response to fasting. Nature. 1996;382:250–2.
33. Oral EA, Simha V, Ruiz E, et al. Leptin-replacement therapy for lipodystrophy. N Engl J Med. 2002;346:570–8.
34. Welt CK, Chan JL, Bullen J, et al. Recombinant human leptin in women with hypothalamic amenorrhea. N Eng J Med. 2004;351:987–7.
35. Sienkiewicz E, Magkos F, Aronis KN, et al. Long-term metreleptin treatment increases bone mineral density and content at the lumbar spine of lean hypoleptinemic women. Metabolism. 2011;60:1211–21.
36. Ozata MI, Ozdemir I, Licinio J. Human leptin deficiency caused by a missense mutation: multiple endocrine defects, decreased sympathetic tone, and immune system dysfunction indicate new targets for leptin action, greater central than peripheral resistance to the effects of leptin, and spontaneous correction of leptin-mediated defects. J Clin Endocrinol Metab. 1999;84:3686–95.
37. Kamohara S, Burcelin R, Halaas JL, Friedman JM, Charron MJ. Acute stimulation of glucose metabolism in mice by leptin treatment. Nature. 1997;389:374–7.
38. Asilmaz E, Cohen P, Miyazaki M, et al. Site and mechanism of leptin action in a rodent form of congenital lipodystrophy. J Clin Invest. 2004;113:414–24.
39. Wang M, Chen L, Clark G, et al. Leptin therapy in insulin-deficient type I diabetes. Proc Natl Acad Sci U S A. 2010;107:4813–9.
40. Halaas JL, Boozer C, Blair-West J, Fidahusein N, Denton D, Friedman JM. Physiological response to long-term peripheral and central leptin infusion in lean and obese mice. Proc Natl Acad Sci USA. 1997;94:8878–83.
41. Maffei M, Halaas J, Ravussin E, et al. Leptin levels in human and rodent: Measurement of plasma leptin and *ob* RNA in obese and weight-reduced subjects. Nature Medicine. 1995;1:1155–61.

42. Bence K, Delibegovic M, Xue B, et al. Neuronal PTP1B regulates body weight, adiposity and leptin action. Nat Med. 2006;12:917–24.
43. Bjorbak C, Lavery HJ, Bates SH, et al. SOCS3 mediates feedback inhibition of the leptin receptor via Tyr985. J Biol Chem. 2000;275:40649–57.
44. Knight ZA, Hannan KS, Greenberg ML, Friedman JM. Hyperleptinemia is required for the development of leptin resistance. PLoS One. 2010;5(6):e11376.
45. Schwartz MW, Peskind E, Raskind M, Boyko EJ, Porte D, Jr. Cerebrospinal fluid leptin levels: Relationship to plasma levels and to adiposity in humans. Nat Med.1996; 2:589–93.
46. Heymsfield S, Greenberg A, Fujioka K, et al. Recombinant leptin for weight loss in obese and lean adults. JAMA. 1999;282:1568–75.
47. Roth J, Roland B, Cole R, et al. Leptin responsiveness restored by amylin agonism in diet-induced obesity: evidence from nonclinical and clinical studies. Proc Natl Acad Sci. 2008;105:7257–62.
48. Farooqi I, Keogh JM, Kamath S, et al. Partial leptin deficiency and human adiposity. Nature. 2001;414:34–5.
49. Ioffe E, Moon B, Connolly E, Friedman JM. Abnormal regulation of the leptin gene in the pathogenesis of obesity. Proc Natl Acad Sci USA.1998;95:11852–7.
50. Turek V, Tevaskis J, Levin B, et al. Mechanisms of amylin/leptin synergy in rodent models. Endocrinology. 2010;151:143–52.
51. Muller T, Sullivan L, Habegger K, et al. Restoration of leptin responsiveness in diet-induced obese mice using an optimized leptin analog in combination with exendin-4 or FGF21. J Pept Sci. 2012;18:383–93.
52. Rubino F, Gagner M, Gentileschi P, et al. The early effect of the Roux-en-Y gastric bypass on hormones involved in body weight regulation and glucose metabolism. Ann Surg. 2004;240:236–42.
53. Fei H, Okano HJ, Li C, et al. Anatomic localization of alternatively spliced leptin receptors (Ob-R) in mouse brain and other tissues. Proc Natl Acad Sci USA. 1997;94: 7001–5.

Preface

Twenty years after its discovery, a recombinant form of human leptin has been approved by the US Food and Drug Administration for the treatment of patients with congenital or acquired lipodystrophy. However, the promise of leptin as a general treatment for human obesity and related disorders has remained largely elusive. Nonetheless, a tremendous amount of knowledge has emerged on the biology of leptin, and additional potential areas of therapeutic application in humans are gradually coming into focus. In rodents leptin inhibits food intake, stimulates energy expenditure, reverses obesity, ameliorates insulin resistance, and accelerates sexual maturation. These potent and diverse effects have stimulated interest in exploring a role for leptin in the treatment of human metabolic disorders. This book presents current understanding of the biology and regulation of leptin, and discusses established and emerging areas of therapeutic application of leptin in humans.

Beginning with a succinct synthesis of the vast amount of work—in experimental models, in vitro systems, and other avenues—that has enriched our understanding of leptin's biology, the focus of this book shifts to a fuller consideration of the regulation and role of leptin in humans. The emphasis on human-level data is a unique feature of this book. The results of numerous studies indicate that leptin is indeed a regulated human hormone that interacts with a vast array of physiological, hormonal, immunological, and inflammatory mediators and targets. The detailed consideration of these interactions expands our understanding of the role of leptin in human metabolic pathophysiology.

Next follows a comprehensive presentation of the therapeutic trials of recombinant leptin replacement in human subjects with congenital leptin deficiency, diagnosed either in childhood or during adulthood; leptin supplementation in lean and obese leptin-replete subjects; leptin therapy in patients with lipodystrophy; and other emerging therapeutic areas, including treatment of hypothalamic amenorrhea and emerging novel combination regimens of leptin and other biogenic peptides. Unanswered questions and future directions in leptin research are highlighted in the Foreword by Dr. Jeffrey Friedman and throughout the volume. A fuller understanding of the regulation of leptin, under physiological and pathological conditions, is a critical prerequisite to its rational deployment in the treatment of diverse human disorders.

The creation of this book would have been impossible without the conceptual insight of Kristopher Spring (Editor, Clinical Medicine) and the logistical support of Susan Westendorf (Development Editor), both at Springer. Much gratitude is owed to them for their professionalism and engagement that resulted in the timely execution of the book project.

Memphis, TN, USA Sam Dagogo-Jack

Contents

Contributors

Denis G. Baskin, PhD Endocrinology and Metabolism, VA Puget Sound Medical Center, Seattle, WA, USA

Rebecca J. Brown, MD, MHSc National Institute of Diabetes and Digestive and Kidney Diseases, National Institutes of Health, Bethesda, MD, USA

Jussara M. do Carmo, PhD Department of Physiology and Biophysics, Mississippi Center for Obesity Research, Cardiovascular-Renal Research Center, University of Mississippi Medical Center, Jackson, MS, USA

Sharon Chou, MD Section of Adult and Pediatric Endocrinology, Diabetes and Metabolism, The University of Chicago, Chicago, IL, USA

Karine Clement, MD, PhD Institute of Cardiometabolism and Nutrition, Pitié-Salpêtrière Hospital, Assistance Publique-Hôpitaux de Paris, Inserm UMR-S1166, Université Pierre et Marie Curie-Paris6, Sorbonne University, Paris, France

Christoffer Clemmensen, PhD Institute for Diabetes and Obesity, Helmholtz Zentrum München and Department of Medicine, Technische Universitat Munchen, Munchen, Germany

Robert V. Considine, PhD Division of Endocrinology, Department of Medicine, Indiana University, Indianapolis, IN, USA

Daniel W. Coyne, MD Division of Nephrology, Washington University School of Medicine, St. Louis, MO, USA

Sam Dagogo-Jack, MD, MBBS Division of Endocrinology, Diabetes and Metabolism, The University of Tennessee Health Science Center, Memphis, TN, USA

Julie Dam, PhD Inserm U1016, Institut Cochin, Paris, France

Stephen N. David, MBBS, FACP Department of Medicine, University of Maryland Medical Center, Baltimore, MD, USA

Patricia Ducy, PhD Department of Pathology and Cell Biology, Columbia University, New York, NY, USA

Elisa Fabbrini, MD, PhD Center for Human Nutrition and Atkins Center of Excellence in Obesity Medicine, Washington University School of Medicine, St. Louis, MO, USA

Brian Finan, PhD Department of Medicine, Institute for Diabetes and Obesity, Helmholtz Zentrum München, Technische Universitat Munchen, Munchen, Germany

Phillip Gordon, MD National Institute of Diabetes and Digestive and Kidney Diseases, National Institutes of Health, Bethesda, MD, USA

Michèle Guerre-Millo, PhD Institute of Cardiometabolism and Nutrition, Pitié-Salpêtrière Hospital, Assistance Publique-Hôpitaux de Paris, Inserm UMR-S1166, Université Pierre et Marie Curie-Paris6, Sorbonne University, Paris, France

John E. Hall, PhD Department of Physiology and Biophysics, Mississippi Center for Obesity Research, Cardiovascular-Renal Research Center, University of Mississippi Medical Center, Jackson, MS, USA

Steven B. Heymsfield, MD Pennington Biomedical Research Center, Baton Rouge, LA, USA

Ralf Jockers, PhD Inserm U1016, Institut Cochin, Université Paris Descartes, Sorbonne Paris Cite, Paris, France

Satya Paul Kalra, PhD Department of Neuroscience, College of Medicine, University of Florida, Gainesville, FL, USA

Samuel Klein, MD Center for Human Nutrition, Washington University School of Medicine, St. Louis, MO, USA

Stavroula Kousteni, PhD Department of Medicine, Columbia University, New York, NY, USA

Department of Physiology and Cellular Biophysics, Columbia University, New York, NY, USA

Elizabeth Mary Lamos, MD Division of Endocrinology, Diabetes and Nutrition, University of Maryland School of Medicine, Baltimore, MD, USA

Julio Licinio, MD Mind and Brain Theme, South Australian Health and Medical Research Institute, Adelaide, SA, Australia

Department of Psychiatry, Flinders University Adelaide, SA, Australia

Hillary Loper, MD Division of Endocrinology, Diabetes and Nutrition, University of Maryland School of Medicine, Baltimore, MD, USA

Margherita Maffei, PhD Department of Clinical and Experimental Medicine, University Hospital of Pisa, Pisa, Italy

CNR Institute of Clinical Physiology, Pisa, Italy

Faidon Magkos, PhD Center for Human Nutrition and Atkins Center of Excellence in Obesity Medicine, Washington University School of Medicine, St. Louis, MO, USA

Christos Mantzoros, MD, DSc Section of Endocrinology, Boston VA Healthcare System, Jamaica Plain, MA, USA

Department of Medicine, Beth Israel Deaconess Medical Center, Harvard Medical School and Boston Medical Center, Boston, MA, USA

Richard D. DiMarchi, PhD Department of Chemistry, Indiana University, Bloomington, IN, USA

Giuseppe Matarese, MD, PhD Dipartimento di Medicina e Chirurgia, Facoltà di Medicina e Chirurgia, Università di Salerno Baronissi Campus, Salerno, Italy

Rachel C. Morgan, MD Division of Endocrinology, Department of Medicine, Indiana University, Indianapolis, IN, USA

Timo D. Muller, PhD Department of Medicine, Institute for Diabetes and Obesity, Helmholtz Zentrum München, Technische Universitat Munchen, Munchen, Germany

Heike Münzberg, PhD Pennington Biomedical Research Center, LSU system, Baton Rouge, LA, USA

Anubha Mutneja, MBBS, MD Division of Nephrology, Washington University, St. Louis, MO, USA

Olorunseun O. Ogunwobi, MD, PhD Department of Biological Sciences, Hunter College of The City University of New York, New York, NY, USA

Richa Pandey, MBBS, MD Division of Nephrology, Washington University, St. Louis, MO, USA

Gilberto Paz-Filho, MD The John Curtin School of Medical Research, Australian National University, Canberra, ACT, Australia

Claudio Procaccini, PhD Laboratorio di Immunologia, Istituto di Endocrinologia e Oncologia Sperimentale, Consiglio Nazionale delle Ricerche (IEOS-CNR), Naples, Italy

Valentina Pucino, MD Dipartimento di Scienze Mediche Traslazionali, Università di Napoli "Federico II", Naples, Italy

Alexandre A. da Silva, PhD Department of Physiology and Biophysics, University of Mississippi Medical Center, Jackson, MS, USA

Marthias H. Tschop, MD Institute for Diabetes and Obesity, Helmholtz Zentrum München and Department of Medicine, Techniche Universitat Munchen, Munchen, Germany

Zhen Wang, PhD Department of Physiology and Biophysics, Mississippi Center for Obesity Research, Cardiovascular-Renal Research Center, University of Mississippi Medical Center, Jackson, MS, USA

Lisa M. Younk, BS Department of Medicine, University of Maryland School of Medicine, Baltimore, MD, USA

Discovery of Leptin and Elucidation of Leptin Gene Expression

1

Margherita Maffei

Pubmed search on "leptin" retrieves over 25,200 entries and there is hardly a biological or medical term that has not been linked to leptin. But there was a time when leptin was not around and this chapter describes how this molecule was first imagined and then actually identified. The discovery of the leptin gene is not one of those processes, common in big step forward in the life sciences, that happen almost by chance. It is indeed a vision, a concept that became hard evidence. In this respect it is more similar to the discovery of new subatomic particles predicted by theoretical physics equations than to biological findings as remarkable as penicillin in which a scientist gave a brilliant interpretation of an unpredicted result.

The Milieu Intérieur and Homeostasis

We start by reviewing the conceptual frame that led to leptin imagination. It is first worth mentioning that the contemporary concept of body weight in the so-called industrialized societies is somewhat different from what might have been only 50–60 years ago. Up to the mid-twentieth century less than 10 % of the US population was obese in contrast to the 68 % that is characterized by obesity or overweight today [1]. Maintenance of body weight was thus the most "normal" phenomenon to observe. It is calculated that coefficients of weight variation in the absence of "obesogenic" environments and over relatively short periods are about 0.5–0.6 % and cross sectional observations indicate that they persist over more extended periods [2].

The idea that higher animals possess complex homeostatic mechanisms to maintain a stable internal environment for their living units, the cells, is a fundamental concept of modern physiology. The great physiologist Claude Bernard first conceptualized the existence of a reaction of the organism to external stimuli in the aim to maintain constant conditions within the body [3]. He coined the term *milieu intérieur* which has been translated into English as "internal environment" as opposed to external environment, often referred to as simply "environment." Bernard asserted that "the fixity of the internal environment is the condition of free, independent, life" [2, 4, 5]. Although he focused most of his attention and studies on the regulation of body temperature and to blood, "which should be maintained in a certain composition in order for the organism to live," the idea that energy stores are also part of the stability of the organism is contained in the concept of milieu intérieur. The pancreas being a major focus of his studies,

M. Maffei, Ph.D. (✉)
Department of Clinical and Experimental Medicine, University Hospital of Pisa, Pisa, Italy

CNR Institute of Clinical Physiology, Pisa, Italy
e-mail: m.maffei@ifc.cnr.it

S. Dagogo-Jack (ed.), *Leptin: Regulation and Clinical Applications*,
DOI 10.1007/978-3-319-09915-6_1, © Springer International Publishing Switzerland 2015

Bernard had a keen interest in glucose homeostasis and also conceived a role for the brain in this regulation: according to his work metabolic regulation is achieved through a series of rapid onset–offset signals that maintain a tight control of energy supplies. Afterwards Walter Bradford Cannon gave eating and drinking an explicit role in stabilizing vital functions: according to his theory organisms "…have somehow learned the methods of maintaining constancy and keeping steady" [5–7] and further "the constant conditions which are maintained in the body might be termed *equilibria*… Cannon coined the term homeostasis to synthesize his theory and applied that also to energy balance "The coordinated physiological systems which maintain most of the steady states in the organism are so complex and so peculiar to living beings—involving as they may brain, nerves, the heart …—that I have suggested a special term for these states, *homeostasis*" [6].

VMH Lesions and the Controller System

Starting from the early 1940s the British Royal Navy financed and planned research on food rations, food needs, and other topics that had been relevant during the Second World War. This research was carried in the department of Experimental Medicine directed by the physiologist McCance at the Addenbrooke's Hospital in Cambridge and led to seminal discoveries on the physiological basis of energy balance regulation [8]. As often happens in science the right combination of factors including expertise, personalities, and random events was key to the advancement of knowledge in this field. We will herein mention some of them starting, from Gordon Kennedy: he conducted pioneer studies on the obesity phenotype resulting from lesions of the ventromedial part of the hypothalamus (VMH) in rodents [9]. Kennedy interpreted the results in terms of a negative feedback loop system controlling food intake in normal animal, and hypothesized that the amount of fat in the body provided the information for the control signal that was targeted to the hypothalamus. This concept is known as lipostatic theory and suggests that the amount of fat in the body is measured and maintained constant. Other theories had been previously formulated to explain energy balance: these included Brobeck's concept [10] postulating body temperature as the main parameter to indicate the status of energy balance and Mayer's glucostatic theory in which the controlled quantity is the difference between arterial and venous plasma concentrations of glucose [11, 12]. Kennedy's concept was further developed by Romaine Hervey, a younger fellow at the Department of Experimental Medicine, who was the first to employ parabiosis in studies concerning energy balance regulation. Parabiosis is the surgical union of two animals to produce a common blood supply and allow the investigation of circulating factors in the regulation of physiological systems [8]. In parabiosis experiments we distinguish a treated animal and a partner: what happens to the partner is the result of some treatment dependent changes in blood borne signals that the animal is able to sense. Hervey applied this technique to VMH lesioned rats. The animals in which the lesions were made showed hyperphagia and obesity. Their parabiotic partners, with normal hypothalami, ate much less, became thin and in some cases starved to death. Hervey concluded "…these results may be evidence for a feedback control of food intake, and may throw some light on the information used in such a system" [13, 14]. These data were in fact taken to imply that the obese rat produced a humoral agent that would normally stimulate the brain to inhibit food intake. Although the lesioned rats could not respond to the signal, the factor had to be carried across the parabiotic union and inhibit the food intake of the normal partner [13, 15]. These results led Hervey to state that maintenance of body weight "requires some precision" and he was the first to express the concept in rigorous thermodynamic terms: "during any period it must be true that energy intake − energy output = energy stores." He thus imagined energy homeostasis as a "controller system" borrowing this concept from a branch of engineering that deals with the behavior of dynamical systems [16]. According to this theory *inputs*, also called reference or afferent signals, are sensed and manipulated by a *controller* in order to obtain

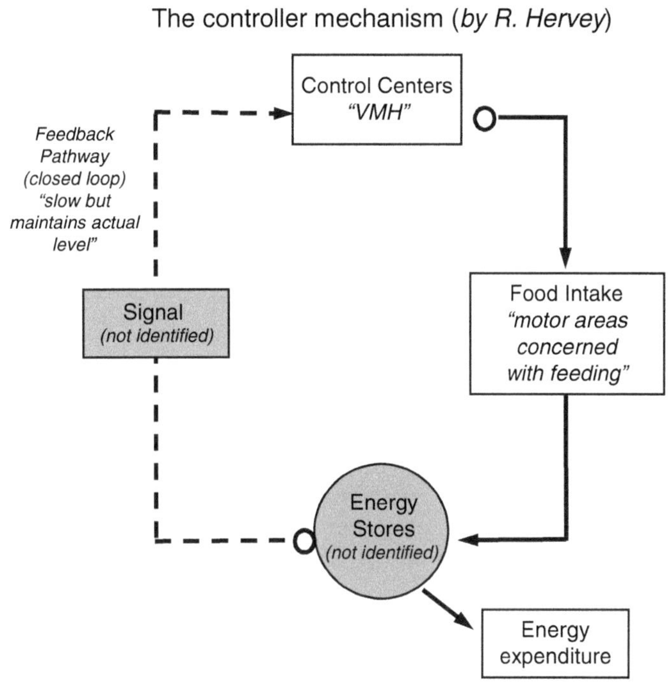

Fig. 1.1 The hypothetical model postulated by Hervey to represent the mechanism regulating energy homeostasis in mammals. Homeostasis can be represented by a controller mechanism, better known as feedback loop: from the energy stores start afferent signals to the center which will in turn produce efferent signals to modulate energy stores. At that stage most of the players were not known. *White box*: known component. *Grey box*: component to be identified

the desired effect on the *output* of the system in a "closed loop system" (Fig. 1.1).

Hervey established the nature of two of the components of this system, namely the VMH as central controller and the output constituted by "motor areas concerned with feeding," while still unknown were "the quantity that the system immediately senses and stabilizes" and the means by which inputs are made to the controller. In the conclusions of the Nature paper published in 1969 Hervey put forward the idea that "regulation of energy balance involves a hormonal feedback signal" and he also discussed the possibility that steroids, already known to affect body weight, could play such a role [16]. The search for the afferent signal had just started.

Douglas Coleman and Parabiosis

VMH lesioned rats are experimental models of obesity obtained by a very drastic and unphysiological treatment: finding the humoral agent hypothesized on the basis of parabiosis results in these models was like looking for a needle in a haystack. But murine models of obesity existed also as a result of spontaneous mutations, and the search was then steered by genetics. In 1949 a few animals in the non-inbred V strain at the Jackson laboratory (Bar Harbor, Maine) were observed to be plump early in life and to become markedly obese and diabetic thereafter. Breeding experiments revealed that the obesity syndrome was caused by a single autosomal recessive gene, *obese* (gene symbol *ob*). The mutation was later transferred on the congenic C57BL/6J background on which it has been propagated since [17, 18]. Dickie and Lane [19] positioned the *ob*6J mutation on proximal chromosome 6 between *Microphthalmia* and *waved-1* loci. The mice were infertile, exhibited hyperphagia and early onset obesity, but on this genetic background only a transient form of hyperglycemia appeared, in association with elevated plasma insulin [20]. A second co-isogenic allele, known as *ob*2J, resulting in a similar obese phenotype, was later identified in the SM/Ckc-Dac mouse strain (Table 1.1).

A few years later in 1965 a new spontaneous obese mutant was identified at the Jackson laboratory [21]. The mutation, arisen on the

Table 1.1 *Ob* and *Db* alleles, genetic background of propagation and effect on glucose metabolism

Allele	Strain of propagation	Obesity	Glucose metabolism
Ob (*obese*) first reported by Ingalls et al. [17]			
Ob	Non-inbred stock	Severe	Diabetes
Ob	C57BL6/J	Severe	Hyperinsulinemia
			Transient
			Hyperglycemia
Ob	C57BL/KsJ	Severe	Severe diabetes
Ob^{2J}	SM/CKc-+^{Dac}	Severe	Hyperinsulinemia
			Transient
			Hyperglycemia
Db (*diabetes*) first reported by Hummel et al. [21]			
Db	C57BL/KsJ	Severe	Severe diabetes
Db	C57BL6/J	Severe	Hyperinsulinemia
			Transient
			Hyperglycemia
Db^{2J}	C57BL/KsJ	Severe	Severe diabetes
Db^{3J}	129/J	Severe	Hyperinsulinemia
			Hypoglycemia
Db^{ad}	C57BL/KsJ	Severe	Severe diabetes

C57BL/ks strain and inherited as an autosomal recessive gene located on chromosome 4, was called *diabetes* (symbol *db*). Mutant mice were characterized by infertility, hyperphagia, and early onset obesity just like the *ob/ob* mutant, but unlike them they developed a severe form of diabetes that reduced their life span. Several alleles of the *db* gene were eventually found on other strains, namely the 2J allele that appeared on the BL6 background and the 3J allele on the 129/J strain. The severity of diabetes differed depending on the background with a stronger phenotype being expressed in the Ks strain [18].

Coleman was intrigued by the differences that the different genetic backgrounds conferred to the expression of the phenotype, especially in terms of the onset and severity of diabetes. He noticed that on the C57BL6 background in which the *ob* original mutation was propagated and in which one of the *db* alleles had spontaneously arisen, the *db/db* and *ob/ob* phenotypes were identical with mild diabetes and markedly elevated plasma insulin sustained throughout a nearly normal life span [22]. Similarly, when he later transferred the *ob* mutant allele to the C57BL/ks background he obtained a mutant with a severe early form of diabetes that compromised its life span, exactly as in the case of the original C57BL/ks *db/db* mutant [23]. Coleman's conclusion was that the wide spectrum of phenotypes observed in *db/db* and *ob/ob* mice depended exclusively on genetic background and that the two genetic defects led to an identical phenotype [24].

The juxtaposition of the two strains of obese mice provided Coleman with a brilliant intuition. He devised a clever set of experiments based on parabiosis experiments (see scheme in Fig. 1.2) that once again were inspired by deductive reasoning, interdisciplinary insights, and of course serendipity. In the first set of parabiosis experiments *db/db* animals were joined to wild type mice. In the very precise Coleman's recollection of his experimental design he explains that this first set was dictated by the need of having parabiosed animals on the same genetic background to minimize vigorous immune rejection [24]. As occasionally observed for partners of VMH lesioned rats, the +/+ members of the pairs expired, their blood glucose decreased to starvation levels and subsequent carcass analysis revealed absence of food remnants in their guts and a liver completely depleted of glycogen. Conversely, the obese *db/db* retained normal blood glucose and presented food in the stomach and in the intestine. These observations led Coleman to a "eureka moment," as he defines it [24]. He postulated that the *db/db* mouse produced a "blood borne factor so powerful that it could induce the normal partner to starve to death," also in consideration of the relatively small portion of blood that is exchanged between two parabiosed animals. Then he parabiosed *ob/ob* with +/+ mice and observed marked improvements in glycaemic control and decreased energy intake in the *ob/ob* mice. When he finally managed to place the two mutations (*ob* and *db*) on the same genetic background he could perform the key experiments by joining the blood circle of *db/db* and *ob/ob* mice. It is interesting, and almost incredible. To read in the Coleman's narrative written for the Lasker Award [24] that in his mind this experiment involving two mice of comparable weight was also aimed at excluding the possibility

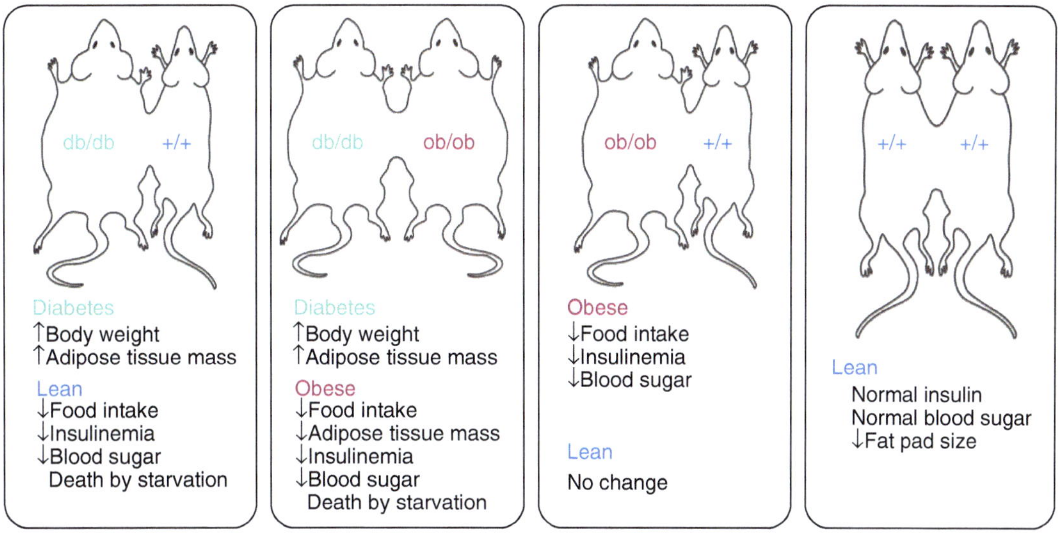

Fig. 1.2 Schematic representation of Coleman's experiments. Reproduced with permission [22]

that in case of union between an obese and a lean animal, the latter was losing weight because of being dragged around by the heavy partner. What Coleman obtained was severe weight loss, hypoglycemia, and in some cases death in the *ob/ob* members of the pairs. Carcass analysis revealed that weight decrease was entirely due to loss of adipose mass. Also in this case *db/db* animals were not affected by parabiosis and kept gaining weight according to their normal growth curve. Coleman's overall conclusion as reported in its own words "…the *db/db* mutant mouse overproduces a satiety factor but cannot respond to it—perhaps owing to a defective receptor—whereas the *ob/ob* mutant recognizes and responds to the factor but cannot produce it. The normal wild type mouse also produces this factor but in insufficient amounts to be lethal."

These findings along with previous knowledge obtained using parabiosis on hypothalamus lesioned rodents laid the basis to build an identikit of the factor missing in the *ob/ob* mouse. The requirements that this factor had to satisfy included the following:

1. A blood borne signal since it is exchanged between parabionts.
2. A bioactive molecule since it causes reduction of food intake and weight.
3. It has to reflect the amount of energy stores since the obese animal overproduces this factor as compared to the lean one.
4. Its receptor is in the hypothalamus since parabiosis performed with rodents carrying lesions in the VMH and in the arcuate nucleus cause starvation and weight loss in the untreated partner, similar to those observed for partners of the *db/db* mouse.

Molecular Genetics: A Novel Approach to Identify the ob Gene

Reverse Genetics and Positional Cloning

Much had been achieved since the theoretical homeostasis and controller models postulated by Cannon and Hervey: there was a factor, a protein, a gene, indeed two, that when altered caused obesity and these molecules had defined features of a satiety signal and its receptor. This was a breakthrough also in the clinical and popular view that had accompanied obesity, considered up to that point a behavioral rather than a physiological problem; instead, science was demonstrating that it was not a matter determined by lack of will or by laziness, but a condition attributable to biological causes yet to be defined. Thus the hunt started. In the years that followed various factors were considered good candidates including cholecystokinin, somatostatin, and pancreatic polypeptide.

Molecular genetics was at its dawn in the 1970s and identifying a gene starting from a mammalian phenotype was almost an impossible task. The subsequent years witnessed a rapid and revolutionary advancement in this discipline, something similar to what was taking place in computer science, with a fruitful mixture of progress in knowledge and technology that led to a real explosion of the field. There are people who start what look like impossible enterprises, because they somewhat view that what appears undoable today will not be such in the near future. These people are called visionaries and sometimes they are considered insane in their pursuit of far too ambitious plans. Jeffrey M Friedman a young MD–PhD at the Rockefeller University was such a person. Dr. Friedman was 30 years old when in 1984 he started his laboratory as a Howard Hughes Medical Institute investigator at the Rockefeller University, focusing his research on the molecular identification of the *ob* and the *db* genes.

Among his first contributions to the genetics of obesity is a paper published in Genomics in 1989, that describes the chromosome mapping of the cholecystokinin (*CCK*) gene [25]. CCK is a peptide hormone, originally found in the small intestine and released in response to nutrient ingestion [26]. The high concentration of this hormone present in the brain and its capability to suppress appetite when peripherally administered to rodents, had led to the hypothesis that CCK could act as the satiety signal missing in the *ob/ob* mice. Friedman and colleagues' work ruled out this possibility by mapping *CCK* locus on murine chromosome 9, whereas the *ob* gene had been previously mapped on chromosome 6.

Friedman and collaborators were aware that the multiple metabolic and physiologic abnormalities present in the *ob/ob* and *db/db* mice made it difficult to separate primary gene effects from secondary metabolic alterations: it was therefore difficult to proceed with classical techniques to isolate the satiety signal on the basis of its being overproduced by the *db/db* mouse or based on its biochemical properties. In addition the site of synthesis of the signal had remained unknown: they then decided to take a completely novel approach that required no specific assumption on the biological nature of the defect, called "reverse genetics" [27]. Nowadays this term defines the studies that investigate which phenotypes arise from a specific sequence but at the time this was how Orkin [28] defined reverse genetics: "the isolation of a gene without reference to a specific protein or without any reagents or functional assays useful in its detection…this requires: first establishing the map position of the gene and then identifying a specific gene within this region in which mutations are strictly correlated with the disease. Restriction fragment length polymorphisms (RFLPs) in combination with cytogenetic methods provide the key to map assignment with a resolution of roughly several million base pairs. Identifying the gene of interest is the practical issue." A few years later a development of reverse research called positional cloning that deals effectively with the "practical issue" was successfully applied by Riordan to identify the gene responsible for cystic fibrosis [29]. Positional cloning was used to identify the *ob* and the *db* genes by Friedman and colleagues: it implies three major steps that will be here first briefly outlined in general and then specifically explained in the case of *ob* (and *db*) identification:

1. Genetic mapping. Based on the assumption that for loci sitting on the same chromosome, and thus not segregating independently, the number of recombination events is inversely related to their physical distance on the DNA, it is possible to map a locus within a DNA region using polymorphic markers. Centimorgan (cM) is the unit that defines this distance: one cM equals a one percent chance that a marker on a chromosome will become separated from a second marker on the same chromosome due to crossing over in a single generation; it is calculated as number of recombination events/number of total meioses × 100.

Although the probability of recombination varies along the genome, 1 cM corresponds on average to one million base pairs on the mammalian genome.
2. Physical mapping. Once that a sufficiently narrow genetic distance between two markers has been established the DNA region can be physically collected using appropriate vectors.
3. Gene identification. Different techniques can be used to identify and characterize the coding candidate genes contained in a given physical DNA region. The presence of mutations in the affected individuals constitutes the ultimate proof that a candidate is the gene responsible for the phenotype under investigation.

Genetic Mapping

Effective genetic mapping implies the existence of several and close polymorphic markers, an issue not so easy to address before the completion of the genome project. The first drafts of the human and mouse genomes were released in 2000 and 2002, respectively. In the early 1990s researchers could only use RFLPs associated with known loci. The probes used to map the *ob* gene were T cell receptor beta (*Tcrb*), carboxypetidase A (*cpa*), met oncogene (*met*), and alpha2 procollagen (*Cola-2*), all having been mapped on chromosome 6. To maximize the variability of these markers Friedman and colleagues established a series of intraspecific and interspecific crosses, a simplification of which is represented in Fig. 1.3a. It is worth mentioning that things were further complicated by sterility of *ob/ob* mice, the impossibility of phenotypically distinguishing between heretozygous +/*ob* and +/+ mice and, last but not least, difficulties in unambiguously assigning the genotype due to the high variance in body weight, fatness and development of type 2 diabetes, depending on the genetic background.

The investigators initially used ovarian transplant to an agouty [30] recipient to set an interspecific cross between *Mus musculus* C57Bl/6J *ob/ob* female and *Mus spretus* male mice and an intraspecific cross between C57Bl/6J *ob/ob* female and DBA/2J +/+mice. The F1 progeny of the two crosses were intercrossed and the distance between a given RFLP and *ob* was determined by scoring the number of obese (*ob/ob*) F2 animals carrying either the *spretus* or the DBA allele. The use of around 750 informative meioses so obtained allowed to position *ob* 11.8 cM proximal to *Tcrb* and 2–4 cM distal to *Met*. Zero (0) recombinants were found for *Cpa* out of 123 scorable animals: the conclusion was that this locus was less than 2.3 cM from *ob* [31]. These same markers were mapped on human chromosome 7q31-34, the region postulated to contain the human *ob* gene [31].

A similar approach was employed in the case of the *db* mutation and permitted to build a genetic map spanning a region of 8 cM [27]. This map places *db* 3 cM distal from *Cjun* and *Ifa* and 5 cM proximal to D4Rp1. The interval defined for *ob* was about 7–8 cM. Physical mapping required a region not larger than 1 cM and this could not be realized without a denser physical map and thus a higher number of markers. To identify additional RFLPs in the *ob* region, the Rockefeller group made use of chromosome microdissection: 19 novel RFLPs were identified one of which did not show any recombinant event across 831 informative meiosis: this marker, named D6Rck13 was used as an entry point for physical mapping of the *ob* mutation [32] together with *Pax4* that was found to be tightly linked to *ob* [33]. Chromosomal microdissection was used in the same way to more finely map the *db* gene [34].

Physical Mapping of the *ob* Gene

So far the discovery of the *ob* and the *db* genes has been treated in parallel. The following paragraphs will be dedicated to the final steps that led to *ob* identification. In contrast to genetic maps, physical maps relate genome positions to each other, using physical distances measured along the DNA helix and expressed in base pairs (bp). Physical mapping make use of intentional fragmentation of genomes that are subsequently

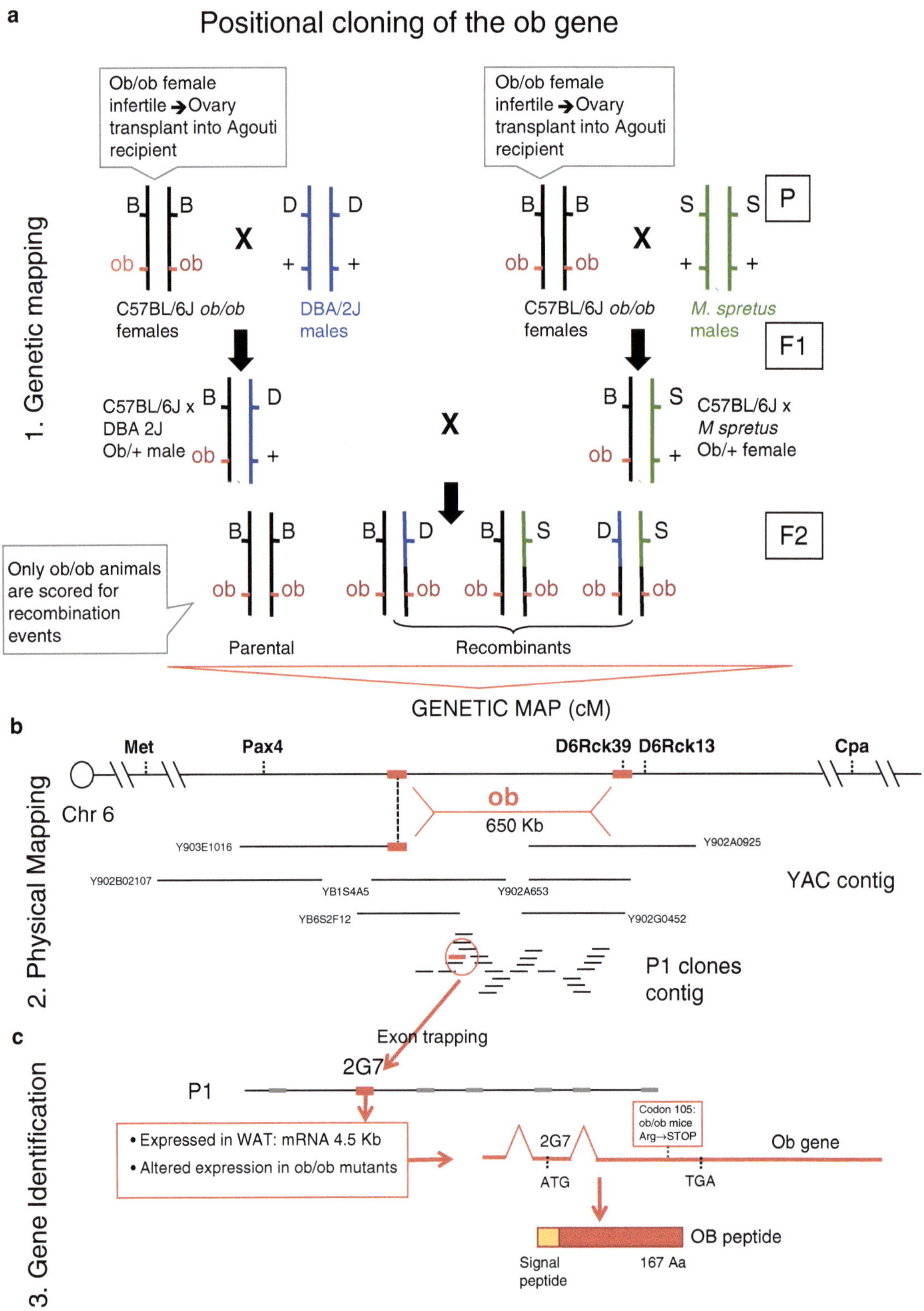

Fig. 1.3 Positional cloning of the *ob* gene is represented following the three phases of its experimental design. The key reagents and steps are represented in *red*. (**a**) Genetic mapping: a representative type of cross (interspecific intercross) is represented. *Mus spretus* (*green allele*) males were mated to C57Bl/6J *ob/ob* ovarian transplants.

cloned into appropriate vectors to build a contig, a contiguous array of overlapping clones. Yeast Artificial Chromosomes (YACs) have been widely used to this purpose since they allow to clone fragments as big as 1,400 Kb. Once that the two entry points (distal and proximal with respect to the centromere) of the gene of interest are isolated, YAC rescued ends are used to walk along the genome by identifying new YACs to cover the whole contig. Importantly YAC ends and YAC subclones sequencing generate new polymorphic markers that are used to narrow down the DNA interval of interest.

In the case of the *ob* gene the entry points to start genome walking were 2 YACs, respectively containing Pax 4 and D6Rck13 (Fig. 1.3b), The strategy explained above allowed to cover the entire region and build a contig with 6 YACs and a series of P1 mouse bacteriophage clones: the handling and amplification of P1s is easier and they can host fragments as large as 100–200 Kb. Animals typing with new polymorphic sequences markers permitted to establish the position of the *ob* gene in an estimated interval of 650 Kb, defined by two markers, each scoring a single recombination event out of 1,606 meioses: one was a novel single strand length polymorphism named D6Rck39 and mapping near named D6Rck13; the other was the distal end of a YAC containing *Pax4*. To facilitate genes identification in the critical 650 Kb region, this was also covered with 24 P1s isolated using YAC ends. In retrospective things were further complicated by the very low rate of recombination (nearly threefold lower than the average for mouse genome) that characterizes the 2.2 Mb critical region where *ob* had been mapped. Indeed, out of 1,606 meioses there were only six recombination events: so that a genetic distance of 1 cM corresponds to about 5.8 Mb in this case [35].

Ob Gene Identification

I joined Friedman's laboratory in the fall of 1993, when the physical map of the *ob* gene had been almost completed: The reader will excuse me if from now on the chapter is written with the addition of some biographical/personal notes. I had just obtained my PhD in Italy with a thesis on population genetics in ancient populations and I was fascinated by the potential that linkage analysis and positional cloning were disclosing: from a disease to its genetic cause. I will never forget my interview with Jeffrey Friedman in his office at the sixth floor of the Rockefeller building. I remember nervously waiting for him and admiring that astonishing view on the East River. He entered and everything was very quick and unusual: Jeff talked fast and for me it was at times hard to understand. Nevertheless he was gentle and friendly; he briefly asked of my PhD work and then started to tell a story of genetically obese mice that had been parabiosed: a word that I learnt that day. He used a precious Montblanc fountain pen to sketch schemes and notes while talking and in front of me pairs of "parabiosed" lean and obese mice were shaped: the Coleman experiment. Then he unexpectedly asked: "So, what do you think?" In rudimentary and uncertain English I answered that it looked like there was a defect in a common signaling pathway, affecting *db/db* and *ob/ob* mice. He seemed satisfied with that

Fig. 1.3 (continued) F1 females (B6 spretus *ob*/+) from this cross were bred to F1 males (B6D2 *ob*/+) generated from a C57Bl/6J *ob/ob* × DBA 2J (*blue allele*) +/+ mating. Only obese animals were used for genetic mapping. Modified from [29] with permission. The *ob* gene was then mapped between *Pax4* and the polymorphic marker D6Rck13 that provided entry points to start the Physical mapping (**b**) of the *ob* gene: a physical contig was built using Yeast Artificial Chromosomes (YACs) and P1 clones. This permitted to isolate novel markers (*in red* the position of the key ones) and to further narrow down the interval to 650 Kb, between the end of YAC Y903E1016 and the marker D6Rck39 (Modified from Zhang et al., 1994). (**c**) Exon trapping on a P1 clone permitted to isolate among others (*in grey*) the 2G7 candidate (*in red*) that proved to be part of the *ob* gene, based on the following evidences: 2G7 is specifically expressed by WAT, its expression is altered in *ob/ob* mice, 2G7 belongs to an open reading frame of a 3 exons gene coding for a 167-Aa peptide that presents a point mutation at codon 105 (Arg → STOP) in C57BL/6J *ob/ob* mice

response, then he asked what my feeling regarding team work was. One week later he offered me a postdoctoral position in his laboratory. I became part of the *ob* team and started to collaborate closely with Yiying Zhang and Ricardo Proenca: my role in the project was to characterize the expression of candidates isolated from the contig by means of exon trapping. This technique, now supplanted by extensive DNA sequencing and bioinformatics tools, allows isolation of exons from large genome DNA fragments and relies on the conservation of sequence at intron–exon boundaries in all eukaryotic species. By cloning a genomic fragment into the intron of an expression vector (pSPL3 in the case of the *ob* gene), exons (if any) encoded in the genomic fragment are spliced into the transcript encoded on the plasmid. Reverse transcriptase polymerase chain reaction (RT-PCR) using primers specific for the vector transcript provides a product for subsequent analysis [36].

Once the putative exons had been isolated from genomic DNA of P1 clones, each of them was sequenced and checked against all sequences present in Genbank. Then Northern blots and reverse transcription PCR were used to screen for the presence of corresponding RNA from a panel of mouse tissues (Tissue Blot) and to analyze candidate expression in *ob/ob* and wild type mice (Mutant Blot). Candidate names followed the cloning strategy code. I remember the first two exons I hybridized to a Northern Blot, named 27 and 28: in their case we were encouraged by some specific expression in the brain (a putative site for ob expression): the signal however was weak and appeared as a smeared band. One Friday (it was early May 1994) I hybridized on the Tissue Blot a ^{32}P labelled probe made out of a candidate named 2G7 that had been just isolated and sequenced, and for which no match in the database had been found. The next Saturday morning, when I developed the film, a sharp very intense and specific band with a size of around 4.5 Kb was visible only in the lane loaded with white adipose tissue (WAT) RNA. My first thought was: "I finally obtained a decent Northern experiment" and the second, "Jeff should see this." When I turned on my back Jeff was there, staring at the film and already very excited about the result. He said something about Coleman having predicted a signal originating in the white adipose tissue (depot of energy stores by definition) and in the minute after listed a series of experiments that needed to be done immediately: the first was the characterization of the 2G7 signal in the *ob/ob* mutants. I was invited to a dear friend's wedding that day, but that did not stop Jeff Friedman, who personally hybridized the same probe used for the Tissue Blot to a blot containing RNA from WAT of two different *ob* mutants. The result was quite clear: 2G7 mRNA was absent in the adipose tissue of SM/Ckc-$+^{Dac}ob^{2J}/ob^{2J}$, present in the lean littermate wild type (SM/Ckc-$+^{Dac}$+/+) and dramatically induced (about 20-fold) in the C57Bl/6 *ob/ob* mutant obese mice as compared to the corresponding lean control (C57Bl/6 +/+). These results were replicated also by RT-PCR [35]. By Sunday afternoon we were reasonably certain that 2G7 was an excellent candidate and the same probe was used to screen a mouse adipose cDNA library in search of the full length gene. 22 complementary clones were isolated and sequence analysis revealed a methionine initiation codon in the 2G7 exon with a 167 aminoacid open reading frame, followed by a long 3′ untranslated region for a total of over 2,800 bp. A database search did not identify any significant homology to any sequence in Genbank. The final confirmation that this sequence was that of the *ob* gene came from sequence analysis (automated and manual) of its open reading frame in cDNA obtained from WAT of C57Bl/6 *ob/ob* mice that overexpressed the transcript: the coding sequence was identical except for one C→T transition that transformed codon 105, coding for arginine, into a stop codon [35]. The hunt, started almost 50 years before had reached an happy end. That evening, before leaving, I left a note on Jeff's desk: "I have no words"; somebody else had left a rose in his office. The laboratory was unusually silent, we all shared a unique moment of intense excitement. I am not religious, but a very religious friend of mine coined a sentence that well describes these feelings: "A discovery is like looking into God's mind. It is why scientists accept to face frustration and failure most of their time."

In the following days we obtained further important and supporting evidences. Southern blot analysis using the 2G7 probe permitted to demonstrate that in SM/Ckc-$+^{Dac}ob^{2J}/ob^{2J}$ mutants absence of *ob* mRNA was associated with a different size of a BgII fragment of genomic DNA. This suggested that this mutation resulted from a deletion/insertion in a regulatory or intronic region. The hypothesis was later confirmed by Moon and Friedman [37] that reported the *ob2J* mutation to be the result of the insertion of a retroviral-like transposon containing several donor and acceptor sites in the first intron of the *ob* gene: this leads to the formation of several chimeric mRNAs, altered splicing and no synthesis of the correct mature *ob* mRNA [37].

The human *ob* gene was cloned by screening an adipose tissue phage cDNA library: as in the case of mouse it predicted a 167-amino-acid open reading frame that was 84 % identical to the murine OB peptide. A high level of evolutionary conservation was revealed also by hybridization of the *ob* cDNA to the genomic DNA of several vertebrates including rat, pig, sheep, cow, cat, chicken, and eel. A more close analysis of both human and mouse OB amino acid sequence revealed the presence of a signal peptide at its N terminus, suggesting that these could be secreted proteins. In vitro transcription and translation experiments in the presence of microsomal membranes confirmed the in silico prediction: the protein coded by the OB gene is a precursor of about 18 kDa that is truncated by 2 kDa and translocated when exposed to a posttranslational processing system. The ob protein fulfilled then one of the most important characteristics of the satiety signal postulated by Kennedy, Hervey, and Coleman: it had the potential to be a circulating peptide, a hormone. These results are represented in Fig. 1.3c.

Elucidation of ob Gene Expression and Bioactivity

All these findings were presented in the first original papers and can be summarized as follows: the murine *ob* gene is expressed by the white adipose tissue and it codes for a 167-amino-acid secreted protein. It is mutated in two independent strains of *ob/ob* mutants and there is a human homologue.

Some relevant questions remained to be addressed and are here briefly outlined with their outcome:

- *Is ob gene expression specifically associated with mature adipocytes and with their terminal differentiation*? The white adipose is composed of two main fractions, namely, a stromal vascular fraction containing preadipocytes, endothelial cells, inflammatory cells and fully mature adipocytes. The use of an established preadipocytes cell line able to undergo adipose conversion (F442A) permitted to positively answer this question. Ob gene expression was in fact typical of the mature adipocyte [38]. This finding by itself paved the way to the concept of adipokine, a molecule secreted by adipocytes, and further, it changed the concept of adipose tissue, not any longer a passive depot of energy storage, but an active endocrine organ [38].
- *What is ob gene regulation in satiety signal resistant mice*? From Hervey's and Coleman's parabiosis experiments we knew that some obese models (*db/db* and VMH lesioned) are resistant to the satiety signal. VMH lesions can be obtained by one intraperitoneal injection of gold-thioglucose (GTG): this causes hyperphagia and in 4 weeks mice double their initial body weight. This model was in place in Friedman's laboratory. Gene expression studies revealed that in both *db/db* and GTG treated mice ob gene expression was upregulated by 20-fold [38]. The data were discussed as follows: "(they) position the *db* gene and the hypothalamus downstream of ob in the pathway that controls body weight…and are consistent with the hypothesis that the ob receptor is encoded by the *db* locus" and further more the increase of ob RNA in GTG mice suggested a non-cell autonomous function of the ob gene product in fat cells, since the overexpression of the wt protein did not prevent obesity in the absence of an intact hypothalamus.
- *Is the ob protein circulating in blood*? Antibodies raised against the recombinant OB

protein allowed to detect a 16 kDa band in the plasma of wild type mice, but not in that of C57Bl/6J *ob/ob* mutants, suggesting that the point mutation caused an unstable truncated protein. The signal was more intense in the lane loaded with the *db/db* plasma [39]. These results established that the OB protein, as postulated by the existence of a signal peptide sequence at its N terminus, was a secreted protein and possibly a hormone.

- *Is the ob protein able to induce satiety and weight loss*? This was obviously one of the most relevant questions. In collaboration with the laboratory of Molecular Biophysics headed by Stephen Burley the OB protein was expressed and renatured. Then administered to *ob/ob*, wild type and *db/db* mice by daily injections. The results obtained in *ob/ob* mice were striking. After 33 days of treatment they had lost 40 % of their initial body weight and had reduced their food intake by 40 % becoming similar to normal wild type animals: importantly their adipose mass was reduced by 50 %, whereas the lean mass was not significantly changed. None of these changes was observed in PBS treated controls. Of note, *ob/ob* mice not treated with the OB protein, but eating the same amount of food intake (pair-fed) lost significantly less weight than animals receiving the recombinant protein, indicating that the input component per se was not the only parameter determining a negative energy balance. Indeed Pelleymounter and colleagues demonstrated that the OB protein is able to increase metabolic rate and locomotor activity [40] and its role in the induction of energy expenditure is now widely acknowledged [41]. Wild type animals treated with the OB protein reduced their food intake and body weight significantly and stabilized both parameters at levels that were respectively 92 % and 88 % those of untreated controls. An impressive reduction in fat mass was observed also in this case with adipose mass accounting for only 0.67 % of total body weight as compared to the 12 % observed in not treated animals. In *db/db* mice no effect was observed, this being consistent with the postulated defect in OB protein receptor [39]. The first "public presentation" of these results was during a lab meeting given by Jeffrey Halaas. In that occasion Friedman announced that we had to pick a name for this novel protein that made mice become thin. He proposed to use the Greek root for thin: leptós. We all agreed to leptin and this name was used for the first time in the Halaas et al. [39] paper published in Science. In the same issue two other important contributions highlighting further aspects of leptin action appeared: weight loss following brain direct administration of very low dosage of the protein suggested that it could act directly on neuronal networks that control feeding and energy balance [42]; Pelleymounter and coworkers demonstrated that the OB protein lowered blood glucose and insulin levels in *ob/ob* mice and that it acted to increase energy expenditure [40].
- *Do leptin levels in plasma reflect the degree of obesity*? We knew that the ob gene mRNA was increased in the WAT of obese models in which the pathway had been interrupted (VMH lesioned *db/db* mice). The same was observed also in mice treated with high fat diet and in old overweight mice [38] but not in three classical models of murine obesity represented by the *Agouti* (A^y/+), the *tubby*, and the *fat* mouse. This was an indication that the transcription machinery in the WAT was not equally induced in all cases: what was important to establish however were the circulating levels of leptin, since all evidences that had been accumulating over time pointed to a hormonal-like biological action with important targets situated in the hypothalamus. The availability of good antibodies permitted first to use a titration method that employed known concentration of the recombinant protein loaded on a Western Blot, and then to develop an ELISA assay (in collaboration with Roger Lallone in Birmingham) for an accurate measurement of plasma leptin in mouse and in humans. The results were very clear: plasma leptin levels were much higher in obese individuals: all rodent models of obesity exhibited dramatically increased level of the circulating

protein as compared to lean controls including also the *Agouti*, *tubby*, and *fat* mouse, for which ob mRNA did not change (see above). In both humans and mouse a positive and highly significant correlation existed between body mass index and plasma leptin, although there was high variability of the circulating protein at each BMI. Consistently weight loss due to food restriction was associated with a decrease in plasma leptin in both humans and mouse [38].

Conclusions

Altogether these results establish that all the characteristics of the OB protein postulated by Coleman were true:

1. It was a circulating signal originating from energy stores (WAT) with the features of a hormone and could thus be exchanged between parabiosed animals.
2. It was a bioactive molecule with a potent anorectic effect and this explained the weight loss in *ob/ob* mice parabiosed to wild type or *db/db* mice and in wild type parabiosed to *db/db*.
3. Its levels reflected the amount of energy stores, now better defined as the white adipose tissue, and thus animals parabiosed to obese models (*db/db* or VMH lesioned) starved to death because they had been receiving very high concentration of the satiety signal.
4. It signals to the hypothalamus. Although *db* subsequent cloning and localization [43, 44] provided the definite confirmation of this hypothesis, at this stage we were already reasonably confident that at least one of leptin targets was in the hypothalamus, based on the following evidences: ob transcriptional levels were increased in mice with VMH lesions, suggesting that a feedback loop is interrupted in this model; leptin direct administration in the brain results in food intake reduction and weight loss even at very low dosage.

In my view a phase of studies on energy balance is concluded by these findings and another is disclosed. Leptin has changed the perspective on weight control problem, by permitting the energy homeostasis field to enter a molecular era. It has been a formidable tool and the heart of the matter to start dissecting the complex mechanisms that regulate feeding behavior and body weight.

Acknowledgements I want to thank: Jeffrey Friedman, who offered me the possibility to be part of this amazing story. When I left his laboratory I brought with me a precious Montblanc fountain pen and a fundamental lesson: to be confident enough in my capacities to be an independent researcher and start my own research. I owe to Jeff also my need to transform into schemes and sketches whatever science issue I am discussing with colleagues and collaborators; Romaine Hervey, with whom I had the privilege of exchanging correspondence recently in search for the very first papers on energy balance regulation and who helped me to better understand the origin of his thoughts on energy balance; my husband Mario Costa, a scientist himself, who moved to New York City in 1993, persuaded me to join him, lived with me during those special years and last but not least spent long hours and long walks along the East River discussing science with me and often giving precious pieces of advice for my experiments.

References

1. Flegal KM, Carroll MD, Ogden CL, Curtin LR. Prevalence and trends in obesity among US adults, 1999–2008. JAMA. 2010;303(3):235–41.
2. Keesey RE, Powley TL. Body energy homeostasis. Appetite. 2008;51(3):442–5.
3. Bernard C. Leçons de physiologie expérimentale appliquée à la médecine, faites au Collège de France. Paris: J.-B. Baillière et fils; 1854.
4. Holmes FL. Claude Bernard, the milieu interieur, and regulatory physiology. Hist Philos Life Sci. 1986; 8(1):3–25.
5. Cooper SJ. From Claude Bernard to Walter Cannon. Emergence of the concept of homeostasis. Appetite. 2008;51(3):419–27.
6. Cannon WB. The wisdom of the body. New York: W.W. Norton & Company; 1932.
7. Booth DA. Physiological regulation through learnt control of appetites by contingencies among signals from external and internal environments. Appetite. 2008;51(3):433–41.
8. Harris RB. Is leptin the parabiotic "satiety" factor? Past and present interpretations. Appetite. 2013;61(1):111–8.
9. Kennedy GC. The hypothalamic control of food intake in rats. Proc R Soc Lond B Biol Sci. 1950; 137(889):535–49.
10. Brobeck JR. Food intake as a mechanism of temperature regulation. Yale J Biol Med. 1948;20(6):545–52.
11. Mayer J. The glucostatic theory of regulation of food intake and the problem of obesity. Bull New Engl Med Cent. 1952;14(2):43–9.

12. Mayer J. Regulation of energy intake and the body weight: the glucostatic theory and the lipostatic hypothesis. Ann N Y Acad Sci. 1955;63(1):15–43.
13. Hervey GR. The effects of lesions in the hypothalamus in parabiotic rats. J Physiol. 1959;145(2):336–52.
14. Hervey GR. Control of appetite. Personal and departmental recollections. Appetite. 2013;61(1):100–10.
15. Harris RB, Hervey E, Hervey GR, Tobin G. Body composition of lean and obese Zucker rats in parabiosis. Int J Obes. 1987;11(3):275–83.
16. Hervey GR. Regulation of energy balance. Nature. 1969;222(5194):629–31.
17. Ingalls AM, Dickie MM, Snell GD. Obese, a new mutation in the house mouse. J Hered. 1950;41:317–8.
18. Herberg L, Coleman DL. Laboratory animals exhibiting obesity and diabetes syndromes. Metabolism. 1977;26(1):59–99.
19. Dickie MM, Lane PW. Plus letter to Roy Robinson 7/7/70. Mouse News Lett. 1957;17:52.
20. Coleman DL, Burkart DL. Plasma corticosterone concentrations in diabetic (db) mice. Diabetologia. 1977;13(1):25–6.
21. Hummel KP, Dickie MM, Coleman DL. Diabetes, a new mutation in the mouse. Science. 1966;153(3740):1127–8.
22. Coleman DL. Obese and diabetes: two mutant genes causing diabetes-obesity syndromes in mice. Diabetologia. 1978;14(3):141–8.
23. Coleman DL, Hummel KP. The influence of genetic background on the expression of the obese (Ob) gene in the mouse. Diabetologia. 1973;9(4):287–93.
24. Coleman DL. A historical perspective on leptin. Nat Med. 2010;16(10):1097–9.
25. Friedman JM, Schneider BS, Barton DE, Francke U. Level of expression and chromosome mapping of the mouse cholecystokinin gene: implications for murine models of genetic obesity. Genomics. 1989;5(3):463–9.
26. Bodanszky M, Tolle JC, Gardner JD, Walker MD, Mutt V. Cholecystokinin (pancreozymin). Synthesis and properties of the N alpha-acetyl-derivative of cholecystokinin 27–33. Int J Pept Protein Res. 1980;16(5):402–11.
27. Bahary N, Leibel RL, Joseph L, Friedman JM. Molecular mapping of the mouse db mutation. Proc Natl Acad Sci U S A. 1990;87(21):8642–6.
28. Orkin SH. Reverse genetics and human disease. Cell. 1986;47(6):845–50.
29. Riordan JR, Rommens JM, Kerem B, Alon N, Rozmahel R, Grzelczak Z, et al. Identification of the cystic fibrosis gene: cloning and characterization of complementary DNA. Science. 1989;245(4922):1066–73.
30. Chua Jr SC, White DW, Wu-Peng XS, Liu SM, Okada N, Kershaw EE, et al. Phenotype of fatty due to Gln269Pro mutation in the leptin receptor (Lepr). Diabetes. 1996;45(8):1141–3.
31. Friedman JM, Leibel RL, Siegel DS, Walsh J, Bahary N. Molecular mapping of the mouse ob mutation. Genomics. 1991;11(4):1054–62.
32. Bahary N, Siegel DA, Walsh J, Zhang Y, Leopold L, Leibel R, et al. Microdissection of proximal mouse chromosome 6: identification of RFLPs tightly linked to the ob mutation. Mamm Genome. 1993;4(9):511–5.
33. Walther C, Guenet JL, Simon D, Deutsch U, Jostes B, Goulding MD, et al. Pax: a murine multigene family of paired box-containing genes. Genomics. 1991; 11(2):424–34.
34. Bahary N, McGraw DE, Shilling R, Friedman JM. Microdissection and microcloning of mid-chromosome 4: genetic mapping of 41 microdissection clones. Genomics. 1993;16(1):113–22.
35. Zhang Y, Proenca R, Maffei M, Barone M, Leopold L, Friedman JM. Positional cloning of the mouse obese gene and its human homologue. Nature. 1994; 372(6505):425–32.
36. Church DM, Stotler CJ, Rutter JL, Murrell JR, Trofatter JA, Buckler AJ. Isolation of genes from complex sources of mammalian genomic DNA using exon amplification. Nature Genetics. 1994;6(1):98–105.
37. Moon BC, Friedman JM. The molecular basis of the obese mutation in ob2J mice. Genomics. 1997;42(1):152–6.
38. Maffei M, Fei H, Lee GH, Dani C, Leroy P, Zhang Y, et al. Increased expression in adipocytes of ob RNA in mice with lesions of the hypothalamus and with mutations at the db locus. Proc Natl Acad Sci U S A. 1995;92(15):6957–60.
39. Halaas JL, Gajiwala KS, Maffei M, Cohen SL, Chait BT, Rabinowitz D, et al. Weight-reducing effects of the plasma protein encoded by the obese gene. Science. 1995;269(5223):543–6.
40. Pelleymounter MA, Cullen MJ, Baker MB, Hecht R, Winters D, Boone T, et al. Effects of the obese gene product on body weight regulation in ob/ob mice. Science. 1995;269(5223):540–3.
41. Friedman JM. Leptin at 14 y of age: an ongoing story. Am J Clin Nutr. 2009;89(3):973S–9.
42. Campfield LA, Smith FJ, Guisez Y, Devos R, Burn P. Recombinant mouse OB protein: evidence for a peripheral signal linking adiposity and central neural networks. Science. 1995;269(5223):546–9.
43. Lee GH, Proenca R, Montez JM, Carroll KM, Darvishzadeh JG, Lee JI, et al. Abnormal splicing of the leptin receptor in diabetic mice. Nature. 1996;379(6566):632–5.
44. Tartaglia LA, Dembski M, Weng X, Deng N, Culpepper J, Devos R, et al. Identification and expression cloning of a leptin receptor, OB-R. Cell. 1995; 83(7):1263–71.

Leptin Receptors and Mechanism of Action

2

Julie Dam, Ralf Jockers, Michèle Guerre-Millo, and Karine Clément

Introduction

The spontaneous apparition of obesity mutant mice at the Jackson Laboratory (Bar Harbor, ME, USA) was a starting point for a long scientific journey, which climaxed in the discovery of leptin. Using these mutants in pioneer parabiosis experiments, DL Coleman proposed that "the *db*/*db* mutant mouse overproduced a satiety factor but could not respond to it—perhaps owing to a defective receptor—whereas the *ob*/*ob* mutant recognized and responded to the factor but could not produce it" (reviewed in [14]). He was right, as proved more than 40 years later when technical progresses in molecular biology allowed cloning the gene of leptin [54, 64] and, 1 year later, the gene of it receptor (LEPR) by virtue of leptin binding [54, 64]. It was then established that LEPR is mutated in various strains of *db*/*db* mice [9, 29–31] and in the *fa*/*fa* Zucker and fa^k/fa^k Koletsky rats [47, 53]. These major breakthroughs were rapidly followed by the identification of rare congenital leptin deficiency and mutations in *LEPR* in subjects with strikingly similar early onset and massive obesity phenotypes as mutant mice [13, 40, 52]. In this chapter, we focus on the genetic abnormalities of *LEPR* gene with dramatic clinical consequences and difficult patient management. In most cases, however, obese patients do not bear mutations in genes related to leptin signaling, but often have abnormally elevated circulating concentrations of leptin. As such, they are considered leptin resistant. Despite a wealth of information on LEPR structure and function, deciphering the molecular mechanisms underlying resistance to leptin remains a challenge. This question is addressed in the first part of this chapter.

LEPR Structure and Mechanism of Action

LEPR Genomic Organization

The genomic organization of the *LEPR* gene is unusual and holds some degree of complexity (Fig. 2.1a). A proximal promoter (P1) produces two distinct transcripts through alternative splicing: *OB-R*, now referred as *LEPR*, and the Leptin Receptor Overlapping Transcript, *LEPROT* [1, 39].

J. Dam, Ph.D. • R. Jockers, Ph.D.
Inserm U1016, Institut Cochin, Université Paris Descartes, Sorbonne Paris Cite, Paris, France

M. Guerre-Millo, Ph.D. • K. Clément, M.D., Ph.D. (✉)
Institute of Cardiometabolism and Nutrition, Pitié-Salpêtrière Hospital, Assistance Publique-Hôpitaux de Paris, Inserm UMR-S1166, Université Pierre et Marie Curie-Paris6, Sorbonne University, Paris, France
e-mail: karine.clement2@gmail.com; karine.clement@psl.aphp.fr

S. Dagogo-Jack (ed.), *Leptin: Regulation and Clinical Applications*,
DOI 10.1007/978-3-319-09915-6_2, © Springer International Publishing Switzerland 2015

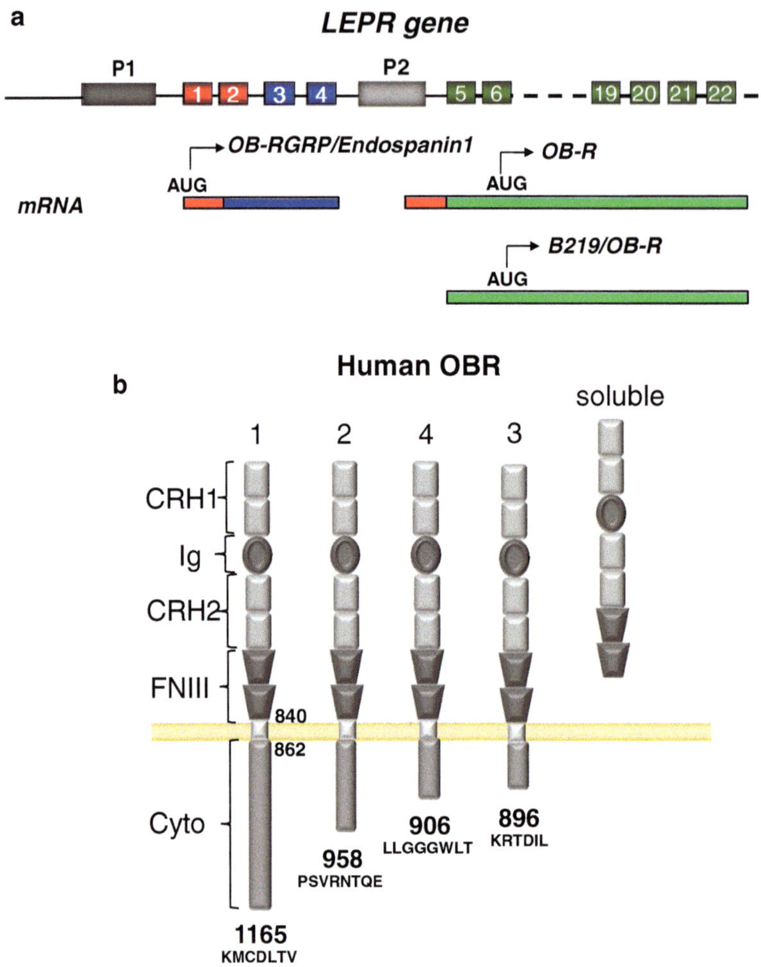

Fig. 2.1 *LEPR* gene and protein organization. (**a**) Schematic representation of the human *LEPR* gene on chromosome 1. LEPR gene expression is controlled by two promoters. The proximal promoter P1 generates two distinct transcripts (Leptin Receptor Overlapping Transcript (LEPROT) and LEPR) through alternative splicing, giving rise to two distinct proteins with no amino acid sequence homology (OB-RGRP/endospanin-1 and LEPR short and long isoforms, respectively). The alternative P2 promoter allows the expression of B219 OBR short isoforms. The AUG initiation codons on the mRNA are indicated by *arrows*. (**b**) Leptin receptor isoforms. There are five different isoforms of LEPR in humans, generated from alternative splicing. All share identical extracellular domains but they differ in the length and sequence of the C-terminal domain. Four of the five isoforms have a transmembrane domain, while the shortest isoform is truncated by proteolysis before the membrane-spanning domain. *CRH* cytokine receptor homology domain, *Ig* immunoglobulin domain, *FNIII* fibronectin III domain. The amino acid sequence at the end of the C-terminal tail is indicated

This overlapping gene structure occurs in humans but is not observed in rodents where the two genes are found distinctly separated. The *LEPR* transcript encodes LEPR protein isoforms (see below), while *LEPROT* transcript encodes LEPR gene-related protein (OB-RGRP) also called endospanin-1. Endospanin-1 is a 4 transmembrane domain-containing protein of 14 kDa with no amino acid sequence in common with LEPR. *LEPR/B219* is a third transcript expressed from the leptin receptor gene using a second internal P2 promoter. This transcript generates different short LEPR isoforms (B219), which are expressed exclusively in hematopoietic cells.

LEPR Isoforms

LEPR belongs to the class I cytokine receptor family and exists in five different isoforms (Fig. 2.1b). Four of them share the first 862 amino acids and display a unique transmembrane domain contained in exon 16. These four isoforms are generated by alternative splicing and differ in the length and sequence of their intracellular carboxyl terminal domain. The fifth isoform, called "soluble" or "secreted" isoform, binds leptin and circulates in the blood stream, but contains no transmembrane domain. Contrary to rodents, the transcript for the soluble isoform does not exist in humans where the soluble LEPR is generated by proteolytic cleavage of the transmembrane isoforms [36]. The long LEPR isoform (isoform 1 or b) is the one with a full-length intracellular domain capable of activating all the known leptin-induced signaling pathways [10, 11, 54]. The function of the short isoform a (or isoform 3) is less understood and may be involved in leptin transport through the blood brain barrier and in leptin clearance [32, 56]. The specific functions of the other short isoforms are still poorly known.

All five LEPR isoforms contain an N-terminal extracellular domain, which is required for ligand binding. This domain is heavily N-glycosylated, with N-glycosylation level reaching up to 1/3 of the total molecular weight of LEPR [21]. The N-terminal part of LEPR is composed of two conserved cytokine receptor homologous domains, CRH1 and CRH2, separated by a conserved immunoglobulin (Ig) domain. Adjacent to the CRH2 domain two fibronectin type 3 (FNIII) domains are located proximal to the transmembrane region.

LEPR Mechanisms of Action

Cell Surface Localization

Leptin binds and activates LEPR at the cell surface. The majority of LEPR is localized in intracellular compartments, including endoplasmic reticulum, *trans*-Golgi apparatus, and endosomes, with only a minor (10–20 %) fraction of LEPR present at the plasma membrane [4]. This subcellular distribution has been attributed to partial retention of the receptors in the biosynthetic pathway, coupled to removal from the plasma membrane via ligand-independent constitutive endocytosis [4]. Whether alteration in LEPR trafficking affects cell surface expression and, in turn, leptin signaling has been scarcely investigated. Experimental evidences suggest that Bardet-Biedl syndrome (BBS) proteins physically interact with LEPR . Moreover, the loss of BBS proteins in mice and in reconstituted cell systems perturbs LEPR trafficking and leptin signaling [15, 26, 50]. In other studies, the endospanin-1 protein encoded by the *LEPROT* transcript has been shown to negatively regulate LEPR cell surface expression by facilitating its lysosomal degradation. Silencing of the protein in mouse hypothalamic arcuate nucleus increases LEPR signaling capacity [15, 51, 57]. Regulation of LEPR trafficking by silencing these proteins or by disrupting their interaction with the receptor represents a possible strategy for improving leptin sensitivity.

Activation

Resonance Energy Transfer experiments in combination with biochemical and modeling studies started to unravel the molecular mechanism of LEPR activation. LEPR is thought to exist as preformed dimers or oligomers at the cell surface [60]. Binding studies in association with site-directed mutagenesis and homology molecular modeling suggest the existence of three different binding sites (I, II, and III) on leptin and support a 2:4 stoichiometry of the leptin–receptor complex [45, 61]. The CRH2 and Ig domains are involved in leptin binding and are required for receptor activation (Fig. 2.2a). Binding site II was shown to be indispensable for high affinity interaction between leptin and CRH2 domain [20, 24]. Engineered leptin mutants with an intact site II but modified site I or site III still bind to the CRH2 domain with strong affinity but are unable to activate the receptor [42, 46, 62]. Binding of two leptin molecules to LEPR triggers a conformational change within the extracellular domain and clustering of receptor dimers to form an hexameric complex (Fig. 2.2a) [45]. Recently, the architecture of the isolated extracellular region of the LEPR in the absence and

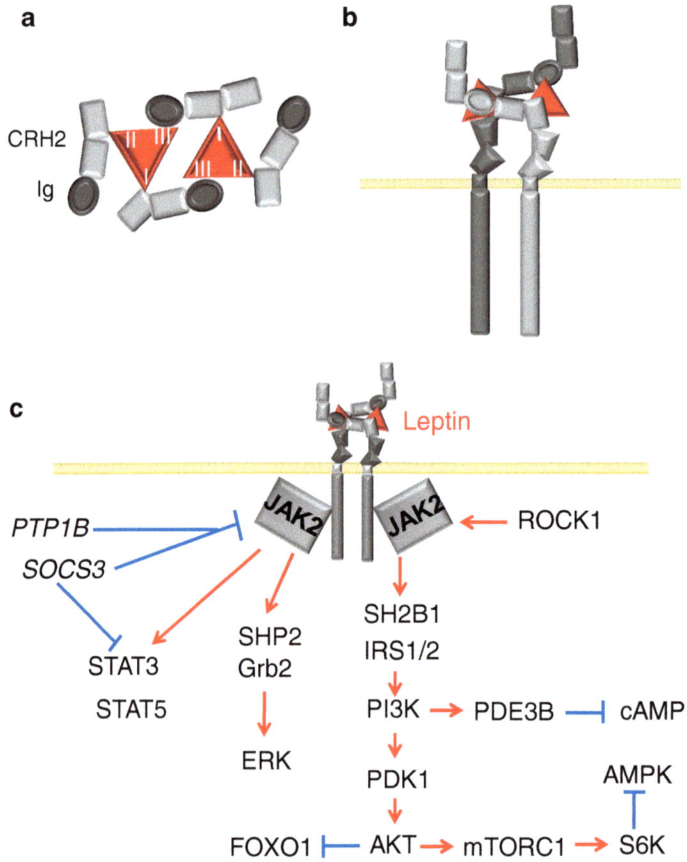

Fig. 2.2 LEPR activation and signaling. (**a**) Leptin–LEPR hexameric complex based on biochemical results and on molecular modeling. The complex contains two molecules of leptin and four LEPR protomers. Each leptin molecule binds three LEPR molecules through the high affinity binding site II (to CRH2) and via the two lower affinity binding sites I (to CRH2) and III (to Ig domain). (**b**) Model for the architecture of leptin/LEPR complex unraveled by single-particle electron microscopy [37]. Leptin employs only epitopes II and III to engage the CHR2 and Ig domain of 2 LEPR protomers, respectively. (**c**) Signaling pathways triggered upon leptin stimulation. Leptin binds to the long isoform LEPR b and activates ROCK1 and JAK2. JAK2 phosphorylates LEPR b on multiple Tyr, which interact with downstream signaling molecules and activate several signaling pathways. LEPR b signaling is regulated negatively by SOCS3 and PTP1B in a feedback loop

presence of leptin has been characterized by single-particle electron microscopy [37]. The results suggest that leptin and LEPR interact in a tetrameric complex with a 2:2 stoichiometry by engaging only leptin sites II and III (Fig. 2.2b). Thus, the role of binding site I and the overall stoichiometry of the leptin :receptor complex still remains elusive, most likely until we obtain structural information of the complex in its membrane-bound form. Additionally, leptin binding rigidifies the flexible hinge of CHR2 and favors a certain orientation of the FNIII domains that is required for LEPR activation [37, 62]. Based on our knowledge of the activation mechanism of other receptors, it is also conceivable that changes in microenvironment (interaction with other proteins, lipid environment) or posttranslational (glycosylation) modifications of LEPR could lead to subtle impairment of activation contributing to leptin resistance.

Signaling Pathways

LEPR is devoid of intrinsic enzymatic activity and its signaling capacity relies on the associated Janus family tyrosine kinase JAK2 [3, 48] (Fig. 2.2c). Upon receptor activation, JAK2 phosphorylates three tyrosine residues in the cytoplasmic domain of the long LEPR -b isoform, leading to the recruitment of signaling proteins of the signal transducer and activator of transcription (STAT) family. The STAT3 pathway is particularly critical and necessary for the effects of leptin on food intake and body weight [2, 41]. STAT3 is recruited to the LEPR-b and is phosphorylated by JAK2 allowing for STAT3 dimerization and translocation to the nucleus to mediate gene transcription. Other intracellular signaling pathways emanating from activated LEPR include the protein tyrosine phosphatase 2 (SHP2)/extracellular regulated kinase (ERK) pathway and the insulin receptor substrate (IRS)/phosphoinositide 3-kinase (PI3K) pathway. The suppressor of cytokine signaling 3 (SOCS3) is induced in response to leptin binding and, in turn, inhibits LEPR signaling via a negative feedback loop ([7, 48], [65]). Other important LEPR inhibitory factors are the protein tyrosine phosphatase-1B (PTP1B) [63] and the T cell protein tyrosine phosphatase TCPTP [35]. Cellular and mouse studies strongly support a role for these factors in leptin resistance at least in rodents [5–8, 35, 63]. Recently, it has been shown that Rho-associated coiled coil-containing protein kinase 1 (ROCK1) activity is required for leptin-induced activation of JAK2 [23]. This finding challenges the common belief that JAK2 is the first kinase activated by leptin. Reciprocal activation of JAK2 and RhoA/ROCK1 brings complexity to the system. Additionally, recent studies highlighted the importance of interacting proteins or lipids for LEPR signaling. Increased association of gangliosides to the LEPR upon leptin stimulation participates in LEPR activation [44]. Low-density lipoprotein receptor-related protein-1 (LRP1) was demonstrated to bind to the leptin–LEPR complex and was shown to be required for LEPR phosphorylation and STAT3 activation [34]. How these intertwined pathways coexist and act to trigger a normal or altered biological response remains elusive.

Genetic Abnormalities in Human LEPR

Mutations in LEPR

The first report describing a mutation in the LEPR in three obese subjects from a Kabilian consanguineous family was published in 1998, 3 years after the identification of the mouse gene. Affected individuals were homozygous for a mutation resulting in abnormal splicing of *LEPR* transcripts and generating a receptor lacking both transmembrane and intracellular domains [13]. Since then, several groups have identified LEPR mutations in extremely obese individuals. In 2007, Farooqi et al. sequenced the LEPR gene in 300 subjects with hyperphagia and severe early-onset obesity and estimated the prevalence of pathogenic *LEPR* mutations in this specific population around 3 % [19]. Other groups discovered LEPR mutations in single families or isolated individuals, such as in two cousins from Egypt [38]. Kakar et al. also identified a homozygous c.1603þ5G>C mutation at the splice donor site of the exon 11-intron 11 junction [25]. This mutation led to out-of-frame skipping of exon 11 and a premature stop codon (p.Arg468Serfs33). Other family cases included the discovery of an homozygous *LEPR* sequence frameshift mutation predicted to generate a truncated protein from a premature stop codon in exon 14 [28]. At variance with other described cases, this mutation was particular in a sense that it was identified in a Caucasian proband with unrelated parents. The father was heterozygous carrier of the mutation and the mother was intriguingly carrying the normal wild type alleles of *LEPR*. Thus the patient inherited from two paternal copies of chromosome 1 (isodisomy). Another genetic anomaly was found in a 7-year old patient with a homozygous 80 kb deletion in the chromosomal 1p31.3 region. The deleted region also comprises the proximal promoter and exons 1 and 2 of the *LEPR* gene and exons 5–19 of the *DNAJC6* gene. The deletion results in the abolishment of DNAJC6 transcript which encodes auxilin-1, a protein required for clathrin-dependent recycling of synaptic vesicles in neurons, but results also in the loss of *LEPROT* transcript. Whereas previously described mutations of the *LEPR* gene in humans concerned all transcripts, the deletion on *LEPR* gene of one of the proximal promoter with the preservation of the second internal promoter, only abolishes the canonical *LEPR* transcripts leaving *LEPR/B219* transcript fully functional [57]. Finally, whole-exome sequencing of 39 unrelated severely obese Pakistani children

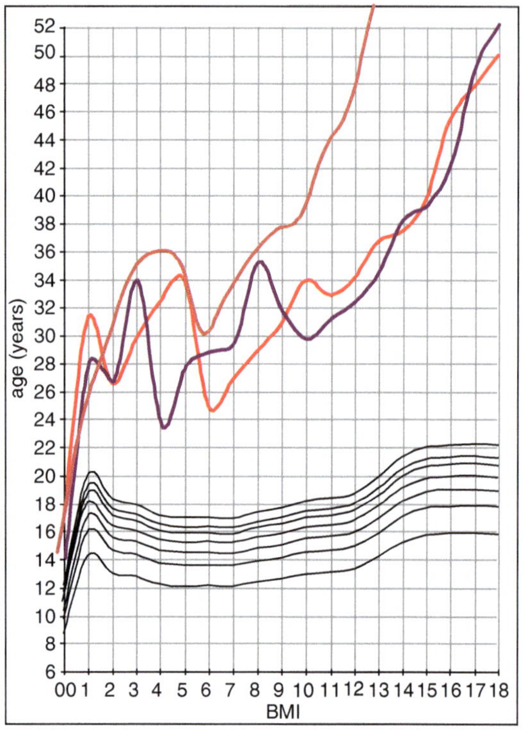

Fig. 2.3 This picture illustrates the very rapid and severe weight gain observed in three French children with *LEPR* mutation [13]. The BMI curves from the mutation carriers are shown in *colors*, compared to the reference curves for French children

revealed two homozygous *LEPR* mutations (an essential splice site mutation in exon 15 (c.2396-1G>T) and a nonsense mutation in exon 10 (c.1675G>A) were discovered in two probands, who were phenotypically indistinguishable from age-matched leptin-deficient subjects from the same population [49].

Clinical Consequences of LEPR Homozygous Mutations

As in leptin-deficient subjects, patients carrying LEPR mutations show an early and dramatic increase in body weight, as illustrated by the weight curve of LEPR deficient subjects (Fig. 2.3). Evaluating body composition in some *LEPR* mutation carriers showed a large amount of total body fat mass (>50 %) but resting energy expenditure was generally related to body corpulence. Feeding behavior is characterized by major hyperphagia and ravenous hunger [33]. Associated with severe early-onset obesity, hypogonadotrophic hypogonadism and thyrotropic insufficiency are frequently observed in *LEP* mutated subjects. It has also been described in some but not all subjects an insufficient somatotrophe secretion, associated with moderate growth delay. It is remarkable to mention that in some individuals with leptin deficiency either due to *LEP* or *LEPR* mutations, there is evidence of spontaneous pubertal development and in general improved endocrine functions with time. The follow-up of the first reported LEPR deficient sisters revealed a normalization of mild thyroid dysfunction and spontaneous puberty [43]. One of these patients was even able to give birth to a healthy son at the age of 26 years. Despite extreme obesity, no major clinical or metabolic complication occurred during pregnancy. This observation of a natural pregnancy in a woman with homozygous mutation of *LEPR* raises questions about the role of leptin signaling in human reproductive functions.

In general, analysis of heterozygous relatives showed that obesity was inconstant and not associated with endocrine abnormalities. An intermediate phenotype was described in rodents [12] and it was discussed that dysregulation of body weight in the *LEPR*$^{+/-}$ heterozygous state might arise from lower expression of the LEPR. If half of functional LEPR is not sufficient to prevent overweight and obesity, it could nevertheless reduce the severity of the phenotype. As described for *MC4R* or *POMC* genes, the penetrance of obesity due to the loss of one copy of *LEPR* gene can be incomplete. Variable clinical expression of the phenotype depends on the localization and the type of mutation, in relation with modulating environmental and genetic factors [18, 22]. Deeper exploration of a sufficient number of patients with one copy of *LEPR* gene is needed to address the relation between heterozygous LEPR mutation and obesity.

Management of Patients

Does the measurement of circulating leptin help in the diagnosis of *LEPR* mutations? Leptin levels were found extremely elevated in some but not all *LEPR* mutation carriers [13, 19, 40]. The specific nature of the first described *LEPR* mutation accounted for very high leptin levels, due to high circulating soluble LEPR shown to be able to trap circulating leptin [27]. Since serum levels of leptin were not disproportionately elevated in patients with other mutation types, it is estimated that serum leptin cannot be used as a marker for leptin-receptor deficiency. Thus, *LEPR* gene screening might be considered in subjects with the association of severe obesity and endocrine dysfunctions but with leptin related to corpulence or moderately elevated [19].

As with most patients with genetic obesity, with the notable exception of leptin-deficient subjects, care of patients with LEPR mutations is difficult and frequently unsuccessful. Factors that could possibly bypass leptin delivery systems are being developed but are not yet available for the treatment of these patients. A first example came with the ciliary neurotrophic factor (CNTF). CNTF activates downstream signaling molecules, such as STAT3, in the hypothalamus area that regulates food intake, even when administered systemically. Treatment with CNTF in humans and animals, including *db/db* mice induced substantial loss of fat mass [59]. The neurotrophic factor, Axokine, an agonist for CNTF receptor, was under development by the Regeneron Company, for the potential treatment of obesity and its metabolic associated complications. But the phase III clinical trials were stopped due to development of antibodies against Axokine in nearly 70 % of the tested subjects after approximately 3 months of treatment. In addition, Axokine treatment had a small positive effect [16].

Regarding other drug therapies, MC4R located downstream of the LEPR is becoming an attractive candidate drug target. Synthetic ligands and small molecule MC4R agonists have been in vitro tested with variable results [17, 58]. But they have to face specific difficulties of possible side effects due to the widespread expression of MC4R in the brain and the already demonstrated role of MC4R in erectile function [17, 58]. Novel pharmacological MC4R agonists are currently under development. Whether patients with mutation in the *LEPR* gene could benefit from this treatment might be considered.

Finally, bariatric surgery is considered as a long-term efficient treatment for severe obesity [55]. The question of such treatment and its potential efficiency is crucial in patients with monogenic obesity. Currently, data on bariatric surgery in patients with genetic obesity are limited and controversial. In one LEPR-deficient patient, vertical gastroplasty was beneficial and sufficient to induce and maintain a 40-kg weight loss (−20 % of the initial weight) over 8 years of regular follow-up [28]. In contrast, a relative failure of surgical therapy was illustrated in a report of rapid weight regain 1 year after bypass in another *LEPR* deficient morbidly obese woman (i.e., the first described patient) [28]. But this patient of low socioeconomic status had extreme difficulties after postsurgical counselling. She was noncompliant with the recommendations provided in this type of purely restrictive surgery and her medical follow-up was very irregular. This report illustrated the important role of environment on the benefice of bariatric surgery especially in case of monogenic obesities or underlined the poor efficiency of bariatric surgery in these patients.

Acknowledgements Teams are supported by grants from the European Union's Seventh Framework Programme (FP7/2007-2013) under grant agreement no. 241592 (to R.J.), the Agence Nationale de la Recherche ANR-12-JSV1-0011 (to J.D.), the "Who am I?" laboratory of excellence no. ANR-11-LABX-0071 funded by the French government through its "Investments for the Future" program operated by the French National Research Agency (ANR) under grant no. ANR-11-IDEX-0005-01 (to J.D. and R.J.) as well as the IHU University/Hospital Institute of Cardiometabolism and Nutrition (ICAN no. ANR-10-IAHU). Institut National de la Santé et de la Recherche Médicale (INSERM), Centre National de la Recherche Scientifique (CNRS), and Programme Hospitalier de Recherche Clinique (AP/HP). The authors thank Mr. Ludovic Le Chat in helping for iconography and paper formatting.

References

1. Bailleul B, Akerblom I, Strosberg AD. The leptin receptor promoter controls expression of a second distinct protein. Nucleic Acids Res. 1997;25:2752–8.
2. Bates SH, Stearns WH, Dundon TA, Schubert M, Tso AWK, Wang Y, Banks AS, Lavery HJ, Haq AK, Maratos-Flier E, Neel BG, Schwartz MW, Myers Jr MG. STAT3 signalling is required for leptin regulation of energy balance but not reproduction. Nature. 2003;421:856–9. doi:10.1038/nature01388.
3. Baumann H, Morella KK, White DW, Dembski M, Bailon PS, Kim H, Lai CF, Tartaglia LA. The full-length leptin receptor has signaling capabilities of interleukin 6-type cytokine receptors. Proc Natl Acad Sci U S A. 1996;93:8374–8.
4. Belouzard S, Delcroix D, Rouillé Y. Low levels of expression of leptin receptor at the cell surface result from constitutive endocytosis and intracellular retention in the biosynthetic pathway. J Biol Chem. 2004;279:28499–508. doi:10.1074/jbc.M400508200.
5. Bjørbaek C, El-Haschimi K, Frantz JD, Flier JS. The role of SOCS-3 in leptin signaling and leptin resistance. J Biol Chem. 1999;274:30059–65.
6. Bjørbaek C, Elmquist JK, El-Haschimi K, Kelly J, Ahima RS, Hileman S, Flier JS. Activation of SOCS-3 messenger ribonucleic acid in the hypothalamus by ciliary neurotrophic factor. Endocrinology. 1999; 140:2035–43. doi:10.1210/endo.140.5.6736.
7. Bjørbaek C, Elmquist JK, Frantz JD, Shoelson SE, Flier JS. Identification of SOCS-3 as a potential mediator of central leptin resistance. Mol Cell. 1998;1: 619–25.
8. Björnholm M, Münzberg H, Leshan RL, Villanueva EC, Bates SH, Louis GW, Jones JC, Ishida-Takahashi R, Bjørbaek C, Myers Jr MG. Mice lacking inhibitory leptin receptor signals are lean with normal endocrine function. J Clin Invest. 2007;117:1354–60. doi:10.1172/JCI30688.
9. Chen H, Charlat O, Tartaglia LA, Woolf EA, Weng X, Ellis SJ, Lakey ND, Culpepper J, Moore KJ, Breitbart RE, Duyk GM, Tepper RI, Morgenstern JP. Evidence that the diabetes gene encodes the leptin receptor: identification of a mutation in the leptin receptor gene in db/db mice. Cell. 1996;84:491–5.
10. Chua Jr SC, Koutras IK, Han L, Liu SM, Kay J, Young SJ, Chung WK, Leibel RL. Fine structure of the murine leptin receptor gene: splice site suppression is required to form two alternatively spliced transcripts. Genomics. 1997;45:264–70. doi:10.1006/geno.1997.4962.
11. Chua Jr SC, White DW, Wu-Peng XS, Liu SM, Okada N, Kershaw EE, Chung WK, Power-Kehoe L, Chua M, Tartaglia LA, Leibel RL. Phenotype of fatty due to Gln269Pro mutation in the leptin receptor (Lepr). Diabetes. 1996;45:1141–3.
12. Chung WK, Belfi K, Chua M, Wiley J, Mackintosh R, Nicolson M, Boozer CN, Leibel RL. Heterozygosity for Lep(ob) or Lep(rdb) affects body composition and leptin homeostasis in adult mice. Am J Physiol. 1998;274:R985–90.
13. Clément K, Vaisse C, Lahlou N, Cabrol S, Pelloux V, Cassuto D, Gourmelen M, Dina C, Chambaz J, Lacorte JM, Basdevant A, Bougnères P, Lebouc Y, Froguel P, Guy-Grand B. A mutation in the human leptin receptor gene causes obesity and pituitary dysfunction. Nature. 1998;392:398–401. doi:10.1038/32911.
14. Coleman DL. A historical perspective on leptin. Nat Med. 2010;16:1097–9. doi:10.1038/nm1010-1097.
15. Couturier C, Sarkis C, Séron K, Belouzard S, Chen P, Lenain A, Corset L, Dam J, Vauthier V, Dubart A, Mallet J, Froguel P, Rouillé Y, Jockers R. Silencing of OB-RGRP in mouse hypothalamic arcuate nucleus increases leptin receptor signaling and prevents diet-induced obesity. Proc Natl Acad Sci U S A. 2007;104:19476–81. doi:10.1073/pnas.0706671104.
16. Doco-Fenzy M, Leroy C, Schneider A, Petit F, Delrue M-A, Andrieux J, Perrin-Sabourin L, Landais E, Aboura A, Puechberty J, Girard M, Tournaire M, Sanchez E, Rooryck C, Ameil A, Goossens M, Jonveaux P, Lefort G, Taine L, Cailley D, Gaillard D, Leheup B, Sarda P, Geneviève D. Early-onset obesity and paternal 2pter deletion encompassing the ACP1, TMEM18, and MYT1L genes. Eur J Hum Genet. 2014;22:471–9. doi:10.1038/ejhg.2013.189.
17. Farooqi IS, Bullmore E, Keogh J, Gillard J, O'Rahilly S, Fletcher PC. Leptin regulates striatal regions and human eating behavior. Science. 2007;317:1355. doi:10.1126/science.1144599.
18. Farooqi IS, Drop S, Clements A, Keogh JM, Biernacka J, Lowenbein S, Challis BG, O'Rahilly S. Heterozygosity for a POMC-null mutation and increased obesity risk in humans. Diabetes. 2006; 55:2549–53. doi:10.2337/db06-0214.
19. Farooqi IS, Wangensteen T, Collins S, Kimber W, Matarese G, Keogh JM, Lank E, Bottomley B, Lopez-Fernandez J, Ferraz-Amaro I, Dattani MT, Ercan O, Myhre AG, Retterstol L, Stanhope R, Edge JA, McKenzie S, Lessan N, Ghodsi M, De Rosa V, Perna F, Fontana S, Barroso I, Undlien DE, O'Rahilly S. Clinical and molecular genetic spectrum of congenital deficiency of the leptin receptor. N Engl J Med. 2007;356:237–47. doi:10.1056/NEJMoa063988.

20. Fong TM, Huang RR, Tota MR, Mao C, Smith T, Varnerin J, Karpitskiy VV, Krause JE, Van der Ploeg LH. Localization of leptin binding domain in the leptin receptor. Mol Pharmacol. 1998;53:234–40.
21. Haniu M, Arakawa T, Bures EJ, Young Y, Hui JO, Rohde MF, Welcher AA, Horan T. Human leptin receptor. Determination of disulfide structure and N-glycosylation sites of the extracellular domain. J Biol Chem. 1998;273:28691–9.
22. Hinney A, Bettecken T, Tarnow P, Brumm H, Reichwald K, Lichtner P, Scherag A, Nguyen TT, Schlumberger P, Rief W, Vollmert C, Illig T, Wichmann H-E, Schäfer H, Platzer M, Biebermann H, Meitinger T, Hebebrand J. Prevalence, spectrum, and functional characterization of melanocortin-4 receptor gene mutations in a representative population-based sample and obese adults from Germany. J Clin Endocrinol Metab. 2006;91:1761–9. doi:10.1210/jc.2005-2056.
23. Huang H, Kong D, Byun KH, Ye C, Koda S, Lee DH, Oh B-C, Lee SW, Lee B, Zabolotny JM, Kim MS, Bjørbæk C, Lowell BB, Kim Y-B. Rho-kinase regulates energy balance by targeting hypothalamic leptin receptor signaling. Nat Neurosci. 2012;15:1391–8. doi:10.1038/nn.3207.
24. Iserentant H, Peelman F, Defeau D, Vandekerckhove J, Zabeau L, Tavernier J. Mapping of the interface between leptin and the leptin receptor CRH2 domain. J Cell Sci. 2005;118:2519–27. doi:10.1242/jcs.02386.
25. Kakar N, Ahmad J, Kubisch C, Borck G. Exon skipping and severe childhood-onset obesity caused by a leptin receptor mutation. Am J Med Genet A. 2013;161:2672–4. doi:10.1002/ajmg.a.36125.
26. Kimber W, Peelman F, Prieur X, Wangensteen T, O'Rahilly S, Tavernier J, Farooqi IS. Functional characterization of naturally occurring pathogenic mutations in the human leptin receptor. Endocrinology. 2008;149:6043–52. doi:10.1210/en.2008-0544.
27. Lahlou N, Clement K, Carel JC, Vaisse C, Lotton C, Le Bihan Y, Basdevant A, Lebouc Y, Froguel P, Roger M, Guy-Grand B. Soluble leptin receptor in serum of subjects with complete resistance to leptin: relation to fat mass. Diabetes. 2000;49:1347–52.
28. Le Beyec J, Cugnet-Anceau C, Pépin D, Alili R, Cotillard A, Lacorte J-M, Basdevant A, Laville M, Clément K. Homozygous leptin receptor mutation due to uniparental disomy of chromosome 1: response to bariatric surgery. J Clin Endocrinol Metab. 2013;98:E397–402. doi:10.1210/jc.2012-2779.
29. Lee G, Li C, Montez J, Halaas J, Darvishzadeh J, Friedman JM. Leptin receptor mutations in 129 db3J/db3J mice and NIH facp/facp rats. Mamm Genome. 1997;8:445–7.
30. Lee GH, Proenca R, Montez JM, Carroll KM, Darvishzadeh JG, Lee JI, Friedman JM. Abnormal splicing of the leptin receptor in diabetic mice. Nature. 1996;379:632–5. doi:10.1038/379632a0.
31. Li C, Ioffe E, Fidahusein N, Connolly E, Friedman JM. Absence of soluble leptin receptor in plasma from dbPas/dbPas and other db/db mice. J Biol Chem. 1998;273:10078–82.
32. Li Z, Ceccarini G, Eisenstein M, Tan K, Friedman JM. Phenotypic effects of an induced mutation of the ObRa isoform of the leptin receptor. Mol Metab. 2013;2:364–75. doi:10.1016/j.molmet.2013.07.007.
33. Licinio J, Caglayan S, Ozata M, Yildiz BO, de Miranda PB, O'Kirwan F, Whitby R, Liang L, Cohen P, Bhasin S, Krauss RM, Veldhuis JD, Wagner AJ, DePaoli AM, McCann SM, Wong M-L. Phenotypic effects of leptin replacement on morbid obesity, diabetes mellitus, hypogonadism, and behavior in leptin-deficient adults. Proc Natl Acad Sci U S A. 2004;101:4531–6. doi:10.1073/pnas.0308767101.
34. Liu Q, Zhang J, Zerbinatti C, Zhan Y, Kolber BJ, Herz J, Muglia LJ, Bu G. Lipoprotein receptor LRP1 regulates leptin signaling and energy homeostasis in the adult central nervous system. PLoS Biol. 2011;9:e1000575. doi:10.1371/journal.pbio.1000575.
35. Loh K, Fukushima A, Zhang X, Galic S, Briggs D, Enriori PJ, Simonds S, Wiede F, Reichenbach A, Hauser C, Sims NA, Bence KK, Zhang S, Zhang Z-Y, Kahn BB, Neel BG, Andrews ZB, Cowley MA, Tiganis T. Elevated hypothalamic TCPTP in obesity contributes to cellular leptin resistance. Cell Metab. 2011;14:684–99. doi:10.1016/j.cmet.2011.09.011.
36. Maamra M, Bidlingmaier M, Postel-Vinay MC, Wu Z, Strasburger CJ, Ross RJ. Generation of human soluble leptin receptor by proteolytic cleavage of membrane-anchored receptors. Endocrinology. 2001;142:4389–93. doi:10.1210/endo.142.10.8442.
37. Mancour LV, Daghestani HN, Dutta S, Westfield GH, Schilling J, Oleskie AN, Herbstman JF, Chou SZ, Skiniotis G. Ligand-induced architecture of the leptin receptor signaling complex. Mol Cell. 2012;48:655–61. doi:10.1016/j.molcel.2012.09.003.
38. Mazen I, El-Gammal M, Abdel-Hamid M, Farooqi IS, Amr K. Homozygosity for a novel missense mutation in the leptin receptor gene (P316T) in two Egyptian cousins with severe early onset obesity. Mol Genet Metab. 2011;102:461–4. doi:10.1016/j.ymgme.2010.12.013.
39. Mercer JG, Moar KM, Hoggard N, Strosberg AD, Froguel P, Bailleul B. B219/OB-R 5'-UTR and leptin receptor gene-related protein gene expression in mouse brain and placenta: tissue-specific leptin receptor promoter activity. J Neuroendocrinol. 2000;12:649–55.
40. Montague CT, Farooqi IS, Whitehead JP, Soos MA, Rau H, Wareham NJ, Sewter CP, Digby JE, Mohammed SN, Hurst JA, Cheetham CH, Earley AR, Barnett AH, Prins JB, O'Rahilly S. Congenital leptin deficiency is associated with severe early-onset obesity in humans. Nature. 1997;387:903–8. doi:10.1038/43185.
41. Myers MG, Cowley MA, Münzberg H. Mechanisms of leptin action and leptin resistance. Annu Rev Physiol. 2008;70:537–56. doi:10.1146/annurev.physiol.70.113006.100707.
42. Niv-Spector L, Gonen-Berger D, Gourdou I, Biener E, Gussakovsky EE, Benomar Y, Ramanujan KV, Taouis M, Herman B, Callebaut I, Djiane J, Gertler A. Identification of the hydrophobic strand in the A-B loop of leptin as major binding site III: implications

for large-scale preparation of potent recombinant human and ovine leptin antagonists. Biochem J. 2005;391:221–30. doi:10.1042/BJ20050457.
43. Nizard J, Dommergues M, Dommergue M, Clément K. Pregnancy in a woman with a leptin-receptor mutation. N Engl J Med. 2012;366:1064–5. doi:10.1056/NEJMc1200116.
44. Nordström V, Willershäuser M, Herzer S, Rozman J, von Bohlen Und Halbach O, Meldner S, Rothermel U, Kaden S, Roth FC, Waldeck C, Gretz N, de Angelis MH, Draguhn A, Klingenspor M, Gröne H-J, Jennemann R. Neuronal expression of glucosylceramide synthase in central nervous system regulates body weight and energy homeostasis. PLoS Biol. 2013;11:e1001506. doi:10.1371/journal.pbio.1001506.
45. Peelman F, Iserentant H, De Smet A-S, Vandekerckhove J, Zabeau L, Tavernier J. Mapping of binding site III in the leptin receptor and modeling of a hexameric leptin. leptin receptor complex. J Biol Chem. 2006;281:15496–504. doi:10.1074/jbc.M512622200.
46. Peelman F, Van Beneden K, Zabeau L, Iserentant H, Ulrichts P, Defeau D, Verhee A, Catteeuw D, Elewaut D, Tavernier J. Mapping of the leptin binding sites and design of a leptin antagonist. J Biol Chem. 2004;279:41038–46. doi:10.1074/jbc.M404962200.
47. Phillips MS, Liu Q, Hammond HA, Dugan V, Hey PJ, Caskey CJ, Hess JF. Leptin receptor missense mutation in the fatty Zucker rat. Nat Genet. 1996;13:18–9. doi:10.1038/ng0596-18.
48. Robertson SA, Leinninger GM, Myers Jr MG. Molecular and neural mediators of leptin action. Physiol Behav. 2008;94:637–42. doi:10.1016/j.physbeh.2008.04.005.
49. Saeed S, Bonnefond A, Manzoor J, Philippe J, Durand E, Arshad M, Sand O, Butt TA, Falchi M, Arslan M, Froguel P. Novel LEPR mutations in obese Pakistani children identified by PCR-based enrichment and next generation sequencing. Obesity (Silver Spring). 2014;22:1112–7. doi:10.1002/oby.20667.
50. Seo S, Guo D-F, Bugge K, Morgan DA, Rahmouni K, Sheffield VC. Requirement of Bardet-Biedl syndrome proteins for leptin receptor signaling. Hum Mol Genet. 2009;18:1323–31. doi:10.1093/hmg/ddp031.
51. Séron K, Couturier C, Belouzard S, Bacart J, Monté D, Corset L, Bocquet O, Dam J, Vauthier V, Lecœur C, Bailleul B, Hoflack B, Froguel P, Jockers R, Rouillé Y. Endospanins regulate a postinternalization step of the leptin receptor endocytic pathway. J Biol Chem. 2011;286:17968–81. doi:10.1074/jbc.M111.224857.
52. Strobel A, Issad T, Camoin L, Ozata M, Strosberg AD. A leptin missense mutation associated with hypogonadism and morbid obesity. Nat Genet. 1998;18:213–5. doi:10.1038/ng0398-213.
53. Takaya K, Ogawa Y, Hiraoka J, Hosoda K, Yamori Y, Nakao K, Koletsky RJ. Nonsense mutation of leptin receptor in the obese spontaneously hypertensive Koletsky rat. Nat Genet. 1996;14:130–1. doi:10.1038/ng1096-130.
54. Tartaglia LA, Dembski M, Weng X, Deng N, Culpepper J, Devos R, Richards GJ, Campfield LA, Clark FT, Deeds J, Muir C, Sanker S, Moriarty A, Moore KJ, Smutko JS, Mays GG, Wool EA, Monroe CA, Tepper RI. Identification and expression cloning of a leptin receptor, OB-R. Cell. 1995;83:1263–71.
55. Ujjainwalla F, Sebhat IK. Small molecule ligands of the human melanocortin-4 receptor. Curr Top Med Chem. 2007;7:1068–84.
56. Uotani S, Bjørbaek C, Tornøe J, Flier JS. Functional properties of leptin receptor isoforms: internalization and degradation of leptin and ligand-induced receptor downregulation. Diabetes. 1999;48:279–86.
57. Vauthier V, Jaillard S, Journel H, Dubourg C, Jockers R, Dam J. Homozygous deletion of an 80 kb region comprising part of DNAJC6 and LEPR genes on chromosome 1P31.3 is associated with early onset obesity, mental retardation and epilepsy. Mol Genet Metab. 2012;106:345–50. doi:10.1016/j.ymgme.2012.04.026.
58. Williamson DA, Ravussin E, Wong M-L, Wagner A, Dipaoli A, Caglayan S, Ozata M, Martin C, Walden H, Arnett C, Licinio J. Microanalysis of eating behavior of three leptin deficient adults treated with leptin therapy. Appetite. 2005;45:75–80. doi:10.1016/j.appet.2005.01.002.
59. Xing D-J, Zhang H-X, Huang N, Wu K-C, Huang X-F, Huang F, Tong Y, Pang C-P, Qu J, Jin Z-B. Comprehensive molecular diagnosis of Bardet-Biedl syndrome by high-throughput targeted exome sequencing. PLoS One. 2014;9:e90599. doi:10.1371/journal.pone.0090599.
60. Zabeau L, Defeau D, Iserentant H, Vandekerckhove J, Peelman F, Tavernier J. Leptin receptor activation depends on critical cysteine residues in its fibronectin type III subdomains. J Biol Chem. 2005;280:22632–40. doi:10.1074/jbc.M413308200.
61. Zabeau L, Defeau D, Van der Heyden J, Iserentant H, Vandekerckhove J, Tavernier J. Functional analysis of leptin receptor activation using a Janus kinase/signal transducer and activator of transcription complementation assay. Mol Endocrinol. 2004;18:150–61. doi:10.1210/me.2003-0078.
62. Zabeau L, Verhee A, Catteeuw D, Faes L, Seeuws S, Decruy T, Elewaut D, Peelman F, Tavernier J. Selection of non-competitive leptin antagonists using a random nanobody-based approach. Biochem J. 2012;441:425–34. doi:10.1042/BJ20110438.
63. Zabolotny JM, Bence-Hanulec KK, Stricker-Krongrad A, Haj F, Wang Y, Minokoshi Y, Kim Y-B, Elmquist JK, Tartaglia LA, Kahn BB, Neel BG. PTP1B regulates leptin signal transduction in vivo. Dev Cell. 2002; 2:489–95.
64. Zhang Y, Proenca R, Maffei M, Barone M, Leopold L, Friedman JM. Positional cloning of the mouse obese gene and its human homologue. Nature. 1994;372: 425–32. doi:10.1038/372425a0.
65. Xu AW1, Ste-Marie L, Kaelin CB, Barsh GS. Inactivation of signal transducer and activator of transcription 3 in proopiomelanocortin (Pomc) neurons causes decreased pomc expression, mild obesity, and defects in compensatory refeeding. Endocrinology. 2007;148(1):72–80. Epub 2006 Oct 5.

3 Leptin Interaction with Brain Orexigenic and Anorexigenic Pathways

Denis G. Baskin

Abbreviations

ARC	Arcuate nucleus
AGRP	Agouti-related peptide
aMSH	Alpha melanocyte stimulation hormone
CART	Cocaine- and amphetamine-regulated transcript
CCK	Cholecystokinin
CNS	Central nervous system
CRH	Corticotropin releasing hormone
CSF	Cerebrospinal fluid
fMRI	Functional magnetic resonance imaging
GABA	Gamma amino butyric acid
JAK2	Janus-activated kinase 2
Lep	Leptin gene
LepR	Leptin receptor
MAPK	Mitogen-activated protein kinase
MCH	Melanin concentrating hormone
MC4r	Melanocortin 4 receptor
NMDR	N-methyl-D-aspartate
NPY	Neuropeptide Y
NTS	Nucleus of the solitary tract
OXr	Oxytocin receptor
PI3K	Phosphatidylinositol 3-OH-kinase
POMC	Proopiomelanocortin
PVN	Paraventricular nucleus
STAT3	Signal transducer and activator of transcription 3
Y1r	Neuropeptide Y Y1 receptor

D.G. Baskin (✉)
Endocrinology and Metabolism, VA Puget Sound Medical Center, Seattle, WA, USA
e-mail: baskindg@uw.edu

Introduction

Obesity, once thought to result from lack of willpower, is now understood to be the result of impaired regulation of energy homeostasis by central nervous system (CNS) circuits that respond to metabolic cues from the periphery and adjust food intake and energy expenditure to maintain a regulated mass of adipose tissue. The neural pathways that regulate food intake and energy expenditure integrate stimuli from sensory and autonomic inputs arising outside the brain, from endocrine signals that arise in the periphery and act on the CNS by crossing the blood–brain barrier, as well as from nutrients that influence the activity of CNS neural function [1]. The preponderance of experimental research in this area has been conducted on animal models; relatively few studies have been conducted on human brain pathways that respond to the anorexigenic signaling provided by leptin, although recent use of imaging techniques is shedding light on the responses of the human brain to leptin.

Central to the hypothesis that the CNS plays a key role in the regulation of body weight is the concept of adiposity signals: a class of physiological signals that circulate in direct proportion to the mass of adipose tissue [2]. As such, they

S. Dagogo-Jack (ed.), *Leptin: Regulation and Clinical Applications*,
DOI 10.1007/978-3-319-09915-6_3,

potentially inform the brain about the relative state of adipose tissue mass and energy homeostasis. Because their mean plasma concentrations are relatively constant over time, reflecting the long term states of energy stores, adiposity signals differ from other hormonal signals that influence food intake and whose levels vary around meals and act on the CNS—either directly or by neural inputs—to influence the timing of meal termination (e.g., satiety signals) or their initiation.

Abundant evidence suggests that adipose tissue mass is a relatively accurate benchmark of the state of energy homeostasis over long periods of time in adult humans, and large changes in weight are primary a consequence of proportional changes in fat stores (adiposity). Thus, body weight can be viewed as the integral of energy consumption (food intake) and energy expenditure (metabolism, activity, and sympathetic nervous system activity); the balance of these processes is what is meant by energy balance or energy homeostasis. A major paradigm in the field of obesity research is that adiposity signals are a critical component of a physiological mechanism for the regulation of energy homeostasis by the CNS. Leptin and insulin are considered to be the major adiposity signals to the brain for the long-term regulation of adipose tissue stores, and thus the identification of CNS cells and pathways that respond to adiposity signals and regulate food intake and body weight has been the focus of intense research.

Leptin and the Brain

The reports of the discoveries of the adipose tissue hormone leptin and its receptors in the mid-1990s changed the landscape of research on body weight regulation and held promise for new treatments of human obesity [3–5]. Looking back with the hindsight of our current understanding of the complexity of obesity and the relative ineffectiveness of leptin-based therapies for obesity, we nevertheless can say that the excitement generated by the discovery of leptin led to a greater understanding of role of the CNS in the regulation of energy homeostasis. It's worth noting that while leptin anorexigenic effects could be elicited by peripheral administration of the hormone, its primary site of anorexigenic action was proposed to be in the brain rather than on peripheral tissues. To understand the reason why investigators looked to a central site for leptin's anorexigenic actions, it's instructive to review the conceptual framework at that time about the role of metabolic hormones on the regulation of food intake and body weight by the brain.

Seminal experiments by Woods and Porte in the late 1970s demonstrated that infusion of insulin directly into brain CSF caused a dose-dependent suppression of food intake in both primates and rodents, leading to the hypothesis that insulin from the pancreas provides a signal to the brain for the regulation of food intake and body weight [6]. The validity of this hypothesis—that insulin enters the brain to regulate adipose mass—was not widely appreciated nor accepted for many years despite a growing body of supportive evidence, in part because of the traditional dogma that viewed insulin as a hormone that mainly acts on peripheral tissues to regulate glucose and lipid metabolism. The notion that a peptide hormone of insulin's molecular size could cross the blood–brain barrier and affect neuronal functions that control eating and energy expenditure did not fit the conventional paradigm of insulin's role in metabolic physiology. This reluctance was in the face of mounting data demonstrating that insulin administered directly into the hypothalamic third ventricle dose-dependently reduces food intake and body weight gain, attenuates the hyperphagia of insulin-deficient type 1 diabetes, and blocks expression of orexigenic neuropeptides in the brain [2, 7, 8].

Nevertheless, the evidence that had accumulated in support of insulin as an adiposity signal to the brain was prophetic as it set the stage for the research community to accept the idea that a peripheral peptide whose plasma levels are directly proportionate to fat mass could do the same. Moreover, the emerging literature had pointed to peptidergic neurons in the hypothalamus, the arcuate nucleus in particular, as being major targets of the adiposity action of insulin in the rat brain. Prophetically, early morphological and histochemical studies on leptin action in the brain demonstrated that arcuate nucleus neurons were also targets of leptin's adiposity actions on food intake and body weight.

Contributing to the slow uptake of accepting insulin to be a CNS adiposity signal were early reports of insulin synthesis by neurons in the brain. This literature confounded the issue, as any CNS actions of insulin related to food intake could accordingly be attributed to neuronal secretion of insulin rather than the action of insulin that had entered the brain from the periphery. While insulin receptors are widely distributed in the CNS [9–11], supporting the hypothesis that the brain is a target of circulating insulin, evidence for synthesis or secretion of insulin in the adult mammalian brain has not been unequivocally demonstrated and is generally believed not to be a factor in the metabolic effects of insulin in the brain. Although occasional articles reporting insulin gene expression in the CNS appear in the literature, it is fair to conclude that while it is possible that some neurons may secrete insulin in very low concentrations for local neural transmission or modulation, such processes would be probably be distinct from the actions of peripheral insulin acting as an adiposity signal for influencing food intake and body weight.

Over the years, studies on animal models had established a key role for the hypothalamus in regulating homeostasis responses to food ingestion. The many observations in rodents as well as the findings in humans that lesions of the ventromedial hypothalamus cause obesity, whereas damage to the lateral hypothalamus results in anorexigenic syndromes, focused the attention of researchers on the hypothalamus as a potential central target of peripheral metabolic signals for regulating energy balance. In the pre-leptin era, neurons expressing neuropeptide Y (NPY) in the hypothalamic arcuate nucleus were implicated in the negative feedback of insulin adiposity signaling. NPY expression in the arcuate nucleus stimulates food intake, an action that can be attenuated by insulin [12–14]. Thus, when leptin was first shown to have an anorexigenic action in the CNS, it was logical for investigators to look to the arcuate nucleus as a site for leptin responsive neurons [8]. A large body of literature has established that specific neurons in the arcuate nucleus are a primary target of leptin and mediate the anorexigenic effects of this adiposity signal. A wealth of histochemical, molecular, behavioral, electrophysiological, and pharmacological data has been published to establish a model of hypothalamic circuitry that responds to leptin.

Leptin Receptors in the CNS

Leptin's effects on cells are mediated by transmembrane leptin receptors (LepR) that are encoded by the *LepR* gene [15]. Mutations of the *LepR* gene in rodents result in obesity phenotypes as a consequence of defective leptin receptor molecules (db/db mouse, fa/fa Zucker rat, fa(k)/fa(k) Koletsky rat) [16]. *LepR* is expressed as at least five alternatively spiced forms in rodents. The LepRb (also called Ob-Rb) splice variant is considered to be the functional isoform responsible for leptin's anorexigenic effects in the CNS [17–19] and is found widely distributed in rodent brains. While LepRb leptin receptors are particularly concentrated in the arcuate nucleus, they are also expressed in other regions of the hypothalamus, including the ventromedial nucleus, dorsomedial nucleus, paraventricular nucleus, and perifornical areas, where they are implicated in leptin's anorexigenic effects on food intake [20–22]. In the hypothalamus, LepRb mRNA and immunoreactive protein are expressed by NPY and POMC neurons in the arcuate nucleus [20, 23–27]. Leptin receptors are also expressed by hypothalamic astrocytes, where they are implicated in regulation of synaptic remodeling and leptin's effects on food intake [28] and by ependymal tanycytes where they are proposed to function in the transport of leptin into the brain [29].

Leptin Actions on Hypothalamic Neurons

Our understanding of the sites of leptin action in the CNS is derived largely from morphological, physiological, and behavioral research on animal models, rodents primarily. While leptin has been shown to have effects, both direct and indirect, on many different CNS cell types, neurons that express NPY and proopiomelanocortin (POMC) genes in the arcuate nucleus are believed to be a primary target of leptin's function as an adiposity signal to the brain [2, 8]. Neuropeptide NPY is a potent CNS stimulator of food intake when injected into the brain third ventricle or directly into the arcuate nucleus, and genetic overexpression of NPY leads to obesity in rodents. Expression of the POMC gene in arcuate nucleus neurons is associated with reductions of food intake and loss of body weight. Genetic knockout of POMC expression results in increased food ingestion and obesity. The POMC posttranslational product, alpha-melanocyte stimulating hormone (aMSH) activates postsynaptic melanocortin-4 receptors (MC4r) on downstream neurons in the paraventricular nucleus and elsewhere that mediate anorexia. Arcuate nucleus POMC neurons also co-express agouti related peptide (AGRP) [30], which is released from POMC terminals in response to leptin, resulting in blockade of postsynaptic MC4r receptors and thereby modulates the anorexigenic action of aMSH. Thus leptin engages a counterregulatory neuronal circuit in the arcuate nucleus: leptin activates anorexigenic POMC (aMSH) gene expression and inhibits orexigenic NPY expression, leading to reductions in food intake that can result in reduced adipose tissue stores. Deficiency of leptin signaling to the arcuate nucleus, such as during fasting, activates a counter-regulatory response by permitting increased expression of NPY and AGRP while inhibiting POMC (aMSH) expression, resulting in increased food intake and body weight. Intracerebroventricular injection of leptin blocks the increased arcuate nucleus NPY mRNA and AGRP mRNA expression that occurs in during fasting and consequently prevents hyperphagia and weight gain. In contrast, intracerebroventricular administration of leptin has the opposite effect on expression of POMC expression in arcuate nucleus neurons, elevating POMC mRNA and resulting in decreased food intake and loss of body weight. It's important to realize that arcuate nucleus neurons that express NPY/AGRP and those that express POMC also secrete other peptides and neurotransmitters that potentially influence diverse neuroendocrine functions including reproduction. Leptin acting via LepRb in neonatal mice also influences the early development of hypothalamic circuits that modulate feeding [31].

Neuronal Responses to Leptin

The binding of leptin to LepRb on arcuate nucleus neurons activates intracellular signaling cascades that lead to alterations in neuronal function. The details of leptin signaling pathways and their effects in CNS neurons are well described and have been demonstrated to be closely related to leptin's effects on energy homeostasis [19, 32, 33]. Leptin acting through LepRb activates Janus-activated kinase (JAK)/signal transducer and activator of transcription 3 (STAT3) signaling in NPY/AGRP and POMC neurons [34] and inhibits NPY and AGRP gene expression through phosphatidylinositol 3-OH-kinase (PI3K) signaling [34, 35]. Leptin and insulin have overlapping actions on NPY and POMC gene expression in the arcuate nucleus and signaling. Both induce post-receptor signals that converge on the PI3K pathway, explaining a possible mechanism for leptin enhancement insulin sensitivity of the arcuate nucleus [35]. Electrophysiological studies reveal that leptin increases the firing rate of POMC neurons, consistent with the role of these neurons as mediators of leptin's anorexigenic actions. This occurs by means of reduced inhibition by GABA, which is released from neighboring NPY neurons upon leptin's activation of the latter cells. Recent reports indicate that diet-induced obesity in mice is associated with the failure of LepRb signaling to reduce neuronal action potential frequencies mediated specifically by Kv2.1 cation channels in arcuate nucleus NPY neurons. The effects of leptin on calcium currents in NPY vs. POMC neurons involve different signaling pathways: leptin decreases high voltage-activated calcium currents in arcuate nucleus NPY neurons via a LepR-JAK2-MAPK pathway, whereas it has the opposite effect on arcuate nucleus POMC neurons by a LepR-JAK2-PI3K pathway [36].

The mechanisms underlying the adaptive response to fasting, which is essentially a starvation signal, involve GABA-ergic and glutaminergic neurotransmitters in the arcuate nucleus. AGRP and NPY expression in the arcuate nucleus are activated by fasting as a response to decreased leptin signaling to the brain, the effect of which is to stimulate brain circuits that promote food intake and weight gain, restoring a regulated level of adiposity. This orexigenic effect of leptin is prevented by deletion of N-methyl-D-aspartate (NMDA) glutamate receptors from AGRP neurons, whereas deleting these excitatory receptors from POMC neurons has no effect on energy homeostasis. Moreover, glutaminergic transmission on AGRP dendritic spines is increased by fasting, suggesting that NMDR receptors play a central role in the fasting mediated cellular responses of NPY/AGRP neurons to leptin [37].

Connections of Leptin Target Neurons

Research on leptin-responsive pathways in the brain until recently has been focused largely on measures of food intake and energy expenditure, processes that classically have been associated with the hypothalamus and hindbrain. Leptin-responsive neurons in the arcuate nucleus, NPY and POMC neurons in particular, send projections to other areas of the hypothalamus and throughout the brain, however, to potentially interact with neural systems that influence reproduction, reward-seeking behavior, and cognitive function [1, 31, 38–47]. Likewise, leptin receptors are expressed in many regions, both in the hypothalamus and elsewhere in the CNS, direct providing targets for leptin in diverse CNS functions.

Within the hypothalamus, leptin-responsive NPY/AGRP and POMC neurons project to the paraventricular nucleus where they interact with neurons in downstream pathways to other brain regions that influence energy homeostasis [2]. They also have connections with the lateral hypothalamus and perifornical areas, the locations of neurons that express melanin concentrating hormone (MCH) and orexins, both of which are powerful stimulators of food intake in rodents. Both orexin and MCH neurons project widely to brain regions that influence food intake and metabolism, and their effects are blocked by leptin. Neurons that synthesize orexins are strongly inhibited by leptin, acting through leptin receptors on arcuate nucleus neurons that project to the lateral hypothalamus and form synapses on orexin neurons. Moreover, leptin completely blocks the expression of receptors for MCH in the brain and thus can produce dramatic anorexigenic actions by acting on MCH neurons via arcuate nucleus projections to the lateral hypothalamus as well as directly in areas of the brain that have MCH responsive neurons [48].

Interaction of Leptin with Satiety Signals

A principal physiological mechanism for the anorexigenic effects of leptin involves inhibition of eating. During the ingestion of a meal, neural and endocrine signals are generated from the gastrointestinal tract and transmit satiety signals to the CNS by both vagal and humoral pathways. Food in the stomach activates gastric stretch receptors that project to the hindbrain, particularly the nucleus tractus solitarius (NTS), which regulates meal size, resulting in termination of feeding [49]. Similarly, food entering the intestine causes secretion of gastrointestinal hormones such as cholecystokinin (CCK) that act on vagal afferents that project to the NTS. The effect of these neural and endocrine "satiety signals" is to cause a meal to be terminated. Abundant evidence from studies on rodent models indicates that a major mechanism underlying leptin's anorexigenic effects is potentiating the effect of satiety signals to the NTS. Basically, satiety signals are more potent in the presence of leptin signaling to the brain and less effective under conditions of relative leptin deficiency (Fig. 3.1). Thus, in the presence of leptin signaling to the brain, satiety signals to the NTS are more effective and meals are terminated early; this results in less food and caloric intake which, if continued over time, results in loss of adipose tissue mass. Conversely, in conditions of leptin deficiency such as fasting or genetic absence of leptin (ob/ob mouse) or leptin receptors

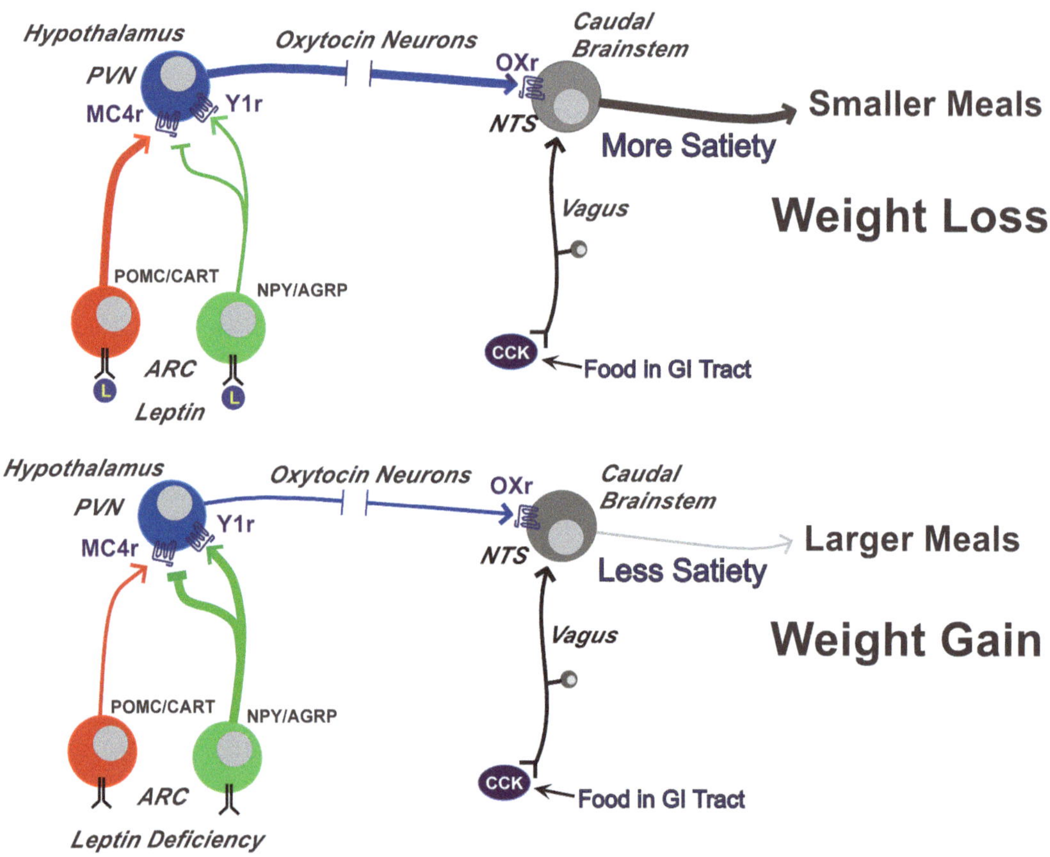

Fig. 3.1 Diagram of a brain pathway for leptin's modulation of satiety and meal size. In the *top panel*, leptin acts on its receptors on ARC/AGRP and NPY/CART neurons in the ARC, resulting in activation of anorexigenic POMC/CART neurons and inhibition of orexigenic NPY/AGRP neurons. aMSH released from POMC/CART terminals in the PVN activate MC4r melanocortin receptors which in turn produce increased signaling of oxytocin to the NTS neurons that respond and integrate vagally mediated CCK-induced satiety signals from the intestine. Oxytocin acting on its receptors (OXr) expressed on NTS neurons increases the effects of satiety signals and results in earlier termination of meals. This pathway produces reduced caloric intake and weight loss if prolonged unchecked. In the *bottom panel*, under conditions of relative leptin deficiency POMC/CART signaling is damped and NPY/POMC signaling stimulated, resulting in increased release of aMSH and AGRP in the PVN. NPY activates orexigenic NPY Y1 receptors and aMSH blocks anorexigenic MC4r receptors that stimulate oxytocin neurons, resulting in reduced oxytocin signaling to the NTS. Accordingly, the satiety effect of CCK satiety signaling from the intestine is less and consequently more food is eaten before meals are terminated. The result if unchecked over long periods of time promotes weight gain and obesity. Long term maintenance of body weight (adiposity) reflects a balance between leptin signaling to the ARC and satiety signals to the NTS. Weight gain or loss potentially results when this homeostatic mechanism is altered

(db/db mouse, fa/fa rat), satiety signals to the NTS are less effective and consequently animals consume larger meals leading to weight gain.

The evidence that the effect of meal-related gastrointestinal (GI) satiety signals could be enhanced by leptin was supported by histochemical studies for the expression of mRNA encoding LepRb receptors as well as LepRb protein by neurons in the NTS; moreover, administration of leptin into either the fourth cerebral ventricle or directly into the dorsal vagal complex (which includes the NTS) suppresses food intake in rats [49]. Thus, the effect of leptin to inhibit food intake is regulated in part by direct action of leptin on hindbrain neural circuits that integrate meal-related GI signals [49–51].

These findings raise the question of the primary CNS site of leptin's physiological action to reduce food ingestion: is this mechanism mediated primarily by leptin target neurons in the hypothalamus or in the NTS, or are both required? Studies using adenoviral gene therapy on the fa(k)/fa(k) Koletsky rat that lacks LepRb receptors and is insensitive to the anorexigenic action of leptin demonstrated that replacing LepRb in the arcuate nucleus (but not the hindbrain) normalized the effect of CCK satiety signaling to the brainstem [52, 53]. Thus, it appears that in the absence of leptin receptors in the hindbrain, leptin signaling to the arcuate nucleus is sufficient to mediate the satiety actions of leptin under experimental conditions.

Neuronal pathways between the hypothalamus and brainstem provide potential anatomic substrates for conveying leptin adiposity signals that activate neurons in the hypothalamus to downstream neurons that regulate food intake and energy expenditure [54]. A key relay center in the hypothalamus for dispersing leptin signaling is the paraventricular nucleus, which has axonal terminals of leptin sensitive arcuate nucleus NPY/AGRP and POMC cell bodies. The PVN in turn has neurons that project widely in the CNS, including oxytocin neurons and corticotropin releasing hormone (CRH) neurons that project directly to the NTS [55]. The population of NTS-projecting oxytocin neurons responds to leptin in the hypothalamus and innervates the region of the NTS that contains neurons that are activated by CCK satiety signals from the GI tract [56, 57]. Catecholaminergic neurons in the NTS have been implicated as participating in this mechanism [58], although they are probably do not respond directly to leptin as they appear not to express LepRb receptors [59]. The phenotypes of hindbrain neurons that integrate leptin-generated signals to the NTS with satiety signals from the GI tract remain largely undefined. Recent evidence suggests that NTS POMC neurons express LepRb receptors, whereas neurons that express cocaine- and amphetamine-regulated transcript (CART), brain-derived neurotrophic factor, neuropeptide Y, nesfatin, catecholamines, GABA, prolactin-releasing peptide, or nitric oxide synthase lack LepRb expression and probably are not direct mediators of leptin action in the NTS [59]. A growing body of research indicates that melanocortin receptors, particularly MC4r, in an arcuate nucleus–oxytocin–NTS neuronal pathway play a key role in modulating leptin's anorexigenic action by limiting the size of meals and potentially increasing energy metabolism [29, 38, 55–57, 60, 61]. However, melanocortin receptors located in the NTS also appear to modulate leptin's anorexigenic effects, which is consistent with the finding of direct anatomical projections of arcuate nucleus POMC neurons to the NTS [62].

Leptin Sensitive Pathways for Regulation of Energy Expenditure

The CNS pathways that mediate leptin's action to increase thermogenesis and energy expenditure also appear to involve neurons in the hypothalamus. Neurons that co-express POMC and CART in the retrochiasmatic area and lateral arcuate nucleus of the hypothalamus activate the sympathetic nervous system by sending projections to sympathetic preganglionic neurons in the thoracic spinal cord. Leptin-sensitive POMC/CART neurons in the arcuate nucleus may also activate sympathetic outflow through their connections with other hypothalamic regions, the PVN and lateral hypothalamus in particular [63]. The mechanisms that underlie leptin's ability to increase thermogenesis are not well understood. Recent evidence indicates that the thermogenic effects of leptin are mediated by GABA-ergic neurons in the arcuate nucleus [64].

CNS Leptin Resistance and Obesity

The observations from rodents that profound obesity results from reduced leptin signaling in the brain in the absence either of functional LepRb leptin receptors or of leptin synthesis contrasts with the elevated leptin levels characteristic of obese animals including humans [7], suggesting that leptin resistance in the brain is a major reason for failure of elevated leptin levels to suppress food intake in states of obesity [17]. The mechanisms of CNS leptin resistance are the subject of intense investigation but still not well understood [19, 65, 66]. High fat diets and inflammatory cytokines are associated with activation of intracellular inflammatory signaling pathways that potentially impair leptin signaling by CNS neurons and neuroglia [67–71]. Impaired leptin transport across the blood–brain barrier in obesity and with high fat diets may contribute to reduced leptin signaling to the brain [29, 72–75], although newly developed leptin analogs may overcome blood–brain barrier leptin resistance [76].

CNS Leptin Action and Diabetes

A central action of leptin that is not well understood is its ability to lower blood glucose levels under conditions of insulin deficiency. It's been shown that adenoviral restoration of LepRb expression in the arcuate nucleus is sufficient to restore normoglycemia in obese diabetic fa(k)/fa(k) Koletsky rats that otherwise lack functional leptin receptors [52]. Genetic restoration of LepRb only to POMC and GABA neurons in the arcuate nucleus has been reported to normalize hyperglycemia in mice otherwise deficient in LepR signaling [77–79]. In mice that are made diabetic by destruction of islet beta cells by streptozotocin, and thus totally devoid of insulin, normoglycemia can be restored by genetically expressing LepRb selectively in hypothalamic POMC and GABA-ergic neurons [80]. Restoring LepRb only to POMC neurons has a minor effect compared to the major effect of restoring LepRb expression to hypothalamic GABA-ergic neurons, whereas restoring LepRb expression to both POMC and GABA-ergic neurons fully corrects the hypoglycemia of insulin-deficient diabetes. Thus, development of drugs targeted to leptin's POMC intracellular signaling pathways hold promise for potential insulin-independent diabetes therapies.

Leptin Actions in Human Brain

Caution is required in making conclusions about brain cellular mechanisms and pathways underlying the role of leptin's regulation of food intake in humans compared to other animal models, as the regulation of food intake and energy expenditure in humans is strongly influenced by reward and psychosocial factors that may play lesser roles in regulation of energy homeostasis in rodent models [17]. Nevertheless, studies on humans utilizing fMRI brain imaging techniques indicate that leptin triggers neuronal activity in regions of the human brain analogous to those that are associated with food intake and satiation as well as reward systems in rodents [81–84], but the identity of specific neurons and pathways as well as the underlying biochemical and molecular mechanisms in humans have not been determined. However, there is an implicit hypothesis in the field of obesity research that the CNS mechanisms that underlie leptin signaling related to energy homeostasis in humans are similar to those of rodent models [85]. As in rodents, human plasma leptin levels are positively correlated with body weight and adipose tissue mass. These clinical observations suggest that leptin expression by adipose tissue in humans is regulated by nutritional status as well as insulin secretion and other hormones, supporting the accepted view that leptin also signals to the brain in humans. Leptin receptors are expressed in the human brain and located in regions homologous to those that express leptin receptors and are involved in energy homeostasis in other mammals [86–88]. Concentrations of leptin in CSF (presumably originating from adipose tissue) of healthy human subjects show diurnal peaks that correlate with CSF POMC level peaks [89], findings that are consistent with an anorexigenic function of leptin in human brain.

In humans, loss-of-function mutations in the leptin gene (analogous to mouse ob/ob mutations) and impaired leptin signaling due to leptin receptor mutations (analogous to mouse db/db mutations) have been reported to be associated with obesity [90]. Little is known about consequence of these mutations to CNS responses to leptin and regulation of energy balance in affected individuals, although developmental abnormalities in energy balance pathways are likely, as leptin has profound effects on development of brain neurocircuits in obese rodents that possess similar mutations. Brain neural activity has been investigated in a few congenital leptin-deficient subjects before and after leptin replacement therapy [81, 82, 91]. These studies indicate that areas of the brain involved in appetitive and reward-seeking behavior have long term responses to visual presentation of food cues in response to leptin.

Mutations in melanocortin receptor genes that mediate leptin's central actions also result in morbid obesity in humans [92]. Humans with these melanocortin receptor mutations become hyperphagic, obese, and usually infertile, as leptin signaling in the brain is also required for development of normal reproductive function [90]. Treatment of obese humans with injections of leptin has not proved to be an effective therapy for weight loss, in part due to CNS leptin resistance, although clinical evidence suggests that leptin injections can prevent weight gain [93]. Attempts to correct obesity and reproductive abnormalities in individuals with loss-of-function leptin mutations by administering recombinant leptin have been successful in a few individuals, but no therapy currently exists to correct deficiencies of leptin signaling to the brain due to loss-of-function leptin receptor gene mutations [90].

The recent applications of functional magnetic resonance imaging (fMRI) in humans receiving leptin therapy are providing clues to neural circuits that respond to leptin in the human brain. An fMRI study in obese humans stimulated by visual food cues after having lost weight discovered that food-related neural activity in brain regions associated with the cognitive and emotional control of eating (including brainstem and hypothalamus) was reversed in subjects that received subcutaneous leptin injections [94]. Administration of leptin to obese subjects that were maintained at 10 % weight loss with leptin repletion produced fMRI images that revealed increased functional connections between the hypothalamus and visual areas as well as decreased functional connections with reward and attention-responsive areas [95]. These findings suggest that leptin may influence brain pathways that affect responses to food cues when humans are in a state of relative negative energy balance, such as during dieting. In an fMRI analysis of food-related brain neural activity in lipodystrophic patients that received leptin therapy, many regions of the brain showed attenuation of postprandial neural activity in regions associated with food intake and reward, including the amygdala, caudate putamen, and nucleus accumbens; however, this effect was not significant in fasting subjects [96]. High resolution techniques for functional brain imaging are now being applied to mechanistic studies of leptin action in brains of genetically obese rodents as well as rats and mice made obese with diets rich in sugars and fats. These studies hold promise for new horizons in understanding how the human brain responds to leptin in obese individuals and for development of effective behavioral and pharmacotherapy to treat obesity in the future.

Acknowledgements This material is based upon work supported by the Research and Development Service, Veterans Health Administration, Department of Veterans Affairs, and the Cellular and Molecular Imaging Core of the Diabetes Research Center at the University of Washington and supported by National Institutes of Health (NIH) grant P30DK017047. Dr. Baskin is the recipient of a VA Senior Research Career Scientist award.

References

1. Berthoud HR, Lenard NR, Shin AC. Food reward, hyperphagia, and obesity. Am J Physiol Regul Integr Comp Physiol. 2011;300(6):R1266–77.
2. Schwartz MW, Woods SC, Porte Jr D, Seeley RJ, Baskin DG. Central nervous system control of food intake. Nature. 2000;404(6778):661–71.
3. Halaas JL, Boozer C, Blair-West J, Fidahusein N, Denton DA, Friedman JM. Physiological response to long-term peripheral and central leptin infusion in lean and obese mice. Proc Natl Acad Sci U S A. 1997;94(16):8878–83.
4. Halaas JL, Gajiwala KS, Maffei M, Cohen SL, Chait BT, Rabinowitz D, et al. Weight-reducing effects of

the plasma protein encoded by the obese gene. Science. 1995;269(5223):543–6.
5. Zhang Y, Proenca R, Maffei M, Barone M, Leopold L, Friedman JM. Positional cloning of the mouse obese gene and its human homologue. Nature. 1994; 372(6505):425–32.
6. Woods SC, Lotter EC, McKay LD, Porte Jr D. Chronic intracerebroventricular infusion of insulin reduces food intake and body weight of baboons. Nature. 1979;282(5738):503–5.
7. Porte Jr D, Baskin DG, Schwartz MW. Insulin signaling in the central nervous system: a critical role in metabolic homeostasis and disease from C. elegans to humans. Diabetes. 2005;54(5):1264–76.
8. Schwartz MW, Baskin DG. Leptin and the brain: then and now. J Clin Invest. 2013;123(6):2344–5.
9. Baskin DG, Figlewicz DP, Woods SC, Porte Jr D, Dorsa DM. Insulin in the brain. Annu Rev Physiol. 1987;49:335–47.
10. Baskin DG, Wilcox BJ, Figlewicz DP, Dorsa DM. Insulin and insulin-like growth factors in the CNS. Trends Neurosci. 1988;11(3):107–11.
11. Marks JL, Porte Jr D, Stahl WL, Baskin DG. Localization of insulin receptor mRNA in rat brain by in situ hybridization. Endocrinology. 1990; 127(6):3234–6.
12. Schwartz MW, Marks JL, Sipols AJ, Baskin DG, Woods SC, Kahn SE, et al. Central insulin administration reduces neuropeptide Y mRNA expression in the arcuate nucleus of food-deprived lean (Fa/Fa) but not obese (fa/fa) Zucker rats. Endocrinology. 1991;128(5): 2645–7.
13. Schwartz MW, Sipols AJ, Grubin CE, Baskin DG. Differential effect of fasting on hypothalamic expression of genes encoding neuropeptide Y, galanin, and glutamic acid decarboxylase. Brain Res Bull. 1993; 31(3–4):361–7.
14. Schwartz MW, Sipols AJ, Marks JL, Sanacora G, White JD, Scheurink A, et al. Inhibition of hypothalamic neuropeptide Y gene expression by insulin. Endocrinology. 1992;130(6):3608–16.
15. Tartaglia LA, Dembski M, Weng X, Deng N, Culpepper J, Devos R, et al. Identification and expression cloning of a leptin receptor, OB-R. Cell. 1995; 83(7):1263–71.
16. Lutz TA, Woods SC. Overview of animal models of obesity. Curr Protoc Pharmacol. ed SJ Enna. 2012; Chapter 5.
17. Ahima RS, Flier JS. Leptin. Annu Rev Physiol. 2000;62:413–37.
18. Munzberg H, Myers Jr MG. Molecular and anatomical determinants of central leptin resistance. Nat Neurosci. 2005;8(5):566–70.
19. Myers MG, Cowley MA, Munzberg H. Mechanisms of leptin action and leptin resistance. Annu Rev Physiol. 2008;70:537–56.
20. Baskin DG, Breininger JF, Schwartz MW. Leptin receptor mRNA identifies a subpopulation of neuropeptide Y neurons activated by fasting in rat hypothalamus. Diabetes. 1999;48(4):828–33.
21. Elmquist JK, Bjorbaek C, Ahima RS, Flier JS, Saper CB. Distributions of leptin receptor mRNA isoforms in the rat brain. J Comp Neurol. 1998;395(4): 535–47.
22. Fei H, Okano HJ, Li C, Lee GH, Zhao C, Darnell R, et al. Anatomic localization of alternatively spliced leptin receptors (Ob-R) in mouse brain and other tissues. Proc Natl Acad Sci U S A. 1997;94(13):7001–5.
23. Baskin DG, Schwartz MW, Seeley RJ, Woods SC, Porte Jr D, Breininger JF, et al. Leptin receptor long-form splice-variant protein expression in neuron cell bodies of the brain and co-localization with neuropeptide Y mRNA in the arcuate nucleus. J Histochem Cytochem. 1999;47(3):353–62.
24. Hakansson ML, Hulting AL, Meister B. Expression of leptin receptor mRNA in the hypothalamic arcuate nucleus—relationship with NPY neurones. Neuroreport. 1996;7(18):3087–92.
25. Baskin DG, Seeley RJ, Kuijper JL, Lok S, Weigle DS, Erickson JC, et al. Increased expression of mRNA for the long form of the leptin receptor in the hypothalamus is associated with leptin hypersensitivity and fasting. Diabetes. 1998;47(4):538–43.
26. Gamber KM, Huo L, Ha S, Hairston JE, Greeley S, Bjorbaek C. Over-expression of leptin receptors in hypothalamic POMC neurons increases susceptibility to diet-induced obesity. PLoS One. 2012;7(1):e30485.
27. Hakansson ML, Brown H, Ghilardi N, Skoda RC, Meister B. Leptin receptor immunoreactivity in chemically defined target neurons of the hypothalamus. J Neurosci. 1998;18(1):559–72.
28. Kim JG, Suyama S, Koch M, Jin S, Argente-Arizon P, Argente J, et al. Leptin signaling in astrocytes regulates hypothalamic neuronal circuits and feeding. Nat Neurosci. 2014;17(7):908–10. doi:10.1038/nn.3725.
29. Balland E, Dam J, Langlet F, Caron E, Steculorum S, Messina A, et al. Hypothalamic tanycytes are an ERK-gated conduit for leptin into the brain. Cell Metab. 2014;19(2):293–301.
30. Hahn TM, Breininger JF, Baskin DG, Schwartz MW. Coexpression of AGRP and NPY in fasting-activated hypothalamic neurons. Nat Neurosci. 1998;1(4):271–2.
31. Bouret SG, Bates SH, Chen S, Myers Jr MG, Simerly RB. Distinct roles for specific leptin receptor signals in the development of hypothalamic feeding circuits. J Neurosci. 2012;32(4):1244–52.
32. Myers Jr MG. Outstanding Scientific Achievement Award Lecture 2010: deconstructing leptin: from signals to circuits. Diabetes. 2010;59(11):2708–14.
33. Elmquist JK, Coppari R, Balthasar N, Ichinose M, Lowell BB. Identifying hypothalamic pathways controlling food intake, body weight, and glucose homeostasis. J Comp Neurol. 2005;493(1):63–71.
34. Banks AS, Davis SM, Bates SH, Myers Jr MG. Activation of downstream signals by the long form of the leptin receptor. J Biol Chem. 2000;275(19): 14563–72.
35. Morrison CD, Morton GJ, Niswender KD, Gelling RW, Schwartz MW. Leptin inhibits hypothalamic Npy

and AGRP gene expression via a mechanism that requires phosphatidylinositol 3-OH-kinase signaling. Am J Physiol Endocrinol Metab. 2005;289(6):E1051–7.
36. Wang JH, Wang F, Yang MJ, Yu DF, Wu WN, Liu J, et al. Leptin regulated calcium channels of neuropeptide Y and proopiomelanocortin neurons by activation of different signal pathways. Neuroscience. 2008;156(1):89–98.
37. Liu T, Kong D, Shah BP, Ye C, Koda S, Saunders A, et al. Fasting activation of AGRP neurons requires NMDA receptors and involves spinogenesis and increased excitatory tone. Neuron. 2012;73(3):511–22.
38. Blevins JE, Baskin DG. Hypothalamic-brainstem circuits controlling eating. Forum Nutr. 2010;63:133–40.
39. Elmquist JK, Ahima RS, Elias CF, Flier JS, Saper CB. Leptin activates distinct projections from the dorsomedial and ventromedial hypothalamic nuclei. Proc Natl Acad Sci U S A. 1998;95(2):741–6.
40. Elmquist JK, Ahima RS, Maratos-Flier E, Flier JS, Saper CB. Leptin activates neurons in ventrobasal hypothalamus and brainstem. Endocrinology. 1997;138(2):839–42.
41. Louis GW, Leinninger GM, Rhodes CJ, Myers Jr MG. Direct innervation and modulation of orexin neurons by lateral hypothalamic LepRb neurons. J Neurosci. 2010;30(34):11278–87.
42. Davis JF, Choi DL, Benoit SC. Insulin, leptin and reward. Trends Endocrinol Metab. 2010;21(2):68–74.
43. Davis JF, Choi DL, Schurdak JD, Fitzgerald MF, Clegg DJ, Lipton JW, et al. Leptin regulates energy balance and motivation through action at distinct neural circuits. Biol Psychiatry. 2011;69(7):668–74.
44. Irving AJ, Harvey J. Leptin regulation of hippocampal synaptic function in health and disease. Philos Trans R Soc Lond B Biol Sci. 2014;369(1633):20130155.
45. Ratra DV, Elias CF. Chemical identity of hypothalamic neurons engaged by leptin in reproductive control. J Chem Neuroanat. 2014;pii: S0891-0618(14)00041-6. doi: 10.1016/j.jchemneu.2014.05.005.
46. Asterholm IW, Rutkowski JM, Fujikawa T, Cho YR, Fukuda M, Tao C, et al. Elevated resistin levels induce central leptin resistance and increased atherosclerotic progression in mice. Diabetologia. 2014;57(6):1209–18.
47. Gautron L, Lazarus M, Scott MM, Saper CB, Elmquist JK. Identifying the efferent projections of leptin-responsive neurons in the dorsomedial hypothalamus using a novel conditional tracing approach. J Comp Neurol. 2010;518(11):2090–108.
48. Kokkotou EG, Tritos NA, Mastaitis JW, Slieker L, Maratos-Flier E. Melanin-concentrating hormone receptor is a target of leptin action in the mouse brain. Endocrinology. 2001;142(2):680–6.
49. Grill HJ, Hayes MR. The nucleus tractus solitarius: a portal for visceral afferent signal processing, energy status assessment and integration of their combined effects on food intake. Int J Obes (Lond). 2009;33 Suppl 1:S11–5.
50. Maniscalco JW, Rinaman L. Systemic leptin dose-dependently increases STAT3 phosphorylation within hypothalamic and hindbrain nuclei. Am J Physiol Regul Integr Comp Physiol. 2014;306(8):R576–85.
51. Grill HJ, Hayes MR. Hindbrain neurons as an essential hub in the neuroanatomically distributed control of energy balance. Cell Metab. 2012;16(3):296–309.
52. Morton GJ, Blevins JE, Williams DL, Niswender KD, Gelling RW, Rhodes CJ, et al. Leptin action in the forebrain regulates the hindbrain response to satiety signals. J Clin Invest. 2005;115(3):703–10.
53. Morton GJ, Niswender KD, Rhodes CJ, Myers Jr MG, Blevins JE, Baskin DG, et al. Arcuate nucleus-specific leptin receptor gene therapy attenuates the obesity phenotype of Koletsky (fa(k)/fa(k)) rats. Endocrinology. 2003;144(5):2016–24.
54. Schwartz GJ. Integrative capacity of the caudal brainstem in the control of food intake. Philos Trans R Soc Lond B Biol Sci. 2006;361(1471):1275–80.
55. Blevins JE, Schwartz MW, Baskin DG. Evidence that paraventricular nucleus oxytocin neurons link hypothalamic leptin action to caudal brain stem nuclei controlling meal size. Am J Physiol Regul Integr Comp Physiol. 2004;287(1):R87–96.
56. Blevins JE, Eakin TJ, Murphy JA, Schwartz MW, Baskin DG. Oxytocin innervation of caudal brainstem nuclei activated by cholecystokinin. Brain Res. 2003;993(1–2):30–41.
57. Matarazzo V, Schaller F, Nedelec E, Benani A, Penicaud L, Muscatelli F, et al. Inactivation of Socs3 in the hypothalamus enhances the hindbrain response to endogenous satiety signals via oxytocin signaling. J Neurosci. 2012;32(48):17097–107.
58. Williams DL, Schwartz MW, Bastian LS, Blevins JE, Baskin DG. Immunocytochemistry and laser capture microdissection for real-time quantitative PCR identify hindbrain neurons activated by interaction between leptin and cholecystokinin. J Histochem Cytochem. 2008;56(3):285–93.
59. Garfield AS, Patterson C, Skora S, Gribble FM, Reimann F, Evans ML, et al. Neurochemical characterization of body weight-regulating leptin receptor neurons in the nucleus of the solitary tract. Endocrinology. 2012;153(10):4600–7.
60. Blevins JE, Morton GJ, Williams DL, Caldwell DW, Bastian LS, Wisse BE, et al. Forebrain melanocortin signaling enhances the hindbrain satiety response to CCK-8. Am J Physiol Regul Integr Comp Physiol. 2009;296(3):R476–84.
61. Blevins JE, Ho JM. Role of oxytocin signaling in the regulation of body weight. Rev Endocr Metab Disord. 2013;14(4):311–29.
62. Zheng H, Patterson LM, Rhodes CJ, Louis GW, Skibicka KP, Grill HJ, et al. A potential role for hypothalamomedullary POMC projections in leptin-induced suppression of food intake. Am J Physiol Regul Integr Comp Physiol. 2010;298(3):R720–8.
63. Elmquist JK. Hypothalamic pathways underlying the endocrine, autonomic, and behavioral effects of leptin. Physiol Behav. 2001;74(4–5):703–8.

64. Kong D, Tong Q, Ye C, Koda S, Fuller PM, Krashes MJ, et al. GABAergic RIP-Cre neurons in the arcuate nucleus selectively regulate energy expenditure. Cell. 2012;151(3):645–57.
65. Levin BE, Dunn-Meynell AA. Reduced central leptin sensitivity in rats with diet-induced obesity. Am J Physiol Regul Integr Comp Physiol. 2002;283(4): R941–8.
66. Munzberg H, Bjornholm M, Bates SH, Myers Jr MG. Leptin receptor action and mechanisms of leptin resistance. Cell Mol Life Sci. 2005;62(6):642–52.
67. Posey KA, Clegg DJ, Printz RL, Byun J, Morton GJ, Vivekanandan-Giri A, et al. Hypothalamic proinflammatory lipid accumulation, inflammation, and insulin resistance in rats fed a high-fat diet. Am J Physiol Endocrinol Metab. 2009;296(5):E1003–12.
68. Guyenet SJ, Nguyen HT, Hwang BH, Schwartz MW, Baskin DG, Thaler JP. High-fat diet feeding causes rapid, non-apoptotic cleavage of caspase-3 in astrocytes. Brain Res. 2013;1512:97–105.
69. Thaler JP, Yi CX, Schur EA, Guyenet SJ, Hwang BH, Dietrich MO, et al. Obesity is associated with hypothalamic injury in rodents and humans. J Clin Invest. 2012;122(1):153–62.
70. Velloso LA, Araujo EP, de Souza CT. Diet-induced inflammation of the hypothalamus in obesity. Neuroimmunomodulation. 2008;15(3):189–93.
71. Ignacio-Souza LM, Bombassaro B, Pascoal LB, Portovedo MA, Razolli DS, Coope A, et al. Defective regulation of the ubiquitin/proteasome system in the hypothalamus of obese male mice. Endocrinology. 2014;155(8):2831–44.
72. Banks WA. Blood-brain barrier and energy balance. Obesity. 2006;14 Suppl 5:234S–7S.
73. Banks WA. Role of the blood-brain barrier in the evolution of feeding and cognition. Ann N Y Acad Sci. 2012;1264:13–9.
74. Banks WA, Farr SA, Morley JE. The effects of high fat diets on the blood-brain barrier transport of leptin: failure or adaptation? Physiol Behav. 2006;88(3): 244–8.
75. Gao Y, Tschop MH, Luquet S. Hypothalamic tanycytes: gatekeepers to metabolic control. Cell Metab. 2014;19(2):173–5.
76. Yi X, Yuan D, Farr SA, Banks WA, Poon CD, Kabanov AV. Pluronic modified leptin with increased systemic circulation, brain uptake and efficacy for treatment of obesity. J Control Release. 2014;pii: S0168-3659(14)00347-2. doi: 10.1016/j.jconrel.2014.05.044.
77. Coppari R, Ichinose M, Lee CE, Pullen AE, Kenny CD, McGovern RA, et al. The hypothalamic arcuate nucleus: a key site for mediating leptin's effects on glucose homeostasis and locomotor activity. Cell Metab. 2005;1(1):63–72.
78. Berglund ED, Vianna CR, Donato Jr J, Kim MH, Chuang JC, Lee CE, et al. Direct leptin action on POMC neurons regulates glucose homeostasis and hepatic insulin sensitivity in mice. J Clin Invest. 2012;122(3):1000–9.
79. Huo L, Gamber K, Greeley S, Silva J, Huntoon N, Leng XH, et al. Leptin-dependent control of glucose balance and locomotor activity by POMC neurons. Cell Metab. 2009;9(6):537–47.
80. Fujikawa T, Berglund ED, Patel VR, Ramadori G, Vianna CR, Vong L, et al. Leptin engages a hypothalamic neurocircuitry to permit survival in the absence of insulin. Cell Metab. 2013;18(3):431–44.
81. Baicy K, London ED, Monterosso J, Wong ML, Delibasi T, Sharma A, et al. Leptin replacement alters brain response to food cues in genetically leptin-deficient adults. Proc Natl Acad Sci U S A. 2007;104(46):18276–9.
82. Farooqi IS, Bullmore E, Keogh J, Gillard J, O'Rahilly S, Fletcher PC. Leptin regulates striatal regions and human eating behavior. Science. 2007;317(5843):1355.
83. Grosshans M, Vollmert C, Vollstadt-Klein S, Tost H, Leber S, Bach P, et al. Association of leptin with food cue-induced activation in human reward pathways. Arch Gen Psychiatry. 2012;69(5):529–37.
84. Schur EA, Kleinhans NM, Goldberg J, Buchwald D, Schwartz MW, Maravilla K. Activation in brain energy regulation and reward centers by food cues varies with choice of visual stimulus. Int J Obes. 2009;33(6):653–61.
85. Wang B, Chandrasekera PC, Pippin JJ. Leptin- and leptin receptor-deficient rodent models: relevance for human type 2 diabetes. Curr Diabetes Rev. 2014;10(2):131–45.
86. Golden PL, Maccagnan TJ, Pardridge WM. Human blood-brain barrier leptin receptor. Binding and endocytosis in isolated human brain microvessels. J Clin Invest. 1997;99(1):14–8.
87. Couce ME, Burguera B, Parisi JE, Jensen MD, Lloyd RV. Localization of leptin receptor in the human brain. Neuroendocrinology. 1997;66(3):145–50.
88. Burguera B, Couce ME, Long J, Lamsam J, Laakso K, Jensen MD, et al. The long form of the leptin receptor (OB-Rb) is widely expressed in the human brain. Neuroendocrinology. 2000;71(3):187–95.
89. Wardlaw SL, Burant CF, Klein S, Meece K, White A, Kasten T, et al. Continuous 24-hour leptin, proopiomelanocortin and amino acid measurements in human cerebrospinal fluid: correlations with plasma leptin, soluble leptin receptor and amino acid levels. J Clin Endocrinol Metab. 2014;99(7):2540–8.
90. Elias CF, Purohit D. Leptin signaling and circuits in puberty and fertility. Cell Mol Life Sci. 2013;70(5): 841–62.
91. Frank S, Heni M, Moss A, von Schnurbein J, Fritsche A, Haring HU, et al. Leptin therapy in a congenital leptin-deficient patient leads to acute and long-term changes in homeostatic, reward, and food-related brain areas. J Clin Endocrinol Metab. 2011;96(8): E1283–7.
92. Farooqi IS, O'Rahilly S. Genetic factors in human obesity. Obesity Rev. 2007;8 Suppl 1:37–40.
93. Rosenbaum M, Goldsmith R, Bloomfield D, Magnano A, Weimer L, Heymsfield S, et al. Low-dose leptin

reverses skeletal muscle, autonomic, and neuroendocrine adaptations to maintenance of reduced weight. J Clin Invest. 2005;115(12):3579–86.
94. Rosenbaum M, Sy M, Pavlovich K, Leibel RL, Hirsch J. Leptin reverses weight loss-induced changes in regional neural activity responses to visual food stimuli. J Clin Invest. 2008;118(7):2583–91.
95. Hinkle W, Cordell M, Leibel R, Rosenbaum M, Hirsch J. Effects of reduced weight maintenance and leptin repletion on functional connectivity of the hypothalamus in obese humans. PLoS One. 2013; 8(3):e59114.
96. Aotani D, Ebihara K, Sawamoto N, Kusakabe T, Aizawa-Abe M, Kataoka S, et al. Functional magnetic resonance imaging analysis of food-related brain activity in patients with lipodystrophy undergoing leptin replacement therapy. J Clin Endocrinol Metab. 2012;97(10):3663–71.

Measurement of Circulating Leptin and Soluble Leptin Receptors

4

Robert V. Considine

Introduction

The lipostasis theory of body weight regulation was proposed by Kennedy in 1953 [1]. In this simple feedback model a peripheral signal is produced in proportion to the amount of adipose tissue in the body. This signal is then compared to a "setpoint" in the central nervous system, and changes in energy intake (appetite) or energy expenditure (physical activity, thermogenesis) initiated to maintain the size of the adipose stores constant. Evidence in support of a circulating factor that regulated body weight was provided by parabiosis experiments. In this technique, two animals are surgically joined along flank incisions running from forelimb to hindlimb, resulting in development of a common vascular network between the two animals. Hervey [2] found that the parabiotic union of a normal rat with an obese rat, made so by lesion of the ventromedial hypothalamus (VMH), resulted in hypophagia and weight loss in the normal animal. The interpretation of this experiment was that the rat with VMH lession could not respond to a circulating signal that was increased as the animal gained weight. The unlesioned animal responded to the increased level of the "satiety signal" and reduced its food intake. Coleman performed parabiosis between a genetically obese *ob*/*ob* mouse and a normal lean mouse and observed a reduction in appetite and weight loss in the obese mouse. This experiment suggested that the *ob*/*ob* mouse was obese because it lacked an adipose related "satiety factor" which was provided in the blood of the lean mouse [3]. Parabiosis of an *ob*/*ob* mouse with a *db*/*db* mouse resulted in weight loss and ultimately death by starvation of the *ob*/*ob* mouse. This experiment provided further evidence that the *ob*/*ob* mouse lacked the body weight regulating signal, and suggested that the *db*/*db* mouse was similar to the VMH lesioned rat which could not respond to its endogenous satiety signal [3]. With the groundbreaking discovery of the *ob* gene by Jeffrey Friedman's group in 1994 [4], leptin appeared to meet the criteria of an adipose tissue "satiety factor" regulating body weight required by the lipostasis theory. Shortly thereafter it was demonstrated that the *db* gene encoded a receptor for leptin (which was defective in *db*/*db* mice) and that several isoforms existed, including a soluble form present in the blood [5, 6]. Thus methods for measurement of leptin and its binding partners in the blood were needed to fully understand the role of leptin to regulate energy intake/expenditure, and to validate the lipostasis theory.

R.V. Considine, PhD (✉)
Division of Endocrinology, Department of Medicine, Indiana University School of Medicine, Indianapolis, IN 46202, USA
e-mail: rconsidi@iu.edu

S. Dagogo-Jack (ed.), *Leptin: Regulation and Clinical Applications*,
DOI 10.1007/978-3-319-09915-6_4, © Springer International Publishing Switzerland 2015

Measurement of Circulating Leptin

The first study to analyze circulating leptin levels utilized a polyclonal antibody to recombinant leptin to immunoprecipitate the protein from rodent and human plasma. The immunoprecipitates were subjected to Western blot and leptin detected with a second antibody directed to the amino terminus of the protein [7]. This study demonstrated that leptin was (1) present in the circulation, (2) significantly increased in genetically obese rodent models, and (3) decreased when mice were fasted for 6 days. In humans plasma leptin correlated with adiposity, was higher in women than in men, and decreased with weight loss. A note added in proof to the study of Maffei et al. [7] described the development of an ELISA that confirmed the findings made using their immunoprecipitation technique.

The first study to focus exclusively on leptin in humans employed a radioimmunoassay to quantitate serum leptin in 136 normal weight and 139 obese subjects [8]. This assay utilized an antibody generated against recombinant human leptin and had a limit of detection of 0.4 ng/ml. Serum leptin was highly correlated with percent body fat, BMI and fasting insulin. Serum leptin was higher in women than in men, but there was no difference when men and women with equivalent percent body fat were compared. Leptin significantly decreased with weight loss over 8–12 weeks, but increased again over 4 weeks of weight maintenance, suggesting that circulating leptin could reflect both the amount of body fat and reductions in caloric intake.

Following the first two publications on leptin levels in humans, a number of additional studies appeared in 1996, many of which utilized a radioimmunoassay developed by Linco Research, Inc (St. Charles, MO). These studies confirmed that leptin was highly correlated with measures of adiposity and was higher in women than in men [9–11]. In addition these early studies suggested that leptin was similar in Mexican Americans with and without type 2 diabetes [9], and that there was no difference in leptin between Caucasians and African Americans [10]. One additional study using a sandwich ELISA found that leptin, corrected for fat mass, declined in post-menopausal women, and suggested that androgens and estrogens likely influenced circulating leptin levels independently of fat mass [12]. Finally, Hosoda et al. showed that human adipose tissue in culture secreted leptin using a radioimmunoassay developed in their laboratory [11].

The number of studies focused on circulating leptin levels increased exponentially over the next several years, with the majority using the Linco radioimmunoassay. Currently there are a number of commercially available ELISA and radioimmunoassays for the measurement of leptin, most of which are in reasonable agreement with respect to the values obtained. Additional information on the relationship of serum leptin with various physiologic and metabolic parameters is presented in detail in other chapters.

Measurement of Soluble Leptin Receptor

In 1995, exactly 1 year following the discovery of the *ob* gene and leptin, the cDNA sequence of the leptin receptor (OB-R) was published [5]. Shortly thereafter Lee et al. [6] reported additional alternatively spliced leptin receptor mRNAs of varying length in mouse brain. One of these receptor isoforms (OB-Re) was identical to the extracellular domain of the other leptin receptors but lacked a transmembrane domain, suggesting that it encoded a protein that could be a soluble leptin binding protein. This suggestion was confirmed by the finding in pregnant mice that leptin was significantly elevated due to an increase in OB-Re expression by the placenta [13]. Additional evidence that the soluble leptin receptor prolonged the half-life of leptin in the circulation was provided by experiments in which adenoviral overexpression of OB-Re led to higher leptin levels in rats and in *ob/ob* mice given exogenous leptin [14]. Transgenic overexpression of soluble leptin receptor to levels approximately twice that in wild type animals results in mice that are thinner and more resistant to weight gain, supporting the concept that greater bound leptin in the circulation results in greater physiologic effects of free leptin [15]. In contrast, the soluble leptin receptor has also been shown to reduce transport of leptin across the blood brain barrier [16] and intracerebroventricular administration of soluble leptin receptor antagonizes leptin signaling in the brain [17]. These findings demonstrate that soluble leptin receptor may be a useful means to regulate leptin action.

Leptin binding activity in human serum was first detected using Sephadex G-100 gel filtration which yielded radiolabeled leptin associated with proteins of 80 and 100 kDa [18]. These 80–100 kDa proteins likely represented a soluble leptin receptor as radiolabeled leptin bound protein could be immunoprecipitated with a polyclonal antibody directed to the extracellular domain of the leptin receptor. In lean subjects a greater percentage of serum leptin was found in the bound form compared to that in obese subjects. Short term fasting decreased free (unbound) leptin in both lean and obese subjects, but fasting had no effect on bound leptin levels. Notably, the effect of fasting to reduce free leptin was greater in the lean subjects. The findings that leptin was associated with binding protein in human serum, and that free unbound leptin was greater in obese subjects, were confirmed shortly thereafter using sucrose gradient centrifugation and ligand blotting to measure bound and free leptin [19]. The observation that short-term fasting lowered free leptin but had no effect on the bound hormone was also confirmed using high performance liquid chromatography to separate free and bound leptin [20, 21]. Additional evidence that the leptin binding protein in human serum could be a soluble leptin receptor was provided by in vitro studies in which the extracellular domain of the human leptin receptor was expressed in COS 7 cells, resulting in a secreted protein that bound leptin with high affinity and that was able to antagonize leptin binding to its receptor on the cell membrane [22].

As antibodies to the leptin receptor were developed and validated, a number of radioimmunoassay and ELISA techniques to measure soluble leptin receptor binding protein were established. Lammert et al. developed an immunofunctional ELISA that detected both leptin and its binding protein [23]. These investigators showed that the soluble leptin receptor was the major leptin binding protein in human serum and that the receptor existed in a glycosylated form. Brabant and colleagues using a radioimmunoassay found that free and bound leptin were not different during pregnancy in women with and without type 1 diabetes [24]. Using an in house [25] and commercially available sandwich ELISA [26–28], a number of laboratories demonstrated that the soluble leptin receptor was higher in women than in men, and inversely correlated with measures of adiposity and leptin. Soluble leptin receptor exhibits a circadian rhythm opposite to that of leptin, with lowest levels in the early morning hours when leptin is at its highest level in the blood [28, 29]. Mantzoros and colleagues coined the term "free leptin index (FLI)", a measure of the biologically active form of leptin derived by dividing total leptin by the amount of soluble leptin receptor, both expressed in ng/ml concentrations [28, 30]. The FLI is significantly greater in obese children [31–33] as it is in adults [25, 28 and others], and FLI is a predictor of liver steatosis in morbidly obese subjects [34]. Soluble leptin receptor levels are predictive of fasting glucose, metabolic syndrome score and measures of adiposity at 2 years follow-up in men, although leptin had a stronger association, suggesting that measures of soluble leptin receptor may not as useful [35]. In subjects from the Nurses' Health Study, higher soluble leptin receptor levels were associated with lower risk of developing type 2 diabetes during a 15 year follow-up period [36].

It is important to note that the source of soluble leptin receptor in humans is different than that in rodents. In humans there are mRNAs that encode the long leptin receptor (OB-Rb using the mouse nomenclature) and a short leptin receptor (OB-Ra) but no evidence for alternative splicing of the leptin receptor gene to yield an mRNA encoding a soluble leptin binding protein [37; and Chap. 2]. In contrast, soluble leptin receptor binding protein is derived by proteolytic cleavage of membrane bound receptors (OB-Ra and OB-Rb) [38, 39]. In addition cultured human subcutaneous adipocytes release appear to release leptin bound to leptin receptor, in addition to free leptin and soluble leptin receptor [40]. Recent work indicates that fatty acids and endoplasmic reticulum stress can induce shedding of leptin receptor extracellular domain from transfected HEK 293 cells, suggesting that these mechanisms could be relevant to generation of soluble leptin receptor binding protein in vivo [41].

Summary and Conclusions

The measurement of leptin and soluble leptin receptor is now routine, with reliable assays commercially available. At least one study suggests that commercially available leptin assays generally measure free leptin, with the soluble leptin receptor interfering with measurement of bound leptin in these assays [25]. Reference ranges for leptin and soluble leptin receptor that meet the Clinical and Laboratory Standards Institute recommendations have not yet been established. Despite this there is agreement that leptin is significantly greater in obese compared to lean subjects, and is greater in women than in men after controlling for body fat content. In contrast, soluble leptin receptor is inversely correlated with adiposity resulting in greater free leptin levels in obese individuals. Although some studies calculate a Free Leptin Index as a measure of bioactive leptin, this has not been a universally accepted practice with most reports simply measuring leptin. Studies in cell models and rodents suggest that the soluble leptin receptor may be used to alter leptin signaling. There are no reports linking endogenous soluble leptin receptor levels to pathology in either rodents or humans.

References

1. Kennedy GR. The role of depot fat in the hypothalamic control of food intake in the rat. Proc R Soc Lond B Biol Sci. 1953;140:578–92.
2. Hervey GR. The effects of lesions in the hypothalamus in parabiotic rats. J Physiol. 1959;145:336–52.
3. Coleman DL. Obese and diabetes: two mutant genes causing diabetes-obesity syndromes in mice. Diabetologia. 1978;14:141–8.
4. Zhang Y, Proenca R, Maffei M, Barone M, Leopold L, Friedman JM. Positional cloning of the mouse *obese* gene and its human homologue. Nature. 1994;372:425–32.
5. Tartaglia LA, Dembski M, Weng X, Deng N, Culpepper J, Devos R, Richards GJ, Campfield LA, Clark FT, Deeds J, Muir C, Sanker S, Moriarty A, Moore KJ, Smutko JS, Mays GG, Wool EA, Monroe CA, Tepper RI. Identification and expression cloning of a leptin receptor, OB-R. Cell. 1995;83:1263–71.
6. Lee GH, Proenca R, Montez JM, Carroll KM, Darvishzadeh JG, Lee JI, Friedman JM. Abnormal splicing of the leptin receptor in diabetic mice. Nature. 1996;379:632–5.
7. Maffei M, Halaas J, Ravussin E, Pratley RE, Lee GH, Zhang Y, Fei H, Kim S, Lallone R, Ranganathan S, Kern PA, Friedman JM. Leptin levels in human and rodent: measurement of plasma leptin and *ob* RNA in obese and weight-reduced subjects. Nat Med. 1995;1:1155–61.
8. Considine RV, Sinha MK, Heiman ML, Kriauciunas A, Stephens TW, Nyce MR, Ohannesian JP, Marco CC, McKee LJ, Bauer TL, Caro JF. Serum immunoreactive-leptin concentrations in normal-weight and obese humans. N Engl J Med. 1996;334:292–5.
9. Haffner SM, Stern MP, Miettinen H, Wei M, Gingerich RL. Leptin concentrations in diabetic and nondiabetic Mexican-Americans. Diabetes. 1996;45:822–4.
10. Ma Z, Gingerich RL, Santiago JV, Klein S, Smith CH, Landt M. Radioimmunoassay of leptin in human plasma. Clin Chem. 1996;42:942–6.
11. Hosoda K, Masuzaki H, Ogawa Y, Miyawaki T, Hiraoka I, Yasuno T, Fujisawa Y, Yoshimasa Y, Nishi S, Yamori Y, Nakao K. Development of a radioimmunoassay for human leptin. Biochem Biophys Res Commun. 1996;221:234–9.
12. Rosenbaum M, Nicolson M, Hirsch J, Heymsfield SB, Gallagher D, Chu F, Leibel RL. Effects of gender, body composition, and menopause on plasma concentrations of leptin. J Clin Endocrinol Metab. 1996;81:3424–7.
13. Gavrilova O, Barr V, Marcus-Samuels B, Reitman M. Hyperleptinemia of pregnancy associated with the appearance of a circulating form of the leptin receptor. J Biol Chem. 1997;272:30546–51.
14. Huang L, Wang Z, Li C. Modulation of circulating leptin levels by its soluble receptor. J Biol Chem. 2001;276:6343–9.
15. Lou PH, Yang G, Huang L, Cui Y, Pourbahrami T, Radda GK, Li C, Han W. Reduced body weight and increased energy expenditure in transgenic mice overexpressing soluble leptin receptor. PLoS One. 2010;5:e11669.
16. Tu H, Kastin AJ, Hsuchou H, Pan W. Soluble receptor inhibits leptin transport. J Cell Physiol. 2008;214:301–5.
17. Zhang J, Scarpace PJ. The soluble leptin receptor neutralizes leptin-mediated STAT3 signalling and anorexic responses in vivo. Br J Pharmacol. 2009;158:475–82.

18. Sinha MK, Opentanova I, Ohannesian JP, Kolaczynski JW, Heiman ML, Hale J, Becker GW, Bowsher RR, Stephens TW, Caro JF. Evidence of free and bound leptin in human circulation. Studies in lean and obese subjects and during short-term fasting. J Clin Invest. 1996;98:1277–82.
19. Houseknecht KL, Mantzoros CS, Kuliawat R, Hadro E, Flier JS, Kahn BB. Evidence for leptin binding to proteins in serum of rodents and humans: modulation with obesity. Diabetes. 1996;45:1638–43.
20. Landt M. Leptin binding and binding capacity in serum. Clin Chem. 2000;46:379–84.
21. Landt M, Horowitz JF, Coppack SW, Klein S. Effect of short-term fasting on free and bound leptin concentrations in lean and obese women. J Clin Endocrinol Metab. 2001;86:3768–71.
22. Liu C, Liu XJ, Barry G, Ling N, Maki RA, De Souza EB. Expression and characterization of a putative high affinity human soluble leptin receptor. Endocrinology. 1997;138:3548–54.
23. Lammert A, Kiess W, Bottner A, Glasow A, Kratzsch J. Soluble leptin receptor represents the main leptin binding activity in human blood. Biochem Biophys Res Commun. 2001;283:982–8.
24. Lewandowski K, Horn R, O'Callaghan CJ, Dunlop D, Medley GF, O'Hare P, Brabant G. Free leptin, bound leptin, and soluble leptin receptor in normal and diabetic pregnancies. J Clin Endocrinol Metab. 1999;84:300–6.
25. van Dielen FM, van't Veer C, Buurman WA, Greve JW. Leptin and soluble leptin receptor levels in obese and weight-losing individuals. J Clin Endocrinol Metab. 2002;87:1708–16.
26. Ogier V, Ziegler O, Méjean L, Nicolas JP, Stricker-Krongrad A. Obesity is associated with decreasing levels of the circulating soluble leptin receptor in humans. Int J Obes Relat Metab Disord. 2002;26:496–503.
27. Shimizu H, Shimomura K, Negishi M, Masunaga M, Uehara Y, Sato N, Shimomura Y, Kasai K, Mori M. Circulating concentrations of soluble leptin receptor: influence of menstrual cycle and diet therapy. Nutrition. 2002;18:309–12.
28. Chan JL, Blüher S, Yiannakouris N, Suchard MA, Kratzsch J, Mantzoros CS. Regulation of circulating soluble leptin receptor levels by gender, adiposity, sex steroids, and leptin: observational and interventional studies in humans. Diabetes. 2002;51:2105–12.
29. Wardlaw SL, Burant CF, Klein S, Meece K, White A, Kasten T, Lucey BP, Bateman RJ. Continuous 24-hour leptin, proopiomelanocortin and amino acid measurements in human cerebrospinal fluid: correlations with plasma leptin, soluble leptin receptor and amino acid levels. J Clin Endocrinol Metab. 2014;99(7):2540–8.
30. Yannakoulia M, Yiannakouris N, Blüher S, Matalas AL, Klimis-Zacas D, Mantzoros CS. Body fat mass and macronutrient intake in relation to circulating soluble leptin receptor, free leptin index, adiponectin, and resistin concentrations in healthy humans. J Clin Endocrinol Metab. 2003;88:1730–6.
31. Reinehr T, Kratzsch J, Kiess W, Andler W. Circulating soluble leptin receptor, leptin, and insulin resistance before and after weight loss in obese children. Int J Obes (Lond). 2005;29:1230–5.
32. Cinaz P, Bideci A, Camurdan MO, Güven A, Gönen S. Leptin and soluble leptin receptor levels in obese children in fasting and satiety states. J Pediatr Endocrinol Metab. 2005;18:303–7.
33. Catli G, Anik A, Tuhan HÜ, Kume T, Bober E, Abaci A. The relation of leptin and soluble leptin receptor levels with metabolic and clinical parameters in obese and healthy children. Peptides. 2014;56:72–6.
34. Medici V, Ali MR, Seo S, Aoki CA, Rossaro L, Kim K, Fuller WD, Vidovszky TJ, Smith W, Jiang JX, Maganti K, Havel PJ, Kamboj A, Ramsamooj R, Török NJ. Increased soluble leptin receptor levels in morbidly obese patients with insulin resistance and nonalcoholic fatty liver disease. Obesity (Silver Spring). 2010;18:2268–73.
35. Hamnvik OP, Liu X, Petrou M, Gong H, Chamberland JP, Kim EH, Christophi CA, Kales SN, Christiani DC, Mantzoros CS. Soluble leptin receptor and leptin are associated with baseline adiposity and metabolic risk factors, and predict adiposity, metabolic syndrome, and glucose levels at 2-year follow-up: the Cyprus Metabolism Prospective Cohort Study. Metabolism. 2011;60:987–93.
36. Sun Q, van Dam RM, Meigs JB, Franco OH, Mantzoros CS, Hu FB. Leptin and soluble leptin receptor levels in plasma and risk of type 2 diabetes in U.S. women: a prospective study. Diabetes. 2010;59:611–8.
37. Chua Jr SC, Koutras IK, Han L, Liu SM, Kay J, Young SJ, Chung WK, Leibel RL. Fine structure of the murine leptin receptor gene: splice site suppression is required to form two alternatively spliced transcripts. Genomics. 1997;45:264–70.
38. Maamra M, Bidlingmaier M, Postel-Vinay MC, Wu Z, Strasburger CJ, Ross RJ. Generation of human soluble leptin receptor by proteolytic cleavage of membrane-anchored receptors. Endocrinology. 2001;142:4389–93.
39. Ge H, Huang L, Pourbahrami T, Li C. Generation of soluble leptin receptor by ectodomain shedding of membrane-spanning receptors in vitro and in vivo. J Biol Chem. 2002;277:45898–903.
40. Brabant G, Nave H, Mayr B, Behrend M, van Harmelen V, Arner P. Secretion of free and protein-bound leptin from subcutaneous adipose tissue of lean and obese women. J Clin Endocrinol Metab. 2002;87:3966–70.
41. Schaab M, Kausch H, Klammt J, Nowicki M, Anderegg U, Gebhardt R, Rose-John S, Scheller J, Thiery J, Kratzsch J. Novel regulatory mechanisms for generation of the soluble leptin receptor: implications for leptin action. PLoS One. 2012;7(4):e34787.

Physiological and Hormonal Factors that Influence Leptin Production

5

Sam Dagogo-Jack

Introduction

Obesity signifies chronic disequilibrium between food consumption and energy expenditure [1–5]. The eventual cloning of the mouse (*ob*) gene and its human homologue [6] in 1994, following insightful predictions from parabiotic experiments by Douglas Coleman two decades previously [7], represents a major milestone in obesity research. The absence of a normal *ob* gene product leads to overfeeding, massive obesity, delayed sexual maturation, endocrinopathies, and immune defects [8] in *ob/ob* mice. The *ob/ob* mutants suffer from hypothermia and exhibit gross endocrine and metabolic features including hypothalamic hypogonadism, hyperinsulinemia, hyperglycemia, and hypercortisolemia [9–13]. Most obese humans appear to have a normal leptin genotype, but rare homozygous mutations of the human leptin gene produce a clinical syndrome similar to the *ob/ob* phenotype [14, 15]. The collective evidence from numerous laboratories indicates that leptin is a regulated hormone that has diverse metabolic and systemic effects. The present chapter discusses the physiological and hormonal factors that influence leptin synthesis and secretion in human beings.

S. Dagogo-Jack, M.D., M.B.B.S. (✉)
Division of Endocrinology, Diabetes and Metabolism, The University of Tennessee Health Science Center, 920 Madison Avenue, Suite 300A, Memphis, TN 38163, USA
e-mail: sdj@uthsc.edu

Circulating Leptin Levels in Humans

Under basal conditions, circulating leptin levels reflect body fat stores, such that obese subjects have hyperleptinemia relative to lean persons [16–20]. Among neonates of full-term pregnancies, cord blood leptin levels are positively correlated with crown-heel length, birth weight and head circumference [21]. Leptin levels are lower in cord blood [22] and neonatal sera [23] in small-for-gestational-age infants compared with larger infants. These observations indicate that the general relationship between leptin and body size is established early during intrauterine life. However, adipocytes may not be the primary source of leptin in fetal life, as indicated by the strong correlation between leptin levels in cord blood and placental weight [22] and the demonstration of leptin production in endometrial tissue, human placenta, and trophoblastic cell cultures [4, 24–27]. Indeed, leptin from placental and trophoblastic sources probably serves as a fetal growth factor [28]. Postnatally, immunoreactive leptin has been detected in low levels in expressed human breast milk, and demonstrated to be absorbable across the gastrointestinal tract of neonatal rodents [29]. Extrapolating from the latter findings, it is likely that circulating leptin levels in suckling infants derive from native as well as maternal sources. The significance of the latter finding is unclear; it is conceivable that maternal leptin absorbed during suckling could play a role in regulating satiety, feeding frequency, and possibly immune function

S. Dagogo-Jack (ed.), *Leptin: Regulation and Clinical Applications*,
DOI 10.1007/978-3-319-09915-6_5, © Springer International Publishing Switzerland 2015

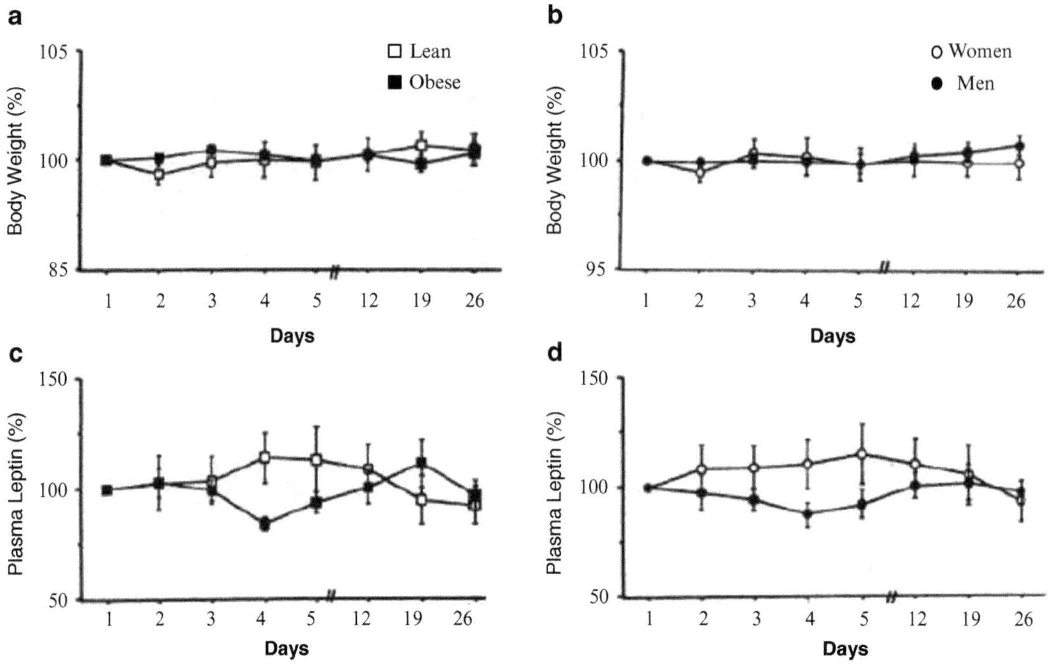

Fig. 5.1 Fasting plasma leptin levels measured daily for 26 days in 20 in lean and obese men and women. Intra-individual leptin levels remained within 80 % and 120 % of baseline values, throughout the 26 days of study. Reproduced from ref. [30] (Liu, Askari, Dagogo-Jack. Endocr Res 25:1–10, 1999), with permission

[8] in infants. Any such metabolic role of maternal leptin transfer is probably of short duration because leptin levels in breast milk obtained from nursing mothers at 6 weeks and 4 months postpartum did not predict anthropometric measures in 118 infants at 2 years [30].

Plasma leptin levels measured in the fasting state are stable and reproducible in lean and obese men and women [31] (Fig. 5.1). In 20 healthy subjects (10 men, 10 women; 10 lean, 10 obese) at stable body weight, blood samples were obtained, after an overnight fast, between 0700 and 0800 on days 1, 2, 3, 4, 5, 12, 19, and 26. Fasting leptin levels on days 2–26 were highly correlated with the baseline levels on day 1 ($R^2=0.9$, $P<0.0001$). Intra-individual leptin levels remained within 80 % and 120 % of baseline values throughout the 26 days of study. Thus, plasma leptin levels are reproducible, with a maximum day-to-day variation of approximately 20 %, in healthy lean and obese persons at stable body weight [31]. Circulating leptin exists in bound and unbound ("free") forms [32–35]. During high performance liquid chromatography, the bound fractions elute as a broad peak (~59–130 kDa) and the free fractions co-elute with monomeric leptin [33]. The soluble leptin receptor is the major leptin binding protein [36]. Bound leptin can be displaced readily by competition from exogenous leptin and by warming sera before chromatography [34].

Physiological Factors

The physiological factors that influence circulating human leptin levels include the amount of body fat [16–20], gender [18, 19, 37], age [37], puberty [38], fasting [39], feeding [40, 41], and exercise [42, 43] (Table 5.1). Leptin levels also show a diurnal pattern, with peak values occurring at night and trough values in the late afternoon [44]. Subsequent studies indicate that the diurnal pattern in plasma leptin levels is entrained to meals rather than the true circadian clock [45].

Table 5.1 Physiological factors that alter leptin levels in humans

Factor	Plasma leptin	Leptin mRNA	References
Gender	F>M	F>M	[18, 19, 21, 37, 46, 47]
Weight gain	Increased	Increased	[16–22, 54, 64]
Weight loss	Decreased	Decreased	[67, 68, 70–72, 75, 76]
Puberty	Increased	ND	[38, 77]
Age	Increased with age	ND	[78, 79]
	Decreased in elderly or post-menopause	ND	[37, 54]
Feeding	Increased	ND	[40, 41, 81]
Fasting	Decreased	ND	[37–39]
Exercise	Decreased	ND	[42, 85–89]

ND no data

Gender and Sex Steroids

In most reports, the female–male ratio in circulating leptin levels approximates 3:1 or greater [18, 19, 37]. The gender dimorphism in plasma leptin levels most likely is explained by the differential effects of androgens and estrogens on adipocyte leptin production. Gender dimorphism is evident at birth: female neonates have significantly higher free leptin and leptin//Ponderal index in cord blood compared to male neonates [21]. The levels of soluble leptin receptor in cord blood were lower in female than male neonates, one mechanism for the higher levels of free or unbound leptin in the female neonates [21]. Compared with eugonadal men, plasma leptin levels were threefold higher in a group of hypogonadal men with testosterone deficiency and relative estrogen excess [46]. The elevated leptin in the hypogonadal men returned to normal male levels within 2 months of testosterone replacement [46]. In another interesting report, male-to-female transvestites, treated with pharmacological doses of estrogen, attained elevated "female" levels of plasma leptin, whereas female-to-male transvestites, given masculizing doses of androgen, showed a significant reduction in circulating leptin levels [47]. Together, these data confirm that opposite effects of testosterone and estradiol on leptin production account for the gender differences in circulating leptin levels. Because testosterone treatment also increases lean muscle mass [48], and women generally have higher percent body fat than men, it is likely that the lower leptin levels in men result from inhibition of leptin synthesis by testosterone coupled with lower leptin output from a smaller fat depot compared to women.

There have been no studies specifically focusing on the effect of progesterone alone on leptin production. However, plasma leptin levels are within the expected range for BMI in women taking a combined estrogen-progestin oral contraceptive medication [49] or postmenopausal hormone replacement therapy [50]. Based on their known androgenic properties, progestins might decrease plasma leptin levels. The neutral effect of combined estrogen-progestin pill on leptin suggests that any pro-androgenic (inhibitory) effect of progesterone on leptin synthesis is counterbalanced by the stimulatory effect of the estrogen component. In summary, women have approximately threefold higher leptin levels than men, a gender disparity that is programmed as early as during intrauterine life. The greater leptin abundance in women reflects higher body fat and the effect of estrogen, and probably subserves important functions in sexual maturation and reproduction. The teleological basis for the markedly lower leptin levels in men is unclear, but low leptin levels could, theoretically, be protective of prostate carcinogenesis [51–53].

Body Fat

Measurement of plasma leptin levels and indices of adiposity in the same individuals consistently documents a very strong correlation ($R^2 \sim 0.7$–0.9) between both measures (Fig. 5.2). Thus, obese and overweight persons generally have higher plasma leptin levels than lean persons [18, 19, 54]. The relationship is a dynamic one, such that short-term weight fluctuations in body fat mass induce same-direction changes in circulating leptin levels. The hyperleptinemia in obese

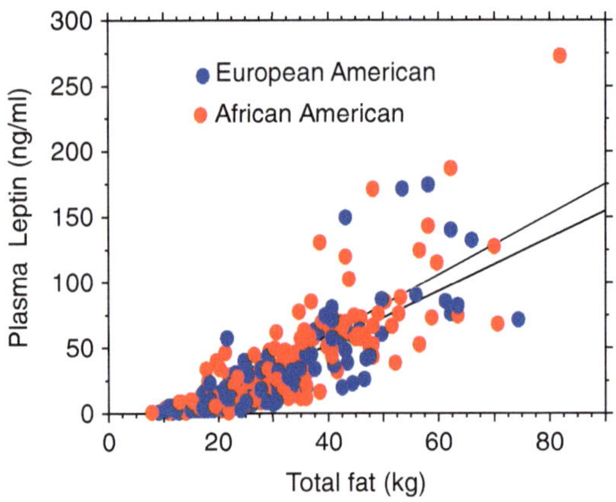

Fig. 5.2 Regression of fasting plasma leptin levels and total body fat in 254 healthy men and women (127 European American, 127 African American), mean age 44.2±10.6 years (±SD). The regression equation is $Y=-29.239+0.002\times X$ ($R^2=0.652$) for European Americans and $Y=-33.447+0.002\times X$ ($R^2=0.659$) for African Americans

humans is associated with increased adipocyte leptin gene expression [16, 17]. White adipose tissue from the subcutaneous compartment has higher leptin production capacity than omental fat or brown adipose tissue [55, 56]. The processes leading to leptin secretion by adipocytes are integrated by the nutrient sensing hexosamine pathway; UDP-N-acetylglucosamine, the end product of the hexosamine biosynthetic pathway, has been identified as an intracellular trigger for leptin secretion [57–59].

The finding of hyperleptinemia in obese persons suggests that human obesity may be a leptin-resistant state; however, the mechanism of such leptin resistance is unclear. In rodent models and rare human examples, leptin-resistant obesity is caused by leptin receptor mutations [60, 61]. Targeted hypothalamic lesions also induced leptin resistance [62]. Since direct infusion of leptin into the cerebral ventricles suppresses appetite and reduces weight more potently than intraperitoneal injection in mice [63], impaired leptin delivery to central sites could be a factor in the development of obesity [20, 64–66]. The subject of leptin resistance is discussed in greater detail in Chap. 6. In summary, fasting or basal leptin levels are in direct proportion to adiposity in humans, reflecting the output of the mass of adipocytes. In that regard, circulating leptin may be considered as a marker of total adipocyte mass or volume ("adipostat").

Weight Loss and Anorexia Nervosa

Decreases in body weight are associated with tandem (and sometimes disproportionate) decreases in circulating leptin levels. In one report, a 10 % decrease in weight resulted in a 30 % decrease in plasma leptin levels [67]. Weight loss also elicits several neuroendocrine and metabolic responses, including suppression of gonadotropins, activation of the hypothalamic–pituitary–adrenal axis, alterations in thyroid hormone regulation and decreases in energy expenditure [67, 68]. The decline in leptin production following weight loss is thus part of an intricate physiological and neuroendocrine adaptation, with the reduced leptin levels serving as a signal of energy deficit or starvation to central effector sites. The lower leptin levels also would disinhibit appetite and stimulate ingestive behavior, to restore body weight to its prior steady state. Indeed, hypoleptinemia has been reported to precede the development of obesity in Pima Indians [69]. Interestingly, administration of recombinant leptin to individuals who had lost 10 % of body weight ameliorated the decline in energy expenditure and corrected the neuroendocrine alterations induced by weight loss [70]. These effects indicate that leptin is not merely an "adipostat," but an active defender of energy homeostasis through its interactions with central integrating sites, particularly during periods of starvation or caloric restriction. Thus, there appears to be a potential therapeutic role for leptin in the prevention of weight regain [67–72] in post-obese subjects. Such an intervention could be an adjunctive approach to the maintenance of weight loss, but the tolerability and durability of such supplemental leptin therapy will need to be established.

The endocrine adaptations in anorexia nervosa, an extreme weight loss state, include suppressed leptin levels; hypothalamic amenorrhea; growth-hormone resistance, leading to low IGF-1 levels; and hypercortisolemia [73, 74]. The severity of the hypoleptinemia in women with anorexia nervosa seems out of proportion to their low BMI, when compared to leptin levels in non-anorectic thin women [75, 76]. The regression line of plasma leptin levels vs. BMI is flat over the BMI range of 10–18 kg/m^2 in women with anorexia nervosa, which suggests a dysregulation of the normal leptin–BMI relationship [76]. Upon successful refeeding, anorectic patients regain body weight and experience restoration of plasma leptin levels and normalization of the linear relationship between leptin and BMI [75, 76]. Clearly, anorexia nervosa is not due to suppression of appetite by excessive leptin production; in fact, there appears to be exaggerated hypoleptinemia, which might be an adaptive mechanism to maximally disinhibit appetite and help kindle ingestive behavior. Curiously, a highly significant positive correlation between plasma levels of leptin and total IGF-I (which disappeared after successful refeeding) has been reported in women with anorexia nervosa; no such correlation was seen among normal-weight controls [76].

Puberty and Age

Serially measured plasma leptin levels are inversely related to age at puberty, and show a peak shortly before pubertal [38, 77]. The reports of increased plasma leptin levels in older individuals compared to younger persons is explained by the higher fat mass in older persons, and possibly also by age-related leptin resistance [78, 79]. In rats, biological responses to leptin (assessed by food intake, oxygen consumption, and hypothalamic NPY expression during 7 days of leptin infusion) appear to decline with age [80]. In humans, Guadalupe-Grau et al. [78] analyzed circulating leptin levels in relation to adiposity measures and vastus lateralis muscle biopsies obtained from BMI-matched subjects from three age groups: 24±4 years ($n=13$), 44±5 years ($n=14$), and 58±8 years ($n=12$). Plasma leptin levels were higher in older compared to younger subjects; body fat also was higher (and lean mass lower) in the older subjects. The expression as well as phosphorylation of leptin receptors in skeletal muscle did not differ significantly by age [78]. However, PTP1B levels were higher and pSTAT3 levels tended to be lower ($P=0.09$) in the oldest age group than in the youngest group. Remarkably, the expression of SOCS (an important mediator of leptin resistance), pJAK2, pAMPKα, and pACCβ showed no age disparities. In a related report, Roszkowska-Gancarz et al. [79] studied 38 young (aged 26.8±3.6 years), 37 elderly (aged 64.7±3.1 years) and 39 long-lived (aged 94.2±3.7 years) healthy, nonobese subjects. Circulating leptin levels and BMI were significantly higher in the older subjects. The expression of leptin receptors (OB-Rb) in peripheral blood mononuclear cells did not differ by age, but that of OB-Ra was lower in the older age groups compared to young subjects. The latter finding was driven mostly by changes observed in women [79]. Thus, the molecular evidence for age-related leptin resistance seems rather modest, which leaves increasing adiposity as the major explanation of the higher leptin levels in older compared to younger persons. A decline in plasma leptin, probably explained by hypoestrogenism, has been reported after the menopause [54]. In another report, an inverse relationship was observed between plasma leptin levels and age in a group of 204 subjects aged 18–80 years, with leptin levels decreasing by ~50 % after age 60 years [37]. The strong relationship between adiposity and leptin suggests that the inclusion of underweight elderly persons probably produced the pattern reported in the latter study [37].

Fasting and Feeding

Plasma leptin levels decreased by ~70 % from baseline values during prolonged (~52 h) fasting [38, 39]. Besides fasting, caloric reduction also downregulates leptin production; in one study, plasma leptin was reduced by 26 % in 5 obese subjects who consumed a 1,000-Cal diet for 10 days [37]. Most of the decline in serum leptin during a 24-h fast is accounted for by a decrease in the free leptin fraction [32]. The marked decline in circulating leptin levels during fasting or caloric reduction is out of proportion to the reduction in body weight or fat mass during these relatively brief fasting periods [39]. The marked hypoleptinemic response to starvation suggests the existence of a rapid leptin response system in defense of acute starvation that is signaled by fasting or reduction of energy intake. The rapid leptin regulatory response system should be contrasted with the slower time course, and more proportionate magnitude, of the decrease in leptin levels that occurs following weight loss. Indeed, the teleological role of leptin is more consistent with that of a peripheral signal for central nervous system adaptation to starvation or energy insecurity rather than an antiobesity hormone.

As a corollary to the fasting-induced hypoleptinemia, plasma leptin levels are stimulated by overfeeding [40, 41], but less so by normal feeding [18, 19]. Kolaczynski et al. [40] investigated the effect of acute and chronic intake of excessive energy on serum leptin in humans. The acute (12-h) protocol consisted of voluntary overfeeding (120 Cal/kg), and the chronic protocol entailed overfeeding to attain 10 % weight gain and maintenance for additional 2 weeks before assessment. In the acute feeding study, circulating leptin levels increased by 40 % over baseline during the final hours of overfeeding, an increase that persisted until the next morning. During chronic overfeeding that resulted in a 10 % weight gain, leptin levels increased more than threefold above baseline values. There was a direct linear relationship between increased leptin levels and weight gain as well as the percent gain of body fat ($r=0.88$; $P<0.01$) [41]. Dietary macro-nutrient components seem to differentially affect leptin levels: 24-h leptin concentrations are lower when three high-fat meals are consumed, compared with high-carbohydrate/low-fat meals that induce larger postprandial glucose excursions and greater insulin secretion [81].

The time course of the postprandial rise in plasma leptin levels is slower, and its magnitude is less robust, compared with the decline in leptin during fasting, which suggests that the physiological purpose of leptin is geared toward maintenance of satiety and prevention of hunger between meals rather than limitation of the size of the index meal. Postprandial leptin increases appear to be attenuated in patients with diabetes, and can be restored by prandial administration of rapid-acting insulin [82]. Thus, the ability of meals to trigger a delayed leptin response might be a counterregulatory mechanism designed to prevent hyperphagia and maintain adequate interpandial intervals. Indeed, the well-known diurnal rhythm in circulating leptin levels (nocturnal peak between midnight and early morning) is entrained to meals rather than the true circadian clock [44, 45]. Appropriate nocturnal rise in leptin might be a mechanism for suppressing appetite during sleep. The nocturnal rise in leptin and the glucocorticoid stimulation of leptin (discussed later) are both abolished by fasting [83, 84].

Exercise

Short-term exercise (≤60 min) of moderate intensity does not acutely alter leptin secretion in healthy men and women, but prolonged strenuous exercise (e.g., marathon running) inhibits leptin secretion significantly [42, 85]. Arteriovenous balance studies in vivo conducted at rest and during 60 min have demonstrated elegantly acute bout of moderate-intensity exercise (50 % VO2 max) does not alter leptin production in abdominal [85]. During prolonged bouts of exercise, decreases in plasma leptin levels have been reported after 1–3 h of running or cycling, but part of this effect has been attributed to diurnal reduction in circulating leptin [86]. Exercise of sufficient intensity that produces significant energy deficits results in suppression of the 24-h mean and amplitude of the diurnal rhythm of leptin [86]. Decreases in leptin levels occur ~48 h after prolonged (≥60 min) aerobic exercise and after ~9 h following prolonged resistance exercise [42, 86]. Exercise training studies have shown variable effects of short-term exercise training (≤12 weeks) on leptin levels, with many studies reporting no change in circulating leptin levels in healthy subjects. In one study, 23 obese women (mean BMI 40.7 ± 6.7 kg/m^2) were enrolled in an exercise program (45-min walking sessions at 60–80 % VO2 max) daily (except weekends) for four weeks (total 20 exercise sessions). Leptin levels were assessed at baseline and at the end of the first, seventh, and twentieth exercise session [87]. Compared with baseline values, plasma leptin level did not change significantly at the end of the first exercise session, but decreased significantly at end of the seventh (59.1 ± 20.1 ng/ml vs. 53.4 ± 21.9 ng/ml, $P=0.003$) and twentieth exercise session (59.1 ± 20.1 ng/ml vs. 51.2 ± 20.5 ng/ml, $P=0.007$), respectively [87]. The authors found no correlation between weight loss during exercise training and the change in leptin levels. Thus, this study of obese women indicated that leptin levels decreased modestly by ~10 % from baseline within 1 week of daily moderate-intensity exercise and by ~13 % within 3 weeks, apparently independently of weight loss [87].

Longer term (>12 weeks) exercise training also has been reported to have variable effects on leptin: some studies report no change in leptin levels beyond the effects predicted by weight loss, while others report residual hypoleptinemia after accounting for weight loss [85]. In a recent report, 97 sedentary individuals (45 men, 52 women) were enrolled in 6 months of supervised exercise training. Blood specimens for leptin assay were obtained at baseline and at 24 h and 72 h after completion of the final training session. Training induced a 1.1-kg decrease in body weight during the 6-month period. Leptin levels decreased by ~10 % at 24 h post-training, but returned to baseline after 72 h [88]. The greatest decrease in leptin was observed among individuals with the highest pre-training leptin levels [88]. The effect of prolonged exercise and exercise training on leptin levels is probably mediated in part by downregulation of leptin mRNA synthesis by catecholamines released during prolonged exercise, variations in energy intake, loss of fat mass, improvements in insulin sensitivity, and alterations in lipid and intermediary metabolism [85–89].

Hormonal Factors

The effects of various hormones on leptin production in humans are summarized in Table 5.2. Insulin, glucocorticoids, and growth hormone (GH) have been reported to increase plasma leptin levels and/or adipocyte leptin mRNA expression in humans. In contrast, catecholamines, insulin-like growth factor-I (IGF-I), and somatostatin appear to decrease leptin production [90, 91]. Besides being regulated by several hormones, leptin also alters the expression of several hormonal axes. For instance, leptin inhibits glucocorticoid secretion in *ob/ob* mice [92] as well as in rat and human adrenocortical cell cultures [93], and modulates insulin secretion [94], insulin action [95], and glucose metabolism [96]. Furthermore, recombinant leptin treatment reverses the neuroendocrine changes induced by weight loss [15, 70], although changes following mild caloric restriction (−500 kcal) appear to be unaffected by leptin [97]. Clearly, there is evidence for modulatory effects of leptin on the hypothalamic-pituitary-adrenal, hypothalamic-pituitary-gonadal, and the hypothalamic-pituitary-thyroid axes [90–97]. What emerges then is a complex hormonal interregulatory system in which leptin production is modulated by several hormones, many of which are, in turn, also modulated by leptin under certain conditions [90–98].

Table 5.2 Hormones that alter leptin levels in humans

Hormone	Plasma leptin	Leptin mRNA	References
Glucocorticoids	Increased	Increased	[120–124, 127, 134, 135]
Insulin	Increased	Increased	[18, 19, 103–105]
Estradiol	Increased	ND	[47]
Testosterone	Decreased	ND	[46, 47]
Growth hormone	Increased (acute)	ND	[142, 145]
	Decreased (chronic)	ND	[143]
IGF-I	Decreased	ND	[142, 144, 145]
Somatostatin	Decreased	ND	[159]

ND no data

Insulin

Fasting plasma leptin levels are strongly correlated with fasting insulin levels ($r \sim 0.6$) [18, 19]. Administration of insulin results in a two- to threefold increase in adipocyte leptin mRNA and circulating levels in rats within 4–6 h [99]. Such an acute effect of insulin on leptin secretion was not seen in humans [19, 100–102]. In vitro, addition of insulin (100 nM) to cultured human adipocytes increased leptin mRNA levels and secretion of leptin protein into the medium after a lag period of 48–72 h [103]. In vivo, a dose-dependent increase in plasma leptin levels occurs following prolonged infusion of insulin under clamped euglycemic conditions [103–105]. An increase of ~50 % above baseline value appears to be the maximum plasma leptin response to insulin in humans [105]. In patients with insulinoma, the elevated leptin levels are normalized after surgical removal of tumor [106], which directly implicates chronic endogenous hyperinsulinemia as a cause of the hyperleptinemia. However, because patients with insulinoma may be driven to eat frequently (in response to hypoglycemia), such overfeeding probably also contributes to the insulinoma-associated hyperleptinemia. The delayed stimulation of human leptin production by insulin is consistent with a transcriptional effect. It would seem physiologically congruent that insulin does not trigger immediate or acute leptin secretion, since such an effect would suppress food intake in a state of insulin abundance, thereby increasing the risk for hypoglycemia. On the other hand, a delayed leptin response to prandial insulin secretion could be a mechanism for restraining hunger and excessive food intake and facilitating substrate disposal [72, 90, 107, 108].

Insulin stimulates leptin synthesis and secretion via a mechanism that involves regulation of glucose metabolism in adipocytes [57, 58]. Alterations in the amount of nutrient flux through the nutrient-sensing hexosamine pathway in the fed or fasting states modulate the levels of UDP-N-acetylglucosamine, which is a key intracellular mediator of the leptin secretion [57, 58]. In vitro studies in isolated adipocytes [57, 109] and in vivo human studies [110] indicate that the stimulatory effect of insulin on leptin production is mediated by increased glucose utilization and metabolism in adipocytes. Diazoxide, an inhibitor of glucose-mediated insulin secretion, decreases plasma leptin levels [111]. The stimulation of leptin production by insulin-mediated glucose metabolism occurs at the transcriptional level [112]; the region of the leptin gene involved in the activation of the leptin promoter lies between −135 and −95 bp and encompasses the binding site for the transcription factor Sp1 [113, 114].

The co-existence of hyperinsulinemia and hyperleptinemia in obese, insulin-resistant persons often presents interpretive difficulties regarding causality. Recall that leptin-deficient, hyperglycemic, and hyperinsulinemic ob/ob mice responded to sub-anorexogenic doses of recombinant leptin (that had no effect on body weight) with normalization of plasma glucose and insulin levels [10, 11]. Similarly, low doses of leptin administered i.v. or into the cerebral ventricles increased glucose utilization in wild type mice [96]. These data characterize leptin as an insulin sensitizer rather than as a mediator of insulin resistance. In fact, leptin can serve as rescue therapy in place of insulin in insulin-deficient mice with experimental type 1 diabetes [108]. To the extent that leptin serves as an endogenous insulin sensitizer, hyperleptinemia may be a compensatory response to insulin resistance, besides being a marker of adiposity, in obese subjects. Studies using euglycemic clamp and other techniques have observed a significant association between fasting plasma leptin levels and insulin sensitivity in lean as well as obese subjects without diabetes [115–117]. In a multivariate regression model, leptin emerged as a strong predictor of insulin sensitivity after controlling for BMI [117]. From regression plots of ISI versus BMI and leptin, a BMI > 27 kg/m^2 and a leptin level > 15 ng/dl strongly predicted decreased insulin sensitivity. Obese persons with fasting leptin levels < 15 ng/ml were 100 % more insulin sensitive than control subjects of similar BMI whose fasting leptin levels are greater than 15 ng/ml [117]. Thus, fasting hyperleptinemia conveys information regarding a possibly compensatory or counterregulatory response to ambient insulin resistance, such that a relatively low leptin level in an obese person signifies relatively preserved insulin sensitivity [117, 118].

Glucocorticoids

Glucocorticoids are potent stimuli for leptin production; the stimulatory action is probably mediated through interaction with glucocorticoid response element in the 5′-regulatory region of the leptin gene [119–125]. In rats, treatment with dexamethasone increases leptin gene expression in adipocytes, accompanied by decreases food intake [126]. In humans, dexamethasone increases leptin mRNA synthesis in adipocytes as well as circulating leptin levels [124, 127, 128]. Cushing's syndrome, an experiment of nature characterized by glucocorticoid excess, is associated with hyperleptinemia [128, 129]. In one report, hyperleptinemia persisted 10 days after transsphenoidal surgery for pituitary Cushing's disease [130], which suggests that adipocyte adaptation to chronic hypercortisolemia is not acutely reversed by surgery. Stress-induced hypercortisolemai during critical illness also is associated with hyperleptinemia [131].

The leptin secretagogue effect appears to be a class property of glucocorticoids, with the notable exception of conflicting reports for methylprednisone. In one placebo-controlled study, conducted in 20 lean men, a 30 min i.v. infusion of methylprednisolone (125 mg) followed by oral administration of methylprednisolone (40 mg/day) for 4 days was reported not to alter plasma leptin levels [132], but another study reported increased leptin following oral administration of methylprednisolone (0.5 mg/kg) daily for 7 days [121]. In contrast to discrepant data with methylprednisolone, other synthetic glucocorticoids, dexamethasone and prednisolone, have consistently stimulatory effects on leptin production [120, 122–124, 127, 133, 134].

To further explore the physiology of glucocorticoid-leptin interaction, we determined the effect of the natural glucocorticoid hydrocortisone on circulating leptin levels and leptin mRNA abundance in human adipose tissue. In the same experiments, we also compared the relative potencies of insulin and hydrocortisone as leptin secretagogues, using a randomized, crossover, placebo-controlled study design [135]. Healthy study subjects (mean age 36.6 ± 1.7 years; BMI 27.6 ± 0.9 kg/m^2) were admitted overnight to the GCRC on three occasions, separated by a 2 week wash-out period. In random fashion, participants were assigned to i.v. infusion of normal saline (placebo), hydrocortisone (3.3 μg/kg.min), or insulin (1 mU/kg.min). Blood glucose was maintained at ~140 mg/dl during the insulin infusion, using variable rate infusion of dextrose (10 %). Hourly blood specimens were obtained for measurement of leptin, insulin and cortisol. Subcutaneous fat biopsies were obtained from a paramedian abdominal region between 0700 and 0800 on day 1 before the infusions, and from the contralateral side on day 2, after the interventions. Total RNA was extracted from fat biopsy specimens and subjected to Northern blot analysis for leptin mRNA expression [135]. Plasma leptin levels were similar at baseline and during the initial 5 h following infusion of placebo, hydrocortisone, or insulin, and showed the expected nocturnal peak (Fig. 5.3). Compared with placebo, infusion of hydrocortisone or insulin resulted in significant increases in plasma leptin levels. Plasma leptin increased from 16.0 ± 3.8 ng/ml to a peak of 42.1 ± 7.0 ng/ml ($P = 0.008$) during hydrocortisone insulin, and from 16.6 ± 2.7 ng/ml to 30.3 ± 4.3 ng/ml ($P = 0.024$) during insulin infusion (Fig. 5.3). The peak change in plasma leptin expressed as a percentage of basal values was 83 ± 12 % during insulin infusion and 163 ± 28 % during hydrocortisone infusion. Compared with insulin, hydrocortisone infusion resulted in a greater ($P = 0.02$) percentage rise in plasma leptin. Leptin mRNA expression in subcutaneous fat (as a ratio of beta-actin abundance) was unchanged after saline infusion, but increased approximately threefold after hydrocortisone infusion [135] (Fig. 5.3). Thus, hydrocortisone (a natural ligand for both types I and II receptors) [136], like dexamethasone (a synthetic type II glucocorticoid receptor-specific ligand), exerts a potent stimulatory effect on leptin production that is more robust than that induced by insulin (Fig. 5.3) [135].

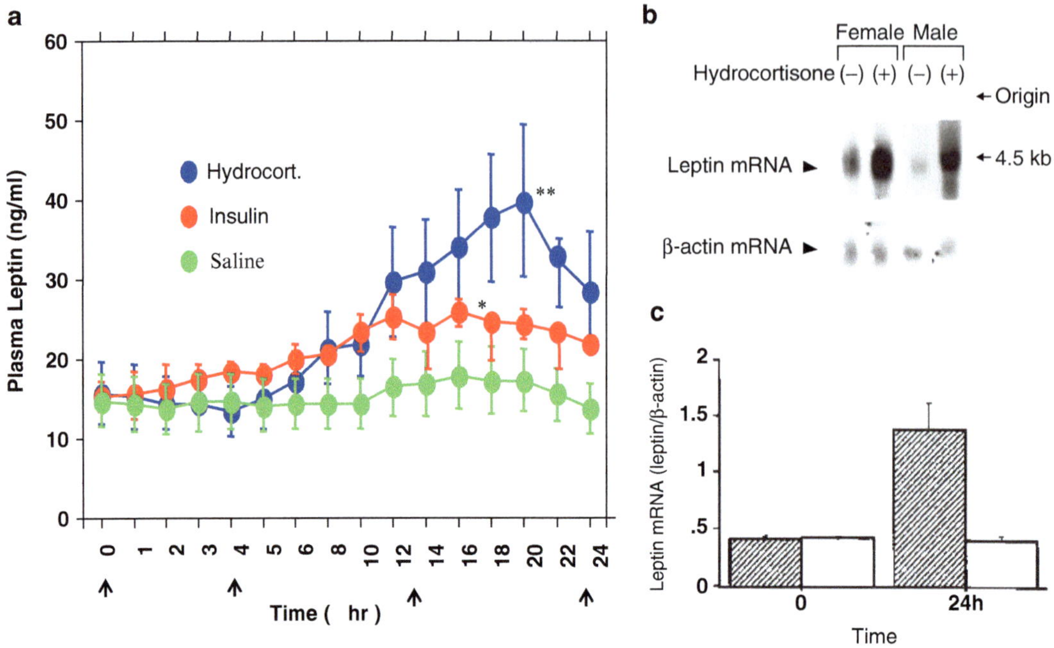

Fig. 5.3 (**a**) Plasma leptin levels during continuous infusion of saline (placebo), insulin, or hydrocortisone for 24 h (0800–0800). $*P=0.024$, $**P=0.008$ compared to saline infusion. Arrows indicate meal times. (**b**) Northern blot analysis of leptin and beta-actin mRNA expression in subcutaneous adipose tissue before (–) and after (+) a 24-h infusion of hydrocortisone in a representative healthy male and female. Thirteen micrograms of total RNA were fractionated on 1 % agarose gel and analyzed. (**c**) Effect of a 24 h infusion of normal saline (*open bars*) or hydrocortisone (*hatched bars*) on adipocyte leptin mRNA abundance relative to abundance of β-actin in healthy subjects. Hydrocortisone infusion resulted in a threefold increase in leptin mRNA abundance. Adapted from Askari H, Liu J, Dagogo-Jack S [135]

Dose–Response

Because early studies had employed mostly pharmacological doses of glucocorticoids to study leptin response, their physiological relevance has been called into question [137].

Subsequent reports have established that the increase in plasma leptin levels following administration of glucocorticoids is dose-related [83], the maximum effect seen with 2–4 mg of dexamethasone (or ~100 mg of hydrocortisone) being a doubling of plasma leptin levels. In a study employing dexamethasone as leptin secretagogue, a linear relationship was observed between the plasma leptin response and plasma dexamethasone levels [122]. In another study, the effects of more physiological doses of hydrocortisone were examined. Healthy volunteers (mean age 36 years, BMI 31 kg/m^2) received i.v. infusion of either saline or two doses of hydrocortisone (30 mg/24 h and 100 mg/24 h) during three overnight admissions to the General Clinical Research Center [83]. The treatments were administered in random order, separated by 1-week "wash-out" periods. Blood samples obtained every 1–2 h were analyzed for leptin levels. During each of the three 24-h periods of experimentation, study subjects consumed a standard diet. The mean 24-h plasma cortisol level (ug/dl) was 6.96 ± 0.89 during saline, 11.43 ± 0.21 ($P<0.001$) during HC (30 mg/24 h), and 23.43 ± 1.06 ($P<0.001$) during HC (100 mg/24 h) infusion, respectively [83]. The peak/baseline plasma leptin levels (ng/ml) were $31.5 \pm 7.7/22.5 + 3.9$ (+40 %) during HC 30-mg/24 h and $45.8 \pm 8.9/24.8 \pm 5.2$ (+85 %, $P<0.01$) during HC 100-mg/24 h infusion [83] (Fig. 5.4). The efficacy of low-dose hydrocortisone (30 mg/day, which is within the physiological range for cortisol production in humans [138]) in

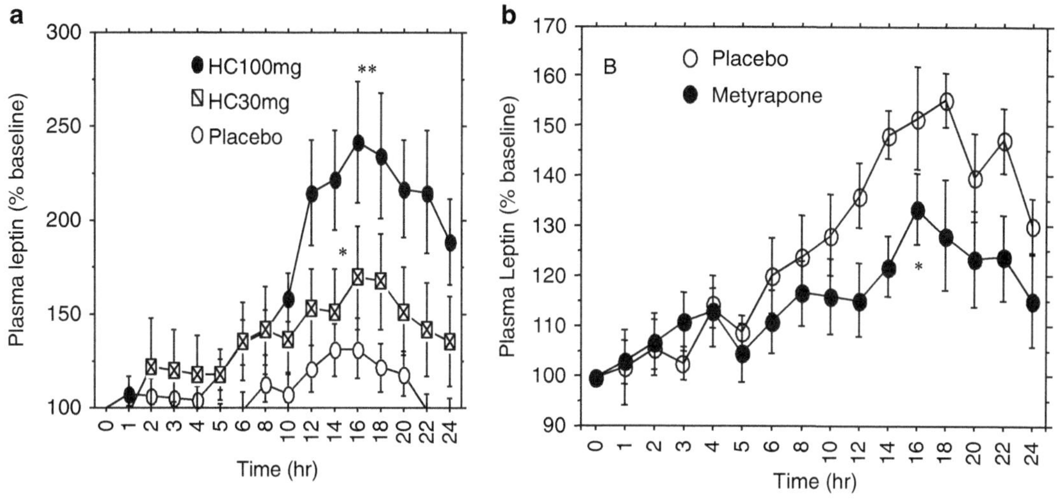

Fig. 5.4 (**a**) Dose–response effect of hydrocortisone (HC) infusion in doses of 30 mg/24 h and 100 mg/ 24 h versus saline (placebo) infusion on plasma leptin levels in healthy subjects. The treatments were administered in random order separated by 1-week "wash-out" periods. The mean 24-h plasma cortisol level (ug/dl) was 6.96±0.89 during saline, 11.43±0.21 ($P<0.001$) during HC (30 mg/24 h), and 23.43±1.06 ($P<0.001$) during HC (100 mg/24 h) infusion, respectively. *$P<0.05$ vs. Placebo; **$P<0.01$ vs. HC30 and Placebo. Adapted from Dagogo-Jack S, Umamaheswaran I, Askari H, Tykodi G [83]. (**b**) Effect of inhibition of cortisol synthesis with metyrapone on circulating leptin levels. The peak nocturnal leptin attained was 55.5±5.4 % above baseline during placebo treatment as compared with 28.5±11.1 % above baseline during metyrapone treatment ($P<0.01$). Adapted from Dagogo-Jack S, Tykodi G, Umamaheswaran I [139]

stimulating leptin secretion rebuts the argument that pharmacological doses of glucocorticoids are required to produce a leptin response [136]. The demonstrated dose–response relationship between hydrocortisone doses and plasma leptin responses (+40 % for 30 mg/day dose and +85 % for 100 mg/day dose) further strengthens the physiological significance of the interactions between glucocorticoids and leptin.

Inhibition of Cortisol Synthesis

The data reviewed in the foregoing sections support the hypothesis that glucocorticoids play a physiological role in the regulation of leptin production. That hypothesis has been tested further by examining the effects of inhibition of endogenous cortisol biosynthesis on leptin secretion [139, 140]. Using a randomized, placebo-controlled, crossover study design (with a 2-week wash-out interval), we studied the effects of administration of metyrapone (750 mg every 4 h for 24 h) or placebo in obese subjects (mean age 30.4±1.56 year, BMI 42.0±1.33 kg/m^2) during overnight admissions to the GCRC [139]. Metyrapone treatment resulted in a significant decrease in plasma cortisol level, which was accompanied by a significant reduction in circulating leptin levels [139]. As pretreatment plasma leptin levels varied markedly among the study subjects (9.2–97.0 ng/ml), values were expressed as percent change from baseline. Compared with placebo, plasma leptin levels decreased significantly within 6 h of metyrapone treatment and the decrease was sustained throughout the study period. Furthermore, the well-known nocturnal rise in plasma leptin between 2000 and 0200 was markedly attenuated during treatment with metyrapone, which implicates cortisol among the mechanisms contributing to the nocturnal rise in leptin. The peak nocturnal leptin level was 55.5±5.4 % above baseline during placebo treatment as compared with 28.5±11.1 % above baseline during metyrapone treatment ($P<0.01$). Thus, treatment with metyrapone (which blocks

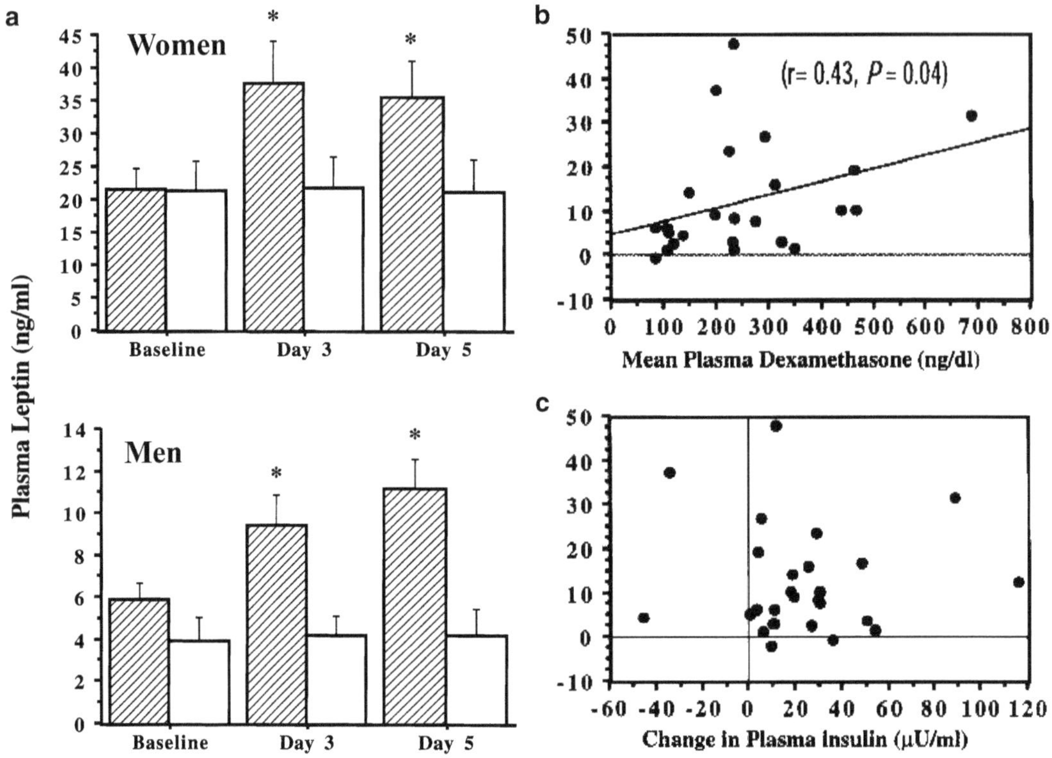

Fig. 5.5 (**a**) Effect of daily treatment with single-dose oral dexamethasone (*hatched bars*) or placebo (*open bars*) on plasma leptin levels in healthy women and men. $*P \leq 0.0001$. (**b**, **c**) Relationship between change in plasma leptin following dexamethasone treatment and plasma dexamethasone concentration (**b**) and change in plasma insulin levels (**c**). Adapted from Dagogo-Jack S, Selke G, Melson AK, Newcomer JW [122]

11-beta-hydroxylase, the final enzyme in cortisol biosynthesis), significantly decreases circulating leptin levels and attenuates the nocturnal rise in leptin by 27 % (Fig. 5.4). Qualitatively similar findings were reported by Laferrere et al. [140]. Interpreted against the backdrop of the numerous reports that show a stimulatory effect of glucocorticoids on leptin synthesis and secretion, the finding that inhibition of endogenous steroidogenesis attenuates circulating leptin levels strengthens the physiological relevance of the glucocorticoid-leptin interaction.

In summary, the evidence for the physiological significance of glucocorticoid regulation of leptin includes (1) the finding that inhibition of endogenous steroidogenesis with metyrapone decreases plasma leptin levels [139, 140] (Fig. 5.4); (2) demonstration of a dose–response relationship between hydrocortisone and plasma leptin response [83] (Fig. 5.4); (3) demonstration of a linear relationship between serum dexamethasone concentration and stimulated leptin levels [122] (Fig. 5.5); (4) modulation of ad libitum food intake by glucocorticoid-induced hyperleptinemia in humans [141]; and (5) the demonstration that fasting abolished the expected leptin response to glucocorticoids [83, 84]. Moreover, unlike the sexual dimorphism observed in basal leptin levels, the leptin response to glucocorticoids (as a percentage of baseline leptin) is similar in men and women [122] (Fig. 5.5). These observations are discussed further in Chap. 15, Dynamic leptin secretion.

GH and IGF-I

Growth hormone replacement has been reported to have opposite effects on plasma leptin, depending on dosage, duration, age, and GH status of recipients. An increased plasma leptin response was reported following GH administration GH-deficient adults [142]. In contrast, decreased plasma leptin levels were observed following GH replacement in GH-deficient children [143]. Treatment with recombinant human IGF-I results in ~30 % decrease in circulating leptin levels [142, 144, 145]. A net increase in plasma leptin was reported during combined treatment with GH and IGF-I for 3 days in adults [145]. The apparent difference in leptin responses to GH among adults and children may be related to age differences in the activity of the GH–IGF-I axis [146]. Because IGF-1 suppresses plasma insulin and GH levels, it is unclear whether the decreased leptin levels [142, 144] are a direct effect of IGF-I or secondary to decreases insulin and/or GH secretion. However, in vitro studies suggest that IGF-I inhibits the stimulatory effect of dexamethasone on leptin mRNA synthesis in rat adipocytes [147].

Florkowski and colleagues [148] reported that treatment with low doses of GH for 3 months was associated with decreased fat stores and plasma leptin levels in GH-deficient adults. Thus, GH might augment circulating leptin levels in the short term but exerts a modest hypoleptinemic effect on chronic therapy, probably due to changes in body composition. An inverse relationship between plasma leptin and the molar ratio of IGF-I to IGF binding protein-3 (IGFBP-3) has been reported [149]. As the IGF-I/IGFBP-3 molar ratio reflects the concentration of "free" or unbound IGF-I in plasma (which is inversely related to adiposity [150]), the finding of an inverse relationship between leptin and "free" IGF-I levels is not unexpected. No significant correlation has been observed between plasma concentrations of leptin and total IGF-I in normal weight or obese individuals [144]. The modest and contrasting effects of GH and IGF-I on leptin production indicate that the known stimulatory effect of hyperinsulinemia on leptin production is not likely mediated by IGF-I receptors on adipocytes [151].

Thyroid Hormone

Valcavi et al. [152] reported that individuals with hypothyroidism show a 50 % reduction in circulating leptin levels, compared with euthyroid controls. The difference persists after adjustments for age, gender, and BMI [152]. In contrast, Sreenan et al. found no significant differences in serum leptin concentrations among subjects with hypothyroidism, compared with euthyroid controls [153]. Plasma leptin levels are generally unaltered by hyperthyroidism [152, 153], and are not acutely affected by treatment with triiodothyronine therapy [98, 154]. Based on these data, it can be inferred that the weight loss that often accompanies hyperthyroidism is not mediated by hyperleptinemia, a conclusion that is also consistent with the increased appetite in hyperthyroidism. On the other hand, the finding of hypoleptinemia in hypothyroid patients suggests a mechanism for the decreased energy expenditure and weight gain associated with hypothyroidism, since thyroid hormone [155, 156] and leptin [156–158] are known inducers of thermogenic uncoupling proteins.

Catecholamines

In rodents as well as human subjects, administration of the beta-adrenergic agonist isoproterenol, which activates adenylate cyclase, results in a dose-dependent decrease in plasma leptin [159, 160]. The time course and magnitude of the decrease in plasma leptin levels during infusion of the beta-adrenergic agonist isoproterenol [159] are similar to those observed following prolonged strenuous exercise [42, 85], which suggests that catecholamines might be involved in the mechanisms underlying exercise-induced hypoleptinemia [161]. In support of the latter, beta-adrenal blockade has been shown to attenuate the exercise-induced fall in leptin levels in rodents [43]. Leptin stimulates sympathetic nerve activity [162, 163]. Thus the frequent finding of decreased activity of the autonomic nervous system in obese subjects [164, 165], despite the ambient hyperleptinemia in obesity, suggests a form of leptin resistance at the sympathoadrenal level.

Somatostatin

Intravenous infusion of somatostatin has been reported to either decrease [159] or have no effect [166] on leptin levels in healthy subjects. In the report showing no effect on plasma leptin levels, somatostatin was infused in a dose of 9 μg/kg/h i.v. over 60 min. In the report by Donahoo et al. [159], plasma leptin decreased by 19 % during the initial 120 min of somatostatin infusion (120 ng/kg/min) and stabilized at that level during an additional 120 min of infusion. Interestingly, physiological replacement doses of insulin (0.07 mU/kg/min), and GH (3 ng/kg/min) were co-infused with somatostatin to achieve the "pancreatic clamp" [159]. Thus, much higher doses of somatostatin, infused over several hours, were required to demonstrate an inhibitory effect on circulating leptin. Because somatostatin potently suppresses several hormonal axes, the reported hypoleptinemic effect could be mediated by suppression of endogenous GH, insulin and, possibly, other hormones. Nonetheless, a direct interaction between leptin and somatostatin is also possible: intracerebroventricular administration of leptin upregulated somatostatin receptors in the rat brain [167].

Hormonal Factors in Uremic Hyperleptinemia

Increased plasma leptin levels have been reported in patients with end-stage renal disease (ESRD) receiving regular hemodialysis [168, 169]. This finding may be due to impaired renal leptin clearance [169, 170]; however, hemodialysis is known to activate the expression of cytokines, which could stimulate leptin production [171, 172]. Notably, ESRD patients treated exclusively by peritoneal dialysis show a marked elevation of plasma leptin levels [173], indicating that hyperleptinemia is a feature of renal failure, not an artifact of the hemodialysis process. The increased immunoreactive leptin concentration in ESRD is not the result of the underlying hypercatabolic state of uremia leading to leptin degradation products [168], nor is it an aberration of binding characteristics [169] in uremic plasma. Impaired renal clearance in ESRD is a contributory mechanism; however, the net renal extraction of leptin (calculated from arteriovenous differences) is only 12–20 % of circulating leptin in normal humans and rodents [169, 170]. Many hormonal substances accumulate in renal failure [174, 175], some of which (e.g., insulin, cortisol, sex steroids, and GH) could be stimuli for leptin production [72, 90, 176]. The subject of leptin and the kidney is treated in detail in Chap. 10.

In conclusion, the collective data from numerous studies in experimental animals and humans indicate that leptin is a regulated hormone, which in turn modulates the expression of several hormones. An increased understanding of the hierarchy, significance, and full ramifications of these intricate hormonal interrelationships would expand knowledge of leptin's physiology and identify potential therapeutic applications.

Acknowledgments The author gratefully acknowledges the sacrifice of research volunteers and the research grants from the National Institutes of Health and the American Diabetes Association that enabled his studies on the metabolic significance of leptin in humans.

References

1. Bray GA. The epidemic of obesity and changes in food intake: the Fluoride Hypothesis. Physiol Behav. 2004;82:115–21.
2. Bray GA, Smith SR, DeJonge L, de Souza R, Rood J, Champagne CM, Laranjo N, Carey V, Obarzanek E, Loria CM, Anton SD, Ryan DH, Greenway FL, Williamson D, Sacks FM. Effect of diet composition on energy expenditure during weight loss: the POUNDS LOST Study. Int J Obes (Lond). 2012;36: 448–55.
3. Hubert HB, Feinleib M, McNamara PM, Castelli WP. Obesity as an independent risk factor for cardiovascular disease: a 26-year follow-up of participants in the Framingham Heart Study. Circulation. 1983; 67:968–77.
4. Ogden CL, Carroll MD, Kit BK, Flegal KM. Prevalence of childhood and adult obesity in the United States, 2011-2012. JAMA. 2014;311: 806–14.
5. Guyenet SJ, Schwartz MW. Clinical review: regulation of food intake, energy balance, and body fat mass: implications for the pathogenesis and treatment of obesity. J Clin Endocrinol Metab. 2012;97: 745–55.
6. Zhang Y, Proenca R, Maffei M, Barone M, Leopold L, Friedman JM. Positional cloning of the mouse obese gene and its human homologue. Nature. 1994;372: 425–32.
7. Coleman DL. Effects of parabiosis of obese with diabetes and normal mice. Diabetologia. 1973;9:294–8.

8. Matarese G. Leptin and the immune system: how nutritional status influences the immune response. Eur Cytokine Netw. 2000;11:7–14.
9. Chehab FF, Lim ME, Lu R. Correction of sterility defect in homozygous obese female mice by treatment with the human recombinant leptin. Nat Genet. 1996;12:318–20.
10. Halaas JL, Gajiwala KS, Maffei M, Cohen SL, Chait BT, Rabinowitz D, Lallone RL, Burley SK, Friedman JM. Weight-reducing effects of the plasma protein encoded by the obese gene. Science. 1995;269:543–6.
11. Pelleymounter MA, Cullen MJ, Baker MB, Hecht R, Winters D, Boone T, Collins F. Effects of the obese gene product on body weight regulation in ob/ob mice. Science. 1995;269:540–3.
12. Campfield LA, Smith FJ, Guisez Y, Devos R, Burn P. Recombinant mouse OB protein: evidence for a peripheral signal linking adiposity and central neural networks. Science. 1995;269:546–9.
13. Weigle DS, Bukowski TR, Foster DC, Holderman S, Kramer JM, Lasser G, Loften-Day CE, Prunkard DE, Raymond C, Kujiper JL. Recombinant ob protein reduces feeding and body weight in the ob/ob mouse. J Clin Invest. 1995;96:2065–70.
14. Montague CT, Faroogi IS, Whitehead JP, Soos MA, Rau H, Wareham NJ, Sewter CP, Digby JE, Mohammed SN, Hurst JA, Cheetham CH, Earley AR, Barnett AH, Prins JB, O'Rahilly S. Congenital leptin deficiency is associated with severe early-onset obesity in humans. Nature. 1997;387:903–8.
15. Licinio J, Caglayan S, Ozata M, Yildiz BO, de Miranda PB, O'Kirwan F, Whitby R, Liang L, Cohen P, Bhasin S, Krauss RM, Veldhuis JD, Wagner AJ, DePaoli AM, McCann SM, Wong ML. Phenotypic effects of leptin replacement on morbid obesity, diabetes mellitus, hypogonadism, and behavior in leptin-deficient adults. Proc Natl Acad Sci U S A. 2004;101:4531–6.
16. Lonnqvist F, Aener P, Nordfors L, Schalling M. Overexpression of the obese (ob) gene in adipose tissue of obese subjects. Nat Med. 1995;1: 950–3.
17. Hamilton BS, Paglia D, Kwan AYM, Deitel M. Increased obese mRNA expression in omental fat cells from massively obese humans. Nat Med. 1995;1:953–6.
18. Considine RV, Sinha MK, Heiman ML, Kriaciunas A, Stephens TW, Nyce MR, Ohannesian JP, Marco CC, McKee LJ, Bauer TL, Caro JF. Serum immunoreactive-leptin concentrations in normal-weight and obese humans. N Engl J Med. 1996;334:292–5.
19. Dagogo-Jack S, Fanelli C, Paramore D, Brothers J, Landt M. Plasma leptin and insulin relationships in obese and nonobese humans. Diabetes. 1996;45: 695–8.
20. Schwartz MW, Peskind E, Boyko EJ, Porte Jr D. Cerebrospinal fluid leptin levels: relationship to plasma levels and to adiposity in humans. Nat Med. 1996;2:589–93.
21. Tennekoon KH, Poopalapillai J, Karunanayake AG, Jayasinghe HD, Kumarasiri JM, De S, Wijesundera AP, Karunanayake EH. Association of cord blood leptin, soluble leptin receptor, insulin-like growth factor-I and insulin-like growth factor-binding protein-1 on birth indices in healthy full-term newborns. Horm Res Paediatr. 2014;81(4):232–8.
22. Koistinen HA, Koivisto VA, Anderson S, Karonen S-L, Kontula K, Oksanen L, Teramo KA. Leptin concentration in cord blood correlates with intrauterine growth. J Clin Endocrinol Metab. 1997;82: 3238–330.
23. Harigaya A, Nagashima K, Nako Y, Morikawa A. Relationship between concentration of serum leptin and fetal growth. J Clin Endocrinol Metab. 1997;82:3281–4.
24. Masuzaki H, Ogawa Y, Sagawa N, Hosoda K, Matsumoto T, Mise H, Nishimura H, Yoshimasa Y, Tanaka I, Mori T, Nakao K. Nonadipose tissue production of leptin: leptin as a novel placenta-derived hormone in humans. Nat Med. 1997;3:1029–33.
25. Mise H, Sagawa N, Matsumoto T, Yura S, Nanno H, Itoh H, Mori T, Masuzaki H, Hosoda K, Ogawa Y, Nakao K. Augmented placental production of leptin in preeclampsia: possible involvement of placental hypoxia. J Clin Endocrinol Metab. 1998;83: 3225–9.
26. Lappas M, Yee K, Permezel M, Rice GE. Release and regulation of leptin, resistin and adiponectin from human placenta, fetal membranes, and maternal adipose tissue and skeletal muscle from normal and gestational diabetes mellitus-complicated pregnancies. J Endocrinol. 2005;186:457–65.
27. Kitawaki J, Koshiba H, Ishihara H, Kusuki I, Tsukamoto K, Honjo H. Expression of leptin receptor in human endometrium and fluctuation during the menstrual cycle. J Clin Endocrinol Metab. 2000;85:1946–50.
28. Chiesa C, Osborn JF, Haass C, Natale F, Spinelli M, Scapillati E, Spinelli A, Pacifico L. Ghrelin, leptin, IGF-1, IGFBP-3, and insulin concentrations at birth: is there a relationship with fetal growth and neonatal anthropometry? Clin Chem. 2008;54:550–8.
29. Casabiell X, Pineiro V, Tome MA, Peino R, Dieguez C, Casanueva FF. Presence of leptin in colostrum and/or breast milk from lactating mothers: a potential role in the regulation of neonatal food intake. J Clin Endocrinol Metab. 1997;82:4270–3.
30. Brunner S, Schmid D, Zang K, Much D, Knoeferl B, Kratzsch J, Amann-Gassner U, Bader BL, Hauner H. Breast milk leptin and adiponectin in relation to infant body composition up to 2 years. Pediatr Obes. 2014. doi: 10.1111/j.2047-6310.2014.222.x.
31. Liu J, Askari H, Dagogo-Jack S. Reproducibility of fasting plasma leptin concentrations in lean and obese humans. Endocr Res. 1999;25:1–10.
32. Sinha MK, Opentanova I, Ohannesian JP, Kolaczynski JW, Heiman ML, Hale J, Becker GW, Bowsher RR, Stephens TW, Caro JF. Evidence of free and bound leptin in human circulation. Studies

in lean and obese subjects and during short-term fasting. J Clin Invest. 1996;98:1277–82.
33. Houseknecht KL, Mantzoros CS, Kuliawat R, Hadro E, Flier JS, Kahn BB. Evidence for leptin binding proteins in serum of rodents and humans: modulation with obesity. Diabetes. 1996;45:1638–43.
34. Landt M. Leptin binding and binding capacity in serum. Clin Chem. 2000;46:379–84.
35. Diamond F, Eichler D, Mayes D, Jorgensen V, Duckett G, Hu C, Cuthbertson D, Root A. Leptin binding activity (LBA) in plasma of nondiabetic and diabetic adolescents and obese children: relation to auxologic and hormonal data. J Pediatr Endocrinol Metab. 2000;13:141–8.
36. Wu Z, Bidlingmaier M, Liu C, De Souza EB, Tschöp M, Morrison KM, Strasburger CJB. Quantification of the soluble leptin receptor in human blood by ligand-mediated immunofunctional assay. J Clin Endocrinol Metab. 2002;87:2931–9.
37. Ostlund Jr RE, Yang JW, Klein S, Gingerich R. Relation between plasma leptin concentration and body fat, gender, diet, age, and metabolic covariates. J Clin Endocrinol Metab. 1996;81:3909–13.
38. Mantzoros CS, Flier JS, Rogol AD. A longitudinal assessment of hormonal and physical alterations during normal puberty in boys. V. Rising leptin levels may signal the onset of puberty. J Clin Endocrinol Metab. 1997;82:1066–70.
39. Boden G, Chen X, Mozzoli M, Ryan I. Effect of fasting on serum leptin in human subjects. J Clin Endocrinol Metab. 1996;81:3419–23.
40. Kolaczynski JW, Ohannesian JP, Considine RV, Marco CC, Caro JF. Response of leptin to short-term and prolonged overfeeding in humans. J Clin Endocrinol Metab. 1996;81:4162–5.
41. Romon M, Lebel P, Velly C, Marcceaux N, Fruchart JC, Dallongeville J. Leptin response to carbohydrate or fat meal and association with subsequent satiety and energy intake. Am J Physiol. 1999;277:E855–61.
42. Landt M, Lawson GM, Helgeson JM, Davila-Roman VG, Ladenson JH, Jaffe AS, Hicker RC. Prolonged exercise decreases serum leptin concentrations. Metabolism. 1997;46:1109–12.
43. Bramlett SB, Zhou J, Harris RB, Hendry SL, Witt TL, Zachwieja JJ. Does beta(3)-adrenoreceptor blockade attenuate acute exercise-induced reductions in leptin mRNA? J Appl Physiol. 1999;87:1678–83.
44. Sinha MK, Ohannesian JP, Heiman ML, Kriauciunas A, Stephens TW, Magosin S, Marco C, Caro JF. Nocturnal rise of leptin in lean, obese, and non-insulin-dependent diabetes mellitus subjects. J Clin Invest. 1996;97:1344–7.
45. Schoeller DA, Cella LK, Sinha MK, Caro JF. Entrainment of the diurnal rhythm of plasma leptin to meal timing. J Clin Invest. 1997;100:1882–7.
46. Jockenhovel F, Blum W, Vogel E, Englaro P, Muller-Wieland D, Reinwein D, Rascher W, Krone W. Testosterone substitution normalizes elevated serum leptin levels in hypogonadal men. J Clin Endocrinol Metab. 1997;82:2510–3.
47. Elbers JMH, Asscheman H, Seidell JC, Frolich M, Meinders AE, Gooren LJG. Reversal of the sex difference in serum leptin levels upon cross-sex hormone administration in transsexuals. J Clin Endocrinol Metab. 1997;82:3267–70.
48. Mooradian AD, Morley JE, Korenman SG. Biological actions of androgens. Endocr Rev. 1997;8:1–28.
49. Nader S, Riad-Gabriel M, Saad MF. The effect of a desogestrel-containing oral contraceptive on glucose tolerance and leptin concentrations in hyperandrogenic women. J Clin Endocrinol Metab. 1977;82:3074–7.
50. Castracane VD, Kraemer RR, Franken MA, Kraemer GR, Gimpel T. Serum leptin concentration in women: effect of age, obesity, and estrogen administration. Fertil Steril. 1998;70:472–7.
51. Stattin P, Söderberg S, Hallmans G, Bylund A, Kaaks R, Stenman UH, Bergh A, Olsson T. Leptin is associated with increased prostate cancer risk: a nested case-referent study. J Clin Endocrinol Metab. 2001;86:1341–5.
52. Hsing AW, Chua Jr S, Gao YT, Gentzschein E, Chang L, Deng J, Stanczyk FZ. Prostate cancer risk and serum levels of insulin and leptin: a population-based study. J Natl Cancer Inst. 2001;93:783–9.
53. Singh SK, Grifson JJ, Mavuduru RS, Agarwal MM, Mandal AK, Jha V. Serum leptin: a marker of prostate cancer irrespective of obesity. Cancer Biomark. 2010;7:11–5.
54. Rosenbaum M, Nicolson M, Hirsch J, Heymsfield SB, Gallagher D, Chu F, Leibel RL. Effects of gender, body composition, and menopause on plasma concentrations of leptin. J Clin Endocrinol Metab. 1996;81:3424–7.
55. Hube F, Lietz U, Igel M, Jensen PB, Tornqvist H, Joost HG, Hauner H. Difference in leptin mRNA levels between omental and subcutaneous abdominal adipose tissue from obese humans. Horm Metab Res. 1996;28:690–3.
56. Oliver P, Picó C, Palou A. Ontogenesis of leptin expression in different adipose tissue depots in the rat. Pflugers Arch. 2001;442:383–90.
57. Mueller WM, Gregoire F, Stanhope KL, Mobbs CV, Mizuno TM, Warden CH, Stern JS, Havel PJ. Evidence that glucose metabolism regulates leptin secretion from cultured adipocytes. Endocrinology. 1998;139:551–8.
58. Patel BK, Koenig JI, Kaplan LM, Hooi SC. Increase in plasma leptin and Lep mRNA concentrations by food intake is dependent on insulin. Metabolism. 1998;47:603–7.
59. Rossetti L. Perspective: hexosamines and nutrient sensing. Endocrinology. 2000;141:1922–5.
60. Chen H, Charlat O, Tartaglia LA, Woolf EA, Weng X, Ellis SJ, Lakey ND, Culpepper J, Moore KJ, Breitbart RE, Duyk GM, Tepper RI, Morgenstern JP. Evidence that the diabetes gene encodes the leptin receptor: identification of a mutation in the leptin receptor gene in db/db mice. Cell. 1996;84:491–5.
61. Lahlou N, Clement K, Carel J-C, Vaisse C, Lotton C, Le Bihan Y, Basdevant A, Lebouc Y, Froguel P,

Roger M, Guy-Grand B. Soluble leptin receptor in serum of subjects with complete resistance to leptin. Diabetes. 2000;49:1347–52.
62. Maffei M, Fei H, Lee G-H, Dani C, Leroy P, Zhang Y, Proenca R, Negrel R, Ailhaud G, Friedman JM. Increased expression in adipocytes of ob RNA in mice with lesions of the hypothalamus and with mutations at the *db* locus. Proc Natl Acad Sci U S A. 1995;92:6957–60.
63. Schwartz MW, Baskin DG, Bukowski TR, Kuijper JL, Foster D, Lasser G, Prunkard DE, Porte Jr D, Woods SC, Seeley RJ, Weigle DS. Specificity of leptin action on elevated blood glucose levels and hypothalamic neuropeptide Y gene expression in *ob/ob* mice. Diabetes. 1996;45:531–5.
64. Caro JF, Kolaczynski JW, Nyce MR, Ohannesian JP, Opentanova I, Goldman WH, Lynn RB, Zhang PL, Sinha MK, Considine RV. Decreased cerebrospinal-fluid/serum leptin ratio in obesity: a possible mechanism for leptin resistance. Lancet. 1996;348:159–61.
65. Zlokovic BV, Jovanovic S, Miao W, Samara S, Verma S, Farrell CL. Differential regulation of leptin transport by the choroid plexus and blood-brain barrier and high affinity transport systems for entry into hypothalamus and across the blood-cerebrospinal fluid barrier. Endocrinology. 2000;141:1434–41.
66. Page-Wilson G, Reitman-Ivashkov E, Meece K, White A, Rosenbaum M, Smiley RM, Wardlaw SL. Cerebrospinal fluid levels of leptin, proopiomelanocortin, and agouti-related protein in human pregnancy: evidence for leptin resistance. J Clin Endocrinol Metab. 2013;98:264–71.
67. Rosenbaum M, Nicolson M, Hirsch J, Murphy E, Chu F, Leibel RL. Effects of weight change on plasma leptin concentrations and energy expenditure. J Clin Endocrinol Metab. 1997;82:3647–54.
68. Leibel RL, Rosenbaum M, Hirsch J. Changes in energy expenditure resulting from altered body weight. N Engl J Med. 1995;332:621–8.
69. Ravussin E, Pratley RE, Maffei M, Wang H, Friedman JM, Bennett PH, Bogardus C. Relatively low plasma leptin concentrations precede weight gain in Pima Indians. Nat Med. 1997;3:238–40.
70. Rosenbaum M, Murphy EM, Heymsfield SB, Matthews DE, Leibel RL. Low dose leptin administration reverses effects of sustained weight-reduction on energy expenditure and circulating concentrations of thyroid hormones. J Clin Endocrinol Metab. 2002;87:2391–4.
71. Nagy TR, Gower BA, Shewchuk RM, Goran MI. Serum leptin and energy expenditure in children. J Clin Endocrinol Metab. 1997;82:4149–53.
72. Dagogo-Jack S. Human leptin regulation and promise in pharmacotherapy. Curr Drug Targets. 2001;2:181–95.
73. Grinspoon S, Gulick T, Askari H, Landt M, Lee K, Anderson E, Ma Z, Vignati L, Bowsher R, Herzog D, Klibanski A. Serum leptin levels in women with anorexia nervosa. J Clin Endocrinol Metab. 1996; 81:3861–3.
74. Misra M, Klibanski A. Endocrine consequences of anorexia nervosa. Lancet Diabetes Endocrinol. 2014. doi: 10.1016/S2213-8587(13)70180-3.
75. Herpertz S, Albers N, Wagner R, Pelz B, Köpp W, Mann K, Blum WF, Senf W, Hebebrand J, Eckert ED, Pomeroy C, Raymond N, Kohler PF, Thuras P, Bowers C. Leptin in anorexia nervosa. Longitudinal changes of circadian leptin, insulin and cortisol plasma levels and their correlation during refeeding in patients with anorexia nervosa. Eur J Endocrinol. 2000;142:373–9.
76. Eckert ED, Pomeroy C, Raymond N, Kohler PF, Thuras P, Bowers CY. Leptin in anorexia nervosa. J Clin Endocrinol Metab. 1998;83:791–5.
77. Matkovic V, Ilich JZ, Skugor M, Badenhop NE, Goel P, Clairmont A, Klisovic D, Nahhas RW, Landoll JD. Leptin is inversely related to age at menarche in humans females. J Clin Endocrinol Metab. 1997;82:3239–45.
78. Guadalupe-Grau A, Larsen S, Guerra B, Calbet JA, Dela F, Helge JW. Influence of age on leptin induced skeletal muscle signalling. Acta Physiol (Oxf). 2014;211:214–28.
79. Roszkowska-Gancarz M, Jonas M, Owczarz M, Kurylowicz A, Polosak J, Franek E, Slusarczyk P, Mossakowska M, Puzianowska-Kuznicka M. Age-related changes of leptin and leptin receptor variants in healthy elderly and long-lived adults. Geriatr Gerontol Int. 2014. doi: 10.1111/ggi.12267.
80. Scarpace PJ, Matheny M, Moore RL, Tumer N. Impaired leptin responsiveness in aged rats. Diabetes. 2000;49:431–5.
81. Havel PJ, Townsend R, Chaump L, Teff K. High-fat meals reduce 24-h circulating leptin concentrations in women. Diabetes. 1999;48:334–41.
82. Griffen SC, Oostema K, Stanhope KL, Graham J, Styne DM, Glaser N, Cummings DE, Connors MH, Havel PJ. Administration of Lispro insulin with meals improves glycemic control, increases circulating leptin, and suppresses ghrelin, compared with regular/NPH insulin in female patients with type 1 diabetes. J Clin Endocrinol Metab. 2006;91:485–91.
83. Dagogo-Jack S, Umamaheswaran I, Askari H, Tykodi G. Leptin response to glucocorticoid occurs at physiological doses and is abolished by fasting. Obes Res. 2003;11:232–7.
84. Laferrère B, Fried SK, Hough K, Campbell SA, Thornton J, Pi-Sunyer FX. Synergistic effects of feeding and dexamethasone on serum leptin levels. J Clin Endocrinol Metab. 1998;83:3742–5.
85. Kraemer RR, Chu H, Castracane VD. Leptin and exercise. Exp Biol Med. 2002;227:701–8.
86. Racette SB, Coppack SW, Landt M, Klein S. Leptin production during moderate-intensity aerobic exercise. J Clin Endocrinol Metab. 1997;82:2275–7.
87. Sari R, Balci MK, Balci N, Karayalcin U. Acute effect of exercise on plasma leptin level and insulin resistance in obese women with stable caloric intake. Endocr Res. 2007;32:9–17.
88. Lowndes J, Zoeller RF, Kyriazis GE, Miles MP, Seip RL, Moyna NM, Visich P, Pescatello L, Gordon P,

Thompson PD, Angelopoulos TJ. Hyperleptinemia is associated with CRP, but not apolipoprotein E, and is reduced by exercise training. Int J Sport Nutr Exerc Metab. 2014 Jan 17. [Epub ahead of print].

89. Perusse L, Collier G, Gagnon J, Leon AS, Rao DC, Skinner JS, Wilmore JH, Nadeau A, Zimmet PZ, Bouchard C. Acute and chronic effects of exercise on leptin levels in humans. J Appl Physiol. 1997; 83:5–10.
90. Dagogo-Jack S. Regulation and possible significance of leptin in humans: leptin in health and disease. Diabetes Rev. 1999;7:23–38.
91. Ahima RS, Saper CB, Flier JS, Elmquist JK. Leptin regulation of neuroendocrine systems. Front Neuroendocrinol. 2000;21:263–307.
92. Stephens TW, Basinski M, Bristow PK, Bue-Valleskey JM, Burgett SG, Craft L, Hale J, Hoffmann J, Hsiung HM, Kriauciunas A, MacKellar W, Rosteck Jr PR, Schoner B, Smith D, Tinsley FC, Zhang X-Y, Heiman M. The role of neuropeptide Y in the antiobesity action of the obese gene product. Nature. 1995;377:530–2.
93. Pralong FP, Roduit R, Waeber G, Castillo E, Mosimann F, Thorens B, Gaillard RC. Leptin inhibits directly glucocorticoid secretion by normal human and rat adrenal gland. Endocrinology. 1998; 139:4264–8.
94. Kieffer TJ, Heller RS, Leech CA, Holz GG, Habener JF. Leptin suppression of insulin secretion by activation of ATP-sensitive K+ channels in pancreatic beta-cells. Diabetes. 1997;46:1087–93.
95. Cohen B, Novick D, Rubinstein M. Modulation of insulin activities by leptin. Science. 1996;274: 1185–8.
96. Kamohara S, Burcelin R, Halaas JL, Friedman JM, Charron MJ. Acute stimulation of glucose metabolism in mice by leptin treatment. Nature. 1997;389:374–7.
97. Shetty GK, Matarese G, Magkos F, Moon H-S, Liu X, Brennan AM, Mylvaganam G, Sykoutri D, DePaoli AM, Mantzoros CS. Leptin administration to overweight and obese subjects for six months increases free leptin concentrations but does not alter circulating hormones of the thyroid and IGF axes during weight loss induced by a mild hypocaloric diet. Eur J Endocrinol. 2011;165:249–54.
98. Orban Z, Bornstein SR, Chrousos GP. The interaction between leptin and the hypothalamic-pituitary-thyroid axis. Horm Metab Res. 1998;30:231–5.
99. Saladin R, De Vos P, Guerre-Millo M, Leturque A, Girard J, Staels B, Auwerx J. Transient increase in obese gene expression after food intake or insulin administration. Nature. 1995;377:527–9.
100. Vidal H, Auboeuf D, De Vos P, Staels B, Riou JP, Auwerx J, Laville M. The expression of ob gene is not acutely regulated by insulin and fasting in human abdominal subcutaneous adipose tissue. J Clin Invest. 1996;98:251–5.
101. Clapham JC, Smith SA, Moore GBT, Hughes MG, Azam H, Scott A, Jung RT. Plasma leptin concentrations and OB gene expression in subcutaneous adipose tissue are not regulated acutely by physiological hyperinsulinemia in lean and obese humans. Int J Obes. 1997;21:179–83.
102. Pratley RE, Nicolson M, Bogardus C, Ravussin E. Effects of acute hyperinsulinemia on plasma leptin concentrations in insulin-sensitive and insulin-resistant Pima Indians. J Clin Endocrinol Metab. 1996;81:4418–21.
103. Kolaczynski JW, Nyce MR, Considine RV, Boden G, Nolan JJ, Henry R, Mudaliar SR, Olefsky J, Caro JF. Acute and chronic effects of insulin on leptin production in humans. Diabetes. 1996;45:699–701.
104. Malmstrom R, Taskinen MR, Karonen SL, Yki-Jarvinen H. Insulin increases plasma leptin concentrations in normal subjects and patients with NIDDM. Diabetologia. 1996;39:993–6.
105. Saad MF, Khan A, Sharma A, Michael R, Riad-Gabriel MG, Boyadjian R, Jinagouda SD, Steil GM, Kamdar V. Physiological insulinemia acutely modulates plasma leptin. Diabetes. 1998;47:544–9.
106. D'Adamo M, Buongiorno A, Maroccia E, Leonetti F, Barbetti F, Giaccari A, Zorretta D, Tamburrano G, Sbraccia P. Increased OB expression leads to elevated plasma leptin concentrations in patients with chronic primary hyperinsulinemia. Diabetes. 1998;47:1625–9.
107. Shimabukuro M, Koyama K, Chen G, Wang MY, Trieu F, Lee Y, Newgard CB, Unger RH. Direct antidiabetic effect of leptin through triglyceride depletion of tissues. Proc Natl Acad Sci U S A. 1996;93:14564–8.
108. Wang MY, Chen L, Clark GO, Lee Y, Stevens RD, Ilkayeva OR, Wenner BR, Bain JR, Charron MJ, Newgard CB, Unger RH. Leptin therapy in insulin-deficient type I diabetes. Proc Natl Acad Sci U S A. 2010;107:4813–9.
109. Mueller WM, Stanhope KL, Gregoire F, Evans JL, Havel PJ. Effects of metformin and vanadium on leptin secretion from cultured rat adipocytes. Obes Res. 2000;8:530–9.
110. Wellhoener P, Fruehwald-Schultes B, Kern W, Dantz D, Kerner W, Born J, Fehm HL, Peters A. Glucose metabolism rather than insulin is a main determinant of leptin secretion in humans. J Clin Endocrinol Metab. 2000;85:1267–71.
111. Standridge M, Alemzadeh R, Zemel M, Koontz J, Moustaid-Moussa N. Diazoxide down-regulates leptin and lipid metabolizing enzymes in adipose tissue of Zucker rats. FASEB J. 2000;14:455–60.
112. Moreno-Aliaga MJ, Stanhope KL, Havel PJ. Transcriptional regulation of the leptin promoter by insulin-stimulated glucose metabolism in 3t3-l1 adipocytes. Biochem Biophys Res Commun. 2001; 283:544–8.
113. Moreno-Aliaga MJ, Swarbrick MM, Lorente-Cebrián S, Stanhope KL, Havel PJ, Martínez JA. Sp1-mediated transcription is involved in the induction of leptin by insulin-stimulated glucose metabolism. J Mol Endocrinol. 2007;38:537–46.

114. Iritani N. Nutritional and insulin regulation of leptin gene expression. Curr Opin Clin Nutr Metab Care. 2000;3:275–9.
115. Segal KR, Landt M, Klein S. Relationship between insulin sensitivity and plasma leptin concentration in lean and obese men. Diabetes. 1996;45:988–91.
116. Nyholm B, Fisker S, Lund S, Møller N, Schmitz O. Increased circulating leptin concentrations in insulin-resistant first-degree relatives of patients with non-insulin-dependent diabetes mellitus: relationship to body composition and insulin sensitivity but not to family history of non-insulin-dependent diabetes mellitus. Eur J Endocrinol. 1997;136:173–9.
117. Askari H, Tykodi G, Liu J, Dagogo-Jack S. Fasting plasma leptin level is a surrogate measure of insulin sensitivity. J Clin Endocrinol Metab. 2010;95:3836–43.
118. Remesar X, Rafecas I, Fernández-López JA, Alemany M. Is leptin an insulin counter-regulatory hormone? FEBS Lett. 1997;402:9–11.
119. Miell JP, Englaro P, Blum WF. Dexamethasone induces an acute and sustained rise in circulating leptin levels in normal human subjects. Horm Metab Res. 1996;28:704–70.
120. Larsson H, Ahren B. Short-term dexamethasone increases plasma leptin independently of changes in insulin sensitivity in healthy women. J Clin Endocrinol Metab. 1996;81:4428–32.
121. Berneis K, Vosmeer S, Keller U. Effects of glucocorticoids and of growth hormone on serum leptin concentration in man. Eur J Endocrinol. 1996;135:663–5.
122. Dagogo-Jack S, Selke G, Melson AK, Newcomer JW. Robust leptin secretory responses to dexamethasone in obese subjects. J Clin Endocrinol Metab. 1997;82:3230–3.
123. Papaspyrou-Rao S, Schneider SH, Petersen RN, Fried SK. Dexamathasone increases leptin expression in humans in vivo. J Clin Endocrinol Metab. 1997;82:1635–7.
124. Kolaczynski JW, Goldstein BJ, Considine RV. Dexamethasone, OB gene, and leptin in humans; effect of exogenous hyperinsulinemia. J Clin Endocrinol Metab. 1997;82:3895–7.
125. Gong D-W, Bi S, Pratley RE, Weintraub BD. Genomic structure and promoter analysis of the human obese gene. J Biol Chem. 1996;271:3971–4.
126. De Vos P, Saladin R, Auwerx J, Staels B. Induction of ob gene expression by corticosteroids is accompanied by body weight loss and reduced food intake. J Biol Chem. 1995;270:15958–61.
127. Considine RV, Nyce MR, Kolaczynski JW, Zhang PL, Ohannesian JP, Moore Jr JH, Fox JW, Caro JF. Dexamethasone stimulates leptin release from human adipocytes: unexpected inhibition by insulin. J Cell Biochem. 1997;65:254–8.
128. Masuzaki H, Ogawa Y, Hosoda K, Miyawaki T, Hanaoka I, Hiraoka J, Yasuno A, Nishimura H, Yoshimasa Y, Nishi S, Nakao K. Glucocorticoid regulation of leptin synthesis and secretion in humans: elevated plasma leptin levels in Cushing's syndrome. J Clin Endocrinol Metab. 1997;82:2542–7.
129. Widjaja A, Schurmeyer TH, Von Zur Muhlenh A, Brabant G. Determinants of serum leptin levels in Cushing's syndrome. J Clin Endocrinol Metab. 1998;83:600–3.
130. Cizza G, Lotsikas AJ, Licinio J, Gold PW, Chrousos GP. Plasma leptin levels do not change in patients with Cushing's disease after correction of hypercortisolism. J Clin Endocrinol Metab. 1997;82:2747–50.
131. Bornstein SR, Licinio J, Tauchnitz R, Negrão AB, Gold P, Chrousos GP. Plasma leptin levels are increased in survivors of acute sepsis: associated loss of diurnal rhythm in cortisol and leptin secretion. J Clin Endocrinol Metab. 1997;83:280–3.
132. Tataranni PA, Pratley R, Maffei M, Ravussin E. Acute and prolonged administration of glucocorticoids (methylprednisolone) does not affect plasma leptin concentration in humans. Int J Obes Relat Metab Disord. 1997;21:327–30.
133. Newcomer JW, Selke G, Melson AK, Gross J, Volger GP, Dagogo-Jack S. Dose-dependent cortisol-induced increases in plasma leptin concentration in healthy humans. Arch Gen Psychiatry. 1998;55:995–1000.
134. Wolthers T, Grofte T, Norrelund H, Poulsen PL, Andreasen F, Christiansen JS, Jorgensen JO. Differential effects of growth hormone and prednisolone on energy metabolism and leptin levels in humans. Metabolism. 1998;47:83–8.
135. Askari H, Liu J, Dagogo-Jack S. Hormonal regulation of human leptin in vivo: effects of hydrocortisone and insulin. Inter J Obes. 2000;24:1254–9.
136. Spencer RL, Young EA, Choo PH, McEwens BS. Adrenal steroid type I and type II receptor binding: estimates of in vivo receptor number, occupancy, and activation with varying levels of steroid. Brain Res. 1990;514:37–48.
137. Torpy DJ, Bornstein SR, Cizza G, Chrousos GP. The effects of glucocorticoids on leptin levels in humans may be restricted to acute pharmacologic dosing. J Clin Endocrinol Metab. 1998;83:1821–2.
138. Cope CL, Black E. The production rate of cortisol in man. Br Med J. 1958;1:1020–4.
139. Dagogo-Jack S, Tykodi G, Umamaheswaran I. Inhibition of cortisol biosynthesis decreases circulating leptin levels in obese humans. J Clin Endocrinol Metab. 2005;90:5333–5.
140. Laferrère B, Abraham C, Awad M, Jean-Baptiste S, Hart AB, Garcia-Lorda P, Kokkoris P, Russell CD. Inhibiting endogenous cortisol blunts the meal-entrained rise in serum leptin. J Clin Endocrinol Metab. 2006;91:2232–8.
141. Askari H, Liu J, Dagogo-Jack S. Energy adaptation to glucocorticoid-induced hyperleptinemia in human beings. Metabolism. 2005;54:876–80.
142. Bianda TL, Glatz Y, Boeni-Schnetzler M, Froesch ER, Schmid C. Effects of growth hormone (GH) and

insulin-like growth factor-I on serum leptin in GH-deficient adults. Diabetologia. 1997;40:363–4.
143. Kristom B, Carlsson B, Rosberg S, Carlsson LM, Albertsson-Wikland K. Short-term changes in serum leptin levels provide a strong metabolic marker for the growth response to growth hormone treatment in children. J Clin Endocrinol Metab. 1998;83: 2735–41.
144. Dagogo-Jack S, Franklin SC, Vijayan A, Liu J, Askari H, Miller SB. Recombinant human insulin-like growth factor-I (IGF-I) therapy decreases plasma leptin concentration in patients with chronic renal insufficiency. Int J Obes. 1998;22:1110–5.
145. Fouque D, Juillard L, Lasna Y, Tabakian A, Laville M, Joly M-O, Laville M. Acute leptin regulation in end-stage renal failure: the role of growth hormone and IGF-1. Kidney Int. 1998;54:932–47.
146. Cara JF, Rosenfield RL, Furlanetto RW. A longitudinal study of the relationship of plasma somatomedic-C concentration to the pubertal growth spurt. Am J Dis Child. 1987;141:562–4.
147. Reul BA, Ongemba LM, Pottier A-M, Henquin J-C, Brichard SM. Insulin and insulin-like growth factor 1 antagonize the stimulation of ob gene expression by dexamethasone in cultured rat adipose tissue. Biochem J. 1997;324:605–10.
148. Florkowski CM, Collier GR, Zimmet PZ, Livesey JH, Espiner EA, Donald RA. Low-dose growth hormone replacement lowers plasma leptin and fat stores without affecting body mass index in adults with growth hormone deficiency. Clin Endocrinol (Oxf). 1996;45:769–73.
149. Paolisso G, Ammendola S, Del Buono A, Gambardella A, Riondino M, Tagliamonte MR, Rizzo MR, Carella C, Varricchio M. Serum levels of insulin-likc growth factor-I (IGF-I) and IGF binding protein-3 in healthy centenarians: relationship with plasma leptin and lipid concentrations, insulin action, and cognitive function. J Clin Endocrinol Metab. 1997;82:2204–9.
150. Frystyk J, Vestbo E, Skjaerbaek C, Mogensen CE, Orskov H. Free insulin-like growth factors in human obesity. Metabolism. 1995; 44 Suppl 4:37–44.
151. King GL, Rechler MM, Kahn CR. Interactions between receptors for insulin and the insulin-like growth factors on adipocytes. J Biol Chem. 1982; 257:10001–6.
152. Valcavi R, Zini M, Peino R, Casanueva FF, Dieguez C. Influence of thyroid status on serum immunoreactive leptin levels. J Clin Endocrinol Metab. 1997; 82:1632–4.
153. Sreenan S, Caro JF, Refetoff S. Thyroid dysfunction is not associated with alterations in serum leptin levels. Thyroid. 1997;7:407–9.
154. Mantzoros CS, Rosen HN, Greenspan SL, Flier JS, Moses AC. Short-term hyperthyroidism has no effect on leptin levels in man. J Clin Endocrinol Metab. 1997;82:497–9.
155. Bianco AC, Silva JE. Intracellular conversion of thyroxine to triiodothyronine is required for the optimal thermogenic function of brown adipose tissue. J Clin Invest. 1987;79:295–300.
156. Gong DW, He Y, Karas M, Reitman M. Uncoupling protein-3 is a mediator of thermogenesis regulated by thyroid hormone, beta3-adrenergic agonists, and leptin. J Biol Chem. 1997;272:24129–32.
157. Zhou T-T, Shimabukuro M, Koyama K, Lee Y, Wang M-Y, Trieu F, Newgard CB, Unger RH. Induction by leptin of uncoupling protein-2 and enzymes of fatty acid oxidation. Proc Natl Acad Sci U S A. 1997;94:6368–90.
158. Mantzoros CS, Frederich RC, Qu D, Lowell BB, Maratos-Flier E, Flier JS. Severe leptin resistance in brown fat-deficient uncoupling protein promoter-driven diphtheria toxin A mice despite suppression of hypothalamic neuropeptide Y and circulating corticosterone concentrations. Diabetes. 1998;47:230–8.
159. Donahoo WT, Jensen DR, Yost TJ, Eckel RH. Isoproterenol and somatostatin decrease plasma leptin in humans: a novel mechanism regulating leptin secretion. J Clin Endocrinol Metab. 1997; 82:4139–43.
160. Mantzoros CS, Qu D, Frederich RC, Susulic VS, Lowell BB, Maratos-Flier E, Flier JS. Activation of beta (3) adrenergic receptors suppresses leptin expression and mediates a leptin-independent inhibition of food intake in mice. Diabetes. 1996; 45:909–14.
161. Christensen NJ, Galbo H. Sympathetic nervous system activity during exercise. Annu Rev Physiol. 1983;45:139–53.
162. Collins S, Kuhn CM, Petro AE, Swick AG, Chruynk BA, Surwit RS. Role of leptin in fat regulation. Nature. 1996;380:677.
163. Haynes WG, Morgan DA, Walsh SA, Mark AL, Sivitz WI. Receptor-mediated regional sympathetic nerve activation by leptin. J Clin Invest. 1997; 100:270–8.
164. Peterson HR, Rothscild M, Weinberg CR, Fell RD, McLeish KR, Pfeiffer MA. Body fat and activity of the autonomic nervous system. N Engl J Med. 1988;318:1077–83.
165. Tataranni PA, Young JB, Bogardus C, Ravussin E. A low sympathoadrenal activity is associated with body weight and development of central adiposity in Pima Indian men. Obes Res. 1997;5:341–7.
166. Rigamonti AE, Sartorio A, Bonomo SM, Giunta M, Grassi G, Perotti M, Cella SG, Müller EE, Pincelli AI. Effect of a somatostatin infusion on circulating levels of adipokines in obese women. Metabolism. 2012;61:1797–802.
167. Perianes-Cachero A, Burgos-Ramos E, Puebla-Jiménez L, Canelles S, Frago LM, Hervás-Aguilar A, de Frutos S, Toledo-Lobo MV, Mela V, Viveros MP, Argente J, Chowen JA, Arilla-Ferreiro E, Barrios V. Acute up-regulation of the rat brain somatostatin receptor-effector system by leptin is related to activation of insulin signaling and may counteract central leptin actions. Neuroscience. 2013;252: 289–301.

168. Merabet E, Dagogo-Jack S, Coyne DW, Klein S, Santiago JV, Hmiel SP, Landt M. Increased plasma leptin concentration in end-stage renal disease. J Clin Endocrinol Metab. 1997;82:847–50.
169. Sharma K, Considine RV, Michael B, Dunn SR, Weisberg LS, Kurnik BRC, Kurnik PB, O'Connor J, Sinha M, Caro JF. Plasma leptin is partly cleared by the kidney and is elevated in hemodialysis patients. Kidney Int. 1997;51:1980–5.
170. Zeng J, Patterson BW, Klein S, Martin DR, Dagogo-Jack S, Kohrt WM, Miller SB, Landt M. Whole body leptin kinetics and renal metabolism in vivo. Am J Physiol. 1997;273:E1102–6.
171. Macdonald C, Rush DN, Bernstein KN, McKenna RM. Production of tumor necrosis factor alpha and hemodialysis. Nephron. 1993;65:273–7.
172. Zumbach MS, Boehme MWJ, Wahl P, Stremmel W, Ziegler R, Nawroth PP. Tumor necrosis factor increases serum leptin levels in humans. J Clin Endocrinol Metab. 1997;82:4080–2.
173. Dagogo-Jack S, Ovalle F, Geary B, Landt M, Coyne DW. Hyperleptinemia in patients with end-stage renal disease treated by continuous ambulatory peritoneal dialysis. Perit Dial Int. 1998;18:34–40.
174. Katz AI, Emmanouel SD. Metabolism of polypeptide hormones by the normal kidney and in uraemia. Nephron. 1978;22:69–80.
175. Mooradian AD, Morley JE. Endocrine dysfunction in chronic renal failure. Arch Intern Med. 1984;144:351–3.
176. Dagogo-Jack S. Uremic hyperleptinemia: adaptive or maladaptive. Kidney Int. 1998;54:997–8.

Leptin, Obesity, and Leptin Resistance

6

Heike Münzberg and Steven B. Heymsfield

Abbreviations

ob/ob mice	Leptin-deficient mice
db/db mice	Leptin receptor-deficient mice
BBB	Blood–brain barrier
LepRb	Long form leptin receptor
CSF	Cerebrospinal fluid
JAK2	Janus-kinase-2
Y985/1077/1138	Tyrosine residues 985/1077/1138
SHP-2	Src homology-2 domain protein
MAPK	Mitogen-activated-protein-kinase
STAT3/5	Signal-transducer-and-activator-of transcription-3/5
pSTAT3	Phosphor-STAT3
SOCS-3	Suppressor-of-cytokine-signaling-3
PTP1B	Phosphotyrosine phosphatase-1B
HFD	High-fat diet
DIO	Diet-induced obesity
ARC	Arcuate nucleus
α-MSH	α-Melanocyte-stimulating hormone
AgRP	Agouti-related protein
LPS	Lipopolysaccharides
CVO	Circumventricular organ
ME	Median eminence
VMH	Ventromedial hypothalamus
ER	Endoplasmatic reticulum

H. Münzberg, Ph.D. (✉) • S.B. Heymsfield, M.D.
Pennington Biomedical Research Center,
LSU system, 6400 Perkins Road, Baton Rouge,
LA 70808, USA
e-mail: Heike.Munzberg@pbrc.edu

Introduction

Long before leptin was cloned in 1994 [1], its presence had been demonstrated in leptin-deficient *ob/ob* and leptin receptor-deficient *db/db* mice. It was understood that *ob/ob* mice were missing a circulating factor that was plentiful in *db/db* mice, and this circulating factor could cure obesity in *ob/ob* mice, while *db/db* mice were unresponsive to it [2]. Thus, initially it was hoped that the discovery of the hormone leptin by cloning would resolve the ongoing increase in the prevalence of human obesity.

Indeed, the powerful effects of leptin were demonstrated in rare cases of leptin-deficient human patients, where daily leptin injections completely corrected obesity and all other associated neuroendocrine abnormalities in the long term [3, 4]. Unfortunately, for the majority of overweight and obese humans, as well as rodents, the increased adipose tissue mass results in

S. Dagogo-Jack (ed.), *Leptin: Regulation and Clinical Applications*,
DOI 10.1007/978-3-319-09915-6_6, © Springer International Publishing Switzerland 2015

elevated circulating leptin levels that are proportional to adipose tissue mass [5, 6] but are unable to reduce body weight and food intake [7]. This condition has been termed leptin resistance, and is still considered a main obstacle for the successful treatment of obesity.

Thus, like other hormone resistance syndromes (e.g., insulin resistance), leptin resistance seems to be triggered by excess availability of leptin itself, resulting in a reduction of its effectiveness. Even though leptin resistance is generally considered a term for a disease, it is not entirely clear weather leptin resistance is indeed a malfunction of the body or rather a naturally occurring, physiologic state that turns into a pathological condition in its chronic appearance in obese individuals. This review outlines our current knowledge of leptin resistance, different triggers, forms and levels of leptin resistance, and the difficulty in evaluating the importance of leptin resistance in the potential treatment of obesity.

Central Leptin Access: Peripheral Leptin Resistance

The main effect of leptin on food intake and body weight is mediated via central leptin action [8, 9]. Thus, leptin has to enter the brain to execute its proper functions. As a 16 kDa peptide, leptin is too large to cross the blood–brain barrier. In order to reach deep brain areas, leptin is transported across the blood–brain barrier (BBB) by a regulated, saturable transport system [10]. Even though the molecular identity of this leptin transporter system is still unclear, it acts independent of the long form leptin receptor (LepRb) [11]. Thus, the first level of leptin resistance takes place at the availability of leptin at its target sites in the brain and has been termed *peripheral leptin resistance* [12].

Indeed, in obese rats the rate of leptin transport is decreased compared to lean animals, demonstrating that obesity decreases the effectiveness of BBB leptin transport [13]. This is also supported by studies showing that direct central leptin injections recover leptin resistance and improve anorexic leptin effects and body weight loss at least partially [14]. On the other hand, basal central leptin concentration in the cerebrospinal fluid (CSF) is significantly elevated in obese vs. lean individuals [5, 13], and it is not entirely clear why elevated CSF leptin levels do not overcome leptin resistance and if this could also contribute to overall leptin resistance. In any case, central leptin application cannot entirely correct leptin resistance in rodents and it is most likely that leptin transport defects may account in part for the observed leptin resistance in obese subjects, but that other cellular mechanisms are likely to contribute [15].

Leptin Receptor Signaling: Cellular Leptin Resistance

Once leptin reaches the brain it binds to LepRb, the isoform that is responsible for the main effects of leptin on energy homeostasis and other neuroendocrine functions [16, 17]. LepRb is a typical class I cytokine receptor without intrinsic kinase activity; instead leptin binding to LepRb allows the recruitment and activation of janus-kinase-2 (JAK2) to LepRb, which propagates phosphorylation of JAK2 itself and three tyrosine residues on LepRb (Y985, Y1077 and Y1138) [18, 19]. Each of these phosphorylation sites induces a specific signaling pathway with distinct physiological leptin functions (Fig. 6.1). For example, Y985 activates src-homology-2 domain protein (SHP-2) and mitogen-activated-protein-kinase (MAPK) signaling, Y1077 activates signal-transducer-and-activator-of-transcription-5 (STAT5) signaling, and Y1138 activates STAT3 signaling [20, 21]. All of these signaling pathways are able to control gene transcription, even though the majority of leptin regulated gene transcripts still remain unknown.

The phosphorylation and activation of the transcription factor STAT3 (pSTAT3) by leptin has been particularly well described in vitro and in vivo, because pSTAT3 is low in the baseline state, but is robustly and reliably activated by leptin. Furthermore, pSTAT3 can be easily *visualized* in vitro and in vivo within single neurons [22–25] (Figs. 6.2 and 6.3). Also, STAT3 signaling is responsible for the majority of physiological

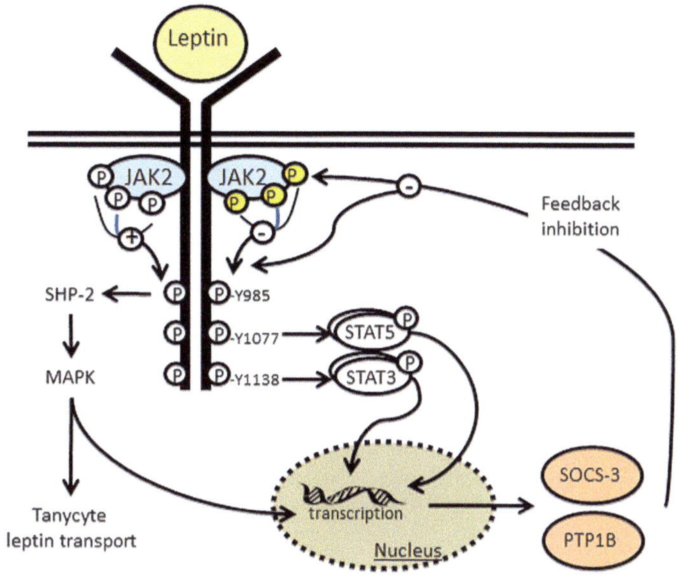

Fig. 6.1 Leptin signaling pathways and cellular leptin resistance. Leptin-induced pSTAT3 is an excellent marker for evaluating leptin sensitivity and resistance. Gene expression of suppressor-of-cytokine-signaling-3 (SOCS3) and phosphotyrosine phosphatase-1B (PTP1B) are regulated by leptin via STAT3 signaling as a negative feedback signal that can mediate leptin resistance

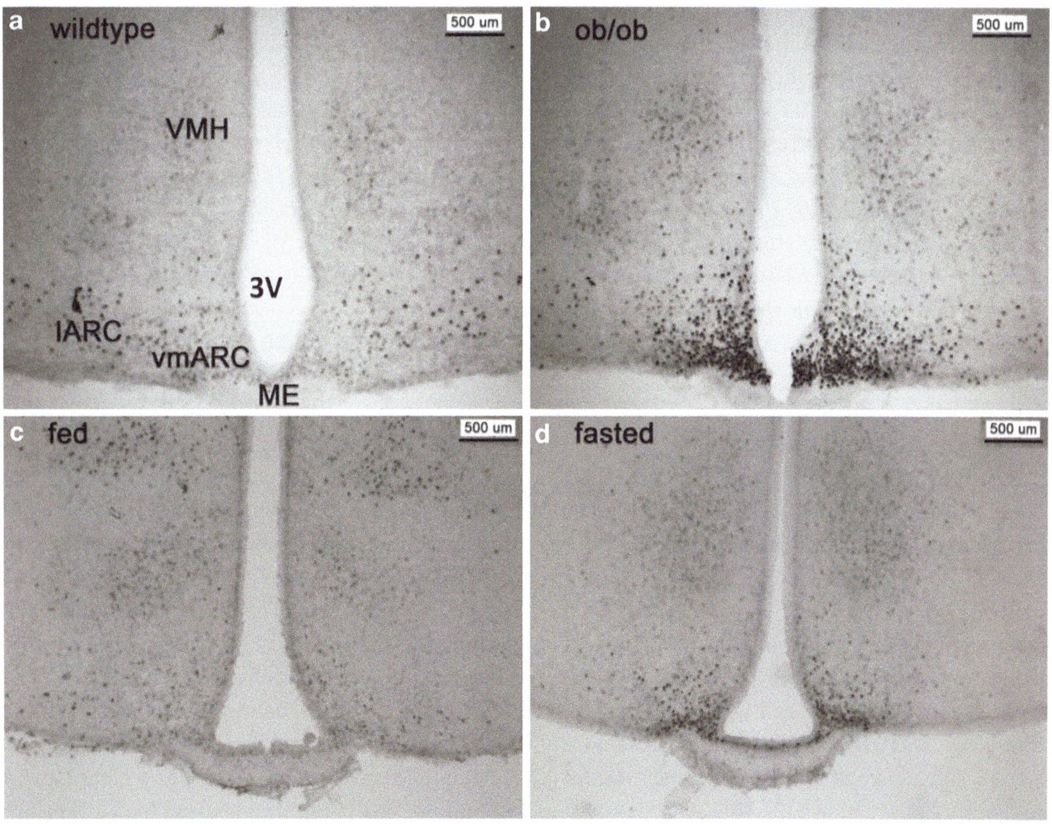

Fig. 6.2 Leptin-induced pSTAT3 correlates with leptin sensitivity. Representative images showing immunohistochemistry for leptin-induced pSTAT3 1 h after peripheral leptin injections (5 mg/kg) of a wild type littermate (**a**) and an *ob*/*ob* mouse (**b**); a fed mouse (**c**); and an overnight fasted mouse (**d**). Decrease in circulating leptin as seen in leptin-deficient *ob*/*ob* mice or fasted mice greatly enhances leptin-induced pSTAT3 signals

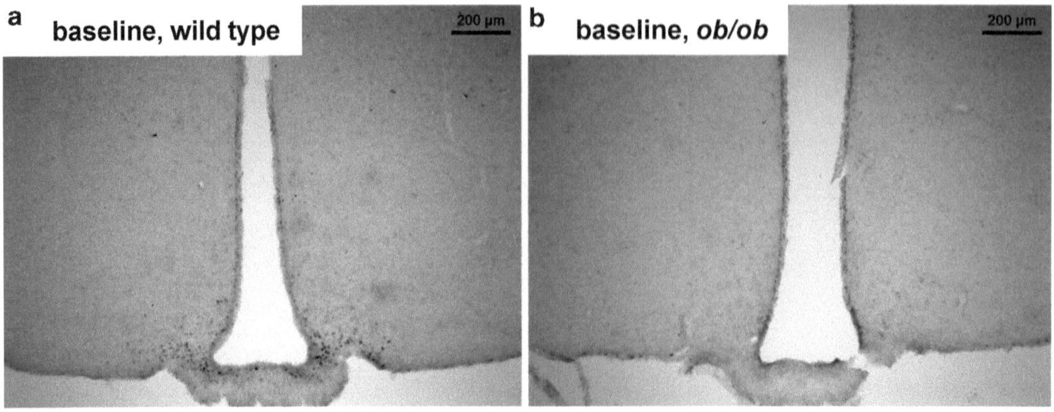

Fig. 6.3 Baseline pSTAT3 correlates with circulating leptin levels. Representative images showing immunohistochemistry for baseline pSTAT3 in an untreated wild type littermate (**a**) and an *ob/ob* mouse (**b**). Note that ob/ob mice lack the baseline pSTAT3 signal in the hypothalamic arcuate nucleus

leptin actions, even though LepRb-associated STAT3 signaling does not regulate leptin's effects on reproduction [15, 26]. Leptin-induced pSTAT3 has also been used to indicate relative changes in leptin sensitivity and the physiological state of leptin resistance (defined as the absence of proper body weight/food intake reduction with leptin) could be recapitulated by decreased STAT3 activation with leptin [14, 27].

Leptin-induced pSTAT3 reflects leptin signal intensity via LepRb, but the underlying mechanisms are based on at least two adaptor molecules: suppressor-of-cytokine-signaling-3 (SOCS-3) and phosphotyrosine phosphatase-1B (PTP1B). SOCS-3 gene expression is increased by leptin-induced pSTAT3 [28, 29] and SOCS-3 peptide binds to Y1077 and JAK2 to block leptin signaling in a classic feedback inhibition pathway [30]. Overexpression of SOCS-3 decreases leptin signaling [28]; conversely, heterozygote SOCS-3 deletions (homozygous animals are embryonic lethal) enhances leptin sensitivity and decreases high-fat-diet (HFD)-induced weight gain [31, 32]. Similarly, PTP1B mRNA is upregulated by STAT3 signaling and PTP1B deficiency results in enhanced leptin action [33, 34], even though the exact interaction of PTP1B with LepRb is not exactly known. Most importantly, leptin resistant mice have increased hypothalamic PTP1B and/or SOCS-3 mRNA expression and contribute to leptin resistance [21, 33, 35, 36]. Furthermore, JAK2 itself is highly regulated and phosphorylated which modulates JAK2 activity and LepRb signal transduction [37–39]. Such a dysregulation at the level of LepRb signal transduction has been termed *cellular leptin resistance* and is distinguished from *peripheral leptin resistance* that is due to leptin transport defects to its central target sites [40, 41].

Physiological Trigger of Leptin Resistance

Cellular and peripheral leptin resistance is well established, and commonly associated with increased adiposity and increased circulating leptin levels. Leptin-deficient *ob/ob* mice are an exception, where severe obesity is not translated into hyperleptinemia. Therefore, leptin deficiency in man and mouse robustly *increases* leptin sensitivity as indicated by enhanced weight loss, food intake, and LepRb signaling in response to exogenous leptin administrations [3, 42–44] (Fig. 6.2).

Leptin resistance is regarded as a pathological condition, based on the idea that human obesity could be successfully cured with leptin if only leptin resistance could be prevented or corrected. The simplicity of this thought is intriguing, but there may be flaws to this hypothesis. *First*, leptin shows little or no effect even in lean, supposedly leptin sensitive, humans [45], thus increasing leptin sensitivity in obese humans may after all not be sufficient to significantly improve leptin mediated weight loss. *Second*, even in lean ad libitum fed mice the anorexic leptin effects are mild. To obtain significant leptin effects injections of large, pharmacological leptin doses are required and animals are often fasted to enhance leptin sensitivity (Fig. 6.2c, d demonstrates fasting enhanced LepRb signaling). Thus, it may not be possible to find a safe leptin dose that could effectively treat obesity even in leptin-sensitized individuals. *Third*, leptin resistance is triggered by many physiological conditions and can be reversed once the physiological change is normalized. Thus, it is not entirely clear if leptin resistance is indeed a pathological or rather a physiological condition. Below we outline some known physiological triggers of leptin resistance.

HFD-Induced Leptin Resistance

In lean and leptin sensitive animals a switch from normal chow diet to a HFD rapidly and progressively induces leptin resistance as early as 1 week after starting HFD feeding [14, 27]. HFD-induced leptin resistance is physiologically measured by a blunted effect of leptin to decrease body weight and food intake, and at the cellular level by a decrease in leptin-induced pSTAT3 activation or increased baseline SOCS-3 or PTP1B expression in the hypothalamus [27, 46]. Also, further downstream events like leptin-stimulated or inhibited release of neuropeptides from the arcuate nucleus (ARC), e.g., alpha-melanocyte-stimulating hormone (alpha-MSH), agouti-related protein (AgRP), and diminished growth of axonal projection, are affected by HFD-induced leptin resistance [46–48]. Diet-induced obesity (DIO) and leptin resistance are fully reversible once food intake is resumed on a chow diet [46, 49] even though genetic predispositions that play a crucial role in the susceptibility for HFD-induced weight gain can result in long term body weight changes [50, 51]. Adiposity, leptin resistance, and hyperleptinemia progress together early on, so that it is unclear if leptin resistance causes obesity or vice versa. Even though it should be noted, if leptin resistance is secondary to obesity, it may still further enhance weight gain.

The concept of cellular leptin resistance is not coherent, because by definition negative feedback mechanisms like SOCS-3 or PTP1B should be counter regulated by changes in pSTAT3 induction. Therefore, high SOCS-3 and PTP1B levels cannot conclusively explain decreased STAT3 activation. The reason for this paradox may lay in the unequal comparison of leptin-induced pSTAT3 versus baseline (unstimulated) SOCS-3 or PTP1B levels. STAT3 is induced by leptin as well as many other factors (e.g., several cytokines), so that leptin-related STAT3 signaling is typically studied after exogenous leptin application, instead of comparing baseline STAT3 levels. Baseline pSTAT3 is observed in the hypothalamic arcuate nucleus and is indeed increased in HFD, hyperleptinemic mice [52–54], which conclusively explains increased baseline SOCS-3 levels in HFD animals [27, 46].

Thus, HFD-induced hyperleptinemia can sufficiently explain increased baseline pSTAT3 and SOCS-3, and is consistent with decreased maximal leptin signaling after exogenous leptin application. Indeed, baseline pSTAT3 signal intensities generally correlate well with circulating leptin levels and baseline pSTAT3 is found in LepRb expressing neurons [43, 55]. For example, leptin-deficient *ob/ob* mice entirely lack baseline pSTAT3 compared to a low, but consistent baseline pSTAT3 level in the ARC of normal wild type mice (Fig. 6.3). Contrary, responsiveness to exogenous leptin is enhanced in mouse models with no or low leptin (*ob/ob* mice or fasted mice) (Fig. 6.2). Thus, baseline pSTAT3 levels are likely proportional to basal circulating leptin and cellular SOCS-3 levels. In contrast, leptin-induced pSTAT3 reflects maximal leptin signaling capacity and depends on baseline SOCS3 or PTP1B levels. Thus, low circulating leptin and cellular SOCS-3 levels (*ob/ob* mice, fasted mice) increase maximal leptin signaling, while high circulating leptin and cellular SOCS-3 levels (HFD-induced obesity) decrease maximal leptin signaling.

Leptin-Induced Leptin Resistance

The question if leptin itself is able to cause leptin resistance is not trivial. In order to treat human obesity safely and efficiently, it would be ill advised if such treatment would further enhance leptin resistance. In order to separate obesity from hyperleptinemia, several studies have explored rodent models of experimentally induced hyperleptinemia, where leptin is infused or virally expressed either in the periphery or centrally [56–60]. All of these studies confirmed that leptin infusion or overexpression initially result in the expected decrease of food intake and body weight, but over time animals became resistant to leptin. This was evident at the physiological level (food intake and body weight) as well as at the cellular level (decreased pSTAT3 induction, dysregulation of hypothalamic neuropeptides). Most importantly, when put on a HFD leptin overexpressing animals gained more weight than vehicle treated (non-leptin resistant) animals on a HFD [41], thus illustrating that hyperleptinemia is sufficient to induce leptin resistance and supporting the idea that leptin resistance indeed enhanced weight gain.

To further test if hyperleptinemia is also required to develop leptin resistance, leptin-deficient *ob/ob* mice were continuously infused with leptin to mimic normal circulating leptin levels and to prevent hyperleptinemia when exposed to HFD feeding. This procedure normalized body weight and food intake in chow fed *ob/ob* mice, but importantly when fed a HFD these mice remained responsive to acute leptin injections as measured by weight loss, anorexia as well as pSTAT3 induction [61]. These data demonstrated that hyperleptinemia is not only sufficient, but also necessary to induce leptin resistance. Surprisingly, HFD feeding in the presence or absence of hyperleptinemia (and therefore leptin resistance) gained similar weight and were hyperphagic. Thus, contrary to other results, indicating that HFD independent of leptin resistance increases body weight. Furthermore, it should be noted that another study showed leptin resistance can develop in the absence of leptin as measured by anorexic leptin actions [35]. Thus, overall there is compelling evidence that hyperleptinemia is an important component in the induction of leptin resistance, but the importance of leptin resistance cannot be conclusively resolved.

Inflammation-Induced Leptin Resistance

Leptin receptors are classic class I cytokine receptors that are similar to IL-6 receptors and both signal via the JAK/STAT signaling pathway. Thus, it is not surprising that inflammation (e.g., induced by lipopolysaccharides (LPS)) also induces hypothalamic pSTAT3 and anorexia [62]. Furthermore, HFD-induced obesity causes low-grade inflammation in peripheral tissues and the brain, with increased circulating and hypothalamic cytokine levels [63]. Interestingly, HFD fed obese animals were also resistant to LPS-induced anorexia and LPS-induced pSTAT3 was blunted, even though LPS-induced fever responses remained intact [54]. Similar to leptin-induced leptin resistance, repeated LPS-injections also cause cellular LPS-resistance and a blunted anorexic LPS response [53]. HFD feeding increases circulating LPS levels, and LPS induces leptin secretion; so that HFD-induced hyperleptinemia may be triggered or enhanced by the inflammatory response to HFD. In any case, LPS and leptin could both contribute to the increased pSTAT3 and SOCS-3 levels at least in the hypothalamic arcuate nucleus to explain the blunted pSTAT3 response to acute leptin or LPS in HFD fed mice [27, 46, 54].

Site-Specific Leptin Resistance

Leptin signaling in the hypothalamus is not uniform and specifically the arcuate nucleus shows particularly strong LepRb expression and leptin signaling such as STAT3 activation and SOCS-3 expression [27, 29]. Cellular leptin resistance is most robustly detected in the ARC, while other hypothalamic and extra-hypothalamic sites remain relatively leptin sensitive [27, 46]. This site-specific leptin resistance is also reflected at the physiological level: leptin resistance almost entirely blocks leptin-induced anorexia, while sympathetic leptin actions (e.g., thermoregulation

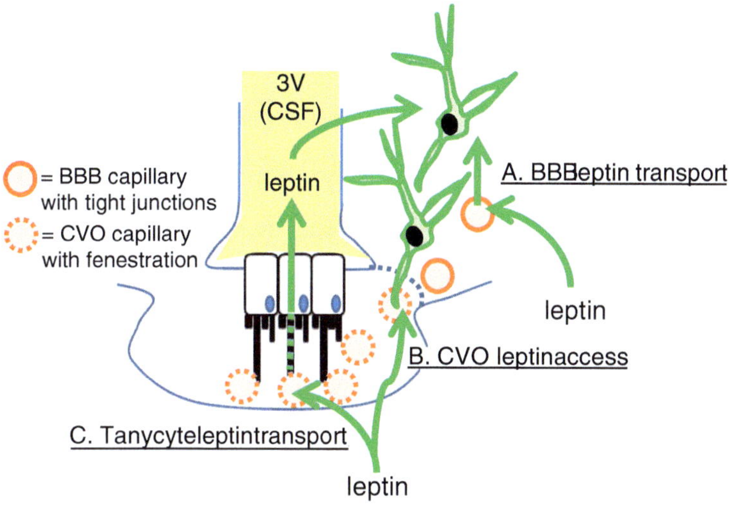

Fig. 6.4 Mechanisms of central leptin access. (A) Leptin is transported across the blood–brain barrier (BBB) via a saturable transporter mechanism, independent of LepRb. (B) LepRb neurons in close proximity to fenestrated capillaries in circumventricular organs (CVO's, e.g., median eminence, area postrema, organum vasculosum) may access leptin directly via projections to fenestrated capillaries. (C) Leptin can be transported via tanycytes that line the border between CVO and BBB to, to enter the cerebrospinal fluid (CSF) in the ventricular space (e.g., the third ventricle, 3V)

and cardiovascular responses) remain leptin responsive [64, 65].

Such a site specific leptin resistance may result from differential access of leptin to ARC LepRb neurons compared to other central sites, thus modulating SOCS-3 or PTP1B levels sites specifically [43]: Peripherally applied leptin acts faster and to lower leptin doses in the ARC compared to other hypothalamic sites. In contrast, centrally applied leptin, that circumvents leptin transport across the BBB, prevented these site-specific differences in leptin action, indicating that leptin reaches ARC LepRb neurons independent of a BBB transport mechanism.

The integrity of a functional BBB in the ARC is well established and indicated by a lack of fenestrated capillaries [66]. Fenestrated capillaries are only found in select sites within the brain and are typically found in close proximity to the ventricular space and are collectively termed circumventricular organs (CV). Indeed, the border between fenestrated capillaries in the median eminence (ME) and ARC is lined by tanycytes, which are highly specialized glial cells connected via tight junctions that shield the ARC from the circulation and the adjacent median eminence [67–69]. The BBB is often seen as rigid barrier and its disruption is associated with illness and unphysiological conditions [70]. However, recent data indicate a less rigid BBB that takes active part to convey metabolic changes to the ARC. During fasting fenestrated capillaries are no longer restricted to the ME and are found in proximal parts of the ARC, which enhances direct access to leptin in at least a subset of ARC neurons [71]. In addition, tanycytes are able to transport leptin into the CVO from where it reaches LepRb target cells [72]. Furthermore, the proximal ARC is connected with the perivascular space of the fenestrated median eminence (Virchow-Robin space) that allows blood-derived substances to reach proximal ARC neurons by perivascular routes [66]. Furthermore, many ARC LepRb neurons project into the ME, from where they can gain direct access to circulating leptin levels [43] (Fig. 6.4). Thus, most LepRb neurons may access leptin via a saturable transport across the BBB, which limits leptin access to these neurons and makes them less susceptible for leptin resistance. However, ARC neurons have direct access to circulating leptin, independent of a BBB transport and respond to changes in circulating leptin levels with increased time- and dose-dependent sensitivity [43] and therefore are prone to leptin resistance. In line with this, tanycyte-mediated leptin transport is sensitive to leptin resistance, while select improvement of tanycyte transport reversed DIO and reinstates leptin sensitivity [72].

Seasonal Leptin Resistance

Seasonal animals are an interesting animal model for obesity research. They undergo annual changes to improve and adapt their physiological performance to environmental challenges, including pronounced fluctuation in body weight and adiposity. Therefore, in seasonal animals a state of obesity is naturally occurring, and is not considered pathologic. In the laboratory seasonal changes are triggered by photoperiods and in the seasonal Siberian hamsters two physiological states are distinguishable based on day/light period duration: Long day (LD = 16 h light) adapted animals are obese with increased adiposity, while short day (SD = 8 h light) adapted animals are lean. LD and SD adapted animals show weight differences up to 10 g [73–75], which is comparable to weight differences in DIO mice after several weeks of HFD feeding compared to chow control animals. Importantly, LD acclimated, obese hamsters also have elevated circulating leptin levels compared to lean SD hamsters and are resistant to body weight reducing effects of leptin, while LD acclimated hamsters remain leptin sensitive. Leptin resistance is also observed on cellular level with decreased leptin-induced pSTAT3 and increased baseline SOCS3 level in the ARC, but not other hypothalamic sites [76–78]. Thus, leptin resistance is an important physiologic, not pathologic, condition that enables seasonal mammals to properly regulate seasonal body weight fluctuation.

Pregnancy/Lactation-Induced Leptin Resistance

Another physiological state of leptin resistance is observed during pregnancy. During pregnancy and lactation the increased energy demands require homeostatic adaptations that are met by increased food intake and facilitation of fat deposition [79, 80]. Increased fat mass, as well as possibly placental leptin production [81], further contribute to elevated circulating leptin levels during pregnancy [82–85]. Consistently, pregnant animals show classic leptin resistance with reduced or absent anorexic leptin effects as well as cellular leptin resistance. However, in contrast to ARC-specific leptin resistance in HFD fed animals and seasonal hamsters, pregnancy results in a select leptin resistance within the hypothalamic ventromedial hypothalamus (VMH) that is mediated by a decrease in LepRb mRNA expression [79]. Therefore, these data further highlight leptin resistance as important physiological adaptation to states of increased energy demand and should be taken into account when evaluating leptin resistance in obese individuals.

Endoplasmic Reticulum Stress-Induced Leptin Resistance

The endoplasmic reticulum (ER) is an important organelle that controls protein translation, folding, maturation, and transport [86, 87]. Physiological insult to the cell (e.g., in form of elevated cytokines (inflammation) and HFD feeding) causes ER stress [86, 88]. ER capacity and ER stress influence the degree of HFD-induced obesity [89, 90]. HFD also increases central ER stress and importantly leptin signaling is potently enhanced by increasing ER capacity, while ER stress robustly induced leptin resistance [91]. Chemical chaperones increase ER function, decrease ER stress and greatly enhance leptin sensitivity and weight loss in HFD fed, leptin resistant mice [91]. Importantly, this first description of potent leptin sensitizer also indicates that improvement of leptin sensitivity indeed would be relevant to support weight loss selectively in leptin resistant individuals. Future clinical trials will have to prove if such leptin sensitizer would represent safe and effective treatment in humans as well.

Conclusion and Perspective

As outlined above there are many factors and mechanisms that would be capable of explaining or at least contributing to leptin resistance in obese humans and may play a role to enhance

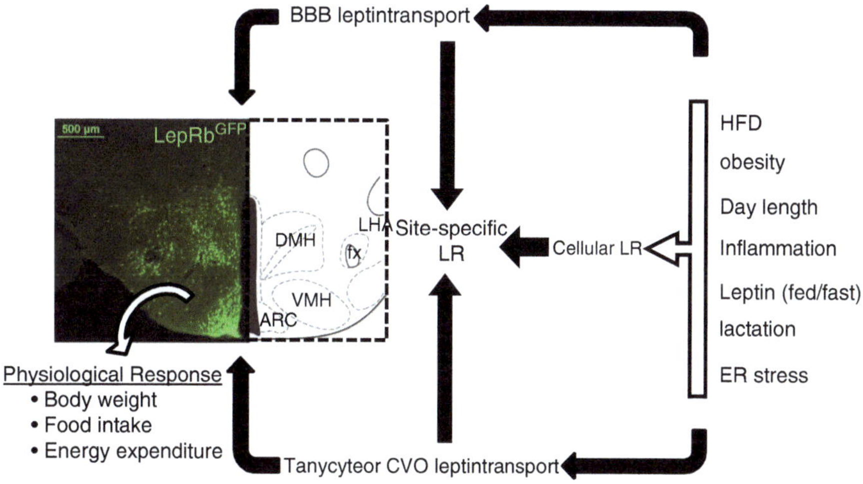

Fig. 6.5 Induction of leptin resistance. Scheme of factors that contribute to the development of leptin resistance

further weight gain (Fig. 6.5). While many data support the physiological necessity of leptin resistance to enhance weight gain and food intake, other data show contradicting results. Thus, the development of drugs or leptin combination therapies to sensitize leptin signaling will have to finally prove the effectiveness and safety of such treatments to improve overall health and quality of life in obese individuals. The described "natural" models of leptin resistance (seasonal animals and during pregnancy) suggests that leptin resistance is not always a pathological condition and requires further studies to test if reversal of leptin resistance in those special conditions may have harmful effects (e.g., reproductive success).

References

1. Zhang Y, Proenca R, Maffei M, Barone M, Leopold L, Friedman JM. Positional cloning of the mouse obese gene and its human homologue. Nature. 1994; 372(6505):425–32.
2. Coleman DL. A historical perspective on leptin. Nat Med. 2010;16(10):1097–9.
3. Farooqi IS, Jebb SA, Langmack G, Lawrence E, Cheetham CH, Prentice AM, et al. Effects of recombinant leptin therapy in a child with congenital leptin deficiency. N Engl J Med. 1999;341(12):879–84.
4. Frank S, Heni M, Moss A, von Schnurbein J, Farooqi S, Haring HU, et al. Long-term stabilization effects of leptin on brain functions in a leptin-deficient patient. PLoS One. 2013;8(6):e65893.
5. Schwartz MW, Peskind E, Raskind M, Boyko EJ, Porte Jr D. Cerebrospinal fluid leptin levels: relationship to plasma levels and to adiposity in humans. Nat Med. 1996;2(5):589–93.
6. Schwartz MW, Seeley RJ. The new biology of body weight regulation. J Am Diet Assoc. 1997;97(1):54–8.
7. Frederich RC, Hamann A, Anderson S, Lollmann B, Lowell BB, Flier JS. Leptin levels reflect body lipid content in mice: evidence for diet-induced resistance to leptin action. Nat Med. 1995;1(12):1311–4.
8. Cohen P, Zhao C, Cai X, Montez JM, Rohani SC, Feinstein P, et al. Selective deletion of leptin receptor in neurons leads to obesity. J Clin Invest. 2001; 108(8):1113–21.
9. Guo K, McMinn JE, Ludwig T, Yu YH, Yang G, Chen L, et al. Disruption of peripheral leptin signaling in mice results in hyperleptinemia without associated metabolic abnormalities. Endocrinology. 2007;148(8):3987–97.
10. Banks WA, Kastin AJ, Huang W, Jaspan JB, Maness LM. Leptin enters the brain by a saturable system independent of insulin. Peptides. 1996;17(2):305–11.
11. Maness LM, Banks WA, Kastin AJ. Persistence of blood-to-brain transport of leptin in obese leptin-deficient and leptin receptor-deficient mice. Brain Res. 2000;873(1):165–7.
12. Scarpace PJ, Tumer N. Peripheral and hypothalamic leptin resistance with age-related obesity. Physiol Behav. 2001;74(4–5):721–7.
13. Banks WA, King BM, Rossiter KN, Olson RD, Olson GA, Kastin AJ. Obesity-inducing lesions of the central nervous system alter leptin uptake by the blood-brain barrier. Life Sci. 2001;69(23):2765–73.
14. El Haschimi K, Pierroz DD, Hileman SM, Bjorbaek C, Flier JS. Two defects contribute to hypothalamic leptin resistance in mice with diet-induced obesity. J Clin Invest. 2000;105(12):1827–32.

15. Bates SH, Stearns WH, Dundon TA, Schubert M, Tso AW, Wang Y, et al. STAT3 signalling is required for leptin regulation of energy balance but not reproduction. Nature. 2003;421(6925):856–9.
16. Chen H, Charlat O, Tartaglia LA, Woolf EA, Weng X, Ellis SJ, et al. Evidence that the diabetes gene encodes the leptin receptor: identification of a mutation in the leptin receptor gene in db/db mice. Cell. 1996; 84(3):491–5.
17. Coleman DL. Diabetes-obesity syndromes in mice. Diabetes. 1982;31(Suppl 1 Pt 2):1–6.
18. Tartaglia LA, Dembski M, Weng X, Deng N, Culpepper J, Devos R, et al. Identification and expression cloning of a leptin receptor, OB-R. Cell. 1995; 83(7):1263–71.
19. Tartaglia LA. The leptin receptor. J Biol Chem. 1997;272(10):6093–6.
20. Banks AS, Davis SM, Bates SH, Myers Jr MG. Activation of downstream signals by the long form of the leptin receptor. J Biol Chem. 2000;275(19): 14563–72.
21. Munzberg H, Bjornholm M, Bates SH, Myers Jr MG. Leptin receptor action and mechanisms of leptin resistance. Cell Mol Life Sci. 2005;62(6):642–52.
22. Munzberg H, Huo L, Nillni EA, Hollenberg AN, Bjorbaek C. Role of signal transducer and activator of transcription 3 in regulation of hypothalamic proopiomelanocortin gene expression by leptin. Endocrinology. 2003;144(5):2121–31.
23. Vaisse C, Halaas JL, Horvath CM, Darnell Jr JE, Stoffel M, Friedman JM. Leptin activation of Stat3 in the hypothalamus of wild-type and ob/ob mice but not db/db mice. Nat Genet. 1996;14(1):95–7.
24. Rosenblum CI, Tota M, Cully D, Smith T, Collum R, Qureshi S, et al. Functional STAT 1 and 3 signaling by the leptin receptor (OB-R); reduced expression of the rat fatty leptin receptor in transfected cells. Endocrinology. 1996;137(11):5178–81.
25. Huo L, Munzberg H, Nillni EA, Bjorbaek C. Role of signal transducer and activator of transcription 3 in regulation of hypothalamic trh gene expression by leptin. Endocrinology. 2004;145(5):2516–23.
26. Bates SH, Dundon TA, Seifert M, Carlson M, Maratos-Flier E, Myers Jr MG. LRb-STAT3 signaling is required for the neuroendocrine regulation of energy expenditure by leptin. Diabetes. 2004;53(12):3067–73.
27. Munzberg H, Flier JS, Bjorbaek C. Region-specific leptin resistance within the hypothalamus of diet-induced obese mice. Endocrinology. 2004;145(11): 4880–9.
28. Bjorbaek C, Elmquist JK, Frantz JD, Shoelson SE, Flier JS. Identification of SOCS-3 as a potential mediator of central leptin resistance. Mol Cell. 1998; 1(4):619–25.
29. Bjorbaek C, El-Haschimi K, Frantz JD, Flier JS. The role of SOCS-3 in leptin signaling and leptin resistance. J Biol Chem. 1999;274(42):30059–65.
30. Bjorbak C, Lavery HJ, Bates SH, Olson RK, Davis SM, Flier JS, et al. SOCS3 mediates feedback inhibition of the leptin receptor via Tyr985. J Biol Chem. 2000;275(51):40649–57.
31. Howard JK, Flier JS. Attenuation of leptin and insulin signaling by SOCS proteins. Trends Endocrinol Metab. 2006;17(9):365–71.
32. Kievit P, Howard JK, Badman MK, Balthasar N, Coppari R, Mori H, et al. Enhanced leptin sensitivity and improved glucose homeostasis in mice lacking suppressor of cytokine signaling-3 in POMC-expressing cells. Cell Metab. 2006;4(2):123–32.
33. Bence KK, Delibegovic M, Xue B, Gorgun CZ, Hotamisligil GS, Neel BG, et al. Neuronal PTP1B regulates body weight, adiposity and leptin action. Nat Med. 2006;12(8):917–24.
34. Zabolotny JM, Bence-Hanulec KK, Stricker-Krongrad A, Haj F, Wang Y, Minokoshi Y, et al. PTP1B regulates leptin signal transduction in vivo. Dev Cell. 2002;2(4):489–95.
35. White CL, Whittington A, Barnes MJ, Wang Z, Bray GA, Morrison CD. HF diets increase hypothalamic PTP1B and induce leptin resistance through both leptin-dependent and -independent mechanisms. Am J Physiol Endocrinol Metab. 2009;296(2):E291–9.
36. Howard JK, Cave BJ, Oksanen LJ, Tzameli I, Bjorbaek C, Flier JS. Enhanced leptin sensitivity and attenuation of diet-induced obesity in mice with haploinsufficiency of Socs3. Nat Med. 2004;10(7): 734–8.
37. Ishida-Takahashi R, Rosario F, Gong Y, Kopp K, Stancheva Z, Chen X, et al. Phosphorylation of Jak2 on Ser(523) inhibits Jak2-dependent leptin receptor signaling. Mol Cell Biol. 2006;26(11):4063–73.
38. Argetsinger LS, Stuckey JA, Robertson SA, Koleva RI, Cline JM, Marto JA, et al. Tyrosines 868, 966, and 972 in the kinase domain of JAK2 are autophosphorylated and required for maximal JAK2 kinase activity. Mol Endocrinol. 2010;24(5):1062–76.
39. Kloek C, Haq AK, Dunn SL, Lavery HJ, Banks AS, Myers Jr MG. Regulation of Jak kinases by intracellular leptin receptor sequences. J Biol Chem. 2002;277(44):41547–55.
40. Myers MG, Cowley MA, Munzberg H. Mechanisms of leptin action and leptin resistance. Annu Rev Physiol. 2008;70:537–56.
41. Scarpace PJ, Zhang Y. Leptin resistance: a predisposing factor for diet-induced obesity. Am J Physiol Regul Integr Comp Physiol. 2009;296(3):R493–500.
42. Harris RB, Zhou J, Redmann Jr SM, Smagin GN, Smith SR, Rodgers E, et al. A leptin dose-response study in obese (ob/ob) and lean (+/?) mice. Endocrinology. 1998;139(1):8–19.
43. Faouzi M, Leshan R, Bjornholm M, Hennessey T, Jones J, Munzberg H. Differential accessibility of circulating leptin to individual hypothalamic sites. Endocrinology. 2007;148(11):5414–23.
44. Montague CT, Farooqi IS, Whitehead JP, Soos MA, Rau H, Wareham NJ, et al. Congenital leptin deficiency is associated with severe early-onset obesity in humans. Nature. 1997;387(6636):903–8.

45. Heymsfield SB, Greenberg AS, Fujioka K, Dixon RM, Kushner R, Hunt T, et al. Recombinant leptin for weight loss in obese and lean adults: a randomized, controlled, dose-escalation trial. JAMA. 1999;282(16):1568–75.
46. Enriori PJ, Evans AE, Sinnayah P, Jobst EE, Tonelli-Lemos L, Billes SK, et al. Diet-induced obesity causes severe but reversible leptin resistance in arcuate melanocortin neurons. Cell Metab. 2007;5(3):181–94.
47. Bouret SG, Gorski JN, Patterson CM, Chen S, Levin BE, Simerly RB. Hypothalamic neural projections are permanently disrupted in diet-induced obese rats. Cell Metab. 2008;7(2):179–85.
48. Bouret SG, Draper SJ, Simerly RB. Trophic action of leptin on hypothalamic neurons that regulate feeding. Science. 2004;304(5667):108–10.
49. Parekh PI, Petro AE, Tiller JM, Feinglos MN, Surwit RS. Reversal of diet-induced obesity and diabetes in C57BL/6J mice. Metabolism. 1998;47(9):1089–96.
50. Levin BE, Dunn-Meynell AA, Banks WA. Obesity-prone rats have normal blood-brain barrier transport but defective central leptin signaling before obesity onset. Am J Physiol Regul Integr Comp Physiol. 2004;286(1):R143–50.
51. Patterson CM, Bouret SG, Dunn-Meynell AA, Levin BE. Three weeks of postweaning exercise in DIO rats produces prolonged increases in central leptin sensitivity and signaling. Am J Physiol Regul Integr Comp Physiol. 2009;296(3):R537–48.
52. Minokoshi Y, Alquier T, Furukawa N, Kim YB, Lee A, Xue B, et al. AMP-kinase regulates food intake by responding to hormonal and nutrient signals in the hypothalamus. Nature. 2004;428(6982):569–74.
53. Borges BC, Rorato R, Avraham Y, da Silva LE, Castro M, Vorobiav L, et al. Leptin resistance and desensitization of hypophagia during prolonged inflammatory challenge. Am J Physiol Endocrinol Metab. 2011;300(5):E858–69.
54. Borges BC, Rorato R, Uchoa ET, Marangon P, da Silva GS, de Paula FJ, et al. High-fat diet induces site-specific unresponsiveness to LPS-stimulated STAT3 activation in the hypothalamus. Am J Physiol Regul Integr Comp Physiol. 2014;306(1):R34–44.
55. Munzberg H. Differential leptin access into the brain—a hierarchical organization of hypothalamic leptin target sites? Physiol Behav. 2008;94(5):664–9.
56. Sahu A. Resistance to the satiety action of leptin following chronic central leptin infusion is associated with the development of leptin resistance in neuropeptide Y neurones. J Neuroendocrinol. 2002;14(10):796–804.
57. Scarpace PJ, Matheny M, Zhang Y, Tumer N, Frase CD, Shek EW, et al. Central leptin gene delivery evokes persistent leptin signal transduction in young and aged-obese rats but physiological responses become attenuated over time in aged-obese rats. Neuropharmacology. 2002;42(4):548–61.
58. Scarpace PJ, Matheny M, Zhang Y, Shek EW, Prima V, Zolotukhin S, et al. Leptin-induced leptin resistance reveals separate roles for the anorexic and thermogenic responses in weight maintenance. Endocrinology. 2002;143(8):3026–35.
59. Martin RL, Perez E, He YJ, Dawson Jr R, Millard WJ. Leptin resistance is associated with hypothalamic leptin receptor mRNA and protein downregulation. Metabolism. 2000;49(11):1479–84.
60. Qiu J, Ogus S, Lu R, Chehab FF. Transgenic mice overexpressing leptin accumulate adipose mass at an older, but not younger, age. Endocrinology. 2001; 142(1):348–58.
61. Knight ZA, Hannan KS, Greenberg ML, Friedman JM. Hyperleptinemia is required for the development of leptin resistance. PLoS One. 2010;5(6):e11376.
62. Hosoi T, Okuma Y, Kawagishi T, Qi X, Matsuda T, Nomura Y. Bacterial endotoxin induces STAT3 activation in the mouse brain. Brain Res. 2004;1023(1):48–53.
63. Thaler JP, Schwartz MW. Minireview: inflammation and obesity pathogenesis: the hypothalamus heats up. Endocrinology. 2010;151(9):4109–15.
64. Mark AL. Selective leptin resistance revisited. Am J Physiol Regul Integr Comp Physiol. 2013;305(6):R566–81.
65. Rahmouni K, Morgan DA, Morgan GM, Mark AL, Haynes WG. Role of selective leptin resistance in diet-induced obesity hypertension. Diabetes. 2005; 54(7):2012–8.
66. Shaver SW, Pang JJ, Wainman DS, Wall KM, Gross PM. Morphology and function of capillary networks in subregions of the rat tuber cinereum. Cell Tissue Res. 1992;267(3):437–48.
67. Bolborea M, Dale N. Hypothalamic tanycytes: potential roles in the control of feeding and energy balance. Trends Neurosci. 2013;36(2):91–100.
68. Langlet F, Mullier A, Bouret SG, Prevot V, Dehouck B. Tanycyte-like cells form a blood-cerebrospinal fluid barrier in the circumventricular organs of the mouse brain. J Comp Neurol. 2013;521(15):3389–405.
69. Rodriguez EM, Blazquez JL, Pastor FE, Pelaez B, Pena P, Peruzzo B, et al. Hypothalamic tanycytes: a key component of brain-endocrine interaction. Int Rev Cytol. 2005;247:89–164.
70. Obermeier B, Daneman R, Ransohoff RM. Development, maintenance and disruption of the blood-brain barrier. Nat Med. 2013;19(12):1584–96.
71. Langlet F, Levin BE, Luquet S, Mazzone M, Messina A, Dunn-Meynell AA, et al. Tanycytic VEGF-A boosts blood-hypothalamus barrier plasticity and access of metabolic signals to the arcuate nucleus in response to fasting. Cell Metab. 2013;17(4):607–17.
72. Balland E, Dam J, Langlet F, Caron E, Steculorum S, Messina A, et al. Hypothalamic tanycytes are an ERK-gated conduit for leptin into the brain. Cell Metab. 2014;19(2):293–301.
73. Rousseau K, Atcha Z, Cagampang FR, Le RP, Stirland JA, Ivanov TR, et al. Photoperiodic regulation of leptin resistance in the seasonally breeding Siberian hamster (Phodopus sungorus). Endocrinology. 2002;143(8):3083–95.

74. Heldmaier G, Klingenspor M, Werneyer M, Lampi BJ, Brooks SP, Storey KB. Metabolic adjustments during daily torpor in the Djungarian hamster. Am J Physiol. 1999;276(5 Pt 1):E896–906.
75. Klingenspor M, Niggemann H, Heldmaier G. Modulation of leptin sensitivity by short photoperiod acclimation in the Djungarian hamster, Phodopus sungorus. J Comp Physiol B. 2000;170(1):37–43.
76. Tups A, Ellis C, Moar KM, Logie TJ, Adam CL, Mercer JG, et al. Photoperiodic regulation of leptin sensitivity in the Siberian hamster, Phodopus sungorus, is reflected in arcuate nucleus SOCS-3 (suppressor of cytokine signaling) gene expression. Endocrinology. 2004;145(3):1185–93.
77. Tups A, Barrett P, Ross AW, Morgan PJ, Klingenspor M, Mercer JG. The suppressor of cytokine signalling 3, SOCS3, may be one critical modulator of seasonal body weight changes in the Siberian hamster, Phodopus sungorus. J Neuroendocrinol. 2006;18(2): 139–45.
78. Tups A, Stohr S, Helwig M, Barrett P, Krol E, Schachtner J, et al. Seasonal leptin resistance is associated with impaired signalling via JAK2-STAT3 but not ERK, possibly mediated by reduced hypothalamic GRB2 protein. J Comp Physiol B. 2012;182(4): 553–67.
79. Ladyman SR, Grattan DR. Region-specific reduction in leptin-induced phosphorylation of signal transducer and activator of transcription-3 (STAT3) in the rat hypothalamus is associated with leptin resistance during pregnancy. Endocrinology. 2004;145(8): 3704–11.
80. Shirley B. The food intake of rats during pregnancy and lactation. Lab Anim Sci. 1984;34(2):169–72.
81. Sagawa N, Yura S, Itoh H, Kakui K, Takemura M, Nuamah MA, et al. Possible role of placental leptin in pregnancy: a review. Endocrine. 2002;19(1):65–71.
82. Garcia MD, Casanueva FF, Dieguez C, Senaris RM. Gestational profile of leptin messenger ribonucleic acid (mRNA) content in the placenta and adipose tissue in the rat, and regulation of the mRNA levels of the leptin receptor subtypes in the hypothalamus during pregnancy and lactation. Biol Reprod. 2000; 62(3):698–703.
83. Grattan DR, Ladyman SR, Augustine RA. Hormonal induction of leptin resistance during pregnancy. Physiol Behav. 2007;91(4):366–74.
84. Phillipps HR, Ladyman SR, Grattan DR. Maintained expression of genes associated with metabolism in the ventromedial hypothalamic nucleus despite development of leptin resistance during pregnancy in the rat. Physiol Rep. 2013;1(6):e00162.
85. Seeber RM, Smith JT, Waddell BJ. Plasma leptin-binding activity and hypothalamic leptin receptor expression during pregnancy and lactation in the rat. Biol Reprod. 2002;66(6):1762–7.
86. Ron D, Walter P. Signal integration in the endoplasmic reticulum unfolded protein response. Nat Rev Mol Cell Biol. 2007;8(7):519–29.
87. Walter P, Ron D. The unfolded protein response: from stress pathway to homeostatic regulation. Science. 2011;334(6059):1081–6.
88. Ozcan U, Ozcan L, Yilmaz E, Duvel K, Sahin M, Manning BD, et al. Loss of the tuberous sclerosis complex tumor suppressors triggers the unfolded protein response to regulate insulin signaling and apoptosis. Mol Cell. 2008;29(5):541–51.
89. Ozcan U, Cao Q, Yilmaz E, Lee AH, Iwakoshi NN, Ozdelen E, et al. Endoplasmic reticulum stress links obesity, insulin action, and type 2 diabetes. Science. 2004;306(5695):457–61.
90. Scheuner D, Vander MD, Song B, Flamez D, Creemers JW, Tsukamoto K, et al. Control of mRNA translation preserves endoplasmic reticulum function in beta cells and maintains glucose homeostasis. Nat Med. 2005;11(7):757–64.
91. Ozcan L, Ergin AS, Lu A, Chung J, Sarkar S, Nie D, et al. Endoplasmic reticulum stress plays a central role in development of leptin resistance. Cell Metab. 2009;9(1):35–51.

Leptin and Intermediary Metabolism: Focus on Glucoregulation and Lipids

7

Rachel C. Morgan and Robert V. Considine

Introduction

As has been discussed in previous chapters, the discovery of leptin opened new areas of investigation into the signaling mechanisms through which body weight is regulated. Shortly following the discovery of the *Lep* gene (originally *ob* gene) and the point mutation resulting in the lack of leptin in *ob/ob* mice [1], recombinant leptin protein was synthesized. The first logical experiments were to administer exogenous leptin to *ob/ob* mice to test if the hormone could reduce hyperphagia and obesity, thus testing the hypothesis that leptin was an adipose tissue-derived hormone that regulated caloric intake and body weight through activation of central neural processes. In studies from three different laboratories published together [2–4] it was definitively established that administration of leptin to obese mice reduced food intake and body weight. It was also observed in these studies that leptin induced-weight loss resulted in lower insulin and glucose levels [2, 3], in line with expectations that significant weight loss improves these metabolic parameters. Interestingly however, it was noted that in *ob/ob* mice treated with the lowest dose of leptin that no weight loss occurred, but surprisingly, insulin and glucose were reduced [2]. This was the first hint that leptin might regulate glucose homeostasis independent of its weight reducing effects. Subsequent work has now strengthened the concept that leptin regulates intermediary metabolism independent of its effects on food intake and body weight. This chapter focuses on the mechanisms through which leptin regulates glucose and lipid metabolism, with findings in rodents distinguished from those made in humans or using human tissue.

Metabolic Effects of Leptin Resulting from Direct Tissue Actions

Blood glucose levels are the result of the complex interaction of a number of processes including digestion and uptake of glucose from the intestine, utilization and storage of glucose by insulin target tissues, and production of glucose by the liver (primarily) during post-absorptive periods. Metabolism and storage of fatty acids and triglycerides also involves coordinated interaction between tissues including, but not limited to,

R.C. Morgan, M.D.
Division of Endocrinology, Department of Medicine, Indiana University, Indianapolis, IN 46202, USA

R.V. Considine, Ph.D. (✉)
Division of Endocrinology, Department of Medicine, Indiana University School of Medicine, Indianapolis, IN 46202, USA
e-mail: rconsidi@iu.edu

S. Dagogo-Jack (ed.), *Leptin: Regulation and Clinical Applications*,
DOI 10.1007/978-3-319-09915-6_7, © Springer International Publishing Switzerland 2015

the liver, muscle, and adipose tissue. With the discovery that leptin receptors were present on many cells outside of the central nervous system (discussed in detail in Chap. 2) early studies addressed the possibility that leptin could act directly to control glucose and lipid metabolism without activating neuronal processes in the brain.

Direct Effects of Leptin on Glucose Utilization

A direct tissue effect of leptin to regulate glucose uptake and metabolism in isolated skeletal muscle and adipocytes has not been reproducibly observed. Some in vitro studies in rodent muscles or clonal C2C12 or L6 cells found that leptin increased basal and or insulin stimulated glucose uptake [5–7], but others found no effect, or that leptin inhibited glucose uptake [8–10]. In rodent adipocytes leptin either impaired insulin-stimulated glucose uptake [11] or had no effect [8, 12, 13]. In human derived cells leptin regulation of glucose uptake is also contradictory, with leptin having no effect in human adipocytes differentiated in vitro [14], but increasing basal and insulin-stimulated glucose uptake in cultured human myotubes [15]. The reasons for the disparate effects described above are not entirely clear but likely due to different leptin preparations and experimental conditions. Importantly it should be noted that all of these studies used leptin at concentrations that were much higher than that measured in the blood of obese rodents or humans, implying that any effects observed should be considered pharmacologic rather than physiologic.

Regulation of Hepatic Glucose Production by Leptin Binding to Hepatocytes

In contrast to the variable effects of leptin on glucose uptake in liver and muscle, the direct effect of leptin binding in the liver is to reduce glucose release. Exposure of isolated rat hepatocytes to leptin for 16 h resulted in a dose-dependent increase in the incorporation of glucose into glycogen [16]. Leptin also inhibited the production of glucose from gluconeogenic substrates provided to isolated hepatocytes in culture [17]. Portal infusion of leptin into rat livers isolated in the postprandial state inhibited epinephrine- and glucagon-induced glycogenolysis [17, 18]. Overall these studies suggest that leptin can decrease blood glucose concentrations via a reduction in hepatic glucose release, independent of effects on weight loss or glucose uptake in muscle and adipose tissue.

Leptin Has Tissue Specific Effects on Lipid Metabolism

Direct tissue effects of leptin on fatty acid metabolism have been more easily demonstrated than effects on glucose metabolism at concentrations of leptin that better approximate physiologic levels. In isolated mouse or rat soleus muscle leptin increases fatty acid oxidation and decreases synthesis of muscle triglyceride. Leptin also attenuates the effects of insulin to decrease β-oxidation and increase triglyceride synthesis in muscle [19–21]. In isolated skeletal muscle preparations from lean humans, leptin increases partitioning of fatty acids toward oxidation and away from storage but is ineffective in muscle preparations from obese humans or diet induced obese rats [21, 22]. These observations suggest that during development of obesity, skeletal muscle becomes resistant to the effects of leptin (see Chap. 6), resulting in accumulation of intramuscular triglyceride, which contributes to insulin resistance in the muscle.

Lipolysis in rodent muscle [21] and adipose tissue [23–25] is also increased by leptin treatment, resulting in reduced triglyceride content of the tissues. This effect of leptin is not detected in adipocytes from *db*/*db* mice or fa/fa rats, which lack functional leptin receptors [24, 25]. Interestingly, leptin induced lipolysis results in release of the glycerol backbone of triglyceride from muscle and adipose tissue, but not the fatty acids, which are oxidized in the tissue [19, 24].

Leptin promotes the oxidation of fatty acids in skeletal muscle by activation of AMP-activated protein kinase (AMPK) [26]. AMPK stimulates fatty acid oxidation by inhibiting acetyl coenzyme A carboxylase (ACC), the enzyme that carboxylates acetyl CoA to malonyl CoA. ACC inhibition leads to suppressed malonyl-CoA production, thereby activating carnitine-palmitoyl transferase 1 activity to increase fatty acid oxidation. The initial activation of AMPK by leptin (15 min) occurs via signaling through skeletal muscle leptin receptors. Longer term leptin effects involve activation of the sympathetic nervous system [26], as discussed in more detail in the section below. The ability of leptin to decrease the fatty acid content of skeletal muscle, which would increase the insulin sensitivity of the tissue, should contribute to effects of leptin to promote glucose uptake when detected.

Liver triglyceride metabolism is responsive to direct regulation by leptin. Adenoviral reconstitution of functional hepatic leptin receptors in *fa/fa* rats results in increased β-oxidation and reduced triglyceride content [27]. When perfused into isolated liver from lean rats, leptin rapidly decreases triglyceride levels, an effect not observed with perfusion of liver from diet-induced obese rats [28]. Acute intravenous infusion of leptin into lean and obese rats increased fatty acid oxidation and reduced triglyceride content of liver only in the lean animals [29]. Leptin did not activate hepatic AMPK in these studies but phosphorylation of the PI3-kinase substrate Akt was increased. The inability of leptin to increase fatty acid oxidation and reduce hepatic triglyceride in obese rats suggests that the liver in these animals is leptin resistant (see Chap. 6 for detailed discussion of leptin resistance).

Leptin Regulates Pancreatic Function

Insulin is the primary hormonal regulator of glucose and lipid metabolism. Leptin could thus influence glucose and lipid metabolism in insulin target tissues indirectly by altering β-cell function and insulin release. Shortly following the identification of the leptin receptor, expression in the pancreas was documented [30], suggesting that leptin could act directly to regulate insulin secretion.

Direct Effects of Leptin on β-Cells

Leptin inhibits basal and glucose-stimulated insulin release in perfused pancreas preparations and isolated islets of *ob/ob* mice, and in rat islets in a dose dependent manner [30–33]. Leptin was ineffective in reducing insulin secretion from perfused pancreas or isolated islets of *fa/fa* rats or *db/db* mice, which lack functional leptin receptors [30]. Leptin also inhibits insulin release from human islet preparations in a dose-dependent manner, but this effect required 16–24 h exposure [32, 34, 35]. Leptin suppresses insulin secretion via a number of mechanisms including reducing glucose transport, cellular ATP levels and activating ATP-sensitive K^+ channels leading to cellular hyperpolarization [31, 34, 36, 37]. Knockdown of leptin receptors on β-cells in transgenic mice results in increased basal insulin release and lower blood sugar [38], although this study could not completely rule out effects mediated by a small reduction in hypothalamic leptin receptor expression in these transgenic mice. As insulin stimulates expansion of adipose tissue and induces leptin synthesis and release from adipocytes, and leptin in turn can inhibit insulin release from β-cells, this adipoinsular axis has been hypothesized to function as a break to slow adipose tissue growth [39]. See Chap. 7 for a detailed discussion of leptin regulation of β-cell function.

Prevention of Islet Lipotoxicity

The triglyceride content of pancreatic islets from Zucker Diabetic Fatty (ZDF) rats is higher than that in their lean littermates. Leptin treatment of isolated islets increased β-oxidation and lowered triglycerides in wild-type, and heterozygous ZDF rats, but had no effect in islets from homozygous rats which fully lack functional leptin receptors [19]. Overexpression of leptin receptor in islets from homozygous ZDF rats followed by leptin treatment resulted in reduced triglyceride and prevention of triglyceride formation from exogenous fatty acids in vitro [40]. Mice with islet specific knockout of leptin receptors exhibit impaired glucose tolerance due in part to blunted acute insulin response to glucose when challenged with a high fat diet. In contrast to wild type mice which experience islet hyperplasia to compensate for insulin resistance with high fat diet, the islet specific leptin receptor knockout mice showed a significantly reduced islet mass. The loss of islets may have resulted from lipotoxicity in the absence of islet leptin receptors [41].

Direct Effects of Leptin on α-Cells

Glucagon promotes glycogenolysis and gluconeogenesis in the fasting state, and hyperglucagonemia can worsen hyperglycemia in diabetes [42]. Leptin receptors are present on glucagon secreting αTC1-9 cells and α-cells in the mouse and human pancreas [43]. Leptin hyperpolarized the membrane potential of α-cells, inhibiting calcium oscillations and glucagon release in αTC1-9 cells and murine α-cells [43]. In contrast leptin had no effect on glucagon release from cultured hamster InR1G9 transfected with murine leptin receptors, despite a robust increase in STAT3 phosphorylation [44]. The reasons for these discrepant findings are not immediately apparent but the lack of an effect in the hamster cells might result from ineffective coupling of intracellular signaling between the transfected leptin receptors and glucagon secretion.

Metabolic Effects of Leptin Mediated by the Central Nervous System

The central nervous system (CNS) mediates the homeostatic regulation of many functions including respiration, body temperature, thirst, and hunger. Thus, it is reasonable to expect that the brain would also participate in the regulation of metabolism. However, following the discoveries that insulin and glucagon were secreted by the pancreas, much of the focus on the regulation of glucose homeostasis has been on the interactions between the pancreas and insulin target tissues, with less emphasis on a role for the CNS. Due in part to the discovery of leptin and its actions in the CNS there is now a greater and growing appreciation for the regulation of metabolism by the brain [45, 46].

Central Effects of Leptin on Glucose Metabolism

Kamohara et al. [47] were the first to observe that intracerebroventricular (icv) administration of leptin acutely enhanced glucose turnover (uptake and oxidation in muscle with concomitant glucose release from the liver) in wild-type C57/BL6 mice. Liu et al. [48] found that icv leptin shifted glucose flux in the liver from glycogenolysis to gluconeogenesis, and proposed that this change limited hepatic triglyceride formation by shunting free fatty acids into the β-oxidation pathway. In *fa/fa* rats and *ob/ob* mice icv leptin increased both insulin inhibition of hepatic glucose production and insulin-stimulated glucose disposal in peripheral tissues [49, 50]. A single injection of leptin into the ventromedial hypothalamus of conscious unrestrained rats increased glucose uptake into brown adipose tissue, heart, and skeletal muscle, but not white adipose tissue, with this effect mediated through the sympathetic nerves innervating these tissues [51, 52]. Adenoviral expression of leptin in the hypothalamus significantly reduced blood glucose in diabetic Akita mice without altering body weight or food intake [53]. Continuous icv administration of leptin to streptozotocin-induced diabetic rats inhibited glucose production in the liver and increased tissue glucose utilization to lower blood glucose levels [54]. These findings are consistent with in vitro studies showing inhibition of glucose release from isolated hepatocytes [16–18]. Recently, icv leptin in sheep increased expression of IGFBP2 and AKT2 phosphorylation in skeletal muscle via the activation of the sympathetic nerves [15]. Blocking IGFBP2 expression in cultured human myotubes attenuated the ability of leptin to increase glucose uptake, identifying a novel mechanism through which leptin may regulate skeletal muscle glucose uptake.

The studies above support the concept that leptin action in the brain regulates glucose homeostasis but there are several limitations to consider. Intracerebroventricular leptin injection can activate neurons in several areas of the brain, and the doses of leptin given, although lower than that provided by intravenous injection, may still be high relative to physiologic levels. Using leptin receptor null allele mice in which leptin receptor expression could be reactivated with adeno associated virus expressing FLPe-recombinase, Coppari et al. [55] demonstrated that neurons within the arcuate nucleus of the hypothalamus mediate the effects of leptin on glucose homeostasis. They found that restoration of leptin receptors on only one side of the brain had a modest effect on body weight and food intake, but markedly improved hyperinsulinemia, and normalized blood glucose and locomotor activity. An important aspect of this study is that leptin receptor expression occurred at physiologic levels only in neurons that normally express leptin receptors. That same year, Morton et al. [56] used adenoviral gene therapy to express leptin receptors in the area of the arcuate nucleus of Koletsky *fa/fa* rats. They found that restoration of leptin signaling in the hypothalamus improved insulin sensitivity beyond that achieved by reductions in food intake or body weight, and that the beneficial effect of restored leptin signaling could be blocked by a PI3 kinase inhibitor.

Huo et al. [57] restored leptin receptor expression in proopiomelanocortin expressing neurons in the arcuate nucleus of *db/db* mice, resulting in marked reductions in food intake and modest reductions in body weight. Importantly, blood glucose was entirely normalized, an effect that could not be replicated by pair feeding *db/db* mice. The mechanism through which blood glucose was improved was not established. Restoring leptin receptor expression only in POMC neurons using a neuron specific *cre* to remove a transcription blocking cassette, Bergland et al. [58] observed a modest reduction in body weight but complete normalization of blood glucose and hepatic insulin sensitivity, with reduced hyperglucagonemia. Of importance in this study, as in Coppari et al. [55], is that only neurons which would normally express leptin receptor, do so after removal of the transcription blocking cassette, which the authors estimate represent only about 30–40 % of the POMC neurons in the arcuate nucleus.

Central Effects of Leptin on Lipid Metabolism

Leptin has remarkable effects on the lipid content of the body by virtue of its ability to decrease caloric intake, increase energy expenditure and reduce body weight, all due to the action of leptin in the brain. Thus it has been more difficult to isolate a centrally mediated effect of leptin on lipid metabolism that is distinct from effects on caloric intake and body weight.

As discussed above, leptin stimulates the oxidation of fatty acids in skeletal muscle by activation of AMPK [22]. The initial activation of AMPK by leptin (15 min) occurs via signaling through skeletal muscle leptin receptors. However, the longer term effect of leptin (1–6 h) involves activation of the sympathetic nervous system. An intrahypothalamic injection of leptin increased the activity of AMPK in soleus muscle, an effect which could be blocked by denervation of the hindlimb or administration of the α-adrenergic antagonist phentolamine [22]. In contrast, an acute 120 min icv infusion of leptin had no effect on hepatic triglyceride content [28]. Gallardo et al. [59] infused leptin icv for 7 days, and pair-fed saline infused animals to the amount eaten by those receiving leptin. ICV leptin reduced plasma triglyceride more than pair feeding and altered the fatty acid composition in the liver. Leptin also increased hepatic expression of transcription factors and enzymes of lipid oxidation (PGC-1α, PPARα, CD36, CPT-1a) and decreased mRNA expression of enzymes in de novo fatty acid synthesis (ACC, FAS, SCD-1). These findings suggest that icv leptin down regulates hepatic de novo lipogenesis and increase fatty acid oxidation. Following icv leptin for 3 days in *ob/ob* mice, similar effects on expression of genes involved in hepatic β-oxidation were found, but changes in liver weight; hepatic steatosis; hepatic lipidemic profile; and circulating free fatty acids, triglycerides, and cholesterol lipoprotein profile were not different from that of pair fed controls [60]. This study thus did not find an effect of central leptin on lipid metabolism separate from its effects on food intake. In contrast Warne et al. [61] infused leptin icv for 7 days into *ob/ob* at a dose that did not alter food intake of body weight. They found that icv leptin decreased expression of lipogenic genes and hepatic TG content. These effects were the result of sympathetic outflow to the liver, as evidenced by an increase in hepatic noradrenalin content.

Leptin Improves Metabolic Defects in Lipodystrophy and in Type 1 Diabetes

Congenital and acquired lipodystrophies are syndromes characterized by deficiency of subcutaneous adipose tissue and result from a number of different genetic defects. Low leptin levels secondary to lack of subcutaneous fat, with ectopic fat deposition in the liver and muscle, contribute to metabolic abnormalities including insulin resistance, dyslipidemia, pancreatitis, microvascular disease, and diabetes [62, 63].

The effect of leptin to improve metabolism was originally assessed in mouse models of lipodystrophy. In mice expressing a truncated SREBP-1c (nSREBP-1c mice), intravenous infusion of leptin for 12 days reduced food intake and lowered insulin and glucose levels to that of wild type mice [64]. A reduction in insulin and glucose was not achieved by food restriction in a separate group of these transgenic mice, suggesting effects of leptin independent of caloric restriction. In the A-ZIP/F-1 mouse, a more severe model of lipoatrophy, peripheral leptin administration at doses similar to that used in nSREBP-1c mice had no effect on elevated glucose and insulin [65]. As discussed above, leptin treatment of obese mice activates β-oxidation and reduces the lipid content of the liver, an effect that can be achieved following central activation of the sympathetic nervous system or by direct leptin action on hepatocytes. In both nSREBP-1c and A-ZIP/F-1 mice icv leptin reduced hepatic triglyceride content at concentrations that were ineffective when given peripherally [66, 67]. In the A-ZIP/F-1 mice icv leptin increased hepatic AMPK activity via the sympathetic nervous system [67].

Recombinant leptin (metreleptin) has been utilized for treatment of lipodystrophy in humans with doses targeted for replacement or slightly higher. Leptin therapy decreases triglyceride levels, fasting glucose, hemoglobin A1C, and hepatic steatosis and is most effective in those subjects with the lowest circulating leptin levels [62, 63, 68]. Leptin significantly reduces caloric intake in lipodystrophic patients [63], and although an effect of leptin to improve lipid and glucose homeostasis independent of effects on food intake is feasible, this has not yet been demonstrated. See Chap. 20 for a detailed discussion of leptin therapy in lipodystrophic states.

Type 1 diabetes is also characterized by a "relative" leptin deficiency due to loss of insulin-stimulated leptin synthesis in adipocytes [69, 70]. Leptin lowers glucose and prolongs survival in both streptozotocin-treated rats and mice, and in Non-Obese Diabetic (NOD) mice. Effects of leptin to improve metabolism in type 1 diabetic rodents occurred via signaling in the central nervous system to reduce food intake, hyperglucagonemia, and tissue lipid content [54, 71–76]. The metabolic improvements that occur with leptin treatment cannot be achieved with pair feeding alone, supporting the concept that leptin can regulate metabolism independent of effects on food intake. Leptin therapy in two patients with type 1 diabetes and lipodystrophy improved glucose and lipids, and significantly reduced insulin requirements [77]. Clinical trials are underway to determine the usefulness of leptin therapy in type 1 diabetics.

Summary and Conclusions

Leptin regulates intermediary metabolism via direct tissue effects in muscle, adipose tissue, and liver, and via activation of central neural pathways that regulate metabolism in these tissues. While direct tissue effects on glucose uptake are not clear cut, leptin reproducibly stimulates β-oxidation in liver, muscle, and adipocytes to reduce the fatty acid content of these tissues. It is important to keep in mind that when considering direct tissue effects of leptin concentrations greater than that measured in the blood of obese rodents or humans are often required. This may be a consequence of studying isolated tissues or cells, or may suggest that central effects of leptin, which occur at lower concentrations, take precedence over direct tissue effects. It is also important to note that deletion of peripheral tissue leptin receptors in liver, adipose tissue, and small intestine had no adverse metabolic effects [78]. In a second study, deletion of hepatic leptin receptors also had no effect on body weight, body composition, or blood glucose levels during mild fasting or in the random-fed state [79]. However, when challenged with high fat diet, lack of hepatic leptin receptors actually protected the mice from glucose intolerance, with the liver exhibiting greater insulin sensitivity [79]. Given that loss of leptin receptor signaling in the brain uniformly results in adverse metabolic outcomes, it is reasonable to conclude that central effects of leptin have a greater impact on metabolic regulation than do direct tissue responses. Of greater importance than the controversy over direct or centrally mediated effects is that leptin may be an effective therapeutic intervention to improve glucose and lipid metabolism, independent of effects on food intake and energy expenditure.

References

1. Zhang Y, Proenca R, Maffei M, Barone M, Leopold L, Friedman JM. Positional cloning of the mouse obese gene and its human homologue. Nature. 1994; 372(6505):425–32.
2. Pelleymounter MA, Cullen MJ, Baker MB, Hecht R, Winters D, Boone T, Collins F. Effects of the obese gene product on body weight regulation in ob/ob mice. Science. 1995;269:540–3.
3. Halaas JL, Gajiwala KS, Maffei M, Cohen SL, Chait BT, Rabinowitz D, Lallone RL, Burley SK, Friedman JM. Weight-reducing effects of the plasma protein encoded by the obese gene. Science. 1995;269: 543–6.
4. Campfield LA, Smith FJ, Guisez Y, Devos R, Burn P. Recombinant mouse OB protein: evidence for a peripheral signal linking adiposity and central neural networks. Science. 1995;269:546–9.
5. Ceddia RB, William Jr WN, Curi R. Leptin increases glucose transport and utilization in skeletal muscle in vitro. Gen Pharmacol. 1998;31(5):799–801.
6. Harris RB. Acute and chronic effects of leptin on glucose utilization in lean mice. Biochem Biophys Res Commun. 1998;245(2):502–9.
7. Berti L, Gammeltoft S. Leptin stimulates glucose uptake in C2C12 muscle cells by activation of ERK2. Mol Cell Endocrinol. 1999;157(1–2):121–30.
8. Zierath JR, Frevert EU, Ryder JW, Berggren PO, Kahn BB. Evidence against a direct effect of leptin on glucose transport in skeletal muscle and adipocytes. Diabetes. 1998;47(1):1–4.
9. Sweeney G, Keen J, Somwar R, Konrad D, Garg R, Klip A. High leptin levels acutely inhibit insulin-stimulated glucose uptake without affecting glucose transporter 4 translocation in l6 rat skeletal muscle cells. Endocrinology. 2001;142(11):4806–12.
10. Hennige AM, Stefan N, Kapp K, Lehmann R, Weigert C, Beck A, Moeschel K, Mushack J, Schleicher E, Häring HU. Leptin down-regulates insulin action through phosphorylation of serine-318 in insulin receptor substrate 1. FASEB J. 2006;20(8):1206–8.
11. Müller G, Ertl J, Gerl M, Preibisch G. Leptin impairs metabolic actions of insulin in isolated rat adipocytes. J Biol Chem. 1997;272(16):10585–93.
12. Mick G, Vanderbloomer T, Fu CL, McCormick K. Leptin does not affect adipocyte glucose metabolism: studies in fresh and cultured adipocytes. Metabolism. 1998;47(11):1360–5.
13. Ranganathan S, Ciaraldi TP, Henry RR, Mudaliar S, Kern PA. Lack of effect of leptin on glucose transport, lipoprotein lipase, and insulin action in adipose and muscle cells. Endocrinology. 1998;139(5):2509–13.
14. Aprath-Husmann I, Röhrig K, Gottschling-Zeller H, Skurk T, Scriba D, Birgel M, Hauner H. Effects of leptin on the differentiation and metabolism of human adipocytes. Int J Obes Relat Metab Disord. 2001;25(10):1465–70.
15. Yau SW, Henry BA, Russo VC, McConell GK, Clarke IJ, Werther GA, Sabin MA. Leptin enhances insulin sensitivity by direct and sympathetic nervous system regulation of muscle IGFBP-2 expression—evidence from non-rodent models. Endocrinology. 2014; 155(6):2133–43.
16. Aiston S, Agius L. Leptin enhances glycogen storage in hepatocytes by inhibition of phosphorylase and exerts an additive effect with insulin. Diabetes. 1999;48(1):15–20.
17. Ceddia RB, Lopes G, Souza HM, Borba-Murad GR, William Jr WN, Bazotte RB, Curi R. Acute effects of leptin on glucose metabolism of in situ rat perfused livers and isolated hepatocytes. Int J Obes Relat Metab Disord. 1999;23(11):1207–12.
18. Nemecz M, Preininger K, Englisch R, Fürnsinn C, Schneider B, Waldhäusl W, Roden M. Acute effect of leptin on hepatic glycogenolysis and gluconeogenesis in perfused rat liver. Hepatology. 1999;29(1):166–72.
19. Shimabukuro M, Koyama K, Chen G, Wang MY, Trieu F, Lee Y, Newgard CB, Unger RH. Direct

antidiabetic effect of leptin through triglyceride depletion of tissues. Proc Natl Acad Sci U S A. 1997;94(9):4637–41.

20. Muoio DM, Dohm GL, Tapscott EB, Coleman RA. Leptin opposes insulin's effects on fatty acid partitioning in muscles isolated from obese ob/ob mice. Am J Physiol. 1999;276(5 Pt 1):E913–21.
21. Steinberg GR, Dyck DJ. Development of leptin resistance in rat soleus muscle in response to high-fat diets. Am J Physiol Endocrinol Metab. 2000;279(6): E1374–82.
22. Steinberg GR, Parolin ML, Heigenhauser GJ, Dyck DJ. Leptin increases FA oxidation in lean but not obese human skeletal muscle: evidence of peripheral leptin resistance. Am J Physiol Endocrinol Metab. 2002;283(1):E187–92.
23. Siegrist-Kaiser CA, Pauli V, Juge-Aubry CE, Boss O, Pernin A, Chin WW, Cusin I, Rohner-Jeanrenaud F, Burger AG, Zapf J, Meier CA. Direct effects of leptin on brown and white adipose tissue. J Clin Invest. 1997;100(11):2858–64.
24. Wang MY, Lee Y, Unger RH. Novel form of lipolysis induced by leptin. J Biol Chem. 1999;274(25): 17541–4.
25. Frühbeck G, Aguado M, Gómez-Ambrosi J, Martínez JA. Lipolytic effect of in vivo leptin administration on adipocytes of lean and ob/ob mice, but not db/db mice. Biochem Biophys Res Commun. 1998;250(1): 99–102.
26. Minokoshi Y, Kim YB, Peroni OD, Fryer LG, Müller C, Carling D, Kahn BB. Leptin stimulates fatty-acid oxidation by activating AMP-activated protein kinase. Nature. 2002;415(6869):339–43.
27. Lee Y, Wang MY, Kakuma T, Wang ZW, Babcock E, McCorkle K, Higa M, Zhou YT, Unger RH. Liporegulation in diet-induced obesity. The antisteatotic role of hyperleptinemia. J Biol Chem. 2001; 276(8):5629–35.
28. Huang W, Dedousis N, Bhatt BA, O'Doherty RM. Impaired activation of phosphatidylinositol 3-kinase by leptin is a novel mechanism of hepatic leptin resistance in diet-induced obesity. J Biol Chem. 2004;279(21):21695–700.
29. Huang W, Dedousis N, Bandi A, Lopaschuk GD, O'Doherty RM. Liver triglyceride secretion and lipid oxidative metabolism are rapidly altered by leptin in vivo. Endocrinology. 2006;147(3):1480–7.
30. Emilsson V, Liu YL, Cawthorne MA, Morton NM, Davenport M. Expression of the functional leptin receptor mRNA in pancreatic islets and direct inhibitory action of leptin on insulin secretion. Diabetes. 1997;46(2):313–6.
31. Kieffer TJ, Heller RS, Leech CA, Holz GG, Habener JF. Leptin suppression of insulin secretion by the activation of ATP-sensitive K+channels in pancreatic beta-cells. Diabetes. 1997;46(6):1087–93.
32. Kulkarni RN, Wang ZL, Wang RM, Hurley JD, Smith DM, Ghatei MA, Withers DJ, Gardiner JV, Bailey CJ, Bloom SR. Leptin rapidly suppresses insulin release from insulinoma cells, rat and human islets and, in vivo, in mice. J Clin Invest. 1997;100(11): 2729–36.
33. Ookuma M, Ookuma K, York DA. Effects of leptin on insulin secretion from isolated rat pancreatic islets. Diabetes. 1998;47(2):219–23.
34. Seufert J, Kieffer TJ, Leech CA, Holz GG, Moritz W, Ricordi C, Habener JF. Leptin suppression of insulin secretion and gene expression in human pancreatic islets: implications for the development of adipogenic diabetes mellitus. J Clin Endocrinol Metab. 1999;84(2):670–6.
35. Lupi R, Marchetti P, Maffei M, Del Guerra S, Benzi L, Marselli L, Bertacca A, Navalesi R. Effects of acute or prolonged exposure to human leptin on isolated human islet function. Biochem Biophys Res Commun. 1999;256(3):637–41.
36. Harvey J, McKenna F, Herson PS, Spanswick D, Ashford ML. Leptin activates ATP-sensitive potassium channels in the rat insulin-secreting cell line, CRI-G1. J Physiol. 1997;504(Pt 3):527–35.
37. Lam NT, Cheung AT, Riedel MJ, Light PE, Cheeseman CI, Kieffer TJ. Leptin reduces glucose transport and cellular ATP levels in INS-1 beta-cells. J Mol Endocrinol. 2004;32(2):415–24.
38. Covey SD, Wideman RD, McDonald C, Unniappan S, Huynh F, Asadi A, Speck M, Webber T, Chua SC, Kieffer TJ. The pancreatic beta cell is a key site for mediating the effects of leptin on glucose homeostasis. Cell Metab. 2006;4(4):291–302.
39. Kieffer TJ, Habener JF. The adipoinsular axis: effects of leptin on pancreatic beta-cells. Am J Physiol Endocrinol Metab. 2000;278(1):E1–14.
40. Wang MY, Koyama K, Shimabukuro M, Newgard CB, Unger RH. OB-Rb gene transfer to leptin-resistant islets reverses diabetogenic phenotype. Proc Natl Acad Sci U S A. 1998;95(2):714–8.
41. Morioka T, Asilmaz E, Hu J, Dishinger JF, Kurpad AJ, Elias CF, Li H, Elmquist JK, Kennedy RT, Kulkarni RN. Disruption of leptin receptor expression in the pancreas directly affects beta cell growth and function in mice. J Clin Invest. 2007;117(10): 2860–8.
42. Holst JJ, Christensen M, Lund A, de Heer J, Svendsen B, Kielgast U, Knop FK. Regulation of glucagon secretion by incretins. Diabetes Obes Metab. 2011;13 Suppl 1:89–94.
43. Tudurí E, Marroquí L, Soriano S, Ropero AB, Batista TM, Piquer S, López-Boado MA, Carneiro EM, Gomis R, Nadal A, Quesada I. Inhibitory effects of leptin on pancreatic alpha-cell function. Diabetes. 2009;58(7):1616–24.
44. Chen L, Philippe J, Unger RH. Glucagon responses of isolated α cells to glucose, insulin, somatostatin, and leptin. Endocr Pract. 2011;17(5):819–25.
45. Lam CK, Chari M, Lam TK. CNS regulation of glucose homeostasis. Physiology (Bethesda). 2009;24: 159–70.
46. Grayson BE, Seeley RJ, Sandoval DA. Wired on sugar: the role of the CNS in the regulation of glucose homeostasis. Nat Rev Neurosci. 2013;14(1):24–37.

47. Kamohara S, Burcelin R, Halaas JL, Friedman JM, Charron MJ. Acute stimulation of glucose metabolism in mice by leptin treatment. Nature. 1997;389:374–7.
48. Liu L, Karkanias GB, Morales JC, Hawkins M, Barzilai N, Wang J, Rossetti L. Intracerebroventricular leptin regulates hepatic but not peripheral glucose fluxes. J Biol Chem. 1998;273:31160–7.
49. Cusin I, Zakrzewska KE, Boss O, Muzzin P, Giacobino JP, Ricquier D, Jeanrenaud B, Rohner-Jeanrenaud F. Chronic central leptin infusion enhances insulin-stimulated glucose metabolism and favors the expression of uncoupling proteins. Diabetes. 1998; 47:1014–9.
50. van den Hoek AM, Teusink B, Voshol PJ, Havekes LM, Romijn JA, Pijl H. Leptin deficiency per se dictates body composition and insulin action in ob/ob mice. J Neuroendocrinol. 2008;20(1):120–7.
51. Minokoshi Y, Haque MS, Shimazu T. Microinjection of leptin into the ventromedial hypothalamus increases glucose uptake in peripheral tissues in rats. Diabetes. 1999;48(2):287–91.
52. Haque MS, Minokoshi Y, Hamai M, Iwai M, Horiuchi M, Shimazu T. Role of the sympathetic nervous system and insulin in enhancing glucose uptake in peripheral tissues after intrahypothalamic injection of leptin in rats. Diabetes. 1999;48(9):1706–12.
53. Ueno N, Inui A, Kalra PS, Kalra SP. Leptin transgene expression in the hypothalamus enforces euglycemia in diabetic, insulin-deficient nonobese Akita mice and leptin-deficient obese ob/ob mice. Peptides. 2006; 27:2332–42.
54. German JP, Thaler JP, Wisse BE, Oh-I S, Sarruf DA, Matsen ME, Fischer JD, Taborsky Jr GJ, Schwartz MW, Morton GJ. Leptin activates a novel CNS mechanism for insulin-independent normalization of severe diabetic hyperglycemia. Endocrinology. 2011;152(2): 394–404.
55. Coppari R, Ichinose M, Lee CE, Pullen AE, Kenny CD, McGovern RA, Tang V, Liu SM, Ludwig T, Chua Jr SC, Lowell BB, Elmquist JK. The hypothalamic arcuate nucleus: a key site for mediating leptin's effects on glucose homeostasis and locomotor activity. Cell Metab. 2005;1(1):63–72.
56. Morton GJ, Gelling RW, Niswender KD, Morrison CD, Rhodes CJ, Schwartz MW. Leptin regulates insulin sensitivity via phosphatidylinositol-3-OH kinase signaling in mediobasal hypothalamic neurons. Cell Metab. 2005;2(6):411–20.
57. Huo L, Gamber K, Greeley S, Silva J, Huntoon N, Leng XH, Bjørbaek C. Leptin-dependent control of glucose balance and locomotor activity by POMC neurons. Cell Metab. 2009;9(6):537–47.
58. Berglund ED, Vianna CR, Donato Jr J, Kim MH, Chuang JC, Lee CE, Lauzon DA, Lin P, Brule LJ, Scott MM, Coppari R, Elmquist JK. Direct leptin action on POMC neurons regulates glucose homeostasis and hepatic insulin sensitivity in mice. J Clin Invest. 2012;122(3):1000–9.
59. Gallardo N, Bonzón-Kulichenko E, Fernández-Agulló T, Moltó E, Gómez-Alonso S, Blanco P, Carrascosa JM, Ros M, Andrés A. Tissue-specific effects of central leptin on the expression of genes involved in lipid metabolism in liver and white adipose tissue. Endocrinology. 2007;148(12):5604–10.
60. Prieur X, Tung YC, Griffin JL, Farooqi IS, O'Rahilly S, Coll AP. Leptin regulates peripheral lipid metabolism primarily through central effects on food intake. Endocrinology. 2008;149(11):5432–9.
61. Warne JP, Alemi F, Reed AS, Varonin JM, Chan H, Piper ML, Mullin ME, Myers Jr MG, Corvera CU, Xu AW. Impairment of central leptin-mediated PI3K signaling manifested as hepatic steatosis independent of hyperphagia and obesity. Cell Metab. 2011; 14(6):791–803.
62. Chong AY, Lupsa BC, Cochran EK, Gorden P. Efficacy of leptin therapy in the different forms of human lipodystrophy. Diabetologia. 2010;53(1):27–35.
63. Oral EA, Chan JL. Rationale for leptin-replacement therapy for severe lipodystrophy. Endocr Pract. 2010;16(2):324–33.
64. Shimomura I, Hammer RE, Ikemoto S, Brown MS, Goldstein JL. Leptin reverses insulin resistance and diabetes mellitus in mice with congenital lipodystrophy. Nature. 1999;401(6748):73–6.
65. Gavrilova O, Marcus-Samuels B, Leon LR, Vinson C, Reitman ML. Leptin and diabetes in lipoatrophic mice. Nature. 2000;403(6772):850.
66. Asilmaz E, Cohen P, Miyazaki M, Dobrzyn P, Ueki K, Fayzikhodjaeva G, Soukas AA, Kahn CR, Ntambi JM, Socci ND, Friedman JM. Site and mechanism of leptin action in a rodent form of congenital lipodystrophy. J Clin Invest. 2004;113(3):414–24.
67. Miyamoto L, Ebihara K, Kusakabe T, Aotani D, Yamamoto-Kataoka S, Sakai T, Aizawa-Abe M, Yamamoto Y, Fujikura J, Hayashi T, Hosoda K, Nakao K. Leptin activates hepatic 5′-AMP-activated protein kinase through sympathetic nervous system and α1-adrenergic receptor: a potential mechanism for improvement of fatty liver in lipodystrophy by leptin. J Biol Chem. 2012;287(48):40441–7.
68. Savage DB, O'Rahilly S. Leptin therapy in lipodystrophy. Diabetologia. 2010;53(1):7–9.
69. Havel PJ, Uriu-Hare JY, Liu T, Stanhope KL, Stern JS, Keen CL, Ahrén B. Marked and rapid decreases of circulating leptin in streptozotocin diabetic rats: reversal by insulin. Am J Physiol. 1998;274(5 Pt 2):R1482–91.
70. Kiess W, Anil M, Blum WF, Englaro P, Juul A, Attanasio A, Dötsch J, Rascher W. Serum leptin levels in children and adolescents with insulin-dependent diabetes mellitus in relation to metabolic control and body mass index. Eur J Endocrinol. 1998;138(5):501–9.
71. Yu X, Park BH, Wang MY, Wang ZV, Unger RH. Making insulin-deficient type 1 diabetic rodents thrive without insulin. Proc Natl Acad Sci U S A. 2008;105(37):14070–5.
72. Chinookoswong N, Wang JL, Shi ZQ. Leptin restores euglycemia and normalizes glucose turnover in insulin-deficient diabetes in the rat. Diabetes. 1999; 48(7):1487–92.

73. Lin CY, Higginbotham DA, Judd RL, White BD. Central leptin increases insulin sensitivity in streptozotocin-induced diabetic rats. Am J Physiol Endocrinol Metab. 2002;282(5):E1084–91.
74. Hidaka S, Yoshimatsu H, Kondou S, Tsuruta Y, Oka K, Noguchi H, Okamoto K, Sakino H, Teshima Y, Okeda T, Sakata T. Chronic central leptin infusion restores hyperglycemia independent of food intake and insulin level in streptozotocin-induced diabetic rats. FASEB J. 2002;16(6):509–18.
75. Kojima S, Asakawa A, Amitani H, Sakoguchi T, Ueno N, Inui A, Kalra SP. Central leptin gene therapy, a substitute for insulin therapy to ameliorate hyperglycemia and hyperphagia, and promote survival in insulin-deficient diabetic mice. Peptides. 2009;30(5):962–6.
76. Fujikawa T, Berglund ED, Patel VR, Ramadori G, Vianna CR, Vong L, Thorel F, Chera S, Herrera PL, Lowell BB, Elmquist JK, Baldi P, Coppari R. Leptin engages a hypothalamic neurocircuitry to permit survival in the absence of insulin. Cell Metab. 2013;18(3):431–44.
77. Park JY, Chong AY, Cochran EK, Kleiner DE, Haller MJ, Schatz DA, Gorden P. Type 1 diabetes associated with acquired generalized lipodystrophy and insulin resistance: the effect of long-term leptin therapy. J Clin Endocrinol Metab. 2008;93(1):26–31.
78. Guo K, McMinn JE, Ludwig T, Yu YH, Yang G, Chen L, Loh D, Li C, Chua Jr S, Zhang Y. Disruption of peripheral leptin signaling in mice results in hyperleptinemia without associated metabolic abnormalities. Endocrinology. 2007;148(8):3987–97.
79. Huynh FK, Levi J, Denroche HC, Gray SL, Voshol PJ, Neumann UH, Speck M, Chua SC, Covey SD, Kieffer TJ. Disruption of hepatic leptin signaling protects mice from age- and diet-related glucose intolerance. Diabetes. 2010;59(12):3032–40.

Pathogenesis of Hepatic Steatosis and Fibrosis: Role of Leptin

8

Faidon Magkos, Elisa Fabbrini, and Samuel Klein

Definition, Diagnosis, and Prevalence of Nonalcoholic Fatty Liver Disease

Nonalcoholic fatty liver disease (NAFLD) encompasses a spectrum of liver abnormalities, ranging from simple steatosis, to steatohepatitis and cirrhosis, in the absence of "excessive" alcohol consumption or any other identifiable cause(s) for liver disease [1]. Histologically, NAFLD can be categorized into: (1) simple steatosis in the absence of hepatocellular injury (nonalcoholic fatty liver, NAFL); and (2) steatohepatitis (nonalcoholic steatohepatitis, NASH), characterized by the presence of steatosis and inflammation with hepatic injury (ballooning), with or without fibrosis [1]. NASH can progress to cirrhosis, liver failure, and rarely liver cancer, whereas the progression to more severe forms of liver disease is minimal in patients with NAFL. Steatosis is the hallmark of NAFL and NAFLD and can be defined chemically, when intrahepatic triglyceride (IHTG) content exceeds 5 % of liver volume or liver weight [2], histologically, when 5 % of hepatocytes contain visible intracellular triglyceride [3], and radiologically, by using magnetic resonance spectroscopy (MRS) [4]. The results from one study in subjects who were considered to be at low-risk for NAFLD (i.e., normal weight, normal fasting serum glucose and alanine aminotransferase concentrations, and absence of diabetes) indicate an upper "normal" amount of IHTG of 5.6 % of liver volume, which represented the 95th percentile in this population [5]. Data from another study found the 95th percentile for IHTG content was 3 % in young lean subjects with normal oral glucose tolerance [6].

NAFLD has become an important public health problem, because of its high prevalence, the potential progression to severe liver disease and its association with serious cardiometabolic abnormalities, such as insulin resistance, type 2 diabetes, and dyslipidemia. The prevalence rate of NAFLD increases with increasing body mass index (BMI) [7] and varies widely based on the population studied and on the tool used to make the diagnosis. An analysis of liver histology from potential liver donors [8, 9], automobile crash victims [10], autopsy findings [11], and clinical liver biopsies [12] suggests that the prevalence of steatosis and steatohepatitis are approximately 15 % and 3 %, respectively, in non-obese individuals, 65 % and 20 %, respectively, in persons

F. Magkos, Ph.D. • E. Fabbrini, M.D., Ph.D.
Center for Human Nutrition and Atkins Center of Excellence in Obesity Medicine, Washington University School of Medicine, St. Louis, MO USA

S. Klein, M.D. (✉)
Center for Human Nutrition, Washington University School of Medicine, 660 South Euclid Avenue, Campus Box 8031, St. Louis, MO 63110, USA
e-mail: sklein@dom.wustl.edu

S. Dagogo-Jack (ed.), *Leptin: Regulation and Clinical Applications*,
DOI 10.1007/978-3-319-09915-6_8, © Springer International Publishing Switzerland 2015

with class I and II obesity (BMI 30.0–39.9 kg/m^2), and 85 % and 40 %, respectively, in extremely obese patients (BMI >40 kg/m^2). The relationship between BMI and NAFLD is influenced by racial/ethnic background and polymorphisms of specific genes [6, 13, 14].

Pathogenesis and Pathophysiology of NAFLD

The liver performs a number of essential biochemical functions which are necessary for whole-body metabolic homeostasis [15]. The liver maintains plasma glucose concentration within a narrow range, by producing glucose derived from glycogenolysis and gluconeogenesis and releasing it into the bloodstream in the postabsorptive state, and taking up glucose to store it as glycogen in the postprandial state. The liver is also central in normal lipid and lipoprotein metabolism, by taking up and synthesizing fatty acids, channeling them towards oxidative or esterification pathways, and secreting lipoproteins into the bloodstream. NAFLD is associated with alterations in most of the liver's metabolic functions.

NAFLD and Glucose Metabolism: Insulin Resistance

Increased IHTG content is associated with insulin resistance in both the liver (decreased ability of insulin to suppress hepatic glucose production) and skeletal muscle (decreased ability of insulin to stimulate muscle glucose uptake), independent of BMI, percent body fat, and visceral fat mass [16–21]. Although the link between insulin resistance and NAFLD is well established, it is not known whether NAFLD causes or is a consequence of insulin resistance, or possibly both. It has been proposed that an increase in intracellular lipid intermediates and inflammation are involved in the pathogenesis of liver insulin resistance in people with NAFLD. An accumulation of hepatic intracellular lipid intermediates generated by fatty acid metabolism, particularly diacylglycerol (DAG) species, identified in NAFLD, can disrupt normal insulin signaling and inhibit insulin-mediated suppression of hepatic glucose production [22–25]. Intrahepatic inflammation provides a potential mechanistic link between NAFLD and insulin resistance not only in the liver but also skeletal muscle. In a rodent model, increased hepatic nuclear factor (NF)-κB activity causes hepatic steatosis and inflammation, and both hepatic and skeletal muscle insulin resistance [26]. However, steatosis does not always coincide with insulin resistance. Data from studies conducted in rodent models have found that genetic [27, 28] or pharmacological [29] induction of hepatic steatosis is not associated with impaired hepatic or skeletal muscle insulin action, and inhibition of IHTG synthesis decreases hepatic steatosis but does not improve insulin sensitivity [30]. Furthermore, an increase in IHTG content in patients with familial hypobetalipoproteinemia, caused by a genetic defect in the liver's ability to export triglycerides as very low-density lipoprotein (VLDL), is not accompanied by hepatic or peripheral insulin resistance [31, 32]. Taken together, these findings suggest that IHTG accumulation, itself, does not necessarily cause insulin resistance, but is an important marker of multi-organ insulin resistance.

NAFLD and Lipid Metabolism

Hepatocellular steatosis develops when the rate of fatty acid input (uptake from plasma and de novo synthesis) is greater than the rate of fatty acid output (oxidation and secretion as triglyceride). Therefore, the amount of triglyceride present in hepatocytes represents the net result of complex metabolic interactions among: (1) hepatic uptake of plasma free fatty acids (FFA), released from hydrolysis of adipose tissue and circulating triglycerides, (2) de novo lipogenesis (i.e., synthesis of fatty acids from simple precursors), (3) fatty acid oxidation, and (4) fatty acid secretion as triglyceride in VLDL particles.

Compared with subjects who have normal IHTG content, NAFLD is associated with greater basal lipolytic rates, independent of BMI [19, 33, 34], and greater impairment of insulin-mediated suppression of adipose tissue lipolysis (indicative of adipose tissue insulin resistance) [16, 19, 33]. Therefore, the daily release of FFA into the circulation during both fasting and fed conditions is likely greater in people with NAFLD than in those without NAFLD. Furthermore, gene expression of proteins that can facilitate uptake of fatty acids in the liver (hepatic lipase, hepatic lipoprotein lipase, and hepatic CD36) are greater in obese subjects with NAFLD than in those without NAFLD [35–37]. These data suggest that NAFLD is associated with a greater delivery and uptake of systemic plasma FFA to the liver, derived from lipolysis of adipose tissue triglycerides and circulating lipoprotein triglycerides, which likely contributes to IHTG accumulation.

Fatty acids in the liver can also be synthesized de novo through a complex polymerization process which ultimately leads to the formation of palmitate (C16:0) from acetyl-CoA (2-carbon precursor) [38]. In normal subjects, de novo lipogenesis accounts for less than 5 % (in the postabsorptive state) or 10 % (in the postprandial state) of fatty acids incorporated in IHTG and VLDL-triglyceride (~1–2 g/day) [39, 40]. However, the contribution of de novo lipogenesis in subjects with NAFLD is much greater and accounts for 15–23 % of the fatty acids in IHTG and VLDL-triglyceride in the fasting state [40, 41]. The results from a study conducted in lean insulin-sensitive and insulin-resistant young adults, who had normal IHTG content, demonstrated that meal ingestion caused a greater increase in hepatic de novo lipogenesis in insulin-resistant than in insulin-sensitive subjects, which suggests an increase in de novo lipogenesis might even precede IHTG accumulation and NAFLD [42].

Alterations in hepatic fatty acid oxidation could also contribute to the pathogenesis of NAFLD. In rodents, genetic or experimentally induced deficiency in mitochondrial enzymes involved in the oxidation of fatty acids leads to an accumulation of IHTG and hepatic steatosis [43, 44], whereas greater expression or activity of these enzymes reduces IHTG content and ameliorates steatosis [45–48]. However, it is unclear whether fatty acid oxidation is defective in human subjects with NAFLD, because there are currently no reliable methods for measuring hepatic fatty acid oxidation in vivo in man. Indirect measures, such as plasma ketone body concentrations and gene expression of hepatic fatty acid oxidative enzymes are either normal or increased in people with NAFLD [18, 19, 49–52]. At present, therefore, there is no adequate evidence to support the notion that decreased hepatic fatty acid oxidation contributes to IHTG accumulation and the pathogenesis of steatosis.

The majority of circulating triglycerides in the postabsorptive state are carried in the hydrophobic core of VLDL particles, which are synthesized and secreted by the liver. Intrahepatocellular fatty acids that are not oxidized are esterified to triglyceride, which can then be incorporated into VLDL and secreted into the circulation, or stored within the liver. Therefore, the assembly and secretion of VLDL provides a mechanism for reducing IHTG content by exporting triglycerides from the liver into the systemic circulation. In fact, results from studies conducted in both human subjects and animal models indicate that impaired hepatic VLDL secretion, caused by genetic defects [53] or pharmacological agents [54], is associated with an increase in IHTG content. The presence of NAFLD is associated with a marked increase in VLDL-triglyceride secretion rate in human subjects, independent of BMI and percent body fat [34, 55]. However, the increased rate of hepatic VLDL-triglyceride secretion is apparently not adequate to compensate for the increase in the rate of IHTG production, and is therefore unable to prevent the development of steatosis.

Role of Leptin in the Pathogenesis of NAFLD

Data from Animal Studies

Animal models with genetic mutations that cause leptin deficiency (*ob/ob*) or a defective leptin receptor (*db/db* and *fa/fa*) are characterized by obesity and hepatic steatosis. Normalizing leptin signaling in these rodent models, either by providing exogenous leptin (in *ob/ob* animals) or by adenovirus-mediated expression of leptin receptors

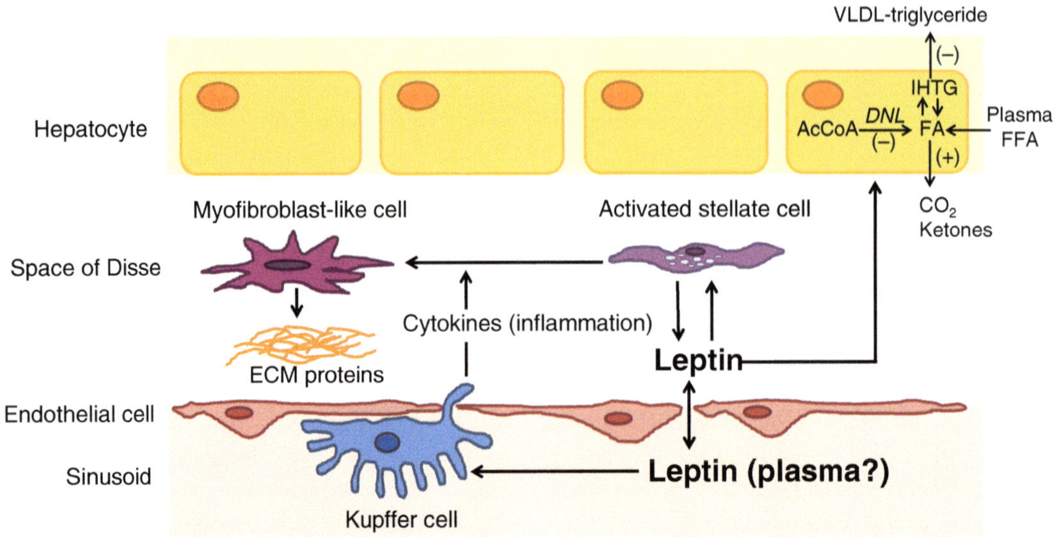

Fig. 8.1 Putative effects of leptin on hepatic steatosis, inflammation, and fibrosis. Although leptin decreases the secretion of very low-density lipoprotein (VLDL)-triglyceride from hepatocytes, leptin facilitates an overall reduction in intrahepatic triglyceride (IHTG) content by increasing fatty acid (FA) oxidation and ketogenesis and by decreasing de novo lipogenesis (DNL). Leptin facilitates the progression of simple steatosis to inflammation and fibrosis; leptin produced by activated hepatic stellate cells, and presumably leptin from plasma, acts on Kupffer cells and increases the production of cytokines that cause inflammation and induce trans-differentiation of stellate cells into myofibroblast-like cells. Myofibroblast cells produce extracellular matrix (ECM) proteins, leading to fibrosis. Leptin can also directly act on stellate cells and induce trans-differentiation into myofibroblast-like cells

(in *db/db* and *fa/fa* animals), decreases body weight and ameliorates steatosis [56–65]. However, providing exogenous leptin to diet-induced obese (DIO) rodent models often does not have marked effects on body weight or IHTG content, because of obesity-induced leptin resistance [66–69]. Alterations in hepatic fatty acid uptake, de novo lipogenesis, fatty acid oxidation, and VLDL-triglyceride secretion are among the proposed mechanisms for leptin-mediated regulation of IHTG balance (Fig. 8.1) [57, 61–63, 66, 68, 70–74]. In leptin-responsive animals, leptin-induced reduction in IHTG content is independent of the decrease in food intake and body weight [57, 72, 73], and occurs within a couple of hours after leptin injection [66, 68]. A reduction in hepatic VLDL-triglyceride secretion and an increase in hepatic fatty acid oxidation and ketogenesis occur rapidly after leptin administration [66, 68], whereas a reduction in hepatic de novo lipogenesis is observed only after chronic leptin treatment [70]. These observations suggest that shunting of hepatic fatty acids towards oxidation and ketone body formation is the primary mechanism for acute leptin-induced reduction in IHTG (Table 8.1).

Table 8.1 Putative metabolic mechanisms for leptin-induced reduction in intrahepatic triglyceride content

↑ Fatty acid oxidation
↑ Ketogenesis
↓ De novo lipogenesis

Data from several studies conducted in rodent models and cell systems suggest that leptin is required for the progression of steatosis to steatohepatitis by facilitating the activation of inflammatory and oxidative stress pathways (Table 8.2). In genetically obese animal models of leptin deficiency (*ob/ob*) or defective leptin action (*db/db* and *fa/fa*), the accumulation of IHTG is not accompanied by hepatic inflammation and fibrosis, particularly when the animals are still young [58, 75–77]. Leptin binding to its functional receptor (long isoform, Ob-Rb) on Kupffer cells from leptin-responsive animal models induces

Table 8.2 Putative mechanisms for the inflammatory and fibrogenic effects of leptin on the liver

Pro-inflammatory mechanisms	*Target cell*
↑ TNF-α	KC
↑ MCP-1	KC
↑ IL-15	KC
↑ Free radicals	KC and HSC
↑ CD14 (KC surface receptor)	KC
Pro-fibrogenic mechanisms	*Target cell*
↑ TGF-β1	KC
↑ HSC proliferation	HSC
↑ Collagen type I	HSC
↑ Procollagen type I	HSC
↑ Smooth muscle actin	HSC
↑ Fibronectin	HSC
↑ TIMP-1	HSC
↓ MMP-1	HSC

TNF-α tumor necrosis factor alpha, *MCP-1* monocyte chemoattractant protein 1, *IL-15* interleukin 15, *TGF-β1* transforming growth factor beta 1, *TIMP-1* tissue inhibitor metalloproteinase-1, *MMP-1* matrix metalloproteinase 1, *KC* Kupffer cells, *HSC* hepatic stellate cells

cytokine release, specifically tumor necrosis factor (TNF)-α, transforming growth factor (TGF)-β1 and interleukin (IL)-15; these effects are much less pronounced in Kupffer cells from leptin receptor-deficient animals [78–80]. Furthermore, leptin causes oxidative stress in hepatic Kupffer and stellate cells from various leptin-responsive animal models and human cell lines [81–84]. Leptin can also facilitate Kupffer cell-mediated inflammation by upregulating CD14 gene expression and protein content. CD14 serves as a surface receptor in Kupffer cells and promotes hyper-reactivity to hepatic insults (e.g., endotoxin), which increases the production of inflammatory cytokines and accelerates the progression of liver inflammation and fibrosis [85].

A recent study conducted in DIO mice, in which steatohepatitis was induced by carbon tetrachloride administration, provides some insights into the mechanisms involved in leptin-mediated hepatic oxidative stress and inflammation [82]. The results from this study showed that carbon tetrachloride administration increased oxidative stress in the liver of DIO mice but not *ob/ob* mice, or DIO mice treated with leptin antibody, and that leptin replacement in *ob/ob* mice restored free radical formation. Free radical formation and expression of the pro-inflammatory cytokines, TNF-α and monocyte chemoattractant protein (MCP)-1, were decreased by inhibiting peroxynitrite, inducible nitric oxide synthase (iNOS), and nicotinamide adenine dinucleotide phosphate (NADPH) oxidase, and by Kupffer cell depletion. Taken together, these data suggest that leptin contributes to the pathogenesis of liver damage by activating NADPH oxidase, which induces iNOS, and stimulates the release of TNF-α and MCP-1 from Kupffer cells through a peroxynitrite-dependent mechanism.

Hepatic fibrosis results from the accumulation of extracellular matrix (ECM) proteins (e.g., fibrillar collagen, fibronectin, laminin, proteoglycans) produced by activated hepatic stellate cells (HSC) that have been transformed to myofibroblast-like cells. Despite extensive hepatic steatosis, leptin-deficient (*ob/ob*) animals exhibit much less hepatic fibrosis than their lean littermates in response to carbon tetrachloride administration [86–89], *Schistosoma mansoni* infection [89, 90], and methionine- and choline-deficient diet feeding [88]. However, fibrotic changes occur as expected when exogenous replacement leptin is co-administered with the fibrotic stimulus [87–89]. Exogenous leptin also augments fibrotic changes that occur in normal animals in response to acute and chronic fibrogenic stimuli (hepatotoxic chemicals such as carbon tetrachloride or thioacetamide) [91]. Furthermore, leptin-resistant animals who have no functional leptin receptors (*fa/fa*) are also resistant to the fibrotic changes that occur in the liver of their lean littermates after thioacetamide administration [92], bile duct ligation [93], pig serum administration [94], or choline-deficient diet feeding [95]. However, leptin-resistant animals that have a functional defect in the long leptin receptor isoform (Ob-Rb) but an intact short leptin receptor isoform (Ob-Ra) (*db/db*) exhibit significant hepatic fibrosis in response to methionine- and choline-deficient diet feeding [96], but have less fibrosis than wild-type littermates in response to thioacetamide administration [97]. These findings suggest that leptin has a permissive role in the fibrogenic pathway in response to liver injury (Table 8.2), and that hepatic leptin signaling [98] through either the long leptin receptor (which is the fully functional isoform) or the short leptin receptor (which is not a fully functional isoform) is sufficient for these changes to occur.

The results from a series of studies conducted in cell systems suggest permissive indirect and direct roles of leptin in the pathogenesis hepatic fibrosis (Fig. 8.1). Leptin is expressed in both rat [92, 99, 100] and human activated HSC [101], but not in quiescent HSC, Kupffer cells, or hepatocytes, which express leptin receptors [92, 99, 100]. Leptin produced by activated HSC acts on Kupffer cells and increases TGF-β1 production in response to fibrogenic stimuli [79, 92, 102]. The increase in TGF-β1 seen normally during fibrogenesis is abolished by leptin deficiency, or dysfunctional leptin signaling [92], but is restored by leptin replacement [88, 89]. TGF-β1 is a major profibrogenic cytokine, and activates type I collagen promoters, upregulates gene expression of ECM proteins, such as collagen and fibronectin [103], and is important in the hepatic wound-healing response, including myofibroblast generation and extracellular matrix deposition [104]. Therefore, attenuated or absent leptin signaling prevents the increase in gene expression of ECM proteins (procollagen type I, collagen type I, fibronectin, smooth muscle actin), and the increase in hepatic hydroxyproline concentration (a marker of collagen content) in response to liver injury, whereas leptin administration abolishes these effects and restores normal fibrogenic responses [88, 89, 91, 94, 105]. Data from studies conducted in both animal and human HSC systems support direct effects of leptin in the pathogenesis of fibrosis by: (1) upregulating collagen type I gene expression and protein production via the Jak-Stat pathway [86, 106, 107]; (2) upregulating tissue inhibitor of metalloproteinase-1 (TIMP-1) and downregulating matrix metalloproteinase (MMP)-1 via the Jak-Stat and ERK and p38 pathways [81, 84, 107–109]; and (3) upregulating gene expression of several proinflammatory cytokines [105, 109], and (4) protecting HSC from apoptosis and increasing their proliferation [79, 97, 110–112]. These observations are consistent with both an indirect effect of leptin in hepatic fibrogenesis by stimulating HSC transdifferentiation into myofibroblast-like cells that produce ECM proteins [79, 113] and an direct effect on HSC, themselves.

Data from Human Studies

The relationship between plasma leptin concentrations and the amount of IHTG or the histological grades of hepatic steatosis, inflammation, and fibrosis has been evaluated in several cross-sectional studies in human subjects. The results from some studies found that plasma leptin concentrations are greater in: (1) obese patients with NAFLD who have moderate-to-severe steatosis than in those with mild steatosis; (2) those with moderate-to-severe lobular and portal inflammation than in those with mild degrees of inflammation; and (3) those with hepatic fibrosis than in those without fibrosis [85, 114–120]. However, BMI and fat mass were also greater in these groups, which might have been responsible for the increase in leptin concentrations [85, 114–120]. In contrast, most, but not all [121–125], studies that matched subject groups on BMI and sex, or body fat, found no significant differences in plasma leptin concentrations: (1) among subjects with NASH or NAFL, or normal IHTG content [126–133]; (2) between NAFLD subjects with different grades of steatosis [134]; (3) between those with simple steatosis and those with steatohepatitis [85, 126, 128, 129, 133, 135]; and (4) between those with and without liver fibrosis [121]. Also, the results from most multivariate analyses have found that plasma leptin concentration is not independently associated with hepatic histopathology after controlling for BMI and sex [114, 117, 121, 122, 128, 135–138]. However, the results from some studies have found independent associations between circulating leptin and steatosis [114, 120, 121, 124] and between free leptin index (ratio of circulating leptin to its soluble receptor) and both steatosis and fibrosis [137]. Baseline plasma leptin concentration is not associated with NAFLD progression in subjects who already have NAFLD [139], and does not predict the future incidence of NAFLD, determined by ultrasound, during a 7-year follow-up among the general population [140]. Collectively, these observations suggest that leptin is not involved in the pathogenesis and progression of NAFLD in people.

Leptin Deficiency

Leptin therapy has profound hepatic effects in people who have absent or very low plasma leptin concentrations caused by genetic leptin deficiency or congenital or acquired lipodystrophy. These patients have severe hepatomegaly and steatosis, which markedly improves or is completely normalized with leptin replacement therapy [141–148]. Moreover, long-term leptin therapy (~2 years) in patients with acquired and congenital generalized and partial lipodystrophies caused a marked decrease in IHTG content, hepatocellular ballooning and the NASH activity score, but did not affect hepatic fibrosis [144, 149]. Nonetheless, leptin therapy is not always effective in people with low plasma leptin concentrations, and we are aware of one study in patients with human immunodeficiency virus (HIV)-associated lipoatrophy and hypoleptinemia [150] and of a case report of an adolescent girl with acquired generalized lipodystrophy and mild steatohepatitis [151], which found leptin replacement therapy did not improve hepatic steatosis or histopathology. The reason why leptin replacement therapy has favorable effects on hepatic inflammation and does not worsen hepatic fibrosis in people, but promotes inflammation and fibrosis in rodent models is not clear, and underscores the limitations of using these models to understand the pathophysiology of NAFLD in people. The composite of these data demonstrate that leptin therapy in human subjects with some form of leptin deficiency improves hepatic steatosis and specific markers of liver injury. The potential therapeutic effect of leptin administration in obese patients with NAFLD, who typically have high plasma leptin concentrations because of obesity, is not known and deserves further study.

Conclusions and Direction for Future Research

Data from studies conducted in rodent models and in both animal and human cell systems demonstrate that leptin prevents or decreases hepatic steatosis, but facilitates hepatic inflammation and fibrosis. The actions of leptin are particularly pronounced in genetically obese animal models that are leptin-deficient or have defective leptin signaling, and in lipodystrophic animals that have very low plasma leptin concentrations. In contrast, the effects of leptin on hepatic pathophysiology are not usually observed in diet-induced obese animal models, which are hyperleptinemic and presumably resistant to leptin. In people, leptin replacement therapy has profound effects on the liver in patients with absolute or relative leptin deficiency. In contrast, the totality of data in people without leptin deficiency does not support an important role of leptin in the development of steatosis or the progression of NAFL to NASH. However, these conclusions are based on the absence of correlations between systemic plasma leptin concentrations and liver pathology. It is possible that leptin acts primarily in an autocrine and/or paracrine fashion in the liver, which cannot be assessed by evaluating circulating leptin. Therefore, the importance of leptin in the pathogenesis of NAFLD in overweight and obese people is still not clear, and requires additional study.

References

1. Chalasani N, Younossi Z, Lavine JE, et al. The diagnosis and management of non-alcoholic fatty liver disease: practice Guideline by the American Association for the Study of Liver Diseases, American College of Gastroenterology, and the American Gastroenterological Association. Hepatology. 2012; 55:2005–23.
2. Hoyumpa Jr AM, Greene HL, Dunn GD, Schenker S. Fatty liver: biochemical and clinical considerations. Am J Dig Dis. 1975;20:1142–70.
3. Kleiner DE, Brunt EM, Van Natta M, et al. Design and validation of a histological scoring system for nonalcoholic fatty liver disease. Hepatology. 2005; 41:1313–21.

4. Fabbrini E, Conte C, Magkos F. Methods for assessing intrahepatic fat content and steatosis. Curr Opin Clin Nutr Metab Care. 2009;12:474–81.
5. Szczepaniak LS, Nurenberg P, Leonard D, et al. Magnetic resonance spectroscopy to measure hepatic triglyceride content: prevalence of hepatic steatosis in the general population. Am J Physiol Endocrinol Metab. 2005;288:E462–8.
6. Petersen KF, Dufour S, Feng J, et al. Increased prevalence of insulin resistance and nonalcoholic fatty liver disease in Asian-Indian men. Proc Natl Acad Sci U S A. 2006;103:18273–7.
7. Ruhl CE, Everhart JE. Determinants of the association of overweight with elevated serum alanine aminotransferase activity in the United States. Gastroenterology. 2003;124:71–9.
8. Lee JY, Kim KM, Lee SG, et al. Prevalence and risk factors of non-alcoholic fatty liver disease in potential living liver donors in Korea: a review of 589 consecutive liver biopsies in a single center. J Hepatol. 2007;47:239–44.
9. Marcos A, Fisher RA, Ham JM, et al. Selection and outcome of living donors for adult to adult right lobe transplantation. Transplantation. 2000;69:2410–5.
10. Hilden M, Christoffersen P, Juhl E, Dalgaard JB. Liver histology in a 'normal' population—examinations of 503 consecutive fatal traffic casualties. Scand J Gastroenterol. 1977;12:593–7.
11. Lee RG. Nonalcoholic steatohepatitis: a study of 49 patients. Hum Pathol. 1989;20:594–8.
12. Gholam PM, Kotler DP, Flancbaum LJ. Liver pathology in morbidly obese patients undergoing Roux-en-Y gastric bypass surgery. Obes Surg. 2002;12:49–51.
13. Romeo S, Kozlitina J, Xing C, et al. Genetic variation in PNPLA3 confers susceptibility to nonalcoholic fatty liver disease. Nat Genet. 2008;40:1461–5.
14. Browning JD, Szczepaniak LS, Dobbins R, et al. Prevalence of hepatic steatosis in an urban population in the United States: impact of ethnicity. Hepatology. 2004;40:1387–95.
15. Fabbrini E, Magkos F. Obesity and the pathogenesis of nonalcoholic fatty liver disease. In: Kushner RF, Bessesen DH, editors. Treatment of the obese patient, 2nd ed. New York, NY: Springer; 2014:121–35.
16. Korenblat KM, Fabbrini E, Mohammed BS, Klein S. Liver, muscle, and adipose tissue insulin action is directly related to intrahepatic triglyceride content in obese subjects. Gastroenterology. 2008;134:1369–75.
17. Seppala-Lindroos A, Vehkavaara S, Hakkinen AM, et al. Fat accumulation in the liver is associated with defects in insulin suppression of glucose production and serum free fatty acids independent of obesity in normal men. J Clin Endocrinol Metab. 2002;87:3023–8.
18. Sanyal AJ, Campbell-Sargent C, Mirshahi F, et al. Nonalcoholic steatohepatitis: association of insulin resistance and mitochondrial abnormalities. Gastroenterology. 2001;120:1183–92.
19. Bugianesi E, Gastaldelli A, Vanni E, et al. Insulin resistance in non-diabetic patients with non-alcoholic fatty liver disease: sites and mechanisms. Diabetologia. 2005;48:634–42.
20. Fabbrini E, Magkos F, Mohammed BS, et al. Intrahepatic fat, not visceral fat, is linked with metabolic complications of obesity. Proc Natl Acad Sci U S A. 2009;106:15430–5.
21. Vega GL, Chandalia M, Szczepaniak LS, Grundy SM. Metabolic correlates of nonalcoholic fatty liver in women and men. Hepatology. 2007;46:716–22.
22. Magkos F, Su X, Bradley D, et al. Intrahepatic diacylglycerol content is associated with hepatic insulin resistance in obese subjects. Gastroenterology. 2012;142:1444.e2–6.e2.
23. Kumashiro N, Erion DM, Zhang D, et al. Cellular mechanism of insulin resistance in nonalcoholic fatty liver disease. Proc Natl Acad Sci U S A. 2011;108:16381–5.
24. Birkenfeld AL, Shulman GI. Nonalcoholic fatty liver disease, hepatic insulin resistance, and type 2 diabetes. Hepatology. 2014;59:713–23.
25. Jornayvaz FR, Shulman GI. Diacylglycerol activation of protein kinase Cepsilon and hepatic insulin resistance. Cell Metab. 2012;15:574–84.
26. Cai D, Yuan M, Frantz DF, et al. Local and systemic insulin resistance resulting from hepatic activation of IKK-beta and NF-kappaB. Nat Med. 2005;11:183–90.
27. Monetti M, Levin MC, Watt MJ, et al. Dissociation of hepatic steatosis and insulin resistance in mice overexpressing DGAT in the liver. Cell Metab. 2007;6:69–78.
28. Minehira K, Young SG, Villanueva CJ, et al. Blocking VLDL secretion causes hepatic steatosis but does not affect peripheral lipid stores or insulin sensitivity in mice. J Lipid Res. 2008;49:2038–44.
29. Grefhorst A, Hoekstra J, Derks TG, et al. Acute hepatic steatosis in mice by blocking beta-oxidation does not reduce insulin sensitivity of very-low-density lipoprotein production. Am J Physiol Gastrointest Liver Physiol. 2005;289:G592–8.
30. Yu XX, Murray SF, Pandey SK, et al. Antisense oligonucleotide reduction of DGAT2 expression improves hepatic steatosis and hyperlipidemia in obese mice. Hepatology. 2005;42:362–71.
31. Amaro A, Fabbrini E, Kars M, et al. Dissociation between intrahepatic triglyceride content and insulin resistance in familial hypobetalipoproteinemia. Gastroenterology. 2010;139:149–53.
32. Visser ME, Lammers NM, Nederveen AJ, et al. Hepatic steatosis does not cause insulin resistance in people with familial hypobetalipoproteinaemia. Diabetologia. 2011;54:2113–21.
33. Fabbrini E, deHaseth D, Deivanayagam S, Mohammed BS, Vitola BE, Klein S. Alterations in fatty acid kinetics in obese adolescents with increased intrahepatic triglyceride content. Obesity (Silver Spring). 2009;17:25–9.

34. Fabbrini E, Mohammed BS, Magkos F, Korenblat KM, Patterson BW, Klein S. Alterations in adipose tissue and hepatic lipid kinetics in obese men and women with nonalcoholic fatty liver disease. Gastroenterology. 2008;134:424–31.
35. Pardina E, Baena-Fustegueras JA, Catalan R, et al. Increased expression and activity of hepatic lipase in the liver of morbidly obese adult patients in relation to lipid content. Obes Surg. 2009;19:894–904.
36. Westerbacka J, Kolak M, Kiviluoto T, et al. Genes involved in fatty acid partitioning and binding, lipolysis, monocyte/macrophage recruitment, and inflammation are overexpressed in the human fatty liver of insulin-resistant subjects. Diabetes. 2007;56: 2759–65.
37. Miquilena-Colina ME, Lima-Cabello E, Sanchez-Campos S, et al. Hepatic fatty acid translocase CD36 upregulation is associated with insulin resistance, hyperinsulinaemia and increased steatosis in non-alcoholic steatohepatitis and chronic hepatitis C. Gut. 2011;60:1394–402.
38. Hellerstein MK, Schwarz JM, Neese RA. Regulation of hepatic de novo lipogenesis in humans. Annu Rev Nutr. 1996;16:523–57.
39. Barrows BR, Parks EJ. Contributions of different fatty acid sources to very low-density lipoprotein-triacylglycerol in the fasted and fed states. J Clin Endocrinol Metab. 2006;91:1446–52.
40. Diraison F, Moulin P, Beylot M. Contribution of hepatic de novo lipogenesis and reesterification of plasma non esterified fatty acids to plasma triglyceride synthesis during non-alcoholic fatty liver disease. Diabetes Metab. 2003;29:478–85.
41. Donnelly KL, Smith CI, Schwarzenberg SJ, Jessurun J, Boldt MD, Parks EJ. Sources of fatty acids stored in liver and secreted via lipoproteins in patients with nonalcoholic fatty liver disease. J Clin Invest. 2005;115:1343–51.
42. Petersen KF, Dufour S, Savage DB, et al. The role of skeletal muscle insulin resistance in the pathogenesis of the metabolic syndrome. Proc Natl Acad Sci U S A. 2007;104:12587–94.
43. Ibdah JA, Perlegas P, Zhao Y, et al. Mice heterozygous for a defect in mitochondrial trifunctional protein develop hepatic steatosis and insulin resistance. Gastroenterology. 2005;128:1381–90.
44. Zhang D, Liu ZX, Choi CS, et al. Mitochondrial dysfunction due to long-chain Acyl-CoA dehydrogenase deficiency causes hepatic steatosis and hepatic insulin resistance. Proc Natl Acad Sci U S A. 2007;104:17075–80.
45. Seo YS, Kim JH, Jo NY, et al. PPAR agonists treatment is effective in a nonalcoholic fatty liver disease animal model by modulating fatty-acid metabolic enzymes. J Gastroenterol Hepatol. 2008;23: 102–9.
46. Xu A, Wang Y, Keshaw H, Xu LY, Lam KS, Cooper GJ. The fat-derived hormone adiponectin alleviates alcoholic and nonalcoholic fatty liver diseases in mice. J Clin Invest. 2003;112:91–100.
47. Stefanovic-Racic M, Perdomo G, Mantell BS, Sipula IJ, Brown NF, O'Doherty RM. A moderate increase in carnitine palmitoyltransferase 1a activity is sufficient to substantially reduce hepatic triglyceride levels. Am J Physiol Endocrinol Metab. 2008;294: E969–77.
48. Savage DB, Choi CS, Samuel VT, et al. Reversal of diet-induced hepatic steatosis and hepatic insulin resistance by antisense oligonucleotide inhibitors of acetyl-CoA carboxylases 1 and 2. J Clin Invest. 2006;116:817–24.
49. Chalasani N, Gorski JC, Asghar MS, et al. Hepatic cytochrome P450 2E1 activity in nondiabetic patients with nonalcoholic steatohepatitis. Hepatology. 2003; 37:544–50.
50. Kotronen A, Seppala-Lindroos A, Vehkavaara S, et al. Liver fat and lipid oxidation in humans. Liver Int. 2009;29:1439–46.
51. Greco D, Kotronen A, Westerbacka J, et al. Gene expression in human NAFLD. Am J Physiol Gastrointest Liver Physiol. 2008;294:G1281–7.
52. Kohjima M, Enjoji M, Higuchi N, et al. Re-evaluation of fatty acid metabolism-related gene expression in nonalcoholic fatty liver disease. Int J Mol Med. 2007;20:351–8.
53. Schonfeld G, Patterson BW, Yablonskiy DA, et al. Fatty liver in familial hypobetalipoproteinemia: triglyceride assembly into VLDL particles is affected by the extent of hepatic steatosis. J Lipid Res. 2003;44:470–8.
54. Cuchel M, Bloedon LT, Szapary PO, et al. Inhibition of microsomal triglyceride transfer protein in familial hypercholesterolemia. N Engl J Med. 2007;356: 148–56.
55. Adiels M, Taskinen MR, Packard C, et al. Overproduction of large VLDL particles is driven by increased liver fat content in man. Diabetologia. 2006;49:755–65.
56. Lee Y, Wang MY, Kakuma T, et al. Liporegulation in diet-induced obesity. The antisteatotic role of hyperleptinemia. J Biol Chem. 2001;276:5629–35.
57. Singh A, Wirtz M, Parker N, et al. Leptin-mediated changes in hepatic mitochondrial metabolism, structure, and protein levels. Proc Natl Acad Sci U S A. 2009;106:13100–5.
58. Baffy G, Zhang CY, Glickman JN, Lowell BB. Obesity-related fatty liver is unchanged in mice deficient for mitochondrial uncoupling protein 2. Hepatology. 2002;35:753–61.
59. Leclercq IA, Vansteenberghe M, Lebrun VB, et al. Defective hepatic regeneration after partial hepatectomy in leptin-deficient mice is not rescued by exogenous leptin. Lab Invest. 2006;86:1161–71.
60. Yang SQ, Lin HZ, Lane MD, Clemens M, Diehl AM. Obesity increases sensitivity to endotoxin liver injury: implications for the pathogenesis of steatohepatitis. Proc Natl Acad Sci U S A. 1997; 94:2557–62.
61. Ge F, Zhou S, Hu C, Lobdell 4th H, Berk PD. Insulin- and leptin-regulated fatty acid uptake plays a key

causal role in hepatic steatosis in mice with intact leptin signaling but not in ob/ob or db/db mice. Am J Physiol Gastrointest Liver Physiol. 2010;299: G855–66.
62. Asilmaz E, Cohen P, Miyazaki M, et al. Site and mechanism of leptin action in a rodent form of congenital lipodystrophy. J Clin Invest. 2004;113: 414–24.
63. Cohen P, Miyazaki M, Socci ND, et al. Role for stearoyl-CoA desaturase-1 in leptin-mediated weight loss. Science. 2002;297:240–3.
64. Stucchi P, Guzman-Ruiz R, Gil-Ortega M, et al. Leptin resistance develops spontaneously in mice during adult life in a tissue-specific manner. Consequences for hepatic steatosis. Biochimie. 2011;93:1779–85.
65. Warne JP, Alemi F, Reed AS, et al. Impairment of central leptin-mediated PI3K signaling manifested as hepatic steatosis independent of hyperphagia and obesity. Cell Metab. 2011;14:791–803.
66. Huang W, Dedousis N, Bandi A, Lopaschuk GD, O'Doherty RM. Liver triglyceride secretion and lipid oxidative metabolism are rapidly altered by leptin in vivo. Endocrinology. 2006;147:1480–7.
67. Huang W, Dedousis N, O'Doherty RM. Hepatic steatosis and plasma dyslipidemia induced by a high-sucrose diet are corrected by an acute leptin infusion. J Appl Physiol. 2007;102:2260–5.
68. Huang W, Metlakunta A, Dedousis N, Ortmeyer HK, Stefanovic-Racic M, O'Doherty RM. Leptin augments the acute suppressive effects of insulin on hepatic very low-density lipoprotein production in rats. Endocrinology. 2009;150:2169–74.
69. Fishman S, Muzumdar RH, Atzmon G, et al. Resistance to leptin action is the major determinant of hepatic triglyceride accumulation in vivo. FASEB J. 2007;21:53–60.
70. Cohen SM, Werrmann JG, Tota MR. 13C NMR study of the effects of leptin treatment on kinetics of hepatic intermediary metabolism. Proc Natl Acad Sci U S A. 1998;95:7385–90.
71. Ferrante Jr AW, Thearle M, Liao T, Leibel RL. Effects of leptin deficiency and short-term repletion on hepatic gene expression in genetically obese mice. Diabetes. 2001;50:2268–78.
72. Cortes VA, Cautivo KM, Rong S, Garg A, Horton JD, Agarwal AK. Leptin ameliorates insulin resistance and hepatic steatosis in Agpat2-/- lipodystrophic mice independent of hepatocyte leptin receptors. J Lipid Res. 2014;55:276–88.
73. Shimabukuro M, Koyama K, Chen G, et al. Direct antidiabetic effect of leptin through triglyceride depletion of tissues. Proc Natl Acad Sci U S A. 1997;94:4637–41.
74. Stenger C, Hanse M, Pratte D, et al. Up-regulation of hepatic lipolysis stimulated lipoprotein receptor by leptin: a potential lever for controlling lipid clearance during the postprandial phase. FASEB J. 2010; 24:4218–28.
75. Trak-Smayra V, Paradis V, Massart J, Nasser S, Jebara V, Fromenty B. Pathology of the liver in obese and diabetic ob/ob and db/db mice fed a standard or high-calorie diet. Int J Exp Pathol. 2011; 92:413–21.
76. Koteish A, Mae DA. Animal models of steatohepatitis. Best Pract Res Clin Gastroenterol. 2002;16: 679–90.
77. Sugihara T, Koda M, Kishina M, et al. Fatty liver Shionogi-ob/ob mouse: a new candidate for a non-alcoholic steatohepatitis model. Hepatol Res. 2013;43:547–56.
78. Shen J, Sakaida I, Uchida K, Terai S, Okita K. Leptin enhances TNF-alpha production via p38 and JNK MAPK in LPS-stimulated Kupffer cells. Life Sci. 2005;77:1502–15.
79. Wang J, Leclercq I, Brymora JM, et al. Kupffer cells mediate leptin-induced liver fibrosis. Gastroenterology. 2009;137:713–23.
80. Li Z, Lin H, Yang S, Diehl AM. Murine leptin deficiency alters Kupffer cell production of cytokines that regulate the innate immune system. Gastroenterology. 2002;123:1304–10.
81. Cao Q, Mak KM, Lieber CS. Leptin represses matrix metalloproteinase-1 gene expression in LX2 human hepatic stellate cells. J Hepatol. 2007;46:124–33.
82. Chatterjee S, Ganini D, Tokar EJ, et al. Leptin is key to peroxynitrite-mediated oxidative stress and Kupffer cell activation in experimental non-alcoholic steatohepatitis. J Hepatol. 2013;58:778–84.
83. Schroyen B, Guimaraes EL, Dolle L, et al. Leptin-mediated reactive oxygen species production does not significantly affect primary mouse hepatocyte functions in vitro. Eur J Gastroenterol Hepatol. 2012;24:1370–80.
84. Cao Q, Mak KM, Ren C, Lieber CS. Leptin stimulates tissue inhibitor of metalloproteinase-1 in human hepatic stellate cells: respective roles of the JAK/STAT and JAK-mediated H2O2-dependant MAPK pathways. J Biol Chem. 2004;279:4292–304.
85. Imajo K, Fujita K, Yoneda M, et al. Hyperresponsivity to low-dose endotoxin during progression to nonalcoholic steatohepatitis is regulated by leptin-mediated signaling. Cell Metab. 2012;16:44–54.
86. Saxena NK, Ikeda K, Rockey DC, Friedman SL, Anania FA. Leptin in hepatic fibrosis: evidence for increased collagen production in stellate cells and lean littermates of ob/ob mice. Hepatology. 2002; 35:762–71.
87. Honda H, Ikejima K, Hirose M, et al. Leptin is required for fibrogenic responses induced by thioacetamide in the murine liver. Hepatology. 2002;36:12–21.
88. Leclercq IA, Farrell GC, Schriemer R, Robertson GR. Leptin is essential for the hepatic fibrogenic response to chronic liver injury. J Hepatol. 2002; 37:206–13.
89. Potter JJ, Rennie-Tankesley L, Mezey E. Influence of leptin in the development of hepatic fibrosis produced in mice by Schistosoma mansoni infection and by chronic carbon tetrachloride administration. J Hepatol. 2003;38:281–8.
90. Potter JJ, Mezey E. Leptin deficiency reduces but does not eliminate the development of hepatic

fibrosis in mice infected with Schistosoma mansoni. Liver. 2002;22:173–7.
91. Ikejima K, Honda H, Yoshikawa M, et al. Leptin augments inflammatory and profibrogenic responses in the murine liver induced by hepatotoxic chemicals. Hepatology. 2001;34:288–97.
92. Ikejima K, Takei Y, Honda H, et al. Leptin receptor-mediated signaling regulates hepatic fibrogenesis and remodeling of extracellular matrix in the rat. Gastroenterology. 2002;122:1399–410.
93. Ding X, Saxena NK, Lin S, Xu A, Srinivasan S, Anania FA. The roles of leptin and adiponectin: a novel paradigm in adipocytokine regulation of liver fibrosis and stellate cell biology. Am J Pathol. 2005;166:1655–69.
94. Sakaida I, Jinhua S, Uchida K, Terai S, Okita K. Leptin receptor-deficient Zucker (fa/fa) rat retards the development of pig serum-induced liver fibrosis with Kupffer cell dysfunction. Life Sci. 2003;73: 2491–501.
95. Kitade M, Yoshiji H, Kojima H, et al. Leptin-mediated neovascularization is a prerequisite for progression of nonalcoholic steatohepatitis in rats. Hepatology. 2006;44:983–91.
96. Sahai A, Malladi P, Pan X, et al. Obese and diabetic db/db mice develop marked liver fibrosis in a model of nonalcoholic steatohepatitis: role of short-form leptin receptors and osteopontin. Am J Physiol Gastrointest Liver Physiol. 2004;287:G1035–43.
97. Qamar A, Sheikh SZ, Masud A, et al. In vitro and in vivo protection of stellate cells from apoptosis by leptin. Dig Dis Sci. 2006;51:1697–705.
98. Zhou J, Lei W, Shen L, Luo HS, Shen ZX. Primary study of leptin and human hepatocellular carcinoma in vitro. World J Gastroenterol. 2008;14:2900–4.
99. Potter JJ, Womack L, Mezey E, Anania FA. Transdifferentiation of rat hepatic stellate cells results in leptin expression. Biochem Biophys Res Commun. 1998;244:178–82.
100. Otte C, Otte JM, Strodthoff D, et al. Expression of leptin and leptin receptor during the development of liver fibrosis and cirrhosis. Exp Clin Endocrinol Diabetes. 2004;112:10–7.
101. Tang M, Potter JJ, Mezey E. Leptin enhances the effect of transforming growth factor beta in increasing type I collagen formation. Biochem Biophys Res Commun. 2002;297:906–11.
102. Ikejima K, Lang T, Zhang YJ, et al. Expression of leptin receptors in hepatic sinusoidal cells. Comp Hepatol. 2004;3 Suppl 1:S12.
103. Penttinen RP, Kobayashi S, Bornstein P. Transforming growth factor beta increases mRNA for matrix proteins both in the presence and in the absence of changes in mRNA stability. Proc Natl Acad Sci U S A. 1988;85:1105–8.
104. Dooley S, ten Dijke P. TGF-beta in progression of liver disease. Cell Tissue Res. 2012;347:245–56.
105. Choi SS, Syn WK, Karaca GF, et al. Leptin promotes the myofibroblastic phenotype in hepatic stellate cells by activating the hedgehog pathway. J Biol Chem. 2010;285:36551–60.
106. Saxena NK, Saliba G, Floyd JJ, Anania FA. Leptin induces increased alpha2(I) collagen gene expression in cultured rat hepatic stellate cells. J Cell Biochem. 2003;89:311–20.
107. Niu L, Wang X, Li J, et al. Leptin stimulates alpha1(I) collagen expression in human hepatic stellate cells via the phosphatidylinositol 3-kinase/Akt signalling pathway. Liver Int. 2007;27:1265–72.
108. Cao Q, Mak KM, Lieber CS. Leptin enhances alpha1(I) collagen gene expression in LX-2 human hepatic stellate cells through JAK-mediated H2O2-dependent MAPK pathways. J Cell Biochem. 2006;97:188–97.
109. Aleffi S, Petrai I, Bertolani C, et al. Upregulation of proinflammatory and proangiogenic cytokines by leptin in human hepatic stellate cells. Hepatology. 2005;42:1339–48.
110. Saxena NK, Titus MA, Ding X, et al. Leptin as a novel profibrogenic cytokine in hepatic stellate cells: mitogenesis and inhibition of apoptosis mediated by extracellular regulated kinase (Erk) and Akt phosphorylation. FASEB J. 2004;18:1612–4.
111. Jiang JX, Mikami K, Shah VH, Torok NJ. Leptin induces phagocytosis of apoptotic bodies by hepatic stellate cells via a Rho guanosine triphosphatase-dependent mechanism. Hepatology. 2008;48: 1497–505.
112. Lang T, Ikejima K, Yoshikawa M, et al. Leptin facilitates proliferation of hepatic stellate cells through up-regulation of platelet-derived growth factor receptor. Biochem Biophys Res Commun. 2004; 323:1091–5.
113. Si HF, Li J, Lu XW, Jin Y. Suppressive effects of leflunomide on leptin-induced collagen I production involved in hepatic stellate cell proliferation. Exp Biol Med (Maywood). 2007;232:427–36.
114. Aller R, De Luis DA, Izaola O, et al. Lys656Asn polymorphism of leptin receptor, leptin levels and insulin resistance in patients with non alcoholic fatty liver disease. Eur Rev Med Pharmacol Sci. 2012;16: 335–41.
115. Ayonrinde OT, Olynyk JK, Beilin LJ, et al. Gender-specific differences in adipose distribution and adipocytokines influence adolescent nonalcoholic fatty liver disease. Hepatology. 2011;53:800–9.
116. Lebensztejn DM, Wojtkowska M, Skiba E, Werpachowska I, Tobolczyk J, Kaczmarski M. Serum concentration of adiponectin, leptin and resistin in obese children with non-alcoholic fatty liver disease. Adv Med Sci. 2009;54:177–82.
117. Lemoine M, Ratziu V, Kim M, et al. Serum adipokine levels predictive of liver injury in non-alcoholic fatty liver disease. Liver Int. 2009;29:1431–8.
118. Machado MV, Coutinho J, Carepa F, Costa A, Proenca H, Cortez-Pinto H. How adiponectin, leptin, and ghrelin orchestrate together and correlate with the severity of nonalcoholic fatty liver disease. Eur J Gastroenterol Hepatol. 2012;24:1166–72.
119. Uygun A, Kadayifci A, Yesilova Z, et al. Serum leptin levels in patients with nonalcoholic steatohepatitis. Am J Gastroenterol. 2000;95:3584–9.

120. Wong VW, Hui AY, Tsang SW, et al. Metabolic and adipokine profile of Chinese patients with nonalcoholic fatty liver disease. Clin Gastroenterol Hepatol. 2006;4:1154–61.
121. Chitturi S, Farrell G, Frost L, et al. Serum leptin in NASH correlates with hepatic steatosis but not fibrosis: a manifestation of lipotoxicity? Hepatology. 2002;36:403–9.
122. Singh DK, Sakhuja P, Rastogi A, Singh A, Gondal R, Sarin SK. Serum leptin levels correlate with body mass index but not with histologic disease severity in Indian patients with non-alcoholic steatohepatitis: a pilot study. Indian J Med Res. 2013;137:986–7.
123. Swellam M, Hamdy N. Association of nonalcoholic fatty liver disease with a single nucleotide polymorphism on the gene encoding leptin receptor. IUBMB Life. 2012;64:180–6.
124. Nobili V, Manco M, Ciampalini P, et al. Leptin, free leptin index, insulin resistance and liver fibrosis in children with non-alcoholic fatty liver disease. Eur J Endocrinol. 2006;155:735–43.
125. Serin E, Ozer B, Gumurdulu Y, Kayaselcuk F, Kul K, Boyacioglu S. Serum leptin level can be a negative marker of hepatocyte damage in nonalcoholic fatty liver. J Gastroenterol. 2003;38:471–6.
126. Chalasani N, Crabb DW, Cummings OW, et al. Does leptin play a role in the pathogenesis of human nonalcoholic steatohepatitis? Am J Gastroenterol. 2003;98:2771–6.
127. Iorio R, Sepe A, Giannattasio A, et al. Immune phenotype and serum leptin in children with obesity-related liver disease. J Clin Endocrinol Metab. 2006;91:341–4.
128. Kashyap SR, Diab DL, Baker AR, et al. Triglyceride levels and not adipokine concentrations are closely related to severity of nonalcoholic fatty liver disease in an obesity surgery cohort. Obesity (Silver Spring). 2009;17:1696–701.
129. Le D, Marks D, Lyle E, et al. Serum leptin levels, hepatic leptin receptor transcription, and clinical predictors of non-alcoholic steatohepatitis in obese bariatric surgery patients. Surg Endosc. 2007;21:1593–9.
130. Boyraz M, Cekmez F, Karaoglu A, Cinaz P, Durak M, Bideci A. Serum adiponectin, leptin, resistin and RBP4 levels in obese and metabolic syndrome children with nonalcoholic fatty liver disease. Biomark Med. 2013;7:737–45.
131. Musso G, Gambino R, Durazzo M, et al. Adipokines in NASH: postprandial lipid metabolism as a link between adiponectin and liver disease. Hepatology. 2005;42:1175–83.
132. Nakamuta M, Tada S, Uchimura K, et al. Serum leptin levels in patients with nonalcoholic chronic liver disease. Hepatogastroenterology. 2001;48:527–32.
133. Pagano C, Soardo G, Esposito W, et al. Plasma adiponectin is decreased in nonalcoholic fatty liver disease. Eur J Endocrinol. 2005;152:113–8.
134. Aller R, de Luis DA, Fernandez L, et al. Influence of insulin resistance and adipokines in the grade of steatosis of nonalcoholic fatty liver disease. Dig Dis Sci. 2008;53:1088–92.
135. Argentou M, Tiniakos DG, Karanikolas M, et al. Adipokine serum levels are related to liver histology in severely obese patients undergoing bariatric surgery. Obes Surg. 2009;19:1313–23.
136. Fitzpatrick E, Dew TK, Quaglia A, Sherwood RA, Mitry RR, Dhawan A. Analysis of adipokine concentrations in paediatric non-alcoholic fatty liver disease. Pediatr Obes. 2012;7:471–9.
137. Medici V, Ali MR, Seo S, et al. Increased soluble leptin receptor levels in morbidly obese patients with insulin resistance and nonalcoholic fatty liver disease. Obesity (Silver Spring). 2010;18:2268–73.
138. Nakao K, Nakata K, Ohtsubo N, et al. Association between nonalcoholic fatty liver, markers of obesity, and serum leptin level in young adults. Am J Gastroenterol. 2002;97:1796–801.
139. Wong VW, Wong GL, Choi PC, et al. Disease progression of non-alcoholic fatty liver disease: a prospective study with paired liver biopsies at 3 years. Gut. 2010;59:969–74.
140. Zelber-Sagi S, Lotan R, Shlomai A, et al. Predictors for incidence and remission of NAFLD in the general population during a seven-year prospective follow-up. J Hepatol. 2012;56:1145–51.
141. Petersen KF, Oral EA, Dufour S, et al. Leptin reverses insulin resistance and hepatic steatosis in patients with severe lipodystrophy. J Clin Invest. 2002;109:1345–50.
142. Misra A, Garg A. Clinical features and metabolic derangements in acquired generalized lipodystrophy: case reports and review of the literature. Medicine (Baltimore). 2003;82:129–46.
143. Javor ED, Cochran EK, Musso C, Young JR, Depaoli AM, Gorden P. Long-term efficacy of leptin replacement in patients with generalized lipodystrophy. Diabetes. 2005;54:1994–2002.
144. Javor ED, Ghany MG, Cochran EK, et al. Leptin reverses nonalcoholic steatohepatitis in patients with severe lipodystrophy. Hepatology. 2005;41:753–60.
145. Beltrand J, Beregszaszi M, Chevenne D, et al. Metabolic correction induced by leptin replacement treatment in young children with Berardinelli-Seip congenital lipoatrophy. Pediatrics. 2007;120: e291–6.
146. von Schnurbein J, Heni M, Moss A, et al. Rapid improvement of hepatic steatosis after initiation of leptin substitution in a leptin-deficient girl. Horm Res Paediatr. 2013;79:310–7.
147. Oral EA, Simha V, Ruiz E, et al. Leptin-replacement therapy for lipodystrophy. N Engl J Med. 2002; 346:570–8.
148. Simha V, Subramanyam L, Szczepaniak L, et al. Comparison of efficacy and safety of leptin replacement therapy in moderately and severely hypoleptinemic patients with familial partial lipodystrophy of the Dunnigan variety. J Clin Endocrinol Metab. 2012;97:785–92.

149. Safar Zadeh E, Lungu AO, Cochran EK, et al. The liver diseases of lipodystrophy: the long-term effect of leptin treatment. J Hepatol. 2013;59:131–7.
150. Mulligan K, Khatami H, Schwarz JM, et al. The effects of recombinant human leptin on visceral fat, dyslipidemia, and insulin resistance in patients with human immunodeficiency virus-associated lipoatrophy and hypoleptinemia. J Clin Endocrinol Metab. 2009;94:1137–44.
151. Kamran F, Rother KI, Cochran E, Safar Zadeh E, Gorden P, Brown RJ. Consequences of stopping and restarting leptin in an adolescent with lipodystrophy. Horm Res Paediatr. 2012;78:320–5.

9 Leptin in Acute Stress

Stephen N. Davis, Elizabeth M. Lamos, Hillary Loper, and Lisa M. Younk

Abbreviations

6-HDA	6-Hydroxydopamine
ACTH	Adrenocorticotropic hormone
AMPT	α-Methyl-p-tyrosine hydroxylase
BAT	Brown adipose tissue
CRH	Corticotropin releasing hormone
EE	Energy expenditure
hCG	Human chorionic gonadotropin
HF	High fat
HPA axis	Hypothalamic–pituitary–adrenal axis
IGF	Insulin-like growth factor
IL	Interleukin
SNA	Sympathetic nerve activity
SNS	Sympathetic nervous system
SOCS3	Suppressor of cytokine signaling 3
TNF	Tumor necrosis factor
UCP	Uncoupling protein
VMH	Ventromedial nucleus of the hypothalamus
WAT	White adipose tissue

Introduction

In the most basic sense, leptin is a signal of energy balance, decreasing in periods of negative energy balance (i.e., fasting, caloric restriction) and increasing in periods of excess energy (i.e., increased adipose tissue). A decline in leptin levels from basal state invokes an increase in appetite and food intake, as well as energy conservation. Reciprocally, increases in leptin levels signal satiety and related metabolic changes, such as an increase in gluconeogenic contribution to hepatic glucose output and an increase in fat mobilization and fatty acid oxidation. Under states of acute stress, the organism adapts via modulation of hormone release and metabolism, suggesting that leptin levels might change (Tables 9.1 and 9.2) during such situations to assist in regulation of energy expenditure, hunger, and shifts in glucose and lipid metabolism.

S.N. Davis, M.B.B.S., F.A.C.P. (✉)
Department of Medicine, University of Maryland Medical Center, 22 South Greene Street N3W42, Baltimore, MD 21201, USA
e-mail: sdavis@medicine.umaryland.edu

E.M. Lamos, M.D.
Division of Endocrinology, Diabetes and Nutrition, University of Maryland School of Medicine, 827 Linden Avenue, 2nd Floor, Baltimore, MD 21201, USA

H. Loper, M.D.
Division of Endocrinology, Diabetes and Nutrition, University of Maryland School of Medicine, 750 Main Street Suite 310, Baltimore, MD 21136, USA

L.M. Younk, B.S.
Department of Medicine, University of Maryland School of Medicine, 3-013 Bressler Research Building, 655 West Baltimore Street, Baltimore, MD 21201, USA

S. Dagogo-Jack (ed.), *Leptin: Regulation and Clinical Applications*,
DOI 10.1007/978-3-319-09915-6_9, © Springer International Publishing Switzerland 2015

Sympathetic Nervous System

The relationship of leptin to the sympathetic nervous system (SNS) is complex (Fig. 9.1). Leptin, via activation of the Ob-Rb receptors, stimulates the hypothalamus to activate the SNS. Satoh et al. were able to demonstrate that leptin administered into the ventromedial nucleus of the hypothalamus (VMH) increased epinephrine and norepinephrine concentrations in a dose-dependent manner [1]. The downstream sympathetic effects on glucose metabolism and thermogenesis appear to be mediated primarily by uncoupling protein (UCP)-1 in brown adipose tissue (BAT) [2] and UCP-2 and UCP-3 in white adipose tissue (WAT) and other peripheral tissues [3]. The activated SNS then provides negative feedback to regulate leptin production from WAT. Consequently, sympathetic stimulation of WAT via fasting, cold or sympathomimetic administration decreases leptin gene expression and leptin levels. The corollary is that adrenergic inhibition appears to increase leptin gene expression and leptin levels.

Ob gene expression and subsequent leptin levels declined under fasting or cold conditions, which can which activate the SNS [4, 5], and isoproterenol infused in humans reduced plasma leptin levels within 2 h [6]. The SNS may regulate circulating leptin levels at multiple targets. Administration of epinephrine, norepinephrine or beta-receptor agonist led to inhibition of *ob* gene expression in white fat in rodents and humans [5, 7], and adrenergic stimulation altered both

Table 9.1 Effects of increased hormone levels on leptin levels in humans

Hormone	Δ Leptin
Catecholamines[a]	↓
Insulin	↑
Cortisol	↔
Glucocorticoids	↑/↔

[a]General increase in sympathetic nervous system activity. However, decreased leptin is not observed in pheochromocytoma

Table 9.2 States of acute stress associated with changes in circulating leptin levels in humans

↓ Leptin	↑ Leptin
Fasting	Adrenergic inhibition
Cold	Acute sepsis
Sympathomimetics	Critical illness
Hypoglycemia	Acute myocardial infarction
Prolonged endurance exercise	Pregnancy (even prior to weight gain)
Abdominal surgery	Preeclampsia
Pediatric cardiac surgery	

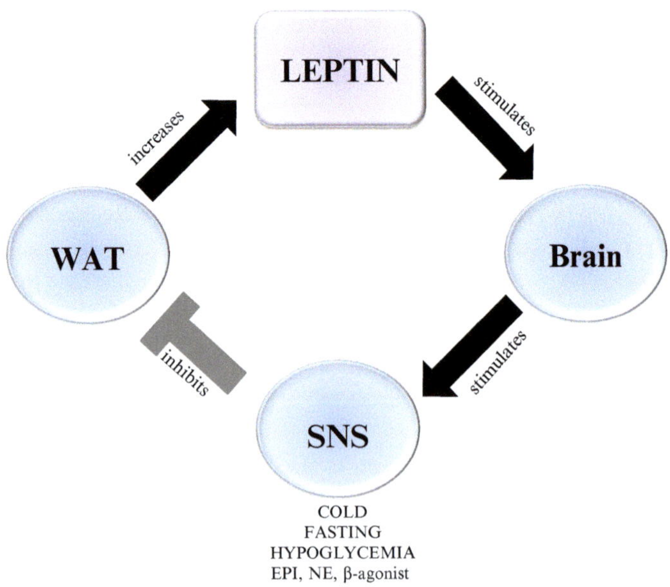

Fig. 9.1 Relationship between the sympathetic nervous system (SNS) and leptin. Increased leptin release from white adipose tissue (WAT) centrally stimulates the SNS. Stimulation of the SNS via exposure to cold, fasting, hypoglycemia, or β-agonists or infusion of epinephrine (EPI) or norepinephrine (NE) inhibits leptin release from WAT

leptin translation (in rodents) and leptin secretion (in humans) [8]. In lean rodents, β_3-adrenoreceptor agonism reduced leptin mRNA in white fat within 4 h and was accompanied by a reduction in plasma leptin levels [9]. In a different study, administration of the combination of propranolol and β_3-receptor antagonist SR 59230A, but neither alone, reversed the reduction in leptin mRNA expression observed with cold exposure [10]. This suggests that the SNS mediates leptin primarily via β_3-adrenoreceptors in animals, however, β_1/β_2-adrenoreceptors may also play a role to some unknown extent. The specific β-receptor subtype(s) involved in leptin control in humans remains unclear. Interestingly, chronically elevated catecholamines observed in pheochromocytoma patients did not suppress leptin levels [11].

Rodent models, in which catecholamine synthesis was blocked using the tyrosine hydroxylase inhibitor, α-methyl-p-tyrosine hydroxylase (AMPT), demonstrated increases in norepinephrine turnover, *ob* gene expression and leptin levels in mice [12]. However, leptin concentrations remained unchanged in both men and women administered AMPT compared to control [13]. Administration of 6-hydroxdopamine (6-HDA), toxic to peripheral sympathetic nerve terminals, had no effect on WAT in rodents, but had similar albeit less robust effects on leptin gene expression and leptin levels as AMPT administration in BAT [14]. AMPT alters both central and peripheral catecholamine synthesis, while 6-HDA has no central or adrenomedullary effect. Therefore, the effect of AMPT administration is likely complex and potentially indicates participation of the adrenal medulla, insulin and/or glucose.

The direct measurement of the effect of leptin on sympathetic nerve activity (SNA) in peripheral tissues was conducted in rodent models using direct microelectrode recordings. Intravenous administration of leptin in rats increased SNA in a dose-dependent manner in BAT (thermogenic), as well as at the kidney, hindlimb and adrenal glands (not classically thermogenic) [15]. Where SNA to BAT is thought to serve thermogenic or metabolic functions, SNA to the kidney is thought to play a part in the cardiovascular effects of leptin [16]. Low dose leptin administration, under conditions of hypothermia (30 °C), potentiated SNA activity in BAT within 30 min in lean Sprague-Dawley rats [17]. Diet-induced obese Sprague-Dawley rats, a model for leptin resistance, exhibited preserved increases in BAT SNA under the same conditions, but the response was not augmented by leptin administration. However, obese Zucker rats, characterized by a leptin receptor defect, failed to demonstrate changes in BAT SNA activity during hypothermia. This suggests that the SNA response to leptin is receptor dependent.

The relationship of leptin to the SNS is incompletely understood. This may be the result of lack of applicability of mouse observations to human physiology [18]. However, in summary, any physiological stimulus leading to sympathetic stimulation of white fat appears to reduce leptin levels. Leptin, in turn, stimulates the SNS. Thus, at the most basic level a regulatory loop between the brain and the adipocyte exists (Fig. 9.1).

Hypothalamic–Pituitary–Adrenal (HPA) Axis

The stress response by the HPA axis is characterized in part by a rise in adrenocorticotropic hormone (ACTH) and cortisol stimulated by corticotropin releasing hormone (CRH). Leptin acts at the level of the hypothalamus via CRH regulation, but this relationship is complex. Leptin infusion in starved *ob/ob* mice resulted in inhibition of CRH mRNA synthesis in the paraventricular nucleus of the hypothalamus [19], and isolated rat hypothalami fail to demonstrate a surge in CRH secretion when provoked with low glucose and subsequently administered leptin [20]. At the same time, ACTH secretion from rat primary cultured pituitary cells remained unchanged, suggesting that the control of glucocorticoid release by leptin occurs at the level of the hypothalamus. In contrast, leptin injected into the third ventricle of starved rats increased CRH production [21] and increased CRH mRNA in normal rats [22]. These conflicting results may reflect differences in the animal model studied and experimental design.

In bovine adrenomedullary cells, leptin inhibited in vitro basal and ACTH-stimulated cortisol release via inhibition of transcription activity [23]. In human adrenal cortex cells, a strong immunohistochemical stain for leptin receptor protein was demonstrated in contrast to the weak signal in the medulla [24]. Leptin inhibited the ACTH-induced secretion of cortisol, among other cortex derived hormones, but had no significant effect on catecholamine release from the medullary chromaffin cells.

Homozygous *ob/ob* mice demonstrated an 85 % higher basal corticosterone level than lean mice, which decreased by>40 % with acute leptin injection [25]. In rodents, surrogate conditions for stress demonstrate that leptin blocks activation of the HPA axis. In starved mice and mice placed in restraint, leptin administration diminishes the rise of ACTH and corticosterone [20, 26]. Chronic administration of leptin to monkeys exposed to a novel unpredictable situation attenuated the expected rise in ACTH and cortisol [27]. However, short-term leptin infusion in the same animal model failed to affect the cortisol response to ACTH administration [28].

Human studies fail to demonstrate a relationship between leptin and the HPA axis as is observed in rodents. Individuals with congenital leptin deficiency demonstrate normal ACTH and cortisol levels [29]. Individuals with leptin receptor defects also demonstrate normal morning ACTH and cortisol levels [30]. Dynamic challenges of the HPA axis with dexamethasone suppression testing in both leptin/receptor deficient groups were also normal. In addition, morning cortisol levels were normal and remain unchanged in leptin deficient children after administration of leptin [31]. Cortisol remains unchanged after leptin administration in healthy individuals who are fasted [32].

However, glucocorticoids do appear to regulate leptin synthesis. Leptin mRNA is induced by dexamethasone in cultured rat adipocytes [33, 34]. This effect is not prevented by protein synthesis inhibitors and suggests that leptin gene expression may be mediated by transcriptional activation perhaps via the glucocorticoid receptor [33]. Additionally, studies using PI3K inhibitors, (MEK inhibitor or rapamycin) in dexamethasone-stimulated rat adipocytes all attenuated leptin secretion [34]. Likely, a complex set of signaling pathways is involved in leptin synthesis and secretion.

In cultured human visceral adipose tissue, *ob* gene expression and leptin secretion increased in a dose-dependent manner when dexamethasone was added to the culture [35]. These leptin responses were four times greater in adipose tissue from obese versus lean individuals. On the other hand, overnight administration of dexamethasone induced no change in leptin levels in normal control individuals [36]. However, in a different study, leptin levels were significantly elevated in lean healthy subjects 24 h after receiving 1 mg of dexamethasone [37]. Obese women demonstrate higher basal leptin levels that increase with small doses of dexamethasone that was not demonstrated in obese men [36]. A study of 17 Cushing's syndrome subjects, found significantly elevated plasma leptin levels compared to obese and healthy subjects [37]. After resection of tumor, cortisol and leptin levels decline. Cushing's syndrome is a state of hypercortisolism that could be recognized as a surrogate for stress. The authors of the study suggested that leptin, which is induced by hypercortisolism, acts as a negative regulator of adrenal cortisol production by its inhibitory effects on the CRH and ACTH production. However, when cortisol was stimulated to physiological stress levels via naloxone, vasopressin, naloxone plus vasopressin or insulin-induced hypoglycemia, plasma leptin levels remained unchanged [38]. This is in contrast to previously discussed studies where leptin was elevated to pharmacologic levels via exogenous glucocorticoids. Interestingly, a significant fall in leptin levels at 60 and 90 min after insulin-induced hypoglycemia may reflect catecholamine response suggesting an overlapping complex interplay of the HPA axis and SNS activation on the regulation of leptin.

Hypoglycemia

Leptin secretion is controlled by competing stimuli under conditions of acute insulin-induced hypoglycemia. In times of prolonged fasting

(6+h), leptin levels begin to fall with a decline in energy availability [39–41]. Hypoglycemia, while not generally as prolonged in research protocols or in clinical scenarios of patients taking insulin, does constitute a more dramatic, immediate need for restoration of glucose levels, suggesting that leptin could play a role in the physiologic counterregulatory response. On the other hand, increased insulin levels cause an increase in leptin under euglycemic conditions. Originally, it was shown that prolonged (>24 h) hyperinsulinemia (infusion rate: 12 pmol/kg/min) was necessary to significantly increase leptin levels in nonobese males [42]. In a later dose-response study in males, the response of leptin to insulin infused at rates of 20, 40, 80, and 400 mU/m^2/min was compared to leptin levels during saline infusion over a time course of 9 h [43]. Compared to the control group, insulin was dose-dependently associated with increases in leptin levels starting in the first 30–60 min of insulin infusion, indicating the effects are more acute than previously observed. Thus, it might be expected that during iatrogenic hypoglycemia leptin could paradoxically increase. However, when blood glucose levels were allowed to fall during hyperinsulinemia (insulin infusion rate: 1.5 mU/kg/min), the rise in leptin levels was both delayed and reduced, indicating that the stimulatory effect of insulin on leptin levels is suppressed in instances of hypoglycemia compared to euglycemia [41]. In fact, in a separate study, when insulin was infused at either a high dose (15 mU/kg/min) or a low dose (1.5 mU/kg/min) and glucose levels were either maintained at euglycemia or hypoglycemia, leptin increased in all four scenarios but the increase was blunted during high and low dose insulin plus hypoglycemia compared to the euglycemia protocols [44]. In a third study, leptin levels actually decreased significantly during the last hour of a 2-h hyperinsulinemic (insulin infusion rate: 1.5 mU/kg/min) hypoglycemic (plasma glucose ~50 mg/dL) glucose clamp in healthy individuals [45]. It has been suggested that the differences in the observed changes in leptin during hypoglycemia in the above two studies may be at least partially due to differences in hypoglycemic protocols (i.e., stepped vs. prolonged moderate hypoglycemia) [45].

The response of leptin to hyperinsulinemic hypoglycemia could be different in type 1 diabetes mellitus as compared to healthy individuals. Basal leptin levels were more than twice as high in type 1 diabetes patients as in healthy controls, likely resulting from insulin therapy, and did not change during two 2-h bouts of hypoglycemia on the same day [45]. Some studies have suggested that catecholamines play a role in the fall in leptin levels during hypoglycemia, and this could be a factor in the differential leptin response to hypoglycemia in type 1 diabetes as the epinephrine response is often blunted in this population. In humans, infusion of isoproterenol during a pancreatic clamp (basal insulin levels) induces a fall in leptin [6]. In a separate study, during a hyperinsulinemic hypoglycemic clamp, leptin levels rose in subjects with type 1 diabetes during hypoglycemia but remained at basal levels in healthy subjects. Upon analysis of the pooled subject data, leptin levels were negatively correlated with the rise in epinephrine and positively correlated with the fall in free fatty acids [46].

It has also been postulated that it is the change in glucose kinetics during changes in glycemia that modulate leptin secretion. Treatment with 2-deoxyglucose or inhibition of glucose transport (using phloretin or cytochalasin-B) or metabolism (using iodoacetate or sodium fluoride) reduces release of leptin in cultured rat adipocytes [47]. Leptin secretion was also reduced after treating cells with metformin. Although metformin enhances glucose uptake and would be expected to increase leptin release, it is also associated with an increase in metabolism of glucose to lactate, suggesting that anaerobic lactate production is not a form of glucose metabolism that causes an increase in leptin [48]. On the other hand, it has also been proposed that insulin-induced changes in glucose metabolism influence leptin release at the transcriptional manner chronically, but that more acute changes in leptin release are mediated by a PI3K-PKBmTOR pathway (and possibly other pathways) [49]. However, during high and low dose insulin infusion at either euglycemia or hypoglycemia, the total amount of dextrose infused was found to be the major predictor of changes in leptin rather than circulating insulin or glucose levels [44].

While the mechanisms of leptin release remain unclear, it seems that during hypoglycemia, changes in glucose metabolism within adipocytes could have an inhibitory effect on leptin release.

The regulatory role of leptin, if any, during hypoglycemia is still unclear. As hypoglycemia represents a period of energy deficit requiring changes in metabolism and an increase in food intake, the presumption could be that leptin would fall in such instances to help drive these responses. The confounding effect of hyperinsulinemia on leptin levels precludes a straightforward examination of the effects of short-term hypoglycemia compared to euglycemia. Moreover, hypoglycemia is accompanied by a robust hormonal response from the sympathetic nervous system, the endocrine pancreas, and the HPA axis, hypothalamic–pituitary–thyroid axis, and the hypothalamic–pituitary–growth axis. With the large fluctuation of so many different hormones and the dramatic changes in substrate metabolism, it would be difficult to tease apart the pathways by which leptin is regulated during hypoglycemia. The large catecholamine response does appear to be one of the factors opposing the stimulatory effects of insulin on leptin levels. The clinical importance of changes in leptin during hypoglycemia also remains to be elucidated. With such powerful counterregulation arising from glucagon and epinephrine, leptin would be expected to be a minor actor during the acute event. Whether or not leptin levels remain altered following hypoglycemia or if changes in leptin exert their effects after a period of recovery is unknown.

Exercise

Exercise is a physiologic stressor on leptin homeostasis that has been widely studied in an attempt to better understand its effect on obesity. While leptin concentrations in humans are known to decrease in response to fasting, many have investigated whether leptin levels might also be modified by exercise-induced negative energy balance. Duration of exercise and variability in energy expenditure (EE) influence changes in plasma leptin concentrations.

In lean and genetically obese (fa/fa) Zucker rats undergoing a single 30 min session of swimming, plasma leptin was decreased by 30 % at the end of exercise in lean animals, but not in obese animals [50]. Leptin changes in lean rats were concomitant with the peak of fatty acid and glycerol release from adipose tissue, suggesting that leptin changes are related to lipolysis. Nine weeks of endurance exercise produced decreased leptin levels, body weight, and food intake in Wistar rats. Endurance exercise also increased Ob-Rb mRNA expression and signaling cascades in the hypothalamus compared with asedentary group [51]. More recently, researchers demonstrated a benefit of exercise on leptin sensitivity in peripheral tissues and the hypothalamus in Sprague Dawley rats given a high fat (HF) diet [52]. Initially, plasma leptin of the HF group was significantly increased compared to that of the control group, and the mRNA expression of Ob-Rb and leptin-related suppressor of cytokine signaling (SOCS3) in the liver and muscle of the HF group was significantly decreased. With initiation of exercise and/or return to a normal diet, HF rats showed decreased plasma leptin levels and increased expression of Ob-Rb and SOCS3 mRNA levels in the hypothalamus, liver, and muscle, which improved leptin sensitivity. Animal models therefore suggest that exercise results in decreased circulating leptin and improved leptin sensitivity in both the hypothalamus and peripheral tissues.

Human studies demonstrate variable results in alterations of leptin metabolism depending on the duration and intensity of exercise. Obese individuals who initiated an aerobic exercise program (45-min walking sessions at 60–80 % of maximum heart rate) showed no change in leptin levels at the end of the first session, but did show improved insulin sensitivity [53]. When sedentary subjects were examined after 20 min of vigorous exercise (70 % VO_{2max}), a statistically significant decrease in leptin levels was seen. However, these levels returned to baseline within an hour of supine recovery [54]. In postmenopausal females, reduced leptin concentrations were seen after 30 min of exercise at 80 % VO_{2max}; however, similar findings were seen with controls and were therefore attributed to diurnal circadian rhythms of leptin [55].

While short periods of exercise do not consistently affect leptin, longer durations of exercise can decrease leptin concentrations. When short duration, maximal intensity (MAX) exercise was compared with a 60-min endurance run at 70 % of VO_{2max} (END) in 9 trained men, energy expenditure was ~200 and ~880 kcal for MAX and END, respectively [56]. Plasma leptin levels did not differ between time points for the MAX run but were significantly lower immediately, 24 h and 48 h post exercise for END. A second study investigating the effects of duration and intensity on leptin levels compared 45 males who participated in one of three competitive endurance races, a half-marathon run (21 km, estimated EE 1,400 kcal), a ski-alpinism race (45 km, estimated EE 5,000 kcal), and an ultra-marathon race (100 km, estimated EE 7,000 kcal) [57]. Pre-race leptin values were significantly correlated with both body mass index and body fat mass. After exercise, serum leptin levels decreased significantly in the ultra-marathon and in the ski-alpinism race, but not in the half-marathon, suggesting that only a prolonged endurance exercise involving a high EE can induce a marked reduction in circulating serum leptin levels. Leptin levels have also been compared in male runners after a rest session (4 h sitting) and an exercise plus rest session (2 h running and 2 h sitting). Leptin concentrations were approximately 30 % lower after the exercise plus rest session as compared to rest alone, which conflicted with many earlier studies [58]. An inverse relationship between leptin levels and glycerol as well as free fatty acid levels was also observed, suggesting a possible role of lipolysis. In conclusion, lowered leptin levels are observed after prolonged exercise that induces lipolysis or with energy expenditure greater than approximately 800 kcal.

In long-term training (≥12 weeks) studies, leptin changes are largely correlated with anthropometric changes, specifically fat mass loss. When 25 obese sedentary premenopausal women underwent a 12-week aerobic exercise program, with intensity corresponding to 50 % of individual maximal oxygen consumption, plasma leptin levels and body weight were reduced [59]. Similar changes have also been observed in trained athletes. Twelve highly trained male rowers were subjected to a 3-week heavy training period followed by a 2-week tapering period. The 3-week training period induced a significant reduction in plasma leptin. While leptin levels increased during the 2-week tapering period, they remained significantly lower than baseline levels [60].

The effect of resistance exercise on leptin concentrations has also been examined. The acute effects of maximum strength (MS), muscular hypertrophy (MH), and strength endurance (SE) resistance exercise protocols on serum leptin were studied in ten young lean men [61]. No differences were found in serum leptin among the MS, MH, SE, and control sessions immediately after exercise and at 30 min of recovery. Despite a reduction in fat mass, no significant decrease in leptin levels was observed in 18 male physical education students after a 6-week strength training program [62]. Leptin changes were examined in sedentary elderly men after a 6 month resistance training program and 6 month detraining period [63]. Participants were randomly assigned to a control, low-intensity, moderate-intensity, or high-intensity training group. Leptin decreased in all groups and was correlated with percent BMI decrease and percent resting metabolic rate increase. Similar to chronic aerobic exercise, leptin changes seem to be correlated to anthropometric changes with long-term resistance training.

Although some results have varied, studies generally suggest that short-term (<60 min) exercise does not affect leptin production. In contrast, exercise that produces a significant energy imbalance (EE>800 kcal) reduces leptin concentrations immediately and at least 48 h after completion. Long-term (≥12 weeks) training programs result in decreased leptin associated with loss of fat mass; however, independent changes are controversial. These reductions in leptin can be attributed to alterations in energy balance and glucoregulatory factors, including improved insulin sensitivity and lipid metabolism, although exact mechanisms remain to be elucidated [64].

Other Clinical Situations

Leptin levels have been studied in various scenarios of clinical stress or inflammation. Leptin has been linked to interleukin (IL)-6 and tumor necrosis factor (TNF)α, both inflammatory cytokines, but the relationship remains incompletely understood. In vitro, leptin was unchanged in the presence of IL-6 [65] and TNFα decreased leptin production [66]. Conversely, during longer-duration exposure to TNFα, leptin levels increased, and in other studies, both cytokines have been found to increase leptin [65, 67]. In addition, IL-6 and TNFα both increase leptin in the presence of dexamethasone perhaps suggesting that the glucocorticoid receptor or cortisol may play a role in the relationship of IL-6 and TNFα and leptin [65, 66]. These differences may reflect the model studied (i.e., adipocyte versus pre-adipocyte) or the duration and type of exposure. However, these findings suggest that leptin may play a role in stress response.

Acute leptin and IL-6 levels are significantly elevated when studied in patients with acute sepsis [68] and critical illness [69]. However, at 24 h a negative correlation of IL-6 to leptin is apparent and the diurnal rhythm of leptin is altered. Additionally, subjects with sepsis or septic shock had leptin concentrations 2 and 4 times greater, respectively, than the control group [70]. In a study of critically ill patients, elevated leptin levels correlated with levels of IL-6 and TNFα [71]. In individuals undergoing abdominal surgery, acute cortisol levels were more than tripled and leptin levels declined by nearly 50 % [72]. Elevated leptin levels are also associated with acute myocardial infarction [73]. In a pediatric cardiac surgery cohort an inverse relationship of IL-6 to leptin levels was observed [74, 75]. The prognostic value of leptin measurement in all critical illness is unclear, but one study did demonstrate that a decline in leptin levels during the prolonged phase of sepsis was not related either to survival or to metabolic and hormonal changes [76].

Pregnancy

Leptin is one of many hormones altered by the physiologic stress of pregnancy. Hyperleptinemia is a hallmark of pregnancy, and leptin production is known to occur in both WAT and the placenta. During gestation, maternal serum leptin levels gradually increase, especially during the second trimester, and fall sharply postpartum [77]. This change is likely due to an increase in bound leptin, as no significant change in free leptin has been observed during 20–30 weeks gestation [78]. In the nongravid state, elevated leptin levels are often attributed to increased adipose tissue with obesity. Increases in leptin levels in early pregnancy before significant weight gain suggest that factors other than simply adiposity are involved [79]. While an increase in leptin levels appears to be ubiquitous in pregnancy, regulation of placental leptin expression and secretion is species specific. In mice, corticosterone-dependent upregulation of leptin secretion from adipose tissue has been observed, whereas leptin is not constitutively secreted by the placenta [80]. In contrast, in baboon [81], bat [82], and human [83], leptin generated by adipose tissue appears to be only partly responsible for the increase in circulating maternal leptin, implicating a role for placental leptin synthesis. Human studies have localized leptin and leptin receptor transcript expression to syncytiotrophoblasts of the placenta [84], and approximately 98 % of leptin produced by the placenta is released into the maternal circulation [85]. Elevated circulating maternal leptin levels during pregnancy can be attributed to varying mechanisms, including placental leptin production, upregulation of adipose leptin production, and production of circulating leptin-binding proteins.

While elevated leptin levels should result in appetite suppression, this is not the case in pregnancy. Animal studies have demonstrated that food intake during pregnancy is increased [86], supporting the increased nutritional demand of fetal growth. This contradiction can be explained by a state of leptin resistance. Though the mechanism of leptin resistance is not entirely clear and seems to vary among species, both placental secretion of leptin binding proteins and reduced hypothalamic response to circulating leptin have been implicated. Mouse models showed dramatically increased expression of the Ob-Re isoform of the leptin receptor mRNA in the placenta at the end of pregnancy, encoding a soluble binding protein that inhibits leptin availability [87]. Researchers also demonstrated a significant reduction of Ob-Rb mRNA levels in the VMH during pregnancy compared with nonpregnant rat controls [88]. Additionally, the number of cells positive for leptin-induced pSTAT3 in the VMH, a measure of signal transduction and transcription activation, was greatly reduced during pregnancy compared with nonpregnant rats, implicating the VMH as a key site involved in pregnancy-induced leptin resistance [88].

Function of Leptin in Pregnancy

If circulating leptin is increased, yet not contributing to hypothalamic regulation of appetite suppression, it must have been preserved for another role. Because of its localization to syncytiotrophoblasts, leptin has been implicated as modulator of endocrine function in the placenta. It is postulated that leptin contributes to placental growth by enhancing mitogenesis, stimulating amino acid uptake and increasing synthesis of extracellular matrix proteins [89]. Mouse studies have shown that leptin is essential for implantation and development of mammary glands but not pregnancy itself [90]. Ramos et al. showed that disruption of leptin signaling resulted in a significant reduction of IL-1 receptor type I, leukemia inhibitory factor, vascular endothelial growth factor receptor 2, and beta3-integrin levels, also suggesting an obligatory role in endometrial receptivity and successful implantation [91]. Recombinant human leptin added to primary cultures of human term placental trophoblast cells stimulated secretion of human chorionic gonadotropin (hCG) and IL-6 and inhibited progesterone secretion [92]. Leptin has also been associated with fetal growth. Cord leptin samples have shown a positive correlation with birth weight independent of insulin-like growth factor (IGF)-1, although the exact mechanism is unknown [93]. Additionally, it has been shown that leptin decreased fetal bone resorption therefore increasing overall bone mass [94].

Leptin in Pathologic Pregnancies

Pathologic states during pregnancy can further stress maternal and fetal leptin homeostasis. Maternal plasma leptin concentrations are similar in pregnant women with type 1 diabetes mellitus and gestational diabetes mellitus as compared to their normoglycemic counterparts when corrected for BMI. However, researchers found that placental leptin mRNA and protein contents were increased threefold and fivefold, respectively, in women requiring chronic insulin therapy during pregnancy [95]. Therefore, alterations in leptin homeostasis in diabetic pregnancies are confined to the fetoplacental unit. Cord leptin was also higher in infants of diabetic mothers, even after birth weight that was corrected for gestational age, supporting an upset in the regulation of fetal growth. Cord leptin levels were strongly correlated with cord IGF-1 levels in the infants of nondiabetic, but not diabetic mothers, suggesting that the latter group has a higher percentage of fat mass in their overall total weight [96].

Leptin changes have also been observed in pregnancies affected by preeclampsia. Plasma leptin levels in preeclamptic women are elevated significantly, compared with gestational age- and BMI-matched normal pregnant women and are reduced to those expected for their body mass indices soon after placental delivery. The rise with preeclampsia correlates with the severity of disease. Leptin secretion was also increased significantly in a human trophoblastic cell line (BeWo cells) cultured under hypoxic conditions (5 % O_2), compared with those cultured under standard conditions (20 % O_2) [97], implicating fetal hypoxia as a stimulator of placental leptin production. In this case, hyperleptinemia may be a compensatory mechanism to increase nutrient delivery to an under perfused placenta [98].

In summary, pregnancy alters leptin homeostasis resulting in increased maternal leptin levels. This increase can largely be attributed to placental leptin production. Similar to obesity, pregnancy creates a state of leptin resistance in part due to downregulation of Ob-Rb receptors in the VMH. In pregnancy, leptin is a modulator of endocrine function in the placenta, directly affecting fetal growth. Leptin homeostasis is further stressed by pathologic states in pregnancy, such as diabetes and preeclampsia.

References

1. Satoh N, Ogawa Y, Katsuura G, Numata Y, Tsuji T, Hayase M, et al. Sympathetic activation of leptin via the ventromedial hypothalamus: leptin-induced increase in catecholamine secretion. Diabetes. 1999;48:1787–93.
2. Scarpace PJ, Matheny M, Pollock BH, Tumer N. Leptin increases uncoupling protein expression and energy expenditure. Am J Physiol. 1997;273: E226–30.
3. Scarpace PJ, Nicolson M, Matheny M. UCP2, UCP3 and leptin gene expression: modulation by food restriction and leptin. J Endocrinol. 1998;159: 349–57.
4. Becker DJ, Ongemba LN, Brichard V, Henquin JC, Brichard SM. Diet- and diabetes-induced changes of ob gene expression in rat adipose tissue. FEBS Lett. 1995;371:324–8.
5. Trayhurn P, Duncan JS, Rayner DV. Acute cold-induced suppression of ob (obese) gene expression in white adipose tissue of mice: mediation by the sympathetic system. Biochem J. 1995;311(Pt 3):729–33.
6. Donahoo WT, Jensen DR, Yost TJ, Eckel RH. Isoproterenol and somatostatin decrease plasma leptin in humans: a novel mechanism regulating leptin secretion. J Clin Endocrinol Metab. 1997;82:4139–43.
7. Carulli L, Ferrari S, Bertolini M, Tagliafico E, Del Rio G. Regulation of ob gene expression: evidence for epinephrine-induced suppression in human obesity. J Clin Endocrinol Metab. 1999;84:3309–12.
8. Ricci MR, Lee MJ, Russell CD, Wang Y, Sullivan S, Schneider SH, et al. Isoproterenol decreases leptin release from rat and human adipose tissue through posttranscriptional mechanisms. Am J Physiol Endocrinol Metab. 2005;288:E798–804.
9. Trayhurn P, Duncan JS, Rayner DV, Hardie LJ. Rapid inhibition of ob gene expression and circulating leptin levels in lean mice by the beta 3-adrenoceptor agonists BRL 35135A and ZD2079. Biochem Biophys Res Commun. 1996;228:605–10.
10. Evans BA, Agar L, Summers RJ. The role of the sympathetic nervous system in the regulation of leptin synthesis in C57BL/6 mice. FEBS Lett. 1999;444: 149–54.
11. Bottner A, Eisenhofer G, Torpy DJ, Ehrhart-Bornstein M, Keiser HR, Chrousos GP, et al. Lack of leptin suppression in response to hypersecretion of catecholamines in pheochromocytoma patients. Metabolism. 1999;48:543–5.
12. Rayner DV, Simon E, Duncan JS, Trayhurn P. Hyperleptinaemia in mice induced by administration of the tyrosine hydroxylase inhibitor alpha-methyl-p-tyrosine. FEBS Lett. 1998;429:395–8.
13. Zimmermann RC, Krahn L, Rahmanie N, Sauer MV. Prolonged inhibition of presynaptic catecholamine synthesis does not alter leptin secretion in normal-weight men and women. Hum Reprod. 1998;13:822–5.
14. Sivitz WI, Fink BD, Morgan DA, Fox JM, Donohoue PA, Haynes WG. Sympathetic inhibition, leptin, and uncoupling protein subtype expression in normal fasting rats. Am J Physiol. 1999;277:E668–77.
15. Haynes WG, Morgan DA, Walsh SA, Mark AL, Sivitz WI. Receptor-mediated regional sympathetic nerve activation by leptin. J Clin Invest. 1997;100: 270–8.
16. Hausberg M, Morgan DA, Chapleau MA, Sivitz WI, Mark AL, Haynes WG. Differential modulation of leptin-induced sympathoexcitation by baroreflex activation. J Hypertens. 2002;20:1633–41.
17. Hausberg M, Morgan DA, Mitchell JL, Sivitz WI, Mark AL, Haynes WG. Leptin potentiates thermogenic sympathetic responses to hypothermia: a receptor-mediated effect. Diabetes. 2002;51:2434–40.
18. Himms-Hagen J. Physiological roles of the leptin endocrine system: differences between mice and humans. Crit Rev Clin Lab Sci. 1999;36:575–655.
19. Huang Q, Rivest R, Richard D. Effects of leptin on corticotropin-releasing factor (CRF) synthesis and CRF neuron activation in the paraventricular hypothalamic nucleus of obese (ob/ob) mice. Endocrinology. 1998;139:1524–32.
20. Heiman ML, Ahima RS, Craft LS, Schoner B, Stephens TW, Flier JS. Leptin inhibition of the hypothalamic-pituitary-adrenal axis in response to stress. Endocrinology. 1997;138:3859–63.
21. Uehara Y, Shimizu H, Ohtani K, Sato N, Mori M. Hypothalamic corticotropin-releasing hormone is a mediator of the anorexigenic effect of leptin. Diabetes. 1998;47:890–3.
22. Schwartz MW, Seeley RJ, Campfield LA, Burn P, Baskin DG. Identification of targets of leptin action in rat hypothalamus. J Clin Invest. 1996;98:1101–6.

23. Bornstein SR, Uhlmann K, Haidan A, Ehrhart-Bornstein M, Scherbaum WA. Evidence for a novel peripheral action of leptin as a metabolic signal to the adrenal gland: leptin inhibits cortisol release directly. Diabetes. 1997;46:1235–8.
24. Glasow A, Haidan A, Hilbers U, Breidert M, Gillespie J, Scherbaum WA, et al. Expression of ob receptor in normal human adrenals: differential regulation of adrenocortical and adrenomedullary function by leptin. J Clin Endocrinol Metab. 1998;83:4459–66.
25. Ahima RS, Prabakaran D, Flier JS. Postnatal leptin surge and regulation of circadian rhythm of leptin by feeding implications for energy homeostasis and neuroendocrine function. J Clin Invest. 1998;101:1020–7.
26. Ahima RS, Prabakaran D, Mantzoros C, Qu D, Lowell B, Maratos-Flier E, et al. Role of leptin in the neuroendocrine response to fasting. Nature. 1996;382:250–2.
27. Wilson ME, Fisher J, Brown J. Chronic subcutaneous leptin infusion diminishes the responsiveness of the hypothalamic-pituitary-adrenal (HPA) axis in female rhesus monkeys. Physiol Behav. 2005;84:449–58.
28. Lado-Abeal J, Mrotek JJ, Stocco DM, Norman RL. Effect of leptin on ACTH-stimulated secretion of cortisol in rhesus macaques and on human adrenal carcinoma cells. Eur J Endocrinol. 1999;141:534–8.
29. Montague CT, Farooqi IS, Whitehead JP, Soos MA, Rau H, Wareham NJ, et al. Congenital leptin deficiency is associated with severe early-onset obesity in humans. Nature. 1997;387:903–8.
30. Clement K, Vaisse C, Lahlou N, Cabrol S, Pelloux V, Cassuto D, et al. A mutation in the human leptin receptor gene causes obesity and pituitary dysfunction. Nature. 1998;392:398–401.
31. Farooqi IS, Matarese G, Lord GM, Keogh JM, Lawrence E, Agwu C, et al. Beneficial effects of leptin on obesity, T cell hyporesponsiveness, and neuroendocrine/metabolic dysfunction of human congenital leptin deficiency. J Clin Invest. 2002;110:1093–103.
32. Chan JL, Heist K, DePaoli AM, Veldhuis JD, Mantzoros CS. The role of falling leptin levels in the neuroendocrine and metabolic adaptation to short-term starvation in healthy men. J Clin Invest. 2003;111:1409–21.
33. De Vos P, Lefebvre AM, Shrivo I, Fruchart JC, Auwerx J. Glucocorticoids induce the expression of the leptin gene through a non-classical mechanism of transcriptional activation. Eur J Biochem. 1998;253:619–26.
34. Bradley RL, Cheatham B. Regulation of ob gene expression and leptin secretion by insulin and dexamethasone in rat adipocytes. Diabetes. 1999;48:272–8.
35. Halleux CM, Servais I, Reul BA, Detry R, Brichard SM. Multihormonal control of ob gene expression and leptin secretion from cultured human visceral adipose tissue: increased responsiveness to glucocorticoids in obesity. J Clin Endocrinol Metab. 1998;83:902–10.
36. Putignano P, Brunani A, Dubini A, Bertolini M, Pasquali R, Cavagnini F, et al. Effect of small doses of dexamethasone on plasma leptin levels in normal and obese subjects: a dose-response study. J Endocrinol Invest. 2003;26:111–6.
37. Masuzaki H, Ogawa Y, Hosoda K, Miyawaki T, Hanaoka I, Hiraoka J, et al. Glucocorticoid regulation of leptin synthesis and secretion in humans: elevated plasma leptin levels in cushing's syndrome. J Clin Endocrinol Metab. 1997;82:2542–7.
38. Nye EJ, Bornstein SR, Grice JE, Tauchnitz R, Hockings GI, Strakosch CR, et al. Interactions between the stimulated hypothalamic-pituitary-adrenal axis and leptin in humans. J Neuroendocrinol. 2000;12:141–5.
39. Korbonits M, Trainer PJ, Little JA, Edwards R, Kopelman PG, Besser GM, et al. Leptin levels do not change acutely with food administration in normal or obese subjects, but are negatively correlated with pituitary-adrenal activity. Clin Endocrinol (Oxf). 1997;46:751–7.
40. Kolaczynski JW, Considine RV, Ohannesian J, Marco C, Opentanova I, Nyce MR, et al. Responses of leptin to short-term fasting and refeeding in humans: a link with ketogenesis but not ketones themselves. Diabetes. 1996;45:1511–5.
41. Schmitz O, Fisker S, Orskov L, Hove KY, Nyholm B, Moller N. Effects of hyperinsulinaemia and hypoglycaemia on circulating leptin levels in healthy lean males. Diabetes Metab. 1997;23:80–3.
42. Boden G, Chen X, Kolaczynski JW, Polansky M. Effects of prolonged hyperinsulinemia on serum leptin in normal human subjects. J Clin Invest. 1997;100:1107–13.
43. Saad MF, Khan A, Sharma A, Michael R, Riad-Gabriel MG, Boyadjian R, et al. Physiological insulinemia acutely modulates plasma leptin. Diabetes. 1998;47:544–9.
44. Wellhoener P, Fruehwald-Schultes B, Kern W, Dantz D, Kerner W, Born J, et al. Glucose metabolism rather than insulin is a main determinant of leptin secretion in humans. J Clin Endocrinol Metab. 2000;85:1267–71.
45. Sandoval DA, Galassetti P, Tate D, Neill A, Davis SN. Leptin responses to antecedent exercise and hypoglycemia in healthy and type 1 diabetes mellitus men and women. J Diabetes Complications. 2003;17:301–6.
46. Fritsche A, Wahl HG, Metzinger E, Renn W, Kellerer M, Haring H, et al. Evidence for inhibition of leptin secretion by catecholamines in man. Exp Clin Endocrinol Diabetes. 1998;106:415–8.
47. Mueller WM, Gregoire FM, Stanhope KL, Mobbs CV, Mizuno TM, Warden CH, et al. Evidence that glucose metabolism regulates leptin secretion from cultured rat adipocytes. Endocrinology. 1998;139:551–8.
48. Mueller WM, Stanhope KL, Gregoire F, Evans JL, Havel PJ. Effects of metformin and vanadium on leptin secretion from cultured rat adipocytes. Obes Res. 2000;8:530–9.
49. Tsai M, Asakawa A, Amitani H, Inui A. Stimulation of leptin secretion by insulin. Indian J Endocrinol Metab. 2012;16:S543–8.

50. Pagano C, Marzolo M, Granzotto M, Ricquier D, Federspil G, Vettor R. Acute effects of exercise on circulating leptin in lean and genetically obese fa/fa rats. Biochem Biophys Res Commun. 1999;255:698–702.
51. Zhao J, Tian Y, Xu J, Liu D, Wang X, Zhao B. Endurance exercise is a leptin signaling mimetic in hypothalamus of Wistar rats. Lipids Health Dis. 2011;10:225.
52. Kang S, Kim KB, Shin KO. Exercise training improves leptin sensitivity in peripheral tissue of obese rats. Biochem Biophys Res Commun. 2013;435:454–9.
53. Sari R, Balci MK, Balci N, Karayalcin U. Acute effect of exercise on plasma leptin level and insulin resistance in obese women with stable caloric intake. Endocr Res. 2007;32:9–17.
54. Legakis IN, Mantzouridis T, Saramantis A, Lakka-Papadodima E. Rapid decrease of leptin in middle-aged sedentary individuals after 20 minutes of vigorous exercise with early recovery after the termination of the test. J Endocrinol Invest. 2004;27: 117–20.
55. Kraemer RR, Johnson LG, Haltom R, Kraemer GR, Hebert EP, Gimpel T, et al. Serum leptin concentrations in response to acute exercise in postmenopausal women with and without hormone replacement therapy. Proc Soc Exp Biol Med. 1999;221:171–7.
56. Olive JL, Miller GD. Differential effects of maximal- and moderate-intensity runs on plasma leptin in healthy trained subjects. Nutrition. 2001;17:365–9.
57. Zaccaria M, Ermolao A, Roi GS, Englaro P, Tegon G, Varnier M. Leptin reduction after endurance races differing in duration and energy expenditure. Eur J Appl Physiol. 2002;87:108–11.
58. Duclos M, Corcuff JB, Ruffie A, Roger P, Manier G. Rapid leptin decrease in immediate post-exercise recovery. Clin Endocrinol (Oxf). 1999;50:337–42.
59. Polak J, Klimcakova E, Moro C, Viguerie N, Berlan M, Hejnova J, et al. Effect of aerobic training on plasma levels and subcutaneous abdominal adipose tissue gene expression of adiponectin, leptin, interleukin 6, and tumor necrosis factor alpha in obese women. Metabolism. 2006;55:1375–81.
60. Jurimae J, Maestu J, Jurimae T. Leptin as a marker of training stress in highly trained male rowers? Eur J Appl Physiol. 2003;90:533–8.
61. Zafeiridis A, Smilios I, Considine RV, Tokmakidis SP. Serum leptin responses after acute resistance exercise protocols. J Appl Physiol (1985). 2003;94:591–7.
62. Ara I, Perez-Gomez J, Vicente-Rodriguez G, Chavarren J, Dorado C, Calbet JA. Serum free testosterone, leptin and soluble leptin receptor changes in a 6-week strength-training programme. Br J Nutr. 2006;96:1053–9.
63. Fatouros IG, Tournis S, Leontsini D, Jamurtas AZ, Sxina M, Thomakos P, et al. Leptin and adiponectin responses in overweight inactive elderly following resistance training and detraining are intensity related. J Clin Endocrinol Metab. 2005;90:5970–7.
64. Kraemer RR, Chu H, Castracane VD. Leptin and exercise. Exp Biol Med (Maywood). 2002;227:701–8.
65. Trujillo ME, Sullivan S, Harten I, Schneider SH, Greenberg AS, Fried SK. Interleukin-6 regulates human adipose tissue lipid metabolism and leptin production in vitro. J Clin Endocrinol Metab. 2004;89:5577–82.
66. Trujillo ME, Lee MJ, Sullivan S, Feng J, Schneider SH, Greenberg AS, et al. Tumor necrosis factor alpha and glucocorticoid synergistically increase leptin production in human adipose tissue: role for p38 mitogen-activated protein kinase. J Clin Endocrinol Metab. 2006;91:1484–90.
67. Zhang HH, Kumar S, Barnett AH, Eggo MC. Tumour necrosis factor-alpha exerts dual effects on human adipose leptin synthesis and release. Mol Cell Endocrinol. 2000;159:79–88.
68. Torpy DJ, Bornstein SR, Chrousos GP. Leptin and interleukin-6 in sepsis. Horm Metab Res. 1998;30: 726–9.
69. Bornstein SR, Licinio J, Tauchnitz R, Engelmann L, Negrao AB, Gold P, et al. Plasma leptin levels are increased in survivors of acute sepsis: associated loss of diurnal rhythm, in cortisol and leptin secretion. J Clin Endocrinol Metab. 1998;83:280–3.
70. Arnalich F, Lopez J, Codoceo R, Jim nez M, Madero R, Montiel C. Relationship of plasma leptin to plasma cytokines and human survival in sepsis and septic shock. J Infect Dis. 1999;180:908–11.
71. Yousef AA, Amr YM, Suliman GA. The diagnostic value of serum leptin monitoring and its correlation with tumor necrosis factor-alpha in critically ill patients: a prospective observational study. Crit Care. 2010;14:R33.
72. Kain ZN, Zimolo Z, Heninger G. Leptin and the perioperative neuroendocrinological stress response. J Clin Endocrinol Metab. 1999;84:2438–42.
73. Meisel SR, Ellis M, Pariente C, Pauzner H, Liebowitz M, David D, et al. Serum leptin levels increase following acute myocardial infarction. Cardiology. 2001;95:206–11.
74. Hoda MR, El-Achkar H, Schmitz E, Scheffold T, Vetter HO, De Simone R. Systemic stress hormone response in patients undergoing open heart surgery with or without cardiopulmonary bypass. Ann Thorac Surg. 2006;82:2179–86.
75. Modan-Moses D, Ehrlich S, Kanety H, Dagan O, Pariente C, Esrahi N, et al. Circulating leptin and the perioperative neuroendocrinological stress response after pediatric cardiac surgery. Crit Care Med. 2001; 29:2377–82.
76. Tzanela M, Orfanos SE, Tsirantonaki M, Kotanidou A, Sotiropoulou C, Christophoraki M, et al. Leptin alterations in the course of sepsis in humans. In Vivo. 2006;20:565–70.
77. Hardie L, Trayhurn P, Abramovich D, Fowler P. Circulating leptin in women: a longitudinal study in the menstrual cycle and during pregnancy. Clin Endocrinol (Oxf). 1997;47:101–6.
78. Lewandowski K, Horn R, O'Callaghan CJ, Dunlop D, Medley GF, O'Hare P, et al. Free leptin, bound leptin, and soluble leptin receptor in normal and diabetic

pregnancies. J Clin Endocrinol Metab. 1999;84: 300–6.

79. Highman TJ, Friedman JE, Huston LP, Wong WW, Catalano PM. Longitudinal changes in maternal serum leptin concentrations, body composition, and resting metabolic rate in pregnancy. Am J Obstet Gynecol. 1998;178:1010–5.
80. Kronfeld-Schor N, Zhao J, Silvia BA, Bicer E, Mathews PT, Urban R, et al. Steroid-dependent up-regulation of adipose leptin secretion in vitro during pregnancy in mice. Biol Reprod. 2000;63:274–80.
81. Hoggard N, Hunter L, Lea RG, Trayhurn P, Mercer JG. Ontogeny of the expression of leptin and its receptor in the murine fetus and placenta. Br J Nutr. 2000; 83:317–26.
82. Kronfeld-Schor N, Zhao J, Silvia BA, Mathews PT, Zimmerman S, Widmaier EP, et al. Hyperleptinemia in pregnant bats is characterized by increased placental leptin secretion in vitro. Endocrine. 2001;14:225–33.
83. Masuzaki H, Ogawa Y, Sagawa N, Hosoda K, Matsumoto T, Mise H, et al. Nonadipose tissue production of leptin: leptin as a novel placenta-derived hormone in humans. Nat Med. 1997;3:1029–33.
84. Henson MC, Swan KF, O'Neil JS. Expression of placental leptin and leptin receptor transcripts in early pregnancy and at term. Obstet Gynecol. 1998;92:1020–8.
85. Linnemann K, Malek A, Sager R, Blum WF, Schneider H, Fusch C. Leptin production and release in the dually in vitro perfused human placenta. J Clin Endocrinol Metab. 2000;85:4298–301.
86. Shirley B. The food intake of rats during pregnancy and lactation. Lab Anim Sci. 1984;34:169–72.
87. Gavrilova O, Barr V, Marcus-Samuels B, Reitman M. Hyperleptinemia of pregnancy associated with the appearance of a circulating form of the leptin receptor. J Biol Chem. 1997;272:30546–51.
88. Ladyman SR, Grattan DR. Suppression of leptin receptor messenger ribonucleic acid and leptin responsiveness in the ventromedial nucleus of the hypothalamus during pregnancy in the rat. Endocrinology. 2005;146:3868–74.
89. Jansson N, Greenwood SL, Johansson BR, Powell TL, Jansson T. Leptin stimulates the activity of the system A amino acid transporter in human placental villous fragments. J Clin Endocrinol Metab. 2003; 88:1205–11.
90. Malik NM, Carter ND, Murray JF, Scaramuzzi RJ, Wilson CA, Stock MJ. Leptin requirement for conception, implantation, and gestation in the mouse. Endocrinology. 2001;142:5198–202.
91. Ramos MP, Rueda BR, Leavis PC, Gonzalez RR. Leptin serves as an upstream activator of an obligatory signaling cascade in the embryo-implantation process. Endocrinology. 2005;146:694–701.
92. Cameo P, Bischof P, Calvo JC. Effect of leptin on progesterone, human chorionic gonadotropin, and interleukin-6 secretion by human term trophoblast cells in culture. Biol Reprod. 2003;68:472–7.
93. Christou H, Connors JM, Ziotopoulou M, Hatzidakis V, Papathanassoglou E, Ringer SA, et al. Cord blood leptin and insulin-like growth factor levels are independent predictors of fetal growth. J Clin Endocrinol Metab. 2001;86:935–8.
94. Ogueh O, Sooranna S, Nicolaides KH, Johnson MR. The relationship between leptin concentration and bone metabolism in the human fetus. J Clin Endocrinol Metab. 2000;85:1997–9.
95. Lepercq J, Cauzac M, Lahlou N, Timsit J, Girard J, Auwerx J, et al. Overexpression of placental leptin in diabetic pregnancy: a critical role for insulin. Diabetes. 1998;47:847–50.
96. Manderson JG, Patterson CC, Hadden DR, Traub AI, Leslie H, McCance DR. Leptin concentrations in maternal serum and cord blood in diabetic and non-diabetic pregnancy. Am J Obstet Gynecol. 2003; 188:1326–32.
97. Mise H, Sagawa N, Matsumoto T, Yura S, Nanno H, Itoh H, et al. Augmented placental production of leptin in preeclampsia: possible involvement of placental hypoxia. J Clin Endocrinol Metab. 1998;83: 3225–9.
98. Tommaselli GA, Pighetti M, Nasti A, D'Elia A, Guida M, Di Carlo C, et al. Serum leptin levels and uterine doppler flow velocimetry at 20 weeks' gestation as markers for the development of pre-eclampsia. Gynecol Endocrinol. 2004;19:160–5.

10 Leptin and the Kidney

Richa Pandey, Anubha Mutneja, Daniel W. Coyne, and Sam Dagogo-Jack

Introduction

Following the discovery of the *obese* (*ob*) gene and its protein product leptin in 1994 [1], studies were performed to determine the role of the kidney in leptin clearance, and the effects of chronic kidney disease (CKD) and end-stage renal disease (ESRD) failure on leptin levels. CKD is defined as a chronic loss of renal function. The severity of CKD is based on glomerular filtration rate (GFR) measured in ml/min/1.73 m^2: stage 1 CKD is defined as GFR >90; stage 2, GFR 60–89; stage 3, GFR 30–59; and stage 4, GFR 15–29. GFR less than 15 (Stage 5 CKD) includes those patients receiving chronic dialysis, and is commonly referred to as ESRD. Circulating levels of numerous proteins and peptide hormones are affected by renal failure [2]. Some patients with CKD and most patients with ESRD also have elevated markers of chronic inflammation, including tumor necrosis factor alpha (TNFα) and various cytokines including interleukin-1 (IL-1), which have been reported to stimulate leptin production [3–5]. Similarly, hyperinsulinemia is common in CKD and dialysis patients, is a risk factor for the development and progression of CKD, while insulin has also been demonstrated to stimulate leptin secretion [6–9]. Consequently, it was hypothesized that ESRD patients might have higher leptin levels due to diminished leptin clearance and increased secretion, as outlined in Fig. 10.1.

R. Pandey, M.B.B.S., M.D. • A. Mutneja, M.B.B.S., M.D.
Division of Nephrology, Washington University, St. Louis, MO, USA

D.W. Coyne, M.D. (✉)
Division of Nephrology, Washington University School of Medicine, 660 S. Euclid Avenue, Campus Box 8129, St. Louis, MO 63110, USA
e-mail: dcoyne@dom.wustl.edu

S. Dagogo-Jack, M.B.B.S., M.D.
Division of Endocrinology, Diabetes and Metabolism, The University of Tennessee Health Science Center, Memphis, TN, USA

Leptin Uptake and Clearance by the Kidney

Early studies in rats outlined the important role of the kidney in leptin clearance. Although extraction of leptin across the renal circulation was high, little intact leptin was detected in the urine, indicating significant intrarenal metabolism [10, 11]. Nephrectomy led to a rapid increase in leptin levels, although the levels fell substantially over time, indicating other mechanisms for leptin metabolism [10]. Kinetic studies suggested that uptake of leptin by the kidney, rather than exclusive glomerular filtration, was the predominant elimination pathway [12]. Other mechanisms affect leptin beyond renal clearance and degrada-

S. Dagogo-Jack (ed.), *Leptin: Regulation and Clinical Applications*,
DOI 10.1007/978-3-319-09915-6_10, © Springer International Publishing Switzerland 2015

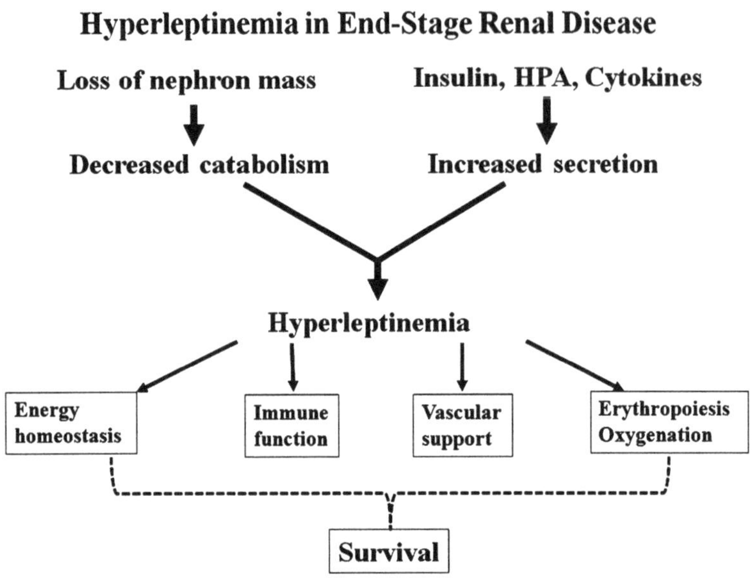

Fig. 10.1 Mechanisms contributing to hyperleptinemia in end-stage renal disease (ESRD) patients, and potential pathways for leptin to affect survival. HPA, hypothalamic–pituitary axis

tion, as a study nephrectomizing rats led to only transient increases in leptin levels [13].

Consistent with animal studies, studies in humans have demonstrated that plasma levels of both free and protein-bound leptin are significantly reduced by passage through the kidney, supporting glomerular filtration and likely uptake and metabolism [14]. The increased leptin levels observed in obese adults with normal renal function can be explained by increased production directly related in adiposity, and not to reduced clearance [15].

Clearance of leptin has now been shown to occur by filtration by the glomerulus, followed by binding by the multiligand receptor megalin in the luminal membrane of the proximal tubules. Megalin-mediated endocytosis of leptin is then followed by degradation in the proximal tubule [16]. Thus, leptin clearance and degradation is mediated by glomerular filtration and tubular uptake. Consequently, as the glomerular filtration rate (GFR) decreases, leptin metabolism through the kidney is impaired. Measuring leptin levels in aortic and renal vein plasma to calculate net leptin extraction by the kidney, Sharma et al. reported that the kidneys in patients with intact renal function extract 12 % of circulating leptin, whereas in patients with renal insufficiency show no measurable uptake of leptin across the renal vasculature [17]. Fruehwald-Schultes et al. found that leptin degradation was impaired in early stages of diabetic nephropathy, leading to elevated levels [18]. In another report, plasma leptin levels correlated inversely with GFR, thus adding to the body of evidence that leptin accumulates with declining GFR [19].

Leptin Levels in ESRD and CKD

In 1997, observational studies in patients on chronic hemodialysis demonstrated significantly higher leptin levels than age- and gender-matched controls with normal renal function, and showed that leptin levels correlated with body mass index (BMI) and fat mass index (see Table 10.1 and Fig. 10.2) [17, 20, 21]. Similarly, in patients receiving peritoneal dialysis, leptin levels were significantly higher than controls [21–25]. Dagogo-Jack and colleagues [23] measured leptin and leptin index (leptin level/BMI) in 36 patients on peritoneal dialysis and noted that leptin index was five-fold higher among men and 7.5-fold higher levels among women, compared to normal controls (Fig. 10.3). Not all ESRD patients have elevated leptin levels; leptin levels lie within the expected normal range for BMI in a significant minority of ESRD patients, and these patients are more likely to be male and nonobese. Major predictors of hyperleptinemia in ESRD patients include female gender, higher BMI, treatment with peritoneal dialysis (compared to hemodialysis) [20, 23–25].

Table 10.1 Major studies examining leptin levels in CKD

Author, year	Number of subjects	Modality	Leptin level ($N \pm$ SD) ng/ml	Comments
Merabet, 1997	141	HD	M 26.8±5.7 F 38.3±5.6	Higher levels than in normal renal function; correlates with BMI.
Sharma, 1997	37	HD	37.6±10.6	Higher than normal after correcting for BMI
Nishizawa, 1998	103	HD	M 5.0±1.2 F 19.3±3.1	Correlation with fat mass index
Dagogo-Jack, 1998	56	PD	M 49.9±18.4 F 220±28.1	7.5-fold elevation as compared to healthy controls when matched for BMI
Parry, 1998	49	PD	M 11 (9–19) F 53 (19–128)	No correlation with CRP, IGF-1, or albumin
Landt, 1999	28	PD	M 18.2±23.6 F 215±120.1	No correlation with CRP and albumin
Heimburger, 1997	PD 16 HD 8	PD and HD	PD 55.6±9.6 HD 72±22.9	Positive correlation between CRP and serum leptin
Johansen, 1998	PD 9 HD 19	PD and HD	PD 10.5 (3.3–266) HD 3.5 (0.8–156)	Negative correlation with albumin and PCR
Fontan, 1999	PD 75 HD 51	PD and HD	PD 36 HD 5.4	Correlation between IGF-1 and leptin
Kagan, 1999	HD 26 PD 20	PD and HD	PD (M 26.1, F 89.4) HD (M 17.7, F 35.6)	High leptin/BMI ratios in CAPD
Nordfors, 1998	Mod 75 Adv RF 104 PD 7	CKD and PD	Mod RF 16.5±1.5 Adv RF 27.7±3.6 PD 39.6±12.6	Positive correlation between serum leptin and CRP
Picoits-Filho, 2002	149	ESRD not on RRT	10 (1.1–220)	Positive correlation with IL-6

In dialysis patients, leptin largely circulates in the free form, rather than protein-bound form [17]. Western blot analysis of samples from ESRD patients and normal controls showed a single band for leptin at 16 kDa in both groups (consistent with the full length protein), without evidence of leptin degradation products [20, 22]. These data are interpreted to indicate that enhanced protein binding or metabolic breakdown products are not accounting for the elevated levels of immunoreactive leptin observed in ESRD [17, 20, 22]. In mice and humans, leptin has been shown to suppress food intake, increase energy expenditure, and alter immunological and metabolic parameters [26–29]. Despite these recognized biologic effects, leptin levels did not correlate with weight changes in ESRD patients during the previous 4 months, which suggests possible leptin resistance in renal failure [22].

Various studies have determined leptin levels in earlier stages of CKD. Menon et al. [30] analyzed serum samples from 798 participants in the Modification of Diet in Renal Disease (MDRD) Study and found that higher leptin levels were associated with older age, female gender, lower GFR, and higher levels of body fat, insulin, and CRP [30]. A 10 % decline in GFR was associated with 6 % increase in leptin level [30]. Being a prospective randomized trial of dietary protein restriction on CKD progression in nondiabetic patients, the MDRD study had baseline leptin levels that were analyzed in relation to renal outcomes. Neither higher leptin levels nor higher CRP levels were independent predictors of progression of CKD [31]. In a recent study of 5,820 adult participants in the multiethnic National Health and Nutrition Examination Survey, higher plasma leptin levels were associated with CKD after adjusting for age, sex, race/ethnicity, education,

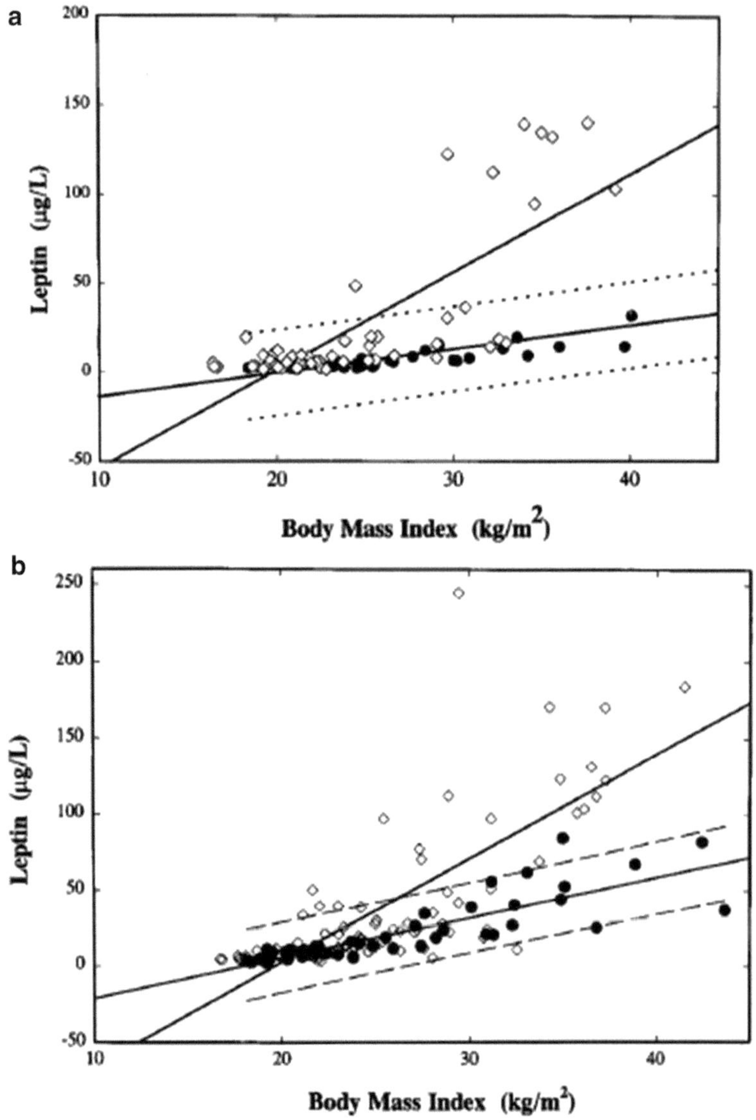

Fig. 10.2 Correlation of plasma leptin levels with BMI. Panel (**a**), Men; Panel (**b**), women. *Diamonds* represent results for ESRD patients, and *circles* show results for control subjects. *Solid lines* are regression curves, and *dotted lines* represent the 95 % confidence interval around the regression lines of normal subjects. From Merabet E et al. J Clin Endo Metab 82:847–850, 1997

smoking, alcohol intake, BMI, and comorbidities (diabetes, hypertension, and dyslipidemia). Individuals in the highest leptin quartile had a threefold increased odds of CKD compared to the referent (quartile 1 of leptin) [32].

The Effect of Dialysis Modalities on Leptin

During hemodialysis, solutes and water are cleared across a semipermeable membrane referred to as a dialyzer. Dialyzer membranes have two major characteristics—permeability and biocompatibility. These membranes based on their composition are categorized into: cellulose, substituted cellulose, cellulosynthetic, and synthetic. Cellulosic dialyzers are more bio-incompatible, and activate the complement cascade and stimulate inflammatory cytokines, while synthetic dialyzers have far less interaction with circulating proteins and blood cells. Thus, studies of hemodialysis patients on different types of dialyzers provide insight into the contribution of the dialysis process to leptin clearance in the setting of differential activation of inflammatory [3, 4].

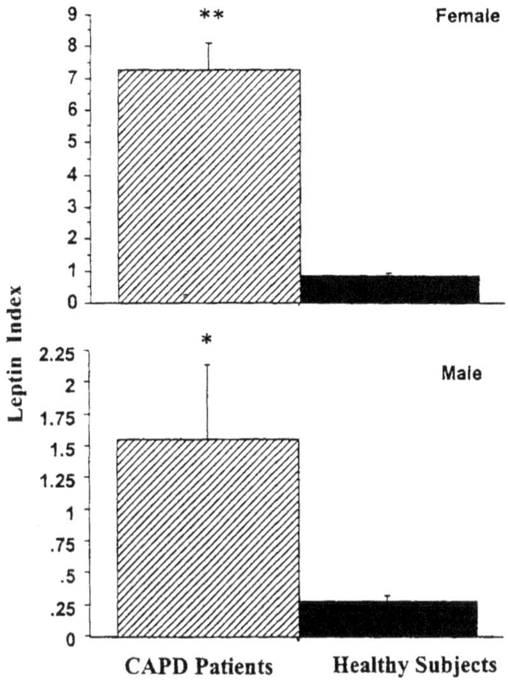

Fig. 10.3 Comparison of leptin index in CAPD-treated patients (*Hatched bars*) and healthy controls (*black bars*). Leptin index was calculated as plasma leptin concentration (ng/mL) divided by body mass index (kg/m^2). ** $p<0.0001$; *$p<0.001$. From Dagogo-Jack S et al. Perit Dial Int 18:34–40, 1998

Dialyzers are also divided into low-flux which provide minimal clearance of middle molecules, generally defined as a molecular weight >10 kDa, and high flux which have significant clearance of molecules with a molecular weight of 10–50 kDa and thus better reflect the clearance provided by the normal glomerular. With a molecular weight of about 16 kDa, clearance of leptin through different dialyzers should vary. Since leptin secretion increases in response to inflammatory cytokines [5, 33], cellulosic membranes were hypothesized to increase leptin levels. As inflammatory markers are increased more by bio-incompatible dialyzers, it was also hypothesized that leptin levels may be higher among patients receiving hemodialysis with cellulosic membranes.

Employing a crossover design, Coyne and colleagues found that use of low-flux cellulosic membranes significantly increased TNF-α levels, but did not alter leptin levels compared to use of low-flux polysulfone dialyzers [34]. In contrast, high-flux dialyzers were more effective in clearing leptin compared to low-flux polysulfone and cellulosic dialyzers, leading to a 30 % reduction in plasma leptin levels (Fig. 10.4) [34]. Clearance of leptin across the dialyzer was also measured,

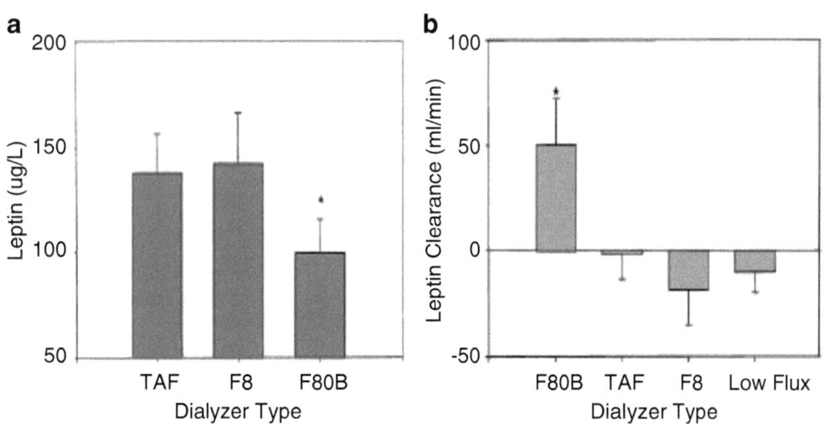

Fig. 10.4 (**a**) Influence of dialyzer type on plasma leptin concentration: Plasma leptin levels were determined weekly while eight patients were dialyzed serially on Terumo low-flux cellulosic dialyzers (TAF), low-flux polysulfone dialyzers (F8), and high-flux polysulfone dialyzers (F80B). The average leptin concentration was significantly lower in the F80B group ($p<0.005$ v TAF; $p<0.02$ v F8). From Coyne DW et al. Amer J Kidney Dis 1998. (**b**) Clearance of leptin by dialyzer type. The pooled data of TAF (a low-flux cellulosic dialyzer) and F8 (a low-flux polysulfone dialyzer) are shown as "low flux." The F80B (high flux polysulfone dialyzer) clearance was significantly higher than the low flux group ($p=0.043$). From Coyne DW et al. Amer J Kidney Dis 1998

and only high flux dialyzers led to significant removal of leptin (Fig. 10.4) [34]. Use of dialyzers with even higher clearance of middle molecules leads to even greater reductions in leptin level [35]. Hemodiafiltration, another form of dialysis frequently employed in Europe, provides the greatest clearance of leptin, but post-dialysis rebound occurs [36]. The latter suggests a multi-compartment distribution of leptin similar to that of beta-2 microglobulin, a well-studied middle molecule [36]. Despite the relationship of the characteristics of dialyzers to leptin levels and leptin clearance, large clinical trials have demonstrated minimal improvement in clinical outcomes when patients are dialyzed using high flux versus low flux dialyzers, or treated with hemodiafiltration versus standard hemodialysis [37, 38]. These trial results suggest leptin levels per se are not a major contributor to the excessively high total and cardiovascular mortality observed in dialysis patients, though none of these modalities normalize leptin levels in the obese patient.

Peritoneal dialysis employs the serosal layer of the peritoneal cavity to achieve clearance of solutes and water. Peritoneal membrane consists of different sized pores—large (20–40 nm), small (4–6 nm), and transcellular (<0.8 nm)—that are responsible for transportation of molecules across the membrane based on their size. A study of patients receiving peritoneal dialysis showed a leptin clearance intermediate to the clearance of the smaller creatinine and larger beta-2 microglobulin [39]. Men on peritoneal dialysis appear to have higher leptin clearance than women [25]. Among ESRD patients, plasma leptin tends to run higher in patients treated with peritoneal dialysis compared with hemodialysis; the disparity has been attributed to lower clearance of leptin by the peritoneal membrane, and possible effects of peritoneal dialysate pH and electrolyte composition on leptin release by local adipocytes [40–42]. To date, no difference in survival rate has been noted between the two modalities of dialysis, despite the consistent observation of higher leptin levels in peritoneal dialysis patients compared to those treated by hemodialysis.

Effect of Renal Transplantation on Leptin

Renal transplantation is performed in patients with stage 5 CKD who may or may not already be receiving chronic dialysis. Transplantation usually results in an increase in eGFR to normal or near normal levels during the first day. Renal transplantation recipients are generally younger, healthier, and less likely to be obese than ESRD patients on dialysis. Landt and colleagues determined changes in leptin levels in 29 adults before and after successful renal transplantation [43]. Mean plasma leptin levels prior to transplant were higher than controls, but this was largely attributable to a few patients with high BMI and very high leptin levels. Six days following renal transplantation, mean leptin levels decreased to control levels, and this normalization was driven by a marked decrease in the obese patients, although even those with normal pre-transplant leptin levels tended to decline. This normalization of leptin persisted for at least 60 days posttransplant [43]. The restoration of renal function leading to a normalization of leptin levels further supports the notion that impaired renal clearance is a major contributor to hyperleptinemia in ESRD. Approximately 6 months onwards following renal transplantation some but not all authors have reported a tendency for plasma leptin levels to increase above the early posttransplant nadir [44–47]. Potential explanations for an increase in leptin in the late posttransplant period include the effects of glucocorticoids [9], insulin therapy for posttransplant diabetes [48, 49], weight gain, and decline in GFR. However, Souza et al. [44] found no correlation between leptin and renal function during 1 year of posttransplant follow-up.

Leptin as a Mediator of End-Organ Damage in CKD and ESRD

Hyperleptinemia has been associated with adverse effects on cardiovascular, renal and vascular remodeling in preclinical studies. Animal studies have shown that leptin caused activation of sympathetic nervous system, attenuated natriuresis, and decreased urinary excretion of nitric oxide [50, 51]. Intracerebroventricular injection of leptin induced a steady increase in mean arterial pressure, and sympathetic nerve activity [50]. However, the leptin-induced increase in sympathetic activity is not always followed by an increase in arterial pressure in animals, and data suggest the leptin-induced production of nitric oxide may modulate any pressor effect of sympathetic activation by leptin [51, 52]. Sodium retention is an early abnormality in CKD and contributes to the presence and severity of hypertension [53]. Progressive decline in GFR is associated with increased risks for hypertension and heart failure. The possible role of leptin (whose levels also increase with declining GFR) in cardiovascular dysfunction among CKD patients remains to be fully elucidated. Leptin's demonstrated effects on hemodynamics and solute retention predict potentially deleterious cardiovascular consequences in CKD. The subject of leptin and hypertension is discussed further in Chap. 14. In animal models, leptin has been reported to mediate adverse cardiovascular effects via increased sympathetic activation, myocyte hypertrophy, and prothrombotic actions [50, 54–56]. Left ventricular hypertrophy increases in frequency and severity with CKD progression and is present in about 50 % of incident dialysis patients [57–59]. The presence of left ventricular hypertrophy also strongly correlates with the risk of cardiovascular events and death in ESRD patients [58, 60].

Progressive loss of GFR resulting in ESRD, despite adequate control of blood pressure and diabetes mellitus, is a frequent problem in CKD patients [61, 62]. Glomerular hyperfiltration may promote progressive glomerular fibrosis via transforming growth factor-β (TGF-β) and other profibrotic inflammatory cytokines [61, 62]. Leptin stimulates cell proliferation and increased synthesis of TGF-β1 and type IV collagen in glomerular endothelial cells, and also increases TGF-β2 receptor expression and glucose transport in glomerular mesangial cells [63, 64]. These changes have been linked to increased extracellular matrix production in the glomerulus and subsequent risk of focal glomerulosclerosis and proteinuria [64]. These animal data implicate hyperleptinemia as a potential mediator of cardiovascular morbidity and progression of renal dysfunction, but corroboration from clinical studies is lacking.

Hyperleptinemia and Clinical Outcomes in ESRD

Nutrition is an important predictor of mortality in CKD patients. In ESRD patients, progressive loss of body weight is associated with increased risk of death, and unlike in the general population, obesity is associated with improved survival [65, 66]. Leptin through its pro-inflammatory action has been postulated to contribute to cachexia and increased morbidity and mortality in CKD and ESRD patients. In this regard, some studies have observed that patients with higher circulating leptin levels in relation to body fat have lower lean mass and increased weight loss over time [67, 68]. In peritoneal dialysis patients, hyperleptinemia was reportedly associated with weight loss [49]; however, Merabet et al. [20] did not observe any correlation between changes in leptin levels and changes in body weight among hemodialyzed patients [20]. In addition to body weight homeostasis, there have been several reports linking leptin to a number of clinical outcomes in patients with CKD and ESRD [69–101].

Anemia

Anemia of CKD and ESRD is another area where a plausible role of leptin has been suggested. The severity of anemia and resistance to exogenous erythropoietin correlate with an increased risk of death in CKD and ESRD patients [69, 70]. The etiology of anemia in CKD and ESRD includes decreased erythropoietin production and inflammation. Leptin receptors are present on hematopoietic cells in the bone marrow; stimulation of rodent bone marrow cells with leptin induces GM-CSF expression, leading to enhanced hematopoiesis [71, 72]. Consonant with these effects, human studies have shown that serum leptin levels correlate positively with higher hemoglobin and improved sensitivity to recombinant erythropoietin [73, 74]. Patients with higher body fat, who also had higher leptin levels, showed increased responsiveness to exogenous erythropoietin [73, 75].

Glucoregulation

Approximately 50 % of patients with ESRD receiving dialysis treatment in the USA have diabetes [76]. Leptin receptors are present on the membranes of pancreatic islet β-cells, where leptin action results in inhibition of insulin secretion [77]. Leptin levels have been found to be higher in lean insulin-resistant individuals as compared to lean insulin-sensitive individuals [78], and higher in obese insulin-resistant persons than obese insulin-sensitive persons [79]. These findings suggest that higher leptin levels might be a compensatory response to ambient insulin resistance, as argued by Dagogo-Jack et al. [79]. In CKD patients, higher leptin levels have been associated with hyperinsulinemia and insulin resistance, independent of body fat [49]. However, it is not known whether hyperleptinemia in CKD patients with diabetes is associated with alteration in glycemic control relative to patients with normoleptinemia.

Metabolic Bone Disease

Metabolic bone disease (MBD) is common in patients with CKD and ESRD, and has unique characteristics compared to patients with normal renal function. To distinguish it from other forms of metabolic bone disease, and to highlight the diverse range of bone and metabolic disturbances, it is now referred to as CKD-MBD. There are several types of bone abnormalities observed in CKD-MBD:osteitis fibrosa, from secondary hyperparathyroidism; osteomalacia, from vitamin D deficiency; and adynamic bone disease [80]. The recognized abnormalities in bone mineral metabolism in patients with CKD and ESRD include secondary hyperparathyroidism, hypocalcemia, hyperphosphatemia, vitamin D deficiency, 1,25-$(OH)_2$-vitamin D (calcitriol) deficiency, and elevated fibroblast growth factor-23 (FGF-23) [80]. All of these abnormalities increase in frequency and severity as GFR declines, and all of these abnormalities have been associated with increased mortality in CKD or ESRD patients [80–89]. In vitro and in vivo studies have indicated that leptin may have osteogenic effects by acting on osteoclasts, osteoblasts, and chondrocytes [90–92]. In a study by Tsuji et al. [93], mice treated with leptin showed increased expression of FGF-23 mRNA in bone, which was associated with a reduction in 1α-hydroxylase and lower levels of calcitriol, calcium, and phosphate.

Leptin has rather interesting correlates with bone parameters in renal-impaired humans [94–96]. In CKD patients, circulating leptin levels correlate inversely with intact PTH, and positively with calcium levels [94–96]. Coen et al. studied 46 hemodialysis patients, using double-tetracycline labeling followed by transiliac bone biopsy, histological, histomorphometric, and histodynamic analyses [94]. The higher leptin levels observed in obese ESRD patients undergoing dialysis treatment were associated with decreased osteoclast numbers and mineral apposition rate and a trend toward decreased osteoblastic activity [94]. However, there was no significant association between leptin levels and low bone turnover disease [94]. The relationship between leptin and bone mineral density has not been well studied in CKD patients and reports from studies in non-CKD populations have been inconsistent [97, 98]. Thus, although leptin appears to have significant interactions with several elements of CKD-MBD, further studies are needed to determine if leptin plays a pathological or beneficial role in bone health in CKD and ESRD patients. The subject of leptin and bone is discussed extensively in Chap. 13.

Leptin and Mortality

ESRD patients have 10–100-fold higher risk of total and cardiovascular mortality compared to age-matched controls. Several factors including cardiovascular disease, malnutrition, inflammation, oxidative stress, and endothelial dysfunction contribute to the increased mortality [66]. The relationship of leptin to mortality in CKD patients has been recently studied. Park et al. [99] studied leptin to adiponectin ratios in PD patients. After adjusting for potential confounders including age, BMI and serum albumin, nondiabetic patients with higher leptin to adiponectin ratio had higher mortality [99]. In hemodialysis patients, low ghrelin levels have been associated with protein energy wasting and higher mortality, especially cardiovascular mortality [100]. Of note, the low ghrelin levels were associated with higher leptin, and CRP levels, which suggests that ghrelin, leptin, and inflammation might be biomarkers of protein energy wasting and higher mortality in ESRD patients. Parenthetically, leptin is a strong stimulant of FGF-23 expression, and circulating FGF-23 levels are markedly elevated in ESRD patients, and correlate with mortality [85, 93].

In contrast, another clinical study examining the relationship of leptin levels to prevalent cardiovascular disease and subsequent mortality found no significant correlation of either cardiovascular disease or mortality with leptin levels or leptin/BMI ratio [101]. Indeed, some studies have associated higher leptin levels with favorable clinical characteristics (including higher serum albumin levels) and improved survival in ESRD patients [102–104]. In a study of 71 hemodialysis patients followed for up to 7 years, Scholze et al. [104] reported that a lower baseline leptin level was associated with 3.8-fold higher risk of mortality than higher leptin levels. Similar paradoxical relationships have been observed between higher levels of cholesterol, blood pressure, or obesity and improved survival in ESRD patients, a phenomenon referred to as "reverse epidemiology" [65, 102]. The observation of higher leptin and higher weight correlating with improved survival in ESRD may reflect confounding health factors which lead to weight loss and lower leptin as patients' clinical condition declines prior to death. Hence, the nutritional impact of leptin in CKD and ESRD patients requires a more exhaustive investigation.

Taken together, these data suggest that hyperleptinemia could be either maladaptive or adaptive in patients with CKD and ESRD, or it may be an innocent bystander that is nevertheless highly associated with other factors mediating progression of CKD and cardiovascular disease [105].

Lowering Leptin Levels in ESRD Patients

Based on current understanding, the rationale for specific intervention to alter circulating leptin levels in patients with CKD or ESRD has not been firmly established. Nonetheless, we here discuss comparative outcomes of different dialysis methods that are associated with differential leptin clearance in ESRD patients. The most effect way to lower leptin levels in ESRD patients appears to be use of high flux dialyzers, or for even greater clearance, use of hemodialfiltration. Notably, a large trial which randomized ESRD patients to low flux or high flux dialyzers found no difference in overall mortality, although secondary analysis of some prespecified cardiac events suggested some benefit [37]. Similarly, a randomized trial assigning ESRD patients to low flux dialyzers versus hemodiafiltration (which would provide even greater reductions in leptin levels), found no difference in mortality [106]. Two other clinical trials that compared high flux dialyzers versus hemodiafiltration have been concluded, with one showing a reduction in mortality in the hemodiafiltration group [107, 108]. Cyclical therapy with recombinant IGF-1 has been reported to decrease serum leptin by ~30 % in patients with pre-terminal (stage 5) CKD, but no clinical outcomes were reported in that study [109].

Thus, although clinical studies aimed specifically at altering leptin have not been performed, the available data do provide indirect insight into the possible impact of leptin manipulation on clinical outcomes in ESRD patients.

Summary

Leptin levels increase in patients with CKD and ESRD due to both reduced clearance/catabolism by the kidneys and likely enhanced production due to stimulation by insulin, glucocorticoids, and inflammatory cytokines. Hyperleptinemia is common in ESRD patients, and is exacerbated by obesity, use of peritoneal versus hemodialysis, and use of low-flux versus high-flux dialyzers for hemodialysis. Renal transplantation leads to normalization of leptin levels within days. While several threads of evidence suggest leptin could be a major pathological contributor to the high incidence of cardiovascular mortality in CKD and ESRD patients, observational data have not strongly linked hyperleptinemia to worse outcomes. Despite ongoing research for almost two decades, major gaps remain in our understanding of the effects of hyperleptinemia in patients with CKD and ESRD.

References

1. Zhang Y, Proenca R, Maffei M, et al. Positional cloning of the mouse obese gene and its human homologue. Nature. 1994;372:425–32.
2. Katz AI, Emmanouel DS. Metabolism of polypeptide hormones by the normal kidney and in uremia. Nephron. 1978;22:69–80.
3. Dinarello CA. Interleukin-1 and tumor necrosis factor and their naturally occurring antagonists during hemodialysis. Kidney Int Suppl. 1992;38:S68–77.
4. Macdonald C, Rush DN, Bernstein KN, et al. Production of tumor necrosis factor alpha and hemodialysis. Nephron. 1993;65:273–7.
5. Zumbach MS, Boehme MW, Wahl P, et al. Tumor necrosis factor increases serum leptin levels in humans. J Clin Endocrinol Metab. 1997;82:4080–2.
6. Kobayashi S, Maesato K, Moriya H, et al. Insulin resistance in patients with chronic kidney disease. Am J Kidney Dis. 2005;45:275–80.
7. Chen J, Muntner P, Hamm LL, et al. Insulin resistance and risk of chronic kidney disease in nondiabetic US adults. J Am Soc Nephrol. 2003;14: 469–77.
8. Kolaczynski JW, Nyce MR, Considine RV, et al. Acute and chronic effects of insulin on leptin production in humans: studies in vivo and in vitro. Diabetes. 1996;45:699–701.
9. Askari H, Liu J, Dagogo-Jack S. Hormonal regulation of human leptin in vivo: effects of hydrocortisone and insulin. Int J Obes Relat Metab Disord. 2000;24:1254–9.
10. Cumin F, Baum HP, Levens N. Mechanism of leptin removal from the circulation by the kidney. J Endocrinol. 1997;155:577–85.
11. Cumin F, Baum HP, Levens N. Leptin is cleared from the circulation primarily by the kidney. Int J Obes Relat Metab Disord. 1996;20:1120–6.
12. Zeng J, Patterson BW, Klein S, et al. Whole body leptin kinetics and renal metabolism in vivo. Am J Physiol. 1997;273(6 Pt 1):E1102–6.
13. Landt M, Martin DR, Zeng J, et al. Plasma leptin concentrations are only transiently increased in nephrectomized rats. Am J Physiol. 1998;275(3 Pt 1):E495–9.
14. Landt M, Ludbrook PA, Billadello JJ. Role of protein binding in renal elimination of leptin. Clin Endocrinol (Oxf). 2003;59:44–8.
15. Klein S, Coppack SW, Mohamed-Ali V, et al. Adipose tissue leptin production and plasma leptin kinetics in humans. Diabetes. 1996;45:984–7.
16. Hama H, Saito A, Takeda T, et al. Evidence indicating that renal tubular metabolism of leptin is mediated by megalin but not by the leptin receptors. Endocrinology. 2004;145:3935–40.
17. Sharma K, Considine RV, Michael B, et al. Plasma leptin is partly cleared by the kidney and is elevated in hemodialysis patients. Kidney Int. 1997;51:1980–5.
18. Fruehwald-Schultes B, Kern W, Beyer J, Forst T, Pfützner A, Peters A. Elevated serum leptin concentrations in type 2 diabetic patients with microalbuminuria and macroalbuminuria. Metabolism. 1999;48:1290–3.
19. Okpechi IG, Pascoe MD, Swanepoel CR, Rayner BL. Microalbuminuria and the metabolic syndrome in non-diabetic black Africans. Diab Vasc Dis Res. 2007;4:365–7.
20. Merabet E, Dagogo-Jack S, Coyne DW, et al. Increased plasma leptin concentration in end-stage renal disease. J Clin Endocrinol Metab. 1997;82: 847–50.
21. Heimbürger O, Lönnqvist F, Danielsson A, Nordenström J, Stenvinkel P. Serum immunoreactive leptin concentration and its relation to the body fat content in chronic renal failure. J Am Soc Nephrol. 1997;8:1423–30.
22. Howard JK, Lord GM, Clutterbuck EJ, Ghatei MA, Pusey CD, Bloom SR. Plasma immunoreactive leptin concentration in end-stage renal disease. Clin Sci (Lond). 1997;93:119–26.
23. Dagogo-Jack S, Ovalle F, Geary B, Landt M, Coyne DW. 1998 Hyperleptinemia in patients with end-stage renal disease treated by continuous ambulatory peritoneal dialysis. Perit Dial Int. 1998;18:34–40.
24. Nordfors L, Lönnqvist F, Heimbürger O, Danielsson A, Schalling M, Stenvinkel P. Low leptin gene expression and hyperleptinemia in chronic renal failure. Kidney Int. 1998;54:1267–75.
25. Landt M, Parvin CA, Dagogo-Jack S, Bryant B, Coyne DW. Leptin elimination in hyperleptinaemic peritoneal dialysis patients. Nephrol Dial Transplant. 1999;14:732–7.
26. Pelleymounter MA, Cullen MJ, Baker MB, et al. Effects of the obese gene product on body weight regulation in ob/ob mice. Science. 1995;269:540–3.
27. Halaas JL, Gajiwala KS, Maffei M, et al. Weight-reducing effects of the plasma protein encoded by the obese gene. Science. 1995;269:543–6.

28. Licinio J, Caglayan S, Ozata M. Phenotypic effects of leptin replacement on morbid obesity, diabetes mellitus, hypogonadism, and behavior in leptin-deficient adults. Proc Natl Acad Sci U S A. 2004;101:4531–6.
29. Farooqi IS, Matarese G, Lord GM, et al. Beneficial effects of leptin on obesity, T cell hyporesponsiveness, and neuroendocrine/metabolic dysfunction of human congenital leptin deficiency. J Clin Invest. 2002;110:1093–103.
30. Menon V, Wang X, Greene T, et al. Factors associated with serum leptin in patients with chronic kidney disease. Clin Nephrol. 2004;61:163–9.
31. Sarnak MJ, Poindexter A, Wang SR, et al. Serum C-reactive protein and leptin as predictors of kidney disease progression in the Modification of Diet in Renal Disease Study. Kidney Int. 2002;62:2208–15.
32. Shankar A, Syamala S, Xiao J, Muntner P. Relationship between plasma leptin level and chronic kidney disease. Int J Nephrol. 2012;2012:269532. doi:10.1155/2012/269532. Epub 2012 May 14.
33. Grunfeld C, Zhao C, Fuller J, Pollack A, Moser A, Friedman J, Feingold KR. Endotoxin and cytokines induce expression of leptin, the ob gene product, in hamsters. J Clin Invest. 1996;97:2152–7.
34. Coyne DW, Dagogo-Jack S, Klein S, Merabet E, Audrain J, Landt M. High-flux dialysis lowers plasma leptin concentration in chronic dialysis patients. Am J Kidney Dis. 1998;32:1031–5.
35. van Tellingen A, Grooteman MP, Schoorl M, ter Wee PM, Bartels PC, Schoorl M, van der Ploeg T, Nubé MJ. Enhanced long-term reduction of plasma leptin concentrations by super-flux polysulfone dialysers. Nephrol Dial Transplant. 2004;19:1198–203.
36. Mandolfo S, Borlandelli S, Imbasciati E. Leptin and beta2-microglobulin kinetics with three different dialysis modalities. Int J Artif Organs. 2006;29:949–55.
37. Eknoyan G, Beck GJ, Cheung AK, et al. Effect of dialysis dose and membrane flux in maintenance hemodialysis. N Engl J Med. 2002;347:2010–9.
38. Cheung AK, Sarnak MJ, Yan G, et al. Cardiac diseases in maintenance hemodialysis patients: results of the HEMO Study. Kidney Int. 2004;65:2380–9.
39. Arkouche W, Juillard L, Delawari E, et al. Peritoneal clearance of leptin in continuous ambulatory peritoneal dialysis. Am J Kidney Dis. 1999;34:839–44.
40. Taskapan MC, Taskapan H, Sahin I, Keskin L, Atmaca H, Ozyalin F. Serum leptin, resistin, and lipid levels in patients with end stage renal failure with regard to dialysis modality. Ren Fail. 2007; 29:147–54.
41. Fontán MP, Rodríguez-Carmona A, Cordido F, García-Buela J. Hyperleptinemia in uremic patients undergoing conservative management, peritoneal dialysis, and hemodialysis: a comparative analysis. Am J Kidney Dis. 1999;34:824–31.
42. Teta D, Maillard M, Tedjani A, Passlick-Deetjen J, Burnier M. The effect of pH-neutral peritoneal dialysis fluids on adipokine secretion from cultured adipocytes. Nephrol Dial Transplant. 2007;22:862–9.
43. Landt M, Brennan DC, Parvin CA, Flavin KS, Dagogo-Jack S, Coyne DW. Hyperleptinaemia of end-stage renal disease is corrected by renal transplantation. Nephrol Dial Transplant. 1998;13: 2271–5.
44. Souza GC, Costa CA, Gonçalves LF, Manfro RC. Leptin serum levels in the first year post-renal transplantation. Transplant Proc. 2007;39:439–40.
45. Kokot F, Adamczak M, Wiecek A, et al. Plasma immunoreactive leptin and neuropeptide Y levels in kidney transplant patients. Am J Nephrol. 1999; 19:28.
46. Kaycan SM, Yildiz A, Kazancioglu R, et al. The changes in serum leptin, body fat mass and insulin resistance after renal transplantation. Clin Transplant. 2003;17:63.
47. El Haggan W, Chauveau P, Barthe N, et al. Serum leptin, body fat, and nutritional markers during the six months post-Kidney transplantation. Metabolism. 2004;53:614.
48. Lane JT, Dagogo-Jack S. Approach to the patient with new-onset diabetes after transplant (NODAT). J Clin Endocrinol Metab. 2011;96:3289–97.
49. Stenvinkel P, Heimbürger O, Lönnqvist F. Serum leptin concentrations correlate to plasma insulin concentrations independent of body fat content in chronic renal failure. Nephrol Dial Transplant. 1997;12:1321–5.
50. Dunbar JC, Hu Y, Lu H. Intracerebroventricular leptin increases lumbar and renal sympathetic nerve activity and blood pressure in normal rats. Diabetes. 1997;46:2040–3.
51. Beltowski J, Wojcicka G, Marciniak A, et al. Oxidative stress, nitric oxide production, and renal sodium handling in leptin-induced hypertension. Life Sci. 2004;74:2987–3000.
52. Fruhbeck G. Pivotal role of nitric oxide in the control of blood pressure after leptin administration. Diabetes. 1999;48:903–8.
53. Hadtstein C, Schaefer F. Hypertension in children with chronic kidney disease: pathophysiology and management. Pediatr Nephrol. 2008;23:363–71.
54. Haynes WG, Morgan DA, Walsh SA, et al. Receptor-mediated regional sympathetic nerve activation by leptin. J Clin Invest. 1997;100:270–8.
55. Selthofer-Relatic K, Radic R, Vizjak V, et al. Hyperleptinemia–non-haemodynamic risk factor for the left ventricular hypertrophy development in hypertensive overweight females. Coll Antropol. 2008;32:681–5.
56. Konstantinides S, Schafer K, Koschnick S, et al. Leptin-dependent platelet aggregation and arterial thrombosis suggests a mechanism for atherothrombotic disease in obesity. J Clin Invest. 2001;108: 1533–40.
57. Paoletti E, Bellino D, Cassottana P, et al. Left ventricular hypertrophy in nondiabetic predialysis CKD. Am J Kidney Dis. 2005;46:320–7.
58. Stack AG, Saran R. Clinical correlates and mortality impact of left ventricular hypertrophy among new

ESRD patients in the United States. Am J Kidney Dis. 2002;40:1202–10.
59. Harnett JD, Parfrey PS, Griffiths SM, et al. Left ventricular hypertrophy in end-stage renal disease. Nephron. 1988;48:107–15.
60. Goodkin DA, Bragg-Gresham JL, Koenig KG, et al. Association of comorbid conditions and mortality in hemodialysis patients in Europe, Japan, and the United States: the Dialysis Outcomes and Practice Patterns Study (DOPPS). J Am Soc Nephrol. 2003;14:3270–7.
61. Bottinger EP. TGF-beta in renal injury and disease. Semin Nephrol. 2007;27:309–20.
62. Eddy AA. Progression in chronic kidney disease. Adv Chronic Kidney Dis. 2005;12:353–65.
63. Wolf G, Chen S, Han DC, et al. Leptin and renal disease. Am J Kidney Dis. 2002;39:1–11.
64. Wolf G, Hamann A, Han DC, et al. Leptin stimulates proliferation and TGF-beta expression in renal glomerular endothelial cells: potential role in glomerulosclerosis. Kidney Int. 1999;56:860–72.
65. Kalantar-Zadeh K, Block G, Humphreys MH, et al. Reverse epidemiology of cardiovascular risk factors in maintenance dialysis patients. Kidney Int. 2003; 63:793–808.
66. Kalantar-Zadeh K, Ikizler TA, Block G, et al. Malnutrition-inflammation complex syndrome in dialysis patients: causes and consequences. Am J Kidney Dis. 2003;42:864–81.
67. Odamaki M, Furuya R, Yoneyama T, et al. Association of the serum leptin concentration with weight loss in chronic hemodialysis patients. Am J Kidney Dis. 1999;33:361–8.
68. Young GA, Woodrow G, Kendall S, et al. Increased plasma leptin/fat ratio in patients with chronic renal failure: a cause of malnutrition? Nephrol Dial Transplant. 1997;12:2318–23.
69. Zhang Y, Thamer M, Stefanik K, et al. Epoetin requirements predict mortality in hemodialysis patients. Am J Kidney Dis. 2004;44:866–76.
70. Szczech LA, Barnhart HX, Inrig JK, et al. Secondary analysis of the CHOIR trial epoetin-alpha dose and achieved hemoglobin outcomes. Kidney Int. 2008;74:791–8.
71. Gainsford T, Willson TA, Metcalf D, et al. Leptin can induce proliferation, differentiation, and functional activation of hemopoietic cells. Proc Natl Acad Sci U S A. 1996;93:14564–8.
72. Umemoto Y, Tsuji K, Yang FC, et al. Leptin stimulates the proliferation of murine myelocytic and primitive hematopoietic progenitor cells. Blood. 1997;90:3438–43.
73. Axelsson J, Qureshi AR, Heimburger O, et al. Body fat mass and serum leptin levels influence epoetin sensitivity in patients with ESRD. Am J Kidney Dis. 2005;46:628–34.
74. Nasri H. Association of serum leptin with anemia in maintenance hemodialysis patients. Saudi J Kidney Dis Transpl. 2006;17:521–5.
75. Kotanko P, Thijssen S, Levin NW. Association between erythropoietin responsiveness and body composition in dialysis patients. Blood Purif. 2008;26:82–9.
76. Dagogo-Jack S. Glycemic control and chronic diabetes complications. In: Umpierrez GE, editor. Therapy for diabetes mellitus and related disorders. 6th ed. Alexandria, VA: American Diabetes Association; 2014. p. 668–95.
77. Emilsson V, Liu YL, Cawthorne MA, et al. Expression of the functional leptin receptor mRNA in pancreatic islets and direct inhibitory action of leptin on insulin secretion. Diabetes. 1997;46:313–6.
78. Segal KR, Landt M, Klein S. Relationship between insulin sensitivity and plasma leptin concentration in lean and obese men. Diabetes. 1996;45:988–91.
79. Askari H, Tykodi G, Liu J, Dagogo-Jack S. Fasting plasma leptin level is a surrogate measure of insulin sensitivity. J Clin Endocrinol Metab. 2010;95: 3836–43.
80. KDIGO. Clinical practice guideline for the diagnosis, evaluation, prevention, and treatment of chronic kidney disease-mineral and bone disorder (CKD-MBD). Kidney Int Suppl. 2009;113:S1–130.
81. Shoben AB, Rudser KD, de Boer IH, et al. Association of oral calcitriol with improved survival in nondialyzed CKD. J Am Soc Nephrol. 2008;19:1613–9.
82. Kovesdy CP, Ahmadzadeh S, Anderson JE, et al. Association of activated vitamin D treatment and mortality in chronic kidney disease. Arch Intern Med. 2008;168:397–403.
83. Gutierrez O, Isakova T, Rhee E, et al. Fibroblast growth factor-23 mitigates hyperphosphatemia but accentuates calcitriol deficiency in chronic kidney disease. J Am Soc Nephrol. 2005;16:2205–15.
84. Teng M, Wolf M, Lowrie E, et al. Survival of patients undergoing hemodialysis with paricalcitol or calcitriol therapy. N Engl J Med. 2003;349:446–56.
85. Gutierrez OM, Mannstadt M, Isakova T, et al. Fibroblast growth factor 23 and mortality among patients undergoing hemodialysis. N Engl J Med. 2008;359:584–92.
86. Isakova T, Xie H, Yang W, et al. Fibroblast growth factor 23 and risks of mortality and end-stage renal disease in patients with chronic kidney disease. JAMA. 2011;305:2432–9.
87. Kalantar-Zadeh K, Kuwae N, Regidor DL, et al. Survival predictability of time-varying indicators of bone disease in maintenance hemodialysis patients. Kidney Int. 2006;70:771–80.
88. Kovesdy CP, Anderson JE, Kalantar-Zadeh K. Outcomes associated with serum phosphorus level in males with non-dialysis dependent chronic kidney disease. Clin Nephrol. 2010;73:268–75.
89. Schumock GT, Andress DL, Marx SE, et al. Association of secondary hyperparathyroidism with CKD progression, health care costs and survival in diabetic predialysis CKD patients. Nephron Clin Pract. 2009;113:c54–61.

90. Martin A, de Vittoris R, David V, et al. Leptin modulates both resorption and formation while preventing disuse-induced bone loss in tail-suspended female rats. Endocrinology. 2005;146:3652–9.
91. Reseland JE, Syversen U, Bakke I, et al. Leptin is expressed in and secreted from primary cultures of human osteoblasts and promotes bone mineralization. J Bone Miner Res. 2001;16:1426–33.
92. Thomas T, Gori F, Khosla S, et al. Leptin acts on human marrow stromal cells to enhance differentiation to osteoblasts and to inhibit differentiation to adipocytes. Endocrinology. 1999;140:1630–8.
93. Tsuji K, Maeda T, Kawane T, et al. Leptin stimulates fibroblast growth factor 23 expression in bone and suppresses renal 1alpha, 25-dihydroxyvitamin D3 synthesis in leptin-deficient mice. J Bone Miner Res. 2010;25:1711–23.
94. Coen G, Ballanti P, Fischer MS, et al. Serum leptin in dialysis renal osteodystrophy. Am J Kidney Dis. 2003;42:1036–42.
95. Zoccali C, Panuccio V, Tripepi G, et al. Leptin and biochemical markers of bone turnover in dialysis patients. J Nephrol. 2004;17:253–60.
96. Ahmadi F, Salari S, Maziar S, et al. Relationship between serum leptin levels and bone mineral density and bone metabolic markers in patients on hemodialysis. Saudi J Kidney Dis Transpl. 2013;24:41–7.
97. Pasco JA, Henry MJ, Kotowicz MA, et al. Serum leptin levels are associated with bone mass in non-obese women. J Clin Endocrinol Metab. 2001;86:1884–7.
98. Kontogianni MD, Dafni UG, Routsias JG, et al. Blood leptin and adiponectin as possible mediators of the relation between fat mass and BMD in perimenopausal women. J Bone Miner Res. 2004;19:546–51.
99. Park JT, Yoo TH, Kim JK, et al. Leptin/adiponectin ratio is an independent predictor of mortality in nondiabetic peritoneal dialysis patients. Perit Dial Int. 2013;33:67–74.
100. Carrero JJ, Nakashima A, Qureshi AR, et al. Protein-energy wasting modifies the association of ghrelin with inflammation, leptin, and mortality in hemodialysis patients. Kidney Int. 2011;79:749–56.
101. Diez JJ, Bossola M, Fernandez-Reyes MJ, et al. Relationship between leptin and all-cause and cardiovascular mortality in chronic hemodialysis patients. Nefrologia. 2011;31:206–12.
102. Kalantar-Zadeh K, Fouque D, Kopple JD. Outcome research, nutrition, and reverse epidemiology in maintenance dialysis patients. J Ren Nutr. 2004;14:64–71.
103. Aguilera A, Bajo MA, Rebollo F, et al. Leptin as a marker of nutrition and cardiovascular risk in peritoneal dialysis patients. Adv Perit Dial. 2002;18:212–7.
104. Scholze A, Rattensperger D, Zidek W, et al. Low serum leptin predicts mortality in patients with chronic kidney disease stage 5. Obesity (Silver Spring). 2007;15(6):1617–22.
105. Dagogo-Jack S. Uremic hyperleptinemia: adaptive or maladaptive. Kidney Int. 1998;54:997–8.
106. Grooteman MP, van den Dorpel MA, Bots ML, et al. Effect of online hemodiafiltration on all-cause mortality and cardiovascular outcomes. J Am Soc Nephrol. 2012;23:1087–96.
107. Ok E, Asci G, Toz H, et al. Mortality and cardiovascular events in online haemodiafiltration (OL-HDF) compared with high-flux dialysis: results from the Turkish OL-HDF Study. Nephrol Dial Transplant. 2013;28:192–202.
108. Maduell F, Moreso F, Pons M, et al. High-efficiency postdilution online hemodiafiltration reduces all-cause mortality in hemodialysis patients. J Am Soc Nephrol. 2013;24:487–97.
109. Dagogo-Jack S, Franklin SC, Vijayan A, Liu J, Askari H, Miller SB. Recombinant human insulin-like growth factor-I (IGF-I) therapy decreases plasma leptin concentration in patients with chronic renal insufficiency. Int J Obes. 1998;22:1110–5.

Leptin, Immune Function, and Inflammation

11

Giuseppe Matarese, Claudio Procaccini,
Valentina Pucino, and Christos Mantzoros

Introduction

Leptin is one of the most important hormones secreted by adipose tissue [1], and its implication in energetic homeostasis at central level has been largely described [2]. The past 20 years of research on adipose tissue has provided important insights into the intricate network that links nutrition, metabolism, and immune homeostasis. In this context leptin works not only as a "fasting hormone" by controlling body weight through the inhibition of food intake and stimulation of energy expenditure by increased thermogenesis [3], but also in the regulation of sexual-reproduction [4], haematopoiesis [5], angiogenesis [6, 7], bone metabolism [8], and glucose homeostasis [9]. Indeed, it has been previously shown, that *ob/ob* and *db/db* mice are not only obese but also show many other immune/endocrine alterations observed during starvation [10–12]. Although an important role of leptin is to regulate body weight through the inhibition of food intake, recent evidence has indicated that leptin is much more than a "fat-o-stat" sensor and it is also involved in the modulation of several innate and adaptive immune responses [13]. Indeed, leptin receptor (LepRb) is expressed by several immune cells, thus suggesting a key role displayed by leptin in the regulation of immune responses [14].

Modulation of the immune system by leptin is exerted at the development, proliferation, anti-apoptotic, maturation, and activation levels [15]. In fact, leptin receptors have been found in neutrophils, monocytes, and lymphocytes, and the leptin receptor belongs to the family of class I cytokine receptors. The overall leptin action in the immune system is a pro-inflammatory effect, activating pro-inflammatory cells, promoting T-helper 1 responses, and mediating the production of the other pro-inflammatory cytokines, such as tumor necrosis factor-α, interleukin (IL)-2, or IL-6.

G. Matarese, M.D., Ph.D. (✉)
Dipartimento di Medicina e Chirurgia, Facoltà di Medicinae Chirurgia, Università di Salerno Baronissi Campus, 84081 Baronissi, Salerno, Italy
e-mail: gmatarese@unisa.it

C. Procaccini, Ph.D.
Laboratorio di Immunologia, Istituto di Endocrinologia e Oncologia Sperimentale, Consiglio Nazionale delle Ricerche (IEOS-CNR), 80131 Naples, Italy

V. Pucino, M.D.
Dipartimento di Scienze Mediche Traslazionali, Università di Napoli "Federico II", 80131 Naples, Italy

C. Mantzoros, M.D., D.Sc.
Section of Endocrinology, Boston VA Healthcare System, Jamaica Plain, MA, USA

Department of Medicine, Beth Israel Deaconess Medical Center, Harvard Medical School and Boston Medical Center, Boston, MA, USA

S. Dagogo-Jack (ed.), *Leptin: Regulation and Clinical Applications*,
DOI 10.1007/978-3-319-09915-6_11, © Springer International Publishing Switzerland 2015

Leptin is therefore able to modulate both innate and adaptive immune response [13]. Moreover, several studies in human revealed that leptin levels associated with autoimmune disorders, infections and endocrine/metabolic diseases, thus suggesting a central role of leptin in immune homeostasis and in the pathogenesis of several inflammatory disorders [16–18]. This chapter analyses the role of leptin in immune homeostasis, and the direct and indirect influences of leptin on inflammation and autoimmunity.

Leptin Regulation of Innate Immunity

Leptin and Monocytes/Macrophages

Studies of several animal models with genetic abnormalities in leptin or leptin receptors revealed obesity-related deficits in macrophage functions in terms of phagocytosis and the expression of proinflammatory cytokines both in vivo and in vitro, whereas on the contrary exogenous leptin upregulates both phagocytosis and the production of cytokines [19] (Table 11.1).

Leptin deficiency increases susceptibility to infectious and inflammatory stimuli and is associated with dysregulation of cytokine production [20]. More specifically, murine leptin deficiency alters Kupffer cell production of cytokines that regulate the innate immune system. In this context, leptin levels increase acutely during infection and inflammation, and may represent a protective component of the host response to inflammation [21]. Elevated circulating IL-18 levels are associated with clinical complications of type 2 diabetes (T2DM) and IL-18 itself regulates cytokine secretion and the function of a number of immune cells, playing a key role in immunity and inflammation. A recent paper has shown that leptin enhances the secretion of interleukin (IL)-18, but not IL-1β from human monocytes via activation of caspase-1; indeed these

Table 11.1 Effects of leptin on the different cell populations of both innate and adaptive immune response

Cell type	Lep receptor	Leptin effects on cell function	Action	References
Monocytes/ macrophages	Yes	Upregulates phagocytic function; upregulates proinflammatory cytokine secretion (TNF-α, IL-6, IL-12) and the expression of activation markers; increases cell motility.	Direct	[19–37]
Dendritic cells	Yes	Promotes survival; increases immature DC migratory performance and the stimulatory capability of allogenic T cells.	Direct	[38–43]
Neutrophils	Unknown	Induces chemotaxis and the release of oxygen radicals	Indirect	[44–53]
NK cells	Yes	Increases the expression of activation marker (CD69); sustains cytotoxic activity and perforin production.	Direct	[54–57]
basophils	Yes	Sustains the migratory capability, enhances their survival rate; leptin increases basophil degranulation	Direct	[58]
eosinophils	Yes	Delays the apoptosis; stimulates the chemokinesis, and induces the release of inflammatory cytokines (IL-1beta and IL-6) and chemokines.	Direct	[59–61]
B cells	Yes	Increases lymphopoiesis and maturation; induces secretion of cytokines, such as IL-6, IL-10, and TNF-α; increases IgG2a production.	Direct	[87–91]
T cells	Yes	Induces the expression of activation markers; increases proliferation of naïve T cells; promotes the switch towards Th1-cell immune responses by increasing IFN-γ and TNF-α secretion; increases the expression of adhesion molecules; promotes the survival of thymic T cells.	Direct	[62–86]
Regulatory T cells	Yes	Constrains their proliferation and suppressive activity, through the activation of the mTOR pathway.	Direct	[69–71]

phenomena were prevented by caspase-1 inhibitor treatment (Ac-YVAD-cmk) [22]. In addition to the increased IL-18 secretion via modulation of the caspase-1 inflammasome function leptin also acts synergistically with ATP in this regard, and therefore contributes to aberrant immune responses in T2DM and other conditions of hyperleptinemia.

Human leptin was found to stimulate proliferation and activation of human circulating monocytes in vitro, promoting the expression of activation markers: CD69, CD25, CD38, and CD71, in addition to increasing the expression of monocytes surface markers, such as HLA-DR, CD11b, and CD11c [23]. Moreover, leptin dose-dependently stimulates the production of pro-inflammatory cytokines by monocytes, (such as TNF-α and IL-6 [25]) and enhances CC-chemokine ligand expression in cultured murine macrophage, through activation of a JAK2-STAT3 pathway [24]. It has been also shown that leptin directly induces the secretion of interleukin 1 receptor antagonist in human monocytes [25] and upregulates IP-10 (interferon-gamma-inducible protein) in monocytic cells [26]. Moreover, in human monocytes it has been shown that leptin increased both free radical and cholesterol productions in vitro [27].

In this context a recent paper by Maya-Monteiro et al. has shown that leptin directly activated macrophages and induced the formation of adipose differentiation-related protein-enriched lipid bodies (lipid droplets), which are emerging as dynamic organelles with roles in lipid metabolism and inflammation. Newly formed lipid bodies were sites of 5-lipoxygenase localization and correlated with an enhanced capacity of leukotriene B(4) production. The authors also showed that these mechanisms were phosphatidylinositol 3-kinase- and mammalian target of rapamycin-dependent, since were inhibited by LY294002 or rapamycin treatment [28]. Another study has demonstrated that leptin accelerates cholesteryl ester accumulation in human monocyte-derived macrophages, by increasing ACAT-1 expression via JAK2 and PI3K, thereby suppressing cholesterol efflux [29].

In alveolar macrophages leptin augments leukotriene synthesis [30] and it plays an important role in regulation of energy homeostasis and the innate immune response against bacterial infections. Indeed *ob/ob* mice exhibit an increased mortality and impaired pulmonary bacterial clearance after intratracheal challenge with Klebsiella pneumoniae. The synthesis of cysteinyl-leukotrienes is reduced and that of PGE(2) enhanced in alveolar macrophage (AMs) of *ob/ob* mice after infection with *K. pneumoniae* in vivo. In the same paper the authors also observed reduced phagocytosis and killing of *K. pneumoniae* in AMs from *ob/ob* mice that was associated with reduced reactive oxygen intermediate production in vitro. On the contrary, cAMP, known to suppress phagocytosis, bactericidal capacity, and reactive oxygen intermediate production, was increased twofold in AMs from *ob/ob* mice [31].

Elevated concentration of leptin in peritoneal fluid may contribute to the pathological process of endometriosis, through activation of peritoneal macrophages. Indeed Wu et al. have shown that treatment of peritoneal macrophages with leptin induced COX-2 expression and the production of prostaglandin F(2alpha) by peritoneal macrophages was increased after leptin stimulation in women with endometriosis [32].

A possible role of leptin as a trophic factor to prevent apoptosis has also been found in serum-depleted human monocytes [33], which is further supporting the role of leptin as a growth factor for the monocytes. Moreover, leptin regulates monocyte function as assessed by in vitro experiments measuring free radical production. Leptin was shown to stimulate the oxidative burst in control monocytes [34], and the binding of leptin at the macrophage cell surface increases lipoprotein lipase expression, through oxidative stress- and PKC-dependent pathways [35].

A recent study on mouse macrophages has demonstrated that leptin is a potent chemoattractant for monocytes and macrophages and that leptin-mediated chemotaxis requires the presence of full-length leptin receptors on migrating cells [36], suggesting that the canonical cell motility machinery is activated upon macrophage exposure to leptin.

Finally a recent report has shown that disrupted leptin signaling in bone marrow-derived cells attenuates the pro-inflammatory conditions that mediate many of the metabolic complications that characterize obesity. Indeed Dib et al. demonstrated that in chimeric C57BL/6J mice reconstituted with leptin receptor-deficient (*db/db*) bone marrow (namely the WT/db mice), gonadal adipose tissue displayed a twofold lower expression of the inflammatory genes *Tnfa*, *Il6*, and *Ccl2* and contained significantly fewer crown-like structures compared with their littermate controls. In addition most of their adipose-resident macrophages expressed galactose-type C type lectin 1 (MGL1) and were C-C chemokine receptor type 2 (CCR2)-negative, indicative of an anti-inflammatory phenotype, which could lead to the greater insulin sensitivity in WT/db mice when compared to WT/WT mice [37].

Leptin and Dendritic Cells

Interesting reports have shown that also dendritic cells (DCs), the major antigen presenting cells (APCs) involved in T lymphocyte priming, are affected by leptin at different levels (Table 11.1). More specifically, leptin deficiency associate with qualitative and quantitative alteration of DC [38]. Indeed it has been shown that DCs from *ob/ob* mice are less potent in stimulation of allogenic T cells in vitro. This impaired functionality is not associated with altered expression of phenotypic markers, but rather with the secretion of immunosuppressive cytokines such as TGF [38]. In this context, Lam et al. have also shown that leptin induces CD40 expression in murine DC and significantly upregulates their immunostimulatory function in driving T cell proliferation. This phenomenon seems to be mediated by the action of Akt, STAT-1alpha, and NF-kappaB; indeed with chromatin immunoprecipitation assay the authors showed that leptin recruits STAT-1alpha, NF-kappaBp65, and RNA polymerase II to the CD40 promoter and enhances histone 4 acetylation in a time-dependent manner [39]. Moreover, Mattioli et al. have shown that leptin induces functional and morphological changes in human DCs, licensing them towards Th1 priming and promoting DC survival [40], by triggering the activation of nuclear factor-kappa B (NF-kappaB) and a parallel upregulation of bcl-2, bcl-XL gene expression and Akt activation [41]. From the same group comes the finding showing that leptin increases immature DC migratory performance both by favoring cytoskeleton dynamics and by upregulating CCR7 surface expression, thus favoring their chemotactic responsiveness [42]. Finally, it has been shown that leptin deficiency impairs maturation of dendritic cells, decreases DC production of IL-12, TNF-α, and IL-6, and sustains DC production of TGF-β. As a consequence of this unique phenotype, DCs generated under leptin-free conditions induced Treg or Th17 cells more efficiently than DCs generated in the presence of leptin [43].

Leptin and Neutrophils

Human polymorphonuclear neutrophils (PMN) have been found to express leptin receptor in vitro and in vivo [44, 45] (Table 11.1). However, Zarkesh-Esfahani et al. [46] demonstrated that neutrophils only express the short form of the leptin receptor, which is enough to signal inside the cell, enhancing the expression of CD11b and preventing apoptosis [45, 46]. From the molecular point of view, leptin seems to delay the cleavage of Bid and Bax, the mitochondrial release of cytochrome c as well as the activation of both caspase-8 and caspase-3 in these cells [45].

Another paper has shown that leptin exhibits anti-apoptotic properties on neutrophils via NF-κB and MEK1/2 MAPK pathway activation, suggesting that leptin may enhance airway inflammation by promoting neutrophil survival [47].

Recently Ubags et al. have demonstrated that pulmonary leptin is induced in injured human and murine lungs and that this cytokine is effective in driving alveolar airspace neutrophilia [48].

In addition Caldefie-Chezet et al. have demonstrated that leptin is able to modulate the functions of this cellular subset. Indeed it promotes neutrophils chemotaxis [49] and the chemoattractant effect is comparable to that of well-known formyl-methionyl-leucyl-phenylalanine (FMLP), also by stimulating intracellular hydrogen peroxide production. Otherwise, when leptin acts as a uremic toxin it interferes with neutrophil chemotaxis [50] and opposite results have shown that leptin is able to inhibit neutrophil migration in response to classical neutrophilic chemoattractants, suggesting that by means of its chemokine-like activity, leptin is capable of inhibiting neutrophil chemotaxis in response to other neutrophilic chemoattractants. Moreover, leptin is required for neutrophil complement-mediated phagocytosis, as neutrophils from leptin-deficient mice exhibited impaired phagocytosis of Klebsiella pneumoniae opsonized with serum containing complement and reduced CD11b expression that could be restored by exogenous leptin replacement [51].

Contrasting results regarding the responsiveness of neutrophils to leptin have been observed in a recent study by Kamp et al., in which with a proteomic approach, the authors showed that leptin did not induce any significant changes in the proteome, but only at very high concentration, leptin induced neutrophil survival but without affecting their chemotactic capability, thus suggesting that this was most likely mediated by an indirect effect [52].

Finally, confirming the critical role of leptin in leukocyte recruitment, a recent paper has shown that mice intraperitoneally injected with a septic dose of lipopolysaccharide (LPS) showed a dramatic increase in the number of neutrophils entering the brain of WT mice. This effect was almost totally abolished in the leptin-deficient mice, which displayed a reduction in the mRNA levels of interleukin-1beta, intracellular adhesion molecule-1 and neutrophil-specific chemokines, a condition reversed by leptin replacement in *ob/ob* mice leading to recovery of neutrophil recruitment into the brain. Similar results have been obtained after 48 h of food deprivation in WT mice or with a single injection of an anti-leptin antiserum 4 h before LPS treatment in WT mice [53].

Leptin and Natural Killer Cells

Human Natural Killer (NK) cells, as other immune cells, constitutively express both long and short forms of Ob receptor, through which leptin can exert its functions (Table 11.1). More specifically, it activates the phosphorylation of STAT3 and then increases the transcription of IL-2 and perforin genes in NK cells, thus sustaining their cytotoxic activity. Consistent with this findings Tian et al. have also shown that the percentage and total amount of NK cells in the liver, spleen, lung, and peripheral blood were decreased in leptin receptor deficient mice (*db/db*) when compared to their littermate controls and the same holds true for the expression of several activation markers. In addition, exogenous leptin treatment increases the basal or enhances the IL-15-induced specific lysis of splenocytes in WT but not in *db/db* mice [54, 55].

In addition to NK cells, leptin seems to have a specific effect also on Invariant natural killer T (iNKT) cells, which are evolutionarily conserved innate T cells able to influence and modulate inflammatory responses. Venken et al. have shown that ObR is expressed also on iNKT cells and that leptin suppresses iNKT cell proliferation and cytokine production in vitro. Indeed leptin-receptor deficiency associates with increased reactivity of iNKT cells, enforcing the role of leptin as an important inhibitor of iNKT cell function [56].

In line with these findings, in vivo blockade of leptin receptor signaling exacerbates ConA-induced hepatitis in wild-type but not in iNKT cell deficient mice, through both Janus kinase (JAK)2 and mitogen-activated protein kinase (MAPK)-dependent mechanisms.

More recently it has been demonstrated that iNKT cells are enriched in human and murine adipose tissue, and that the increase in obesity degree is associated with a reduction of iNKT cells, correlating with pro-inflammatory macrophage infiltration [57]. On the contrary, iNKT cell numbers is restored in mice and humans after weight loss.

Confirming the cross talk between adipose tissue and iNKT, mice lacking iNKT cells had enhanced weight gain, larger adipocyte size, and developed insulin resistance on a high-fat diet. Interestingly, the adoptive transfer of iNKT cells into obese mice decreased body fat, triglyceride levels, leptin, and improved insulin sensitivity through the sustained anti-inflammatory cytokine production by adipose-derived iNKT cells.

Leptin and Basophils

Basophils are the rarest leukocytes subset in human blood, but they play a central role as immunomodulatory as well as effector cells in the control and modulation of allergic inflammation. Recent papers have shown that human basophils express leptin receptor (ObR) at both the mRNA and surface protein levels, and its expression is upregulated by IL-33 treatment (Table 11.1). Suzukawa and collaborators also demonstrated that leptin sustains the migratory capability of human basophils, and enhances their survival rate. Moreover, leptin is also able to upregulate the expression of CD63, which is one of the most studied and better characterized basophil activation marker. All these effects are inhibited by ObR-neutralizing antibodies treatment. The same authors also showed that leptin increases and primes human basophil degranulation in response to FcεRI aggregation and induces Th2-type cytokines production, thus possibly exacerbating allergic inflammation [58].

Leptin and Eosinophils

A recent paper by Conus et al. has shown that leptin delays the apoptotic rate of mature eosinophils in vitro (Table 11.1). More specifically, it delays the cleavage of protein Bax, as well as the mitochondrial release of cytochrome c and second mitochondria-derived activator of caspase, suggesting that it is able to interfere with the apoptotic pathways proximal to mitochondria [59].

On eosinophils, leptin upregulates cell surface expression of adhesion molecules such as ICAM-1 and CD18 but suppresses ICAM-3 and L-selectin. Moreover, leptin can also modulate migratory capability of eosinophils; indeed Wong et al. have shown that this hormone can stimulate the chemokinesis of eosinophils and induce the release of inflammatory cytokines (including IL-1beta and IL-6) and chemokines (such as IL-8, growth-related oncogene-alpha, and MCP-1) [60]. In addition it has been recently demonstrated that leptin induces eosinophil chemotaxis through the rapid phosphorylation of ERK1/2 and p38 mitogen-activated protein kinase, but not through calcium mobilization, and it also amplifying their responses to eotaxin [61].

Leptin Activation of Adaptive Immunity

Leptin and T Cells

Leptin regulation of adaptive immune responses has been strongly studied on human and mouse $CD4^+$ T cells. Indeed, leptin plays a key role in T cell biology by promoting $CD4^+$ T-cell proliferation, cytokine secretion and migration of these immune cells to sites of inflammation [10, 11, 62] (Table 11.1). In particular, leptin has different effects on human naive ($CD45RA^+$) and memory ($CD45RO^+$) $CD4^+$ T cells both of which express the long form of the leptin receptor (LepRb). Specifically leptin promotes naïve T cells proliferation by enhancing their secretion of IL-2 and through the activation of the mitogen-activated protein kinase (MAPK) and phosphatidylinositol-3-kinase (PI3-K) pathway [10]. On memory T cells, leptin promotes the switch towards T helper (Th)1-cell immune responses by increasing proinflammatory cytokine such as interferon-γ (IFN-γ) and TNF-α and the IgG2a production from B cells. Furthermore, leptin increases the expression of adhesion molecules, such as intercellular adhesion molecule 1 (ICAM1, CD54) and very late antigen 2 (VLA2, CD49B), by $CD4^+$ T cells, possibly through the induction of IFN-γ thus inducing their migration to inflammatory sites [10]. The effect of leptin on $CD4^+$ T cell homeostasis is specific as it has been recently shown by Matarese et al. in randomized, double-blinded, placebo-controlled trial of recombinant methionyl-human leptin (metreleptin) administration in replacement doses in women affected by hypothalamic amenorrhea with acquired chronic hypoleptinemia. Metreleptin restored both CD4+ T-cell counts and their in vitro proliferative responses in these women [63]. Recent evidence indicates that leptin inhibits thymic T cells apoptosis, thus supporting their generation, maturation, and survival [64]. Indeed, acute caloric deprivation causes a rapid decrease of serum leptin concentration accompanied by reduced delayed t-type-hypersensitivity DTH responses and thymic atrophy, which are reversible with administration of leptin [10, 11, 64]. Some authors have suggested that leptin also plays a pivotal role in T-cell polarization. Indeed, the induction of cytokine-producing Th1 or Th2 cells from naive CD4+ T cells under polarizing conditions in vitro was generally decreased in cells from leptin-deficient *ob/ob* mice compared with wild-type mice [65]. It has been recently shown that these mice were protected by developing oxazolone-induced colitis, when compared to wild-type mice with normal circulating levels of leptin. In particular *ob/ob* mice had decreased expression of the key transcription factors for Th1 and Th2 polarization, T-bet and GATA-3, and also lower levels of Th2 cytokine such as IL-13 than their littermates [65].

Moreover, leptin promotes lymphocyte survival in human and mouse, by upregulating lymphocyte surface expression of glucose transporters, such as GLUT1 and GLUT4 [66], the anti-apoptotic proteins BCL-2 and BCL-XL and also by modulating autophagy. (which protect T cells from apoptosis and thymocytes from glucocorticoid-induced apoptosis) [67, 68].

Interestingly, leptin has been demonstrated to exert opposite effects on human regulatory CD4+CD25+ (Treg) and conventional CD4+CD25− (Tconv) T cells which both express LepR and produce leptin. Indeed leptin inhibits Treg cell proliferation [69], on the one side, whereas it enhances Tconv proliferation, on the other [70] (Fig. 11.1). This is effect is secondary to the activation of the mammalian target of rapamycin (mTOR) pathway [71]. mTOR is a molecular sensor of cellular nutritional status and integrates signals from the environment to the nucleus for the regulation of cell metabolism, proliferation, and survival. Particularly, on Tconv cells the enhancement in their proliferation associated with inflammatory cytokine secretion, whereas leptin neutralization determined the inhibition of their responses, thus suggesting a key role of this adipocytokine in Tconv cells homeostasis and function and in pathogenesis of several inflammatory and autoimmune disease [72, 73]. It is now well accepted how the regulation of nutrient uptake and utilization together with cytokines and co-stimulatory molecules, including leptin, is critically important for the control of immune cell function and that and how the metabolic state can impact T cell differentiation by regulating the important balance between functionally divergent T-helper 17 (Th17) or T-regulatory (Treg) cell lineages. Interestingly, during activation, T lymphocytes take on a metabolic profile profoundly distinct from that of their quiescent and anergic counterparts; thus, T cell metabolism is highly dynamic and has a strong impact on the ability of T cell to grow, activate, and differentiate [74–76].

Since Th17 cells play an important role in the development and maintenance of inflammation and autoimmunity, several authors also studied the possible link between metabolism/nutrition and susceptibility to autoimmunity via leptin modulation of Th17 cells responses. Indeed it has been described a link between leptin and IL-17 both at the molecular and cellular levels. In *ob/ob* mice, it has been shown a reduced frequency of Th17 cells; this effects was restored to levels comparable to those found in wild-type (WT) animals after administration of exogenous leptin. The same group also found that leptin facilitated Th17 responses by inducing RORγt transcription in CD4+ T cells [77] and in the same study they showed that leptin was able to enhance Th17 responses in (NZB 3 NZW)F1 lupus-prone mice, whereas its neutralization in those mice inhibited Th17 responses [77]. Other authors found that neither the percentage of Th17 cells nor the level of Th17 cell-specific transcription factor RORγt correlated with plasma leptin, but the percentage of Th17 cells or the level of RORγt correlated positively with CD4+ T cell-derived leptin in patients with Hashimoto's thyroiditis [78].

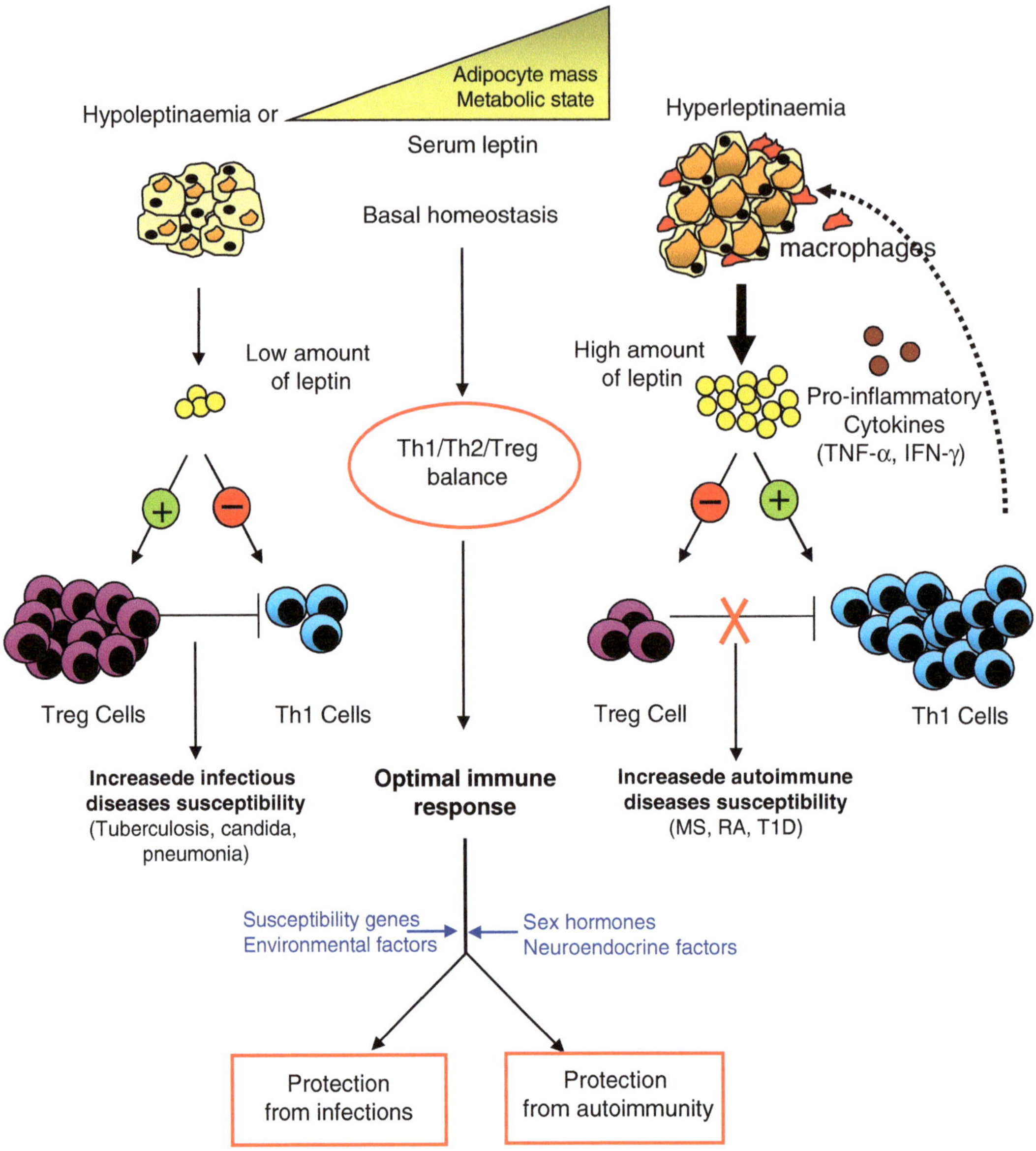

Fig. 11.1 Model of the peripheral leptin signaling in the control of T cell function. In normal subjects, secretion of adipocyte-derived leptin associates with a normal control of metabolic functions and with a balance between the number of Th1 cells and Th2/Treg cells, which are functionally able to suppress immune and autoimmune responses. Indeed leptin contributes to protection from infectious agents, on the one hand, but also to loss of tolerance and autoimmunity, on the other hand. Reduction of the level of circulating leptin [e.g., owing to protein–energy malnutrition (PEM), anorexia nervosa or genetic leptin deficiency (*ob*/*ob*)] results in impaired Th1 response and induction of Treg cells, thus reducing the immunocompetence in humans and mice and increasing susceptibility to infection. Conversely, the high amount of leptin secreted by adipocytes [e.g., obesity or genetic leptin-receptor deficiency (*db*/*db*)], accounts for an altered control of metabolic functions, often associated with insulin-resistance, a high frequency and expansion of Th1 cells and increased secretion of pro-inflammatory cytokines, on one side, and a low proportion and proliferation of Treg cells infiltrating adipose tissue, on the other. Along with the increased numbers of Th1 cells in adipose tissue, higher number of CD8+ T cells, macrophages and mast cells have been reported

Several studies in humans have clearly delineated the role of leptin also in activation of CD8$^+$ lymphocytes which also express LepRb on surface. Indeed, leptin when co-administered with other nonspecific immune-stimulants, results in induction of early (CD69) and late activation markers (CD25, CD71) in both CD4$^+$ and CD8$^+$ lymphocytes [79]. Other authors also demonstrated that leptin is able to regulate the secretion of several cytokines from peripheral CD8$^+$ cells. Specifically, leptin enhances the secretion of IL-2 and IFN-γ and inhibits the production of IL-4 and IL-10 [80]. Furthermore, it was found that in nonagenarians (≥90 years old) leptin plays a key role to sustain naïve CD8$^+$ T cell functions [81]. Some evidence has suggested that leptin also promotes CD8$^+$ T cells activation chronic obstructive pulmonary disease. Indeed, in leptin-deficient *ob/ob* mice (C57BL/6) and in leptin receptor-deficient *db/db* mice (C57BKS), in a model of cigarette smoke (CS)-induced pulmonary inflammation, there was an evident decrease in T cell number and frequency (CD4$^+$ and CD8$^+$) compared to their littermates [82].

Exogenous leptin administration completely restored the skewed inflammatory profile in *ob/ob* mice, thus suggesting a key role of this adipocytokine in the pathogenesis of inflammatory lung diseases. At the immune level, it has been shown that mTOR is able to program the generation of CD8$^+$ effector, to control T cell trafficking, and T cell activation versus anergy, thus suggesting that mTOR provides a direct link between T cell metabolism and function [83–85]. Moreover, leptin contributes to CD8$^+$ T cells activation in a mouse model of environment-linked nonalcoholic steatohepatitis (NASH) [86].

Leptin and B Cells

A great impact of leptin deficiency has been found on the B cell compartment (Table 11.1). Indeed Claycombe et al. have shown that *ob/ob* mice displayed a significant reduction in lymphopoiesis, as testified by 70 % fewer B cells than normal controls, as well as a reduction in the absolute number of pre-B and immature B cells. Seven days of provision of recombinant leptin promoted a twofold increase in B cells number in the bone marrow of the obese mice, while doubling and tripling, respectively, the numbers of pre-B and immature B cells [87]. Similar results have been also detected in the bone marrow of fasted mice, in which intracerebroventricular leptin injection was sufficient to prevent the alteration of B-cell development [88]. Furthermore, leptin promotes B-cell homeostasis by inhibiting apoptosis and by inducing cell cycle entry through the activation of expressions of B-cell CLL/lymphoma 2 (Bcl-2) and cyclin D1 [89]. Moreover, leptin activates human B cells to secrete cytokines, such as IL-6, IL-10, and TNF-α, via activation of JAK2/STAT3 and p38MAPK/ERK1/2 signaling pathways, which may contribute to its inflammatory and immunoregulatory properties [90]. Moreover, the same group showed that leptin-induced B cell-derived proinflammatory cytokines may play a role in chronic inflammation associated with human aging [91]. More specifically, they suggested that leptin induces significantly greater amount of pro-inflammatory cytokines such as IL-6, TNF-α, and IL-10 by B cells from aged humans than young controls. This effect is secondary to the activation leptin-LepRb-STAT3 activation as suggested by increase in the P-STAT3 (signal transducer and activator of transcription-3) levels in B cells from aged humans as compared to young subjects [91]. Finally B lymphocytes appear to be more susceptible to the antiapoptotic effects of leptin, and they show higher surface expression of ObR, compared with T cells [62].

Concluding Remarks

Since its discovery in 1994, leptin has attracted increasing interest in the scientific community for its pleiotropic functions. In immune cells, leptin acts as a proinflammatory cytokine that promotes Th1 responses on one side and inhibits Treg cell expansion on the other, setting the basis for exaggerated, immunoinflammatory responses to altered self or nonself and leading to autoimmunity in subjects with autoimmunity risk factors (i.e., genetic predisposition, HLA, environment, etc.). Future studies are needed to identify the precise relationship among leptin, metabolic state, and Treg cells in the context of autoimmune disease susceptibility. In this context, recent studies from Fontana et al. [92] have shown that caloric restriction and consequent lowering of serum leptin are able in humans to significantly reduce inflammatory parameters (such as IL-6 and CRP), suggesting that the nutritional intervention is able to dampen inflammatory responses. In view of its influence on food intake and metabolism, leptin situates at the interface between metabolism and immunity in modulating not only inflammation but also immune and autoimmune reactivity. Recently, molecules with orexigenic activity such as ghrelin and NPY [13, 93] have been shown to mediate effects opposite to leptin in the hypothalamic control of food intake and on peripheral immune responses. For example, ghrelin blocks leptin-induced secretion of proinflammatory cytokines by human T cells, and NPY ameliorates clinical score and progression of EAE [13, 93]. Thus, several metabolic regulators including leptin might broadly influence vital functions not only by tuning caloric balance but also by affecting immune responses.

Acknowledgements G.M. is supported by grants from Fondazione Italiana Sclerosi Multipla (FISM) 2012/R/11, the European Union IDEAS Programme European Research Council Starting Grant "menTORingTregs" 310496, the Ministero della Salute Grant GR-2010-2315414 and Grant CNR "Medicina Personalizzata." This work is dedicated to the memory of Eugenia Papa and Serafino Zappacosta.

References

1. Zhang Y, Proenca R, Maffei M, Barone M, Leopold L, Friedman JM. Positional cloning of the mouse obese gene and its human homologue. Nature. 1994;372: 425–32.
2. Flier JS. The adipocyte: storage depot or node on the energy information superhighway? Cell. 1995;80:15–8.
3. Friedman JM, Halaas JL. Leptin and the regulation of body weight in mammals. Nature. 1998;395:763–70.
4. Chehab F, Lim M, Lu R. Correction of the sterility defect in homozygous obese female mice by treatment with the human recombinant leptin. Nat Genet. 1996;12:318–20.
5. Bennett BD, Solar GP, Yuan JQ, Mathias J, Thomas GR, Matthews W. A role for leptin and its cognate receptor in hematopoiesis. Curr Biol. 1996;6: 1170–80.
6. Sierra-Honigmann MR, Nath AK, Murakami C, García-Cardeña G, Papapetropoulos A, Sessa WC, et al. Biological action of leptin as an angiogenic factor. Science. 1998;281:1683–6.
7. Pucino V, De Rosa V, Procaccini C, Matarese G. Regulatory T cells, leptin and angiogenesis. Chem Immunol Allergy. 2014;99:155–69.
8. Ducy P, Amling M, Takeda S, Priemel M, Schilling AF, Beil FT, et al. Leptin inhibits bone formation through a hypothalamic relay: a central control of bone mass. Cell. 2000;100:197–207.
9. Berti L, Gammeltoft S. Leptin stimulates glucose uptake in C2C12 muscle cells by activation of ERK2. Mol Cell Endocrinol. 1999;157:121–30.
10. Lord GM, Matarese G, Howard JK, Baker RJ, Bloom SR, Lechler RI. Leptin modulates the T-cells immune response and reverses starvation-induced immunosoppression. Nature. 1998;394:897–901.
11. Lord GM, Matarese G, Howard JK, Lechler RI. The bioenergetics of the immune system. Science. 2001; 292:855–6.
12. Fraser DA, Thoen J, Reseland JE, Førre O, Kjeldsen-Kragh J. Decreased CD4+ lymphocyte activation and increased interleukin-4 production inperipheral blood of rheumatoid arthritis patients after acute starvation. Clin Rheumatol. 1999;18:394–401.
13. La Cava A, Matarese G. The weight of leptin in immunity. Nat Rev Immunol. 2004;4(5):371–9.
14. Procaccini C, Jirillo E, Matarese G. Leptin as an immunomodulator. Mol Aspects Med. 2012;33:35–45.
15. Stofkova A. Leptin and adiponectin: from energy and metabolic dysbalance to inflammation and autoimmunity. Endocr Regul. 2009;43:157–68.
16. Gómez R, Conde J, Scotece M, Gómez-Reino JJ, Lago F, Gualillo O. What's new in our understanding of the role of adipokines in rheumatic diseases? Nat Rev Rheumatol. 2011;7:528–36.
17. Matarese G, Sanna V, Lechler RI, Sarvetnick N, Fontana S, Zappacosta S, et al. Leptin accelerates autoimmune diabetes in female NOD mice. Diabetes. 2002;51:1356–61.
18. Matarese G, Di Giacomo A, Sanna V, Lord GM, Howard JK, Di Tuoro A, et al. Requirement for leptin in the induction and progression of autoimmune encephalomyelitis. J Immunol. 2001;166:5909–16.
19. Loffreda S, Yang SQ, Lin HZ, Karp CL, Brengman ML, Wang DJ, et al. Leptin regulates proinflammatory immune responses. FASEB J. 1998;12:57–65.
20. Faggioni R, Feingold KR, Grunfeld C. Leptin regulation of the immune response and the immunodeficiency of malnutrition. FASEB J. 2001;15:2565–71.
21. Sarraf P, Frederich RC, Turner EM, Ma G, Jaskowiak NT, Rivet 3rd DJ, et al. Multiple cytokines and acute inflammation raise mouse leptin levels: potential role in inflammatory anorexia. J Exp Med. 1997;185: 171–5.

22. Jitprasertwong P, Jaedicke KM, Nile CJ, Preshaw PM, Taylor JJ. Leptin enhances the secretion of interleukin (IL)-18, but not IL-1β, from human monocytes via activation of caspase-1. Cytokine. 2014;65:222–30.
23. Santos-Alvarez J, Goberna R, Sánchez-Margalet V. Human leptin stimulates proliferation and activation of human circulating monocytes. Cell Immunol. 1999;194:6–11.
24. Kiguchi N, Maeda T, Kobayashi Y, Fukazawa Y, Kishioka S. Leptin enhances CC-chemokine ligand expression in cultured murine macrophage. Biochem Biophys Res Commun. 2009;384:311–5.
25. Gabay C, Dreyer M, Pellegrinelli N, Chicheportiche R, Meier CA. Leptin directly induces the secretion of interleukin 1 receptor antagonist in human monocytes. J Clin Endocrinol Metab. 2001;86:783–91.
26. Meier CA, Chicheportiche R, Dreyer M, Dayer JM. IP-10, but not RANTES, is upregulated by leptin in monocytic cells. Cytokine. 2003;21:43–7.
27. Balogh Z, Fóris G, Kosztáczky B, Paragh Jr G, Seres I, Zsíros E, et al. The concentration dependent biphasic effect of leptin on endogenous cholesterol synthesis in human monocytes. Peptides. 2007;28:2081–3.
28. Maya-Monteiro CM, Almeida PE, D'Avila H, Martins AS, Rezende AP, Castro-Faria-Neto H, et al. Leptin induces macrophage lipid body formation by a phosphatidylinositol 3-kinase- and mammalian target of rapamycin-dependent mechanism. J Biol Chem. 2008; 283:2203–10.
29. Hongo S, Watanabe T, Arita S, Kanome T, Kageyama H, Shioda S, et al. Leptin modulates ACAT1 expression and cholesterol efflux from human macrophages. Am J Physiol Endocrinol Metab. 2009;297:E474–82.
30. Mancuso P, Canetti C, Gottschalk A, Tithof PK, Peters-Golden M. Leptin augments alveolar macrophage leukotriene synthesis by increasing phospholipase activity and enhancing group IVC iPLA2 (cPLA2gamma) protein expression. Am J Physiol Lung Cell Mol Physiol. 2004;287:L497–502.
31. Mancuso P, Myers Jr MG, Goel D, Serezani CH, O'Brien E, Goldberg J, et al. Ablation of leptin receptor-mediated ERK activation impairs host defense against Gram-negative pneumonia. J Immunol. 2012;189:867–75.
32. Wu MH, Huang MF, Chang FM, Tsai SJ. Leptin on peritoneal macrophages of patients with endometriosis. Am J Reprod Immunol. 2010;63:214–21.
33. Najib S, Sánchez-Margalet V. Human leptin promotes survival of human circulating blood monocytes prone to apoptosis by activation of p42/44 MAPK pathway. Cell Immunol. 2002;220:143–9.
34. Sánchez-Pozo C, Rodriguez-Baño J, Domínguez-Castellano A, Muniain MA, Goberna R, Sánchez-Margalet V. Leptin stimulates the oxidative burst in control monocytes but attenuates the oxidative burst in monocytes from HIV-infected patients. Clin Exp Immunol. 2003;134:464–9.
35. Maingrette F, Renier G. Leptin increases lipoprotein lipase secretion by macrophages: involvement of oxidative stress and protein kinase C. Diabetes. 2003;52: 2121–8.
36. Gruen ML, Hao M, Piston DW, Hasty AH. Leptin requires canonical migratory signaling pathways for induction of monocyte and macrophage chemotaxis. Am J Physiol Cell Physiol. 2007;293:C1481–8.
37. Dib LH, Ortega MT, Fleming SD, Chapes SK, Melgarejo T. Obesity is characterized by an increased Bone marrow leptin signaling mediates obesity-associated adipose tissue inflammation in male mice. Endocrinology. 2014;155:40–6.
38. Macia L, Delacre M, Abboud G, Ouk TS, Delanoye A, Verwaerde C, et al. Impairment of dendritic cell functionality and steady-state number in obese mice. J Immunol. 2006;177:5997–6006.
39. Lam QL, Zheng BJ, Jin DY, Cao X, Lu L. Leptin induces CD40 expression through the activation of Akt in murine dendritic cells. J Biol Chem. 2007; 282:27587–97.
40. Mattioli B, Straface E, Quaranta MG, Giordani L, Viora M. Leptin promotes differentiation and survival of human dendritic cells and licenses them for Th1 priming. J Immunol. 2005;174:6820–8.
41. Mattioli B, Giordani L, Quaranta MG, Viora M. Leptin exerts an anti-apoptotic effect on human dendritic cells via the PI3K-Akt signaling pathway. FEBS Lett. 2009;583:1102–6.
42. Mattioli B, Straface E, Matarrese P, Quaranta MG, Giordani L, Malorni W, et al. Leptin as an immunological adjuvant: enhanced migratory and CD8+ T cell stimulatory capacity of human dendritic cells exposed to leptin. FASEB J. 2008;22:2012–22.
43. Moraes-Vieira PM, Larocca RA, Bassi EJ, Peron JP, Andrade-Oliveira V, Wasinski F, et al. Leptin deficiency impairs maturation of dendritic cells and enhances induction of regulatory T and Th17 cells. Eur J Immunol. 2014;44:794–806.
44. Caldefie-Chezet F, Poulin A, Tridon A, Sion B, Vasson MP. Leptin: a potential regulator of polymorphonuclear neutrophil bactericidal action? J Leukoc Biol. 2001;69:414–8.
45. Bruno A, Conus S, Schmid I, Simon HU. Apoptotic pathways are inhibited by leptin receptor activation in neutrophils. J Immunol. 2005;174:8090–6.
46. Zarkesh-Esfahani H, Pockley AG, Wu Z, Hellewell PG, Weetman AP, Ross RJ. Leptin indirectly activates human neutrophils via induction of TNF-alpha. J Immunol. 2004;172:1809–14.
47. Sun Z, Dragon S, Becker A, Gounni AS. Leptin inhibits neutrophil apoptosis in children via ERK/NF-κB-dependent pathways. PLoS One. 2013;8: e55249I.
48. Ubags ND, Vernooy JH, Burg E, Hayes C, Bement J, Dilli E, et al. The role of leptin in the development of pulmonary neutrophilia in infection and acute lung injury. Crit Care Med. 2014;42:e143–51.
49. Caldefie-Chezet F, Poulin A, Vasson MP. Leptin regulates functional capacities of polymorphonuclear neutrophils. Free Radic Res. 2003;37:809–14.
50. Ottonello L, Gnerre P, Bertolotto M, Mancini M, Dapino P, Russo R, et al. Leptin as a uremic toxin interferes with neutrophil chemotaxis. J Am Soc Nephrol. 2004;15:2366–23672.

51. Moore SI, Huffnagle GB, Chen GH, White ES, Mancuso P. Leptin modulates neutrophil phagocytosis of Klebsiella pneumoniae. Infect Immun. 2003;71:4182–5.
52. Kamp VM, Langereis JD, van Aalst CW, van der Linden JA, Ulfman LH, Koenderman L. Physiological concentrations of leptin do not affect human neutrophils. PLoS One. 2013;8:e73170.
53. Rummel C, Inoue W, Poole S, Luheshi GN. Leptin regulates leukocyte recruitment into the brain following systemic LPS-induced inflammation. Mol Psychiatry. 2010;15:523–34.
54. Tian Z, Sun R, Wei H, Gao B. Impaired natural killer (NK) cell activity in leptin receptor deficient mice: leptin as a critical regulator in NK cell development and activation. Biochem Biophys Res Commun. 2002;298:297–302.
55. Zhao Y, Sun R, You L, Gao C, Tian Z. Expression of leptin receptors and response to leptin stimulation of human natural killer cell lines. Biochem Biophys Res Commun. 2003;300:247–52.
56. Venken K. A bidirectional crosstalk between iNKT cells and adipocytes mediated by leptin modulates susceptibility for T cell mediated hepatitis. J Hepatol. 2014;60:175–82.
57. Lynch L, Nowak M, Varghese B, Clark J, Hogan AE, Toxavidis V, et al. Adipose tissue invariant NKT cells protect against diet-induced obesity and metabolic disorder through regulatory cytokine production. Immunity. 2012;37:574–87.
58. Suzukawa M, Nagase H, Ogahara I, Han K, Tashimo H, Shibui A, et al. Leptin enhances survival and induces migration, degranulation, and cytokine synthesis of human basophils. J Immunol. 2011;186:5254–60.
59. Conus S, Bruno A, Simon HU. Leptin is an eosinophil survival factor. J Allergy Clin Immunol. 2005;116:1228–34.
60. Wong CK, Cheung PF, Lam CW. Leptin-mediated cytokine release and migration of eosinophils: implications for immunopathophysiology of allergic inflammation. Eur J Immunol. 2007;37:2337–48.
61. Kato H, Ueki S, Kamada R, Kihara J, Yamauchi Y, Suzuki T, et al. Leptin has a priming effect on eotaxin-induced human eosinophil chemotaxis. Int Arch Allergy Immunol. 2011;155:335–44.
62. Papathanassoglou E, El-Haschimi K, Li XC, Matarese G, Strom T, Mantzoros C. Leptin receptor expression and signaling in lymphocytes: kinetics during lymphocyte activation, role in lymphocyte survival, and response to high fat diet in mice. J Immunol. 2006;176:7745–52.
63. Matarese G, La Rocca C, Moon HS, Huh JY, Brinkoetter MT, Chou S, et al. Selective capacity of metreleptin administration to reconstitute CD4+ T-cell number in females with acquired hypoleptinemia. Proc Natl Acad Sci U S A. 2013;110:E818–27.
64. Howard JK, Lord GM, Matarese G, Vendetti S, Ghatei MA, Ritter MA, et al. Leptin protects mice from starvation induced lymphoid atrophy and increases thymic cellularity in *ob*/*ob* mice. J Clin Invest. 1999;104:1051–9.
65. Batra A, Okur B, Glauben R, Erben U, Ihbe J, Stroh T, et al. Leptin: a critical regulator of CD4$^+$ T-cell polarization in vitro and in vivo. Endocrinology. 2010;151:56–62.
66. Sivitz WI, Walsh SA, Morgan DA, Thomas MJ, Haynes WG. Effects of leptin on insulin sensitivity in normal rats. Endocrinology. 1997;138:3395–401.
67. Galgani M, Procaccini C, De Rosa V, Carbone F, Chieffi P, La Cava A, et al. Leptin modulates the survival of autoreactive CD4+ T cells through the nutrient/energy-sensing mammalian target of rapamycin signaling pathway. J Immunol. 2010;185:7474–9.
68. Cassano S, Pucino V, La Rocca C, Procaccini C, De Rosa V, Marone G, Matarese G. Leptin modulates autophagy in human CD4(+)CD25(-) conventional T cells. Metabolism. 2014 Jun 19.
69. De Rosa V, Procaccini C, Calì G, Pirozzi G, Fontana S, Zappacosta S, et al. Key role of leptin in the control of regulatory T cells proliferation. Immunity. 2007;26:241–55.
70. Procaccini C, De Rosa V, Galgani M, Carbone F, Cassano S, Greco D, et al. Leptin-induced mTOR activation defines a specific molecular and transcriptional signature controlling CD4+ effector T cell responses. J Immunol. 2012;189:2941–53.
71. Procaccini C, De Rosa V, Galgani M, Abanni L, Calì G, Porcellini A, et al. An oscillatory switch in mTOR Kinase activity sets regulatory T cell responsiveness. Immunity. 2010;33:1–13.
72. Matarese G. Leptin and immune system: how nutritional status influences the immune response. Eur Cytokine Netw. 2000;11:7–13.
73. Procaccini C, Pucino V, De Rosa V, Marone G, Giuseppe Matarese G. Neuro-endocrine networks controlling immune system in health and disease. Front Immunol. 2014;5:143.
74. Matarese G, Colamatteo A, De Rosa V. Metabolic fuelling of proper T cell functions. Immunol Lett. 2014;161:174–8.
75. Pearce EL, Poffenberger MC, Chang CH, Jones RG. Fueling immunity: insights into metabolism and lymphocyte function. Science. 2013;342:1242454.
76. Matarese G, Procaccini C, De Rosa V. At the crossroad of T cells, adipose tissue, and diabetes. Immunol Rev. 2012;249:116–34.
77. Yu Y, Liu Y, Shi FD, Zou H, Matarese G, La Cava A. Cutting edge: leptin-induced RORγt expression in CD4+ T cells promotes Th17 responses in systemic lupus erythematosus. J Immunol. 2013;190:3054–8.
78. Wang S, Baidoo SE, Liu Y, Zhu C, Tian J, Ma J, et al. T cell-derived leptin contributes to increased frequency of T helper type 17 cells in female patients with Hashimoto's thyroiditis. Clin Exp Immunol. 2013;171:63–8.
79. Martín-Romero C, Santos-Alvarez J, Goberna R, Sánchez-Margalet V. Human leptin enhances activation and proliferation of human circulating T lymphocytes. Cell Immunol. 2000;199:15–24.
80. Rodríguez L, Graniel J, Ortiz R. Effect of leptin on activation and cytokine synthesis in peripheral blood

lymphocytes of malnourished infected children. Clin Exp Immunol. 2007;148:478–85.
81. Chen J, Li J, Lim FC, Wu Q, Douek DC, Scott DK, Ravussin E, et al. Louisiana Healthy Aging Study. Maintenance of naïve CD8 T cells in nonagenarians by leptin, IGFBP3 and T3. Mech Ageing Dev. 2010; 131:29–37.
82. Vernooy JH, Bracke KR, Drummen NE, Pauwels NS, Zabeau L, van Suylen RJ, et al. Leptin modulates innate and adaptive immune cell recruitment after cigarette smoke exposure in mice. J Immunol. 2010; 184:7169–77.
83. Araki K, Turner AP, Shaffer VO, Gangappa S, Keller SA, Bachmann M, et al. MTOR regulates memory CD8 T-cell differentiation. Nature. 2009;460:108–12.
84. Rao RR, Li Q, Odunsi K, Shrikant PA. The mTOR kinase determines effector versus memory CD8+ T cell fate by regulating the expression of transcription factors T-bet and Eomesodermin. Immunity. 2010; 32:67–78.
85. Pearce EL, Walsh MC, Cejas PJ, Harms GM, Shen H, Wang LS, et al. Enhancing CD8 T-cell memory by modulating fatty acid metabolism. Nature. 2009;460: 103–7.
86. Seth RK, Das S, Kumar A, Chanda A, Kadiiska MB, et al. CYP2E1-dependent and leptin-mediated hepatic CD57 expression on CD8+ T cells aid progression of environment-linked nonalcoholic steatohepatitis. Toxicol Appl Pharmacol. 2014;274:42–54.
87. Claycombe K, King LE, Fraker PJ. A role for leptin in sustaining lymphopoiesis and myelopoiesis. Proc Natl Acad Sci U S A. 2008;105:2017–21.
88. Tanaka M, Suganami T, Kim-Saijo M, Toda C, Tsuiji M, Ochi K, Kamei Y, Minokoshi Y, Ogawa Y. Role of central leptin signaling in the starvation-induced alteration of B-cell development. J Neurosci. 2011;31:8373–80.
89. Lam QL, Wang S, Ko OK, Kincade PW, Lu L. Leptin signaling maintains B-cell homeostasis via induction of Bcl-2 and Cyclin D1. Proc Natl Acad Sci U S A. 2010;107:13812–27.
90. Agrawal S, Gollapudi S, Su H, Gupta S. Leptin activates human B cells to secrete TNF-α, IL-6, and IL-10 via JAK2/STAT3 and p38MAPK/ERK1/2 signaling pathway. J Clin Immunol. 2011;31:472–8.
91. Gupta S, Agrawal S, Gollapudi S. Increased activation and cytokine secretion in B cells stimulated with leptin in aged humans. Immun Ageing. 2013;10:3.
92. Fontana L, Eagon JC, Trujillo ME, Scherer PE, Klein S. Visceral fat adipokine secretion is associated with systemic inflammation in obese humans. Diabetes. 2007;56:1010–3.
93. Tilg H, Moschen AR. Adipocytokines: mediators linking adipose tissue, inflammation and immunity. Nat Rev Immunol. 2006;6:772–83.

Leptin and Bone

12

Patricia Ducy and Stavroula Kousteni

Introduction

In striking opposition with the "Halloweenish" view of the skeleton as a dead structure, bone is a remarkably dynamic organ. For instance during growth, chondrocytes located at the growth plate cartilage proliferate at one of the fastest pace seen in the post-developmental organism [1]. Growth also requires a considerable elongation of most skeletal elements as well as their widening, a process called bone modeling [1, 2]. This is achieved though apposition of newly formed bone by a specialized cell type, the osteoblast, which lay down a fibrillar extracellular matrix rich in type I collagen that is subsequently mineralized, while another bone-specific cell type, the osteoclast, carves out the marrow space by resorbing the mineralized matrix [3]. Once growth is completed, a similar cycle of bone formation and resorption, termed bone remodeling, ceaselessly continues throughout the skeleton [4, 5]. This is required to repair the widespread micro-fractures constantly caused by daily life activities to the key structural network that our skeleton represents. Indeed, dysregulation of this process eventually leads to fractures and immobilization, life threatening conditions before the most recent centuries because they impaired the ability to evade dangers, reach for food, and hunt.

This necessity to grow and maintain a sturdy skeleton for proper survival can explain why bone modeling and remodeling appeared during vertebrate evolution despite the expensive energetic investment that the constant succession of destruction and formation they entail represents for the body. By the same token, it is not far-fetched to assume that mechanisms also evolved to limit this sizeable energetic cost, and thereby bone growth and remodeling, when energy intake becomes scarce. Hence, effector(s) of these mechanisms should be involved in the regulation of appetite and/or energy expenditure. This assumption was the first clue toward the identification of leptin as a regulator of bone remodeling. A second one came from an evolutionary perspective. On the scale of evolution the vertebrate skeleton, and more so bone remodeling, are quite recent innovations. Remarkably, whereas adipocyte-equivalent cells are present in other phyla than vertebrates the appearance of leptin

P. Ducy (✉)
Departments of Pathology and Cell Biology, Columbia University, 701 west 168th Street - 1616A HHSC, New York, NY 10032, USA
e-mail: pd2193@columbia.edu

S. Kousteni
Department of Medicine, Columbia University, New York, USA

Department of Physiology and Cellular Biophysics, Columbia University, New York, NY, USA
e-mail: sk2836@columbia.edu

S. Dagogo-Jack (ed.), *Leptin: Regulation and Clinical Applications*,
DOI 10.1007/978-3-319-09915-6_12, © Springer International Publishing Switzerland 2015

during evolution concurs only with the latter [6]. The last clue came from three clinical observations. It has been shown that anorexia halts growth, i.e., modeling, during childhood and causes osteoporosis in adults while bone mineral density at all sites of the skeleton is increased in life-long overweight patients [7–10]. Conversely, menopause, i.e., sex steroid deprivation following gonadal failure, is the most frequent cause of osteoporosis in the western hemisphere [11]. Combining these 3 observations in an integrative manner led to the hypothesis that *bone mass accrual, appetite and/or energy metabolism, and reproduction could be coordinated by the same regulator(s)* [12]. Given that these three functions are strongly influenced by hormones, such regulatory mechanisms were most likely to be endocrine. This was also consistent with the fact that these hypothetical regulator(s) would need to reach all bones of the skeleton although they are distributed throughout the body. At the time this hypothesis was formulated, only one hormone was known to significantly impact both energy metabolism/appetite and reproduction: leptin [13–15]. Analyzing leptin-deficient (*ob/ob*) and leptin receptor-deficient (*db/db*) mouse strains [16, 17] was the first step to test this hormone potential role as a regulator bone mass accrual.

Leptin Negatively Regulates Bone Mass Accrual

Increased Bone Mass in Absence of Leptin Signaling

Both the *ob/ob* and *db/db* mice are obese and hypogonadic [16–18]. If one abides by the clinical observations mentioned above, these mice should have a high bone density because they are largely overweight yet they should abnormally loose bone because they are hypogonadic. These antagonistic conditions should, at best, cause a mild bone loss phenotype. Instead, both mutant strains display a high bone mass phenotype [12, 19]. Indeed, when analyzed by histomorphometry the network of trabeculae that composed the cancellous part of all bones and that is most potently affected by bone remodeling is denser in absence of leptin signaling. As a result these mice have an increase in bone volume and their long bones are more resistant to facture upon mechanical loading. Using the same histological techniques, this high bone mass phenotype can also be observed in mice treated with a leptin antagonist, in *fa/fa* rats (Fig. 12.1—T. Holzmann and M. Amling, original data), and in a newly developed model of leptin knockout rats [20, 21]. Most importantly, such increase in bone mass accrual is consistent with the advanced bone age observed in patients with a deficiency in serum leptin levels (see below, section "Leptin Actions on Bone Remodeling and Human Bone Biology").

An increase in bone mass can result from an increase in bone formation or a decrease in bone resorption or a combination of both mechanisms. Consistent with their hypogonadism, *ob/ob* and *db/db* mice have an increase in bone resorption [12]. It is, however, milder than their innate and permanent sex steroid depletion would have predicted because, by itself, leptin deficiency has a negative effect on bone resorption through its action on the sympathetic tone (see below, section "Efferent Mediators of Leptin's Central Regulation of Bone Remodeling"). Yet the most striking features of mice deficient in leptin signaling is their increase in bone formation by osteoblasts despite their elevated levels of cortisol, one of the most potent inhibitor of bone formation [12, 22–24]. Thus, that *ob/ob* and *db/db* mice have a high bone mass phenotype in presence of two conditions, hypogonadism and hypercortisolemia, which are the two most common causes of osteoporosis, emphasize the importance of the leptin function in regulating bone mass accrual.

Leptin Affects Bone Mass Accrual Independently of its Effect on Body Weight

Mechanical loading is well known for its positive effect on bone mass [25]. Since the absence of leptin dramatically increases body weight, and therefore loading of bones, it is legitimate to

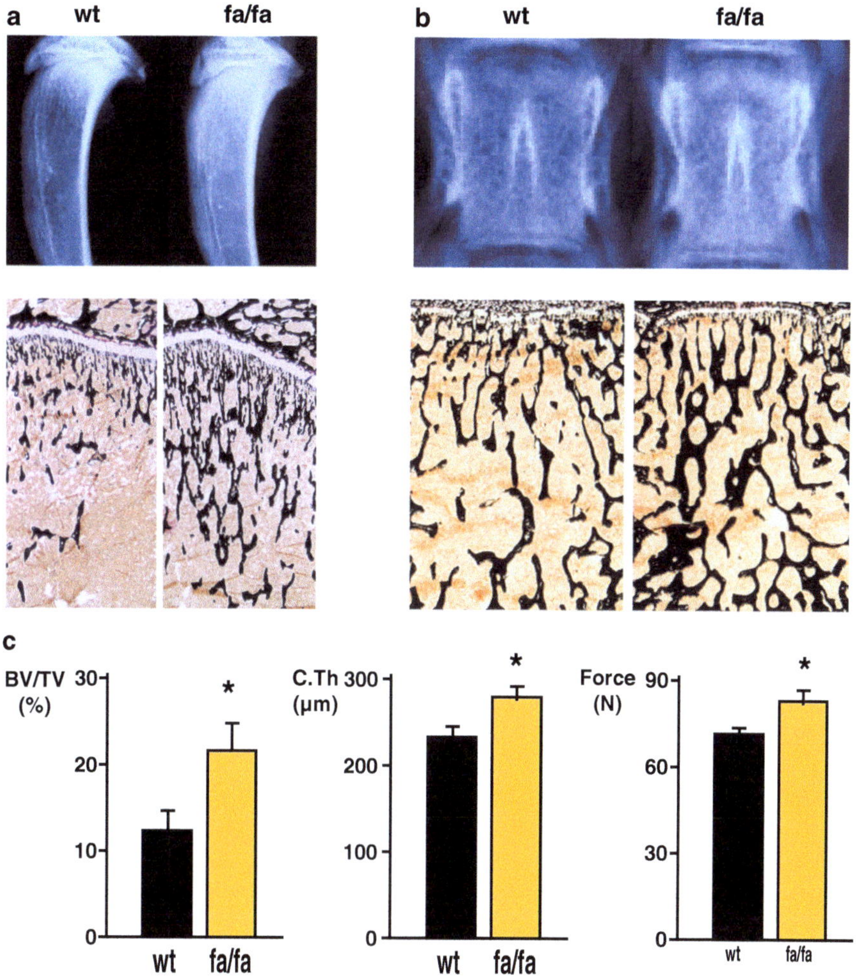

Fig. 12.1 Increased bone mass in leptin signaling deficient *fa/fa* rats. (**a**, **b**) *upper panels*, X-ray micrographs of the tibia (**a**) and vertebrae (**b**). The whiter aspect in *fa/fa* rats indicates a higher bone density. (**a**, **b**) *lower panels*, Cross-sections through undecalcified tibia (**a**) and vertebrae (**b**) stained by the von Kossa–Van Gieson reagents. The amount of mineralized bone trabeculae (in *black*) is increased in *fa/fa* rats. (**c**) Quantification of bone volume (BV/TV, *left panel*), cortical thickness (C.Th, *middle panel*) and strength on a 3-points bending test (*right panel*). *fa/fa* rats show an increase in all three parameters. *, $p > 0.05$

question whether the high bone mass phenotype observed in leptin-deficient rodents is caused by their increased weight or by the absence of leptin itself. Many lines of evidence acquired in various mice engineered to display a dissociation between body weight and leptin levels have validated the latter option (Table 12.1). For instance, mice with an obesity not directly caused by a lack of leptin signaling do not display a bone phenotype (Agouti Yellow (Ay) mice) or show an increase in bone mass caused by a different mechanism (MC4R-deficient mice) involving an isolated decrease of bone resorption without an overt increase in bone formation [12, 26]. Conversely, mice with a deficiency in leptin signaling but that are not obese display an increase in bone formation similar to the one of the *ob/ob* mice. Indeed, very young *ob/ob* mice fed a low fat diet or *ob/+* mice have a normal weight but show an increase in bone mass accrual [12]. Likewise, transgenic mice rendered lipodystrophic through expression of a dominant negative protein blocking the activity

Table 12.1 Changes in bone mass and remodeling parameters correlate with levels of leptin signaling but not with body weight

	Body weight	Serum leptin	Bone mass	Formation	Resorption
ob/ob	+++	0	+	+	–
db/db	+++	±	+	+	–
Mc4r+/– (–/–)	++	–	–	=	+
Ay/+	++	±	=	ND	ND
Young ob/ob on LFD	=	0	+	+	–
ob/+	=	–	+	+	–
A-ZIP transgenic	–	–––	+	+	–

+, increase; + normal level; ±, resistance; –, decrease; 0, absence; ND, not done

Table 12.2 Dissociation between the central effects of leptin signaling on body weight and bone mass accrual

	Central leptin signaling	Body weight	Bone mass	Formation	Resorption
ob/ob	0	+++	+	+	–
l/l	+	=	–	–	+
ob/ob+leptin icv	+	–	–	–	+
wt+MSG	±	=	=	=	=
wt+GTG	±	–	–	–	+
ob/ob+MSG+leptin icv	±	=	–	–	+
ob/ob+GTG+leptin icv	±	–	+	+	–

+, increase; + normal level; ±, partial; –, decrease; 0, absence

of adipocyte differentiation factors display a near complete absence of leptin and a high bone mass phenotype although they are lean [12, 27]. Importantly, this phenotype can be fully corrected by increasing the levels of circulating leptin indicating that it is caused the absence of this hormone but not by the lack of other adipokine [12, 28].

Mechanism of Leptin's Regulation of Bone Remodeling

Leptin Acts Centrally to Regulate Bone Remodeling

Leptin regulation of appetite, energy expenditure and fertility occurs centrally [18, 29]. Thus, it does not come as a surprise that leptin's effect on bone mass accrual also relies on a central action. This was first established through classical experiments of intracerebroventricular infusion (icv) of recombinant leptin, then was confirmed using central injections of leptin-expressing viruses and neuron lesioning [12, 30–34]. When leptin is infused icv in *ob/ob* mice, even at a concentration low enough to avoid leakage to the blood stream, they loose both weight and bone mass at a dramatic pace [12, 34]. As a matter of fact, bone loss can still be observed at icv doses of leptin that do not elicit a significant loss of weight [30], in agreement with the fact that the mechanisms mediating leptin's effect on these two functions are different and thus can have different thresholds. Indeed, chemical lesioning experiments showed that destruction of monosodium glutamate-sensitive neurons of the hypothalamic arcuate nuclei (ARC) affects body weight while bone mass accrual is predominantly affected when neurons of the ventromedial hypothalamus nuclei (VMH) are destroyed using gold thioglucose [33]. That Ay mice loose bone but not weight when infused icv with leptin while *ob/ob* mice infused icv with a MC3R/MC4R agonist loose weigh but not bone further established that leptin's anorexigenic and anti-osteogenic effects rely on distinct signaling events [33] (Table 12.2). Another argument in favor of different mechanism of action between these two functions came from

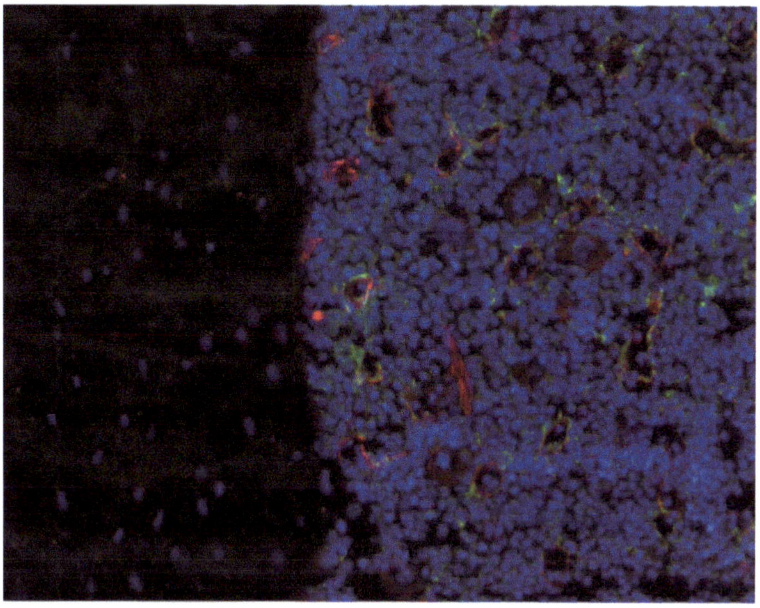

Fig. 12.2 The leptin receptor is not expressed in osteoblasts in vivo. *Lepr-Cre* recombination of a loxP-EYFP reporter in bone sections. Expression of the reporter (*green*) can be detected in perisinusoidal stromal cells in the bone marrow (*red* Meca32 positive cells) but not in osteoblasts or haematopoietic cells (Adapted from Ding et al. Nature 481,457–462, 2012)

the analysis of the *l/l* mice, a gain-of-function model of the leptin receptor. In these mice *LepR* encodes a form of this recpetor mutated on Tyr985 that disrupts its interaction with the SHP2/SOCS3 inhibitory complex [35, 36]. While the *l/l* mice fed a regular chow have a normal body weight, energy expenditure and fertility they show a mirror image of the *db/db* phenotype, i.e., low bone mass, decreased bone formation and increased bone resorption [30, 36].

When injected or infused peripherally leptin can also influence bone remodeling. For instance, transgenic mice with a modest, twofold to fourfold, increase in serum concentration of leptin show a lower bone mass than non-transgenic controls [28, 33]. Importantly, overexpressing *Leptin* in the liver to raise its serum concentration to approximately 1.2 μg/ml (i.e., 250-fold) also induces bone loss although with a much smaller amplitude and a slower pace than icv infusion. This observation suggests that, as it is the case for its control of body weight, leptin's regulation of bone remodeling could be blunted and/or blocked by a resistance mechanism when its serum concentration becomes too high [37–39]. Such a leptin resistance would explain the beneficial effect on bone mass accrual reported in studies using peripheral injections of massive doses of leptin (50 μg/day, i.e., 700-fold the amount used in icv studies) [40, 41]. It is in fact conceivable that, as much as leptin centrally affects bone mass accrual at a lower threshold than it affects body weight, the effect of leptin on bone remodeling is also more quickly impacted by a leptin resistance mechanism. Hence, massive doses of this hormone injected peripherally could still cause weight loss, as some of the above mentioned studies reported, while already eliciting a leptin resistance that will cause a gain of bone mass similar to the one observed in absence of leptin signaling.

In any case, several arguments indicate that leptin does not act on either arms of the bone remodeling process via a direct action on bone cells. First, whether through analyses of gene expression in bone tissue or isolated osteoblasts by Northern blot and PCR or via lineage tracing studies using a Leptin receptor (Lepr)-YFP reporter transgene expression of the leptin receptor cannot be detected in osteoblasts (Fig. 12.2) [12, 42]. Second, when cultured ex-vivo osteoblasts derived from wild type or *db/db* mice proliferate and differentiate similarly. Third, and these are the most decisive points, neither expression of leptin in osteoblasts or the conditional inactivation of *Lepr* specifically in osteoblasts cause a bone phenotype in mice [30, 33]. In contrast, inactivating this gene in neurons induces the same high bone mass phenotype than the one observed in *db/db* mice [30, 43].

Leptin Uses a Serotonin Relay to Regulate Bone Remodeling

While the chemical lesioning experiments points toward the VMH as the relay of leptin antiosteogenic effect in the brain, deletion of the leptin receptor in these same neurons do not cause a bone phenotype [43, 44]. This conundrum stems from the fact that leptin uses a serotonin relay to acts on the VMH neurons of the hypothalamus [43, 45, 46]. Indeed, the signaling form of the leptin receptor is expressed in the neurons of the dorsal and median raphe nuclei that also express *Tph2*, the gene encoding the rate-limiting enzyme in the synthesis of serotonin [43, 47–49]. Upon binding to these neurons leptin exerts a negative effect on the production of serotonin as evidenced by the presence of high levels of serotonin in the brain of *ob/ob* and *db/db* mice and by their decrease upon leptin icv infusion in wild type mice [43]. In agreement with this inhibitory effect, *Tph2*-deficient mice, i.e., lacking brain serotonin, show a low bone mass phenotype mirroring the one observed in *ob/ob* mice. More importantly, if the brain content of the *ob/ob* mice is normalized by inactivating one allele of *Tph2*, their bone phenotype is corrected [43]. Conversely, when *LepR* is specifically inactivated in the *Tph2*-expressing neurons of the brainstem mice develop a bone phenotype similar to the one presented by *db/db* mice [43]. Hence, brain serotonin is a positive regulator of bone mass accrual whose synthesis is inhibited by leptin signaling to brainstem neurons (Fig. 12.3).

Serotonin Signals to VMH Neurons via Htr2c and CREB to Mediate Leptin's Regulation of Bone Mass Accrual

Consistent with the lesioning experiments that identified the VMH nuclei as mediating leptin anti-osteogenic action, dextran anterograde and retrograde neuron tracing studies showed that serotonergic neurons project from the brainstem to the VMH nuclei [43]. Serotonin then signals to VMH neurons via the Htr2c receptor to regulate bone mass accrual. Indeed, depleting this receptor globally causes a low bone mass phenotype with decreased bone formation and increased bone resorption, as the absence of brain serotonin does, and reactivating its expression specifically in VMH neurons corrects this phenotype [43]. That *Tph2+/–*; *Htr2c+/–* compound heterozygous mice have a similar bone phenotype as *Tph2–/–* mice indicates that this receptor is the main, if not the only, of the 14 known serotonin receptors mediating brain serotonin regulation of bone mass accrual [43].

Htr2c, a G protein-coupled receptor (GPCR), can signal though multiple intracellular cascades depending of the isoform generated via RNA editing [50–54]. To mediate serotonin action on bone mass accrual, Htr2c uses Ca^{2+} as a second messenger and a cascade of CaM kinases [55]. By in situ hybridization the genes encoding CaMKKβ, CaMKIIa and CaMKIV are the most highly expressed in the Sf1 positive neurons of the VMH that are known to mediate the leptin-dependent regulation of bone mass accrual [33, 55]. However, treatment of P19 cells differentiated into neurons or of hypothalamic explants with serotonin induces the phosphorylation of only CaMKKβ and CaMKIV, indicating that CaMKII does not mediates its activity [55]. The connection between serotonin, CaMKKβ/CaMKIV expression in the VMH, and bone remodeling is supported by the existence of a bone phenotype of similar nature as the one observed in absence of *Tph2–/–* in mice deficient in *CaMKKβ* (or *CaMKIV*) in VMH neurons or, as it was the case for *Tph2+/–*; *Htr2c+/–* mice, in mice double heterozygous for *Tph2* and *CaMKKβ* (or *CaMKIV*) in VMH neurons [55].

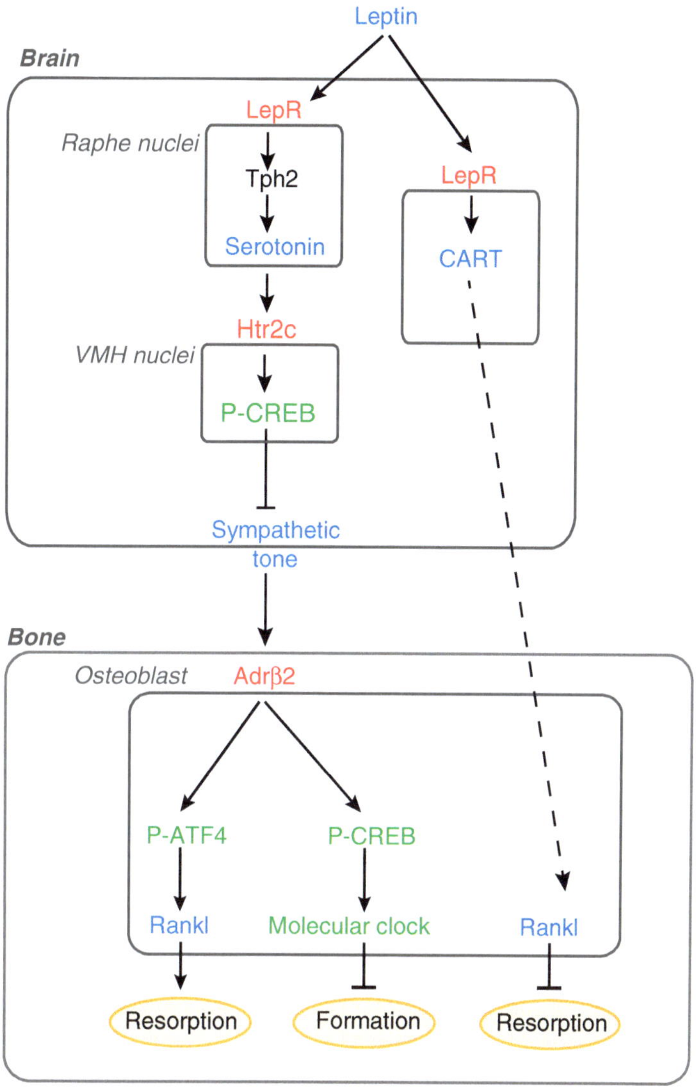

Fig. 12.3 Schematic representation of the leptin regulatory cascade on bone mass accrual. Receptors are in *red*, transcription factors in *green* and secreted molecules are in *blue*. *Dotted lines* indicate that an unknown number of intermediary steps may exist

A common target of Ca^{2+} signaling and of neuron activation is the transcription factor CREB. Both in vitro and in vivo evidence indicates that this factor is a major mediator of serotonin regulation of bone mass accrual [55]. First, addition of serotonin to cultures of differentiated P19 cells or to wild type hypothalamic explants, but not to *Htr2c–/–* explants, induces CREB phosphorylation on Ser133, i.e., its activation. Second, in the explant assay, phosphorylation of CREB and CaMKIV co-localize in the same neurons upon serotonin treatment. Third, mice with an inactivation of *Creb* ($Creb_{VHM}$–/–) or heterozygous compound for *Creb* and *Htr2c* ($Creb_{VHM}$–/–; *Htr2c*+/–) or for *Creb* and *CaMKIV* ($Creb_{VHM}$+/–; $CaMKIV_{VHM}$+/–) in VMH neurons only all show a low bone mass phenotype characterized by decreased bone formation and increased bone resorption [55]. Thus, the negative regulation of bone remodeling by leptin relies on its inhibition of brainstem serotonergic neurons, which normally signals to VMH neurons via an Htr2c→CaMKKβ→CaMKIV→CREB cascade to increased bone formation and decrease bone resorption (Fig. 12.3).

Efferent Mediators of Leptin's Central Regulation of Bone Remodeling

How could the VMH regulate the function of bone cells? Two modes of action can transfer a central signal to peripheral cells: inducing the release of a blood-borne factor or relaying the information via the peripheral nervous system. As it turned out leptin's regulation of bone mass accrual uses both these mechanisms.

The Sympathetic Tone Relays Leptin's Action on Both Bone Formation and Bone Resorption

The first evidence that leptin central action on bone is mediated by a nervous relay came from a variant of the classical parabiosis experiment that identified the *ob* gene as encoding a circulating factor [56]. Instead of connecting an *ob/ob* with a wild type mouse, two *ob/ob* mice are connected and one of them receives a dose of leptin icv low enough not to leak into the general circulation [33]. As expected given the negative impact of leptin on bone mass accrual, the mouse receiving leptin loses bone within a month. The contralateral mouse, however, despite sharing its blood content with the infused mouse does not lose bone (although it loses weight). This observation, and the fact that bone is among the most innervated organ, suggested that leptin most likely uses a nervous relay as its main effector on bone cells.

A significant decrease of the sympathetic tone is one of the many features of the *ob/ob* and *db/db* mice [57] suggesting that the sympathetic nervous system could play such a role. Indeed, in all models engineered to define leptin's central regulation of bone remodeling changes in the sympathetic tone correlates with the bone phenotype observed (Table 12.3). For example, mice without leptin signaling in neurons or more specifically in brainstem neurons all have a decrease in sympathetic tone [30, 43]. Conversely, mice in which leptin activity is increased directly (*l/l* mice) or indirectly (*Tph2–/–*, *Htr2b–/–* or *Creb*$_{VMH}$*–/–* mice) show increased sympathetic output [30, 43, 55]. As a matter of fact, one of the genes downregulated in the hypothalamus of these three mouse strains encodes Tyrosine hydroxylase, the enzyme responsible for the first step in the synthesis of catecholamines [55]. A direct confirmation that leptin acts on bone remodeling via the sympathetic nervous system comes from two key genetic experiments.

Both the synthesis of epinephrine and norepinephrine, two catecholamines mediating many peripheral functions of the sympathetic tone, depends on the enzymatic transformation of dopamine by the Dopamine β-hydroxylase (Dbh). In Dbh-deficient mice, bone mass is increased and leptin icv cannot corrects this phenotype as it does in *ob/ob* mice [33]. At the bone cell level, osteoblasts, which mediate both the sympathetic tone action on bone formation and on bone resorption (see below, section "Molecular Mediators of Leptin-Activated Signaling in Bone"), express the β2 adrenergic receptor (Adrβ2) and its inactivation in these or all cells causes a high bone mass phenotype associated with increased bone formation and decreased bone resorption that cannot be corrected by icv infusion of leptin [33, 58]. Conversely, *ob/ob* mice treated with isoproterenol, a β-adrenergic agonist, lose bone [33]. The same effect can be observed in wild type mice or rats [33, 59–61]. More importantly from a biomedical point of view, wild-type mice or rats treated with the β-blocker propranolol, gain bone to such an extent that it can prevent the deleterious consequence of ovariectomy, a model of postmenopausal bone loss [33, 62, 63]. This finding provides a molecular explanation for the decreased risk of fracture associated with the treatment of patients with some β-blockers (see below, section "Leptin Actions on Bone Remodeling and Human Bone Biology").

Table 12.3 Correlation between leptin signaling, brain serotonin, sympathetic output, and bone remodeling

	Central leptin signaling	Brain serotonin	Sympathetic output	Bone mass
ob/ob	0	+	–	+
db/db	0	+	–	+
$LepR_{BS}$–/–	±	+	–	+
$LepR_{ARC}$–/–	±	–	+	–
$LepR_{VMH}$–/–	±	–	+	–
wt+leptin icv	+	–	+	–
$LepR_{BS}$–/–+leptin icv	±	+	–	+
Tph2–/–	=	0	+	–
ob/ob; *Tph2*+/–	0	=	=	=
Htr2c–/–	=	=	+	–
Tph2+/–; *Htr2c*+/–	=	–	+	–
$CaMKK\beta_{VMH}$–/–	=	=	+	–
Htr2c+/–;$CaMKK\beta_{VMH}$+/–	=	=	+	–
$CaMKIV_{VMH}$–/–	=	=	+	–
Htr2c+/–; $CaMKIV_{VMH}$+/–	=	=	+	–
$Creb_{VMH}$–/–	=	=	+	–
Htr2c+/–; $Creb_{VMH}$+/–	=	=	+	–
Dbh–/–	=	=	–	+

+, increase; + normal level; ±, partial; –, decrease; 0, absence
BS, inactivation in brainstem SERT expressing neurons, ARC, inactivation in arcuate POMC expressing neurons, VMH, inactivation in VMH Sf1 expressing neurons

Leptin's Regulation of *Cart* Expression in the Hypothalamus Affects Bone Resorption

A second, less potent and far less understood, mode of action of leptin on bone mass accrual involves the cocaine amphetamine regulated transcript CART, a neuropeptide present in brain but also in the general circulation [64–66]. *Cart* expression is increased by leptin and is low in the brain of *ob/ob* mice [67–69]. In absence of *Cart* mice develop a late onset low bone mas phenotype characterized by a sole increase in bone resorption indicating that CART acts as an inhibitor of bone resorption [70]. When the *Cart–/–* mice are infused icv with leptin they loose bone faster than wild-type mice due to a more pronounced increase in bone resorption [70]. This is due to the fact that leptin's positive regulation of bone resorption by the sympathetic nervous system occurs normally but is not mitigated by an increase in CART levels. Of note, an increase in CART expression and/or circulating levels explains the high bone mass bone/low bone resorption phenotype of observed in *Mc4R-deficient* mice as well as in patients heterozygous for inactivating mutations in this gene [26, 70].

If CART mediates, at least in part, leptin's effect on bone mass accrual, why was not its effect observed in *ob/ob* mice and, more importantly, in the parabiosis experiment described above? At the present time, and since the identity of the CART receptor is not know, one can only speculate that in either case the role of leptin in regulating fertility and thereby the levels of circulating sex steroid hormones might be interfering. Indeed, in the case of *ob/ob* mice bone resorption is markedly increased due to the lack of estrogen. Hence, in these mice the decreased level of CART, which causes a slow increase in bone resorption, is only a minor component of their high bone resorption phenotype (Fig. 12.4a). In the *ob/ob-ob/ob*+leptin icv parabiosis experiment, the opposite effect takes place (Fig. 12.4b). Activation of *Cart* expression and increased levels of sex steroid hormones in the leptin-receiving mice [29, 71]

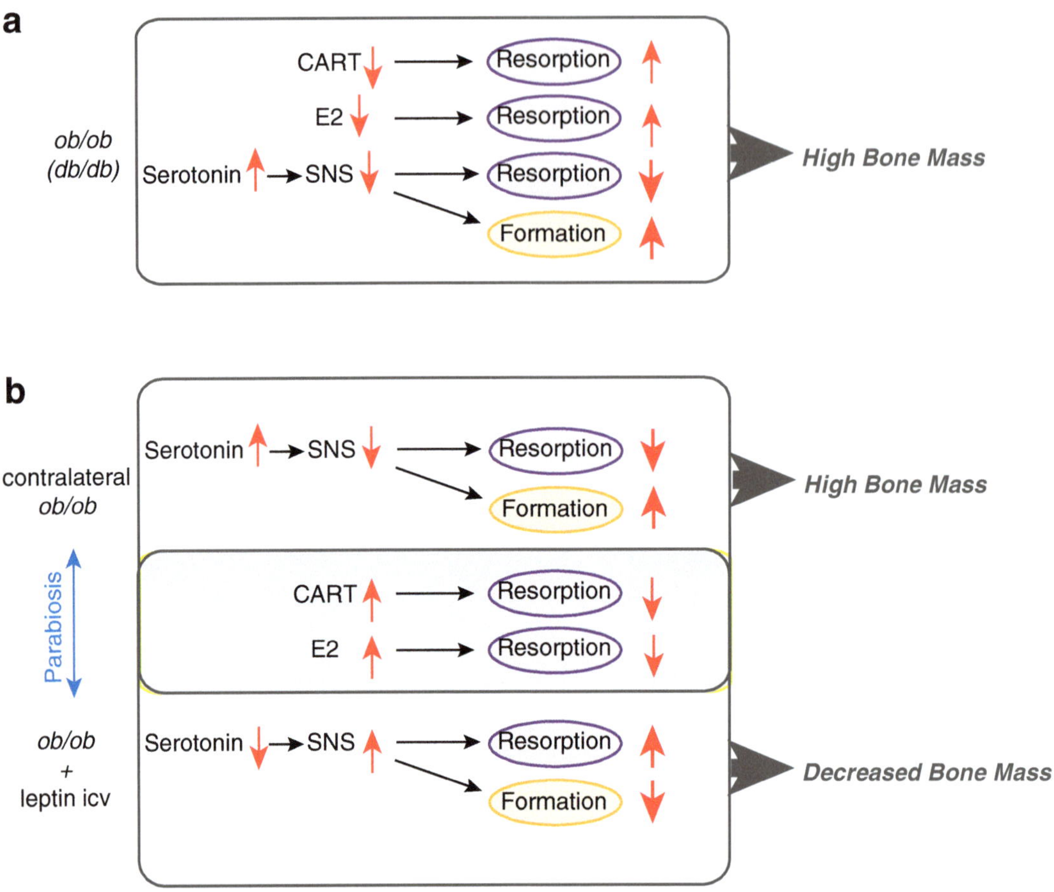

Fig. 12.4 Consequences on bone mass accrual of the absence and presence of leptin. (**a**) Schematic representation of the different influences on bone remodeling caused by the absence of leptin. (**b**) Schematic representation of the influence on bone remodeling of leptin icv infusion in the receiving and contralateral mouse of a pair of parabiosed *ob*/*ob* mice. The region highlighted in *blue* indicates shared signals between the two mice

both decrease bone resorption while the blockade of serotonin production causes an increase in sympathetic output, i.e., an increase in bone resorption and a decrease in bone formation. The end result is a mitigated increase in bone resorption and a decrease in bone formation, resulting in bone loss. In the contralateral mouse, however, the sympathetic tone remains low causing a high bone mass phenotype that, within the 1 month time-frame of this experiment, is not significantly affected by blood-borne effectors such as CART and estrogens.

Molecular Mediators of Leptin-Activated Signaling in Bone

Leptin delivers its double compromising signal to bone mass accrual by concomitantly suppressing bone formation by osteoblasts and increasing bone resorption by osteoclasts. Both effects, however, are mediated by centrally derived signals on osteoblasts only. Indeed, as detailed below, once it reaches the osteoblasts, the sympathetic tone recruits several transcriptional regulators including CREB and ATF4 and components of the molecular clock to inhibit these cells proliferation and thereby decrease bone formation (Fig. 12.3). In parallel, sympathetic tone signaling in osteoblasts also increases the expression of *RankL*, a most powerful osteoclastogenic cytokine [4] and thus favors bone resorption. The same mode of action is used by CART, the other leptin-activated signal, to regulate bone resorption (Fig. 12.3).

Leptin Regulates Bone Formation Through Adrβ2 Signaling in Osteoblasts

As mentioned above, *Adrβ2* is expressed in osteoblasts where it mediates leptin-activated sympathetic signals. Indeed, mice lacking these gene either globally or in osteoblasts only display a high bone mass phenotype in vertebrae and long bones characterized by increased bone formation and decreased bone resorption [58, 70]. The latter effect is more pronounced than the one observed in *ob*/*ob* mice since *Adrβ2*-deficient mice are fertile and have normal sex steroid hormone levels. Of note, although *Adrβ2*-deficient mice have high bone mass, mice deficient for both the *Adrβ2* and *Adrβ1* genes have low bone mass, potentially implying that signaling through Adrβ1 counteracts signaling through Adrβ2 in bone remodeling [72]. Yet, on its own, *Adrβ1* inactivation does not cause bone loss [70]. In contrast, mice without all three β-adrenergic receptors exhibit high bone mass through mechanisms that have not yet been described [73]. The function of the Adrβ1 and Adrβ3 receptors in osteoblasts may not be mediating leptin's regulation of bone remodeling, however, since icv leptin infusions do not cause bone loss in absence of Adrβ2 in all cells or specifically in osteoblasts [58, 70].

Beta-adrenergic receptors are GPCR signaling through the cAMP pathway [74]. Accordingly, cAMP production is induced by isoproterenol (a potent β-adrenergic receptor agonist) in primary osteoblast cultures derived from wild type but not *Adrb2*-deficient mice or in mouse and human osteoblasts treated with the β-blocker propranolol [33, 70]. Upon phosphorylation on Ser133 the transcription factor CREB, a common target of cAMP signaling and a key player in regulating osteoblast biology [58, 75, 76], then relays the Adrβ2/cAMP signal to the nucleus to regulate bone formation through an increase in osteoblast proliferation. The importance of CREB in mediating leptin's effect on bone formation is exemplified by the fact that leptin icv infusion fails to decrease bone formation in mice deficient in this transcription factor in osteoblasts only [58]. That in these same mice the expression of Cyclin genes, of *Myc* and of *Period* (*Per*)*1*, a component of the molecular clock, is affected provided the molecular bases of the role of leptin on bone formation [58].

It was reported decades ago that the secretion of α1(I) collagen and osteocalcin, the two most abundant proteins made by osteoblasts, have circadian variations, suggesting that bone remodeling can be regulated in a circadian manner [77–79]. Accordingly, all the components of the molecular clock are expressed in osteoblasts and their expression is regulated by the sympathetic tone [80]. Prompted by these observations, and in order to understand the mechanism of reduced bone formation by sympathetic signaling, Fu et al. demonstrated that mice lacking genes that encode major components of the molecular clock proteins in all cells or specifically in osteoblasts (*Per1–/–*; *Per2–/–* mice and *Cryptochrome* (*Cry*)*1–/–*; *Cry2–/–* mice) have high bone mass with increased bone formation [80]. Moreover, these mice are resistant to central effects of leptin. In fact, ICV administration of leptin to *Per1–/–*; *Per2m/m* (deletion of PAS domain of Per2) mice could not decrease bone mass but instead resulted in an elevated vertebral bone volume and osteoblast numbers, which is in stark contrast to the result in wild-type mice [80]. Osteoblasts from molecular clock-deficient mice proliferate more rapidly than wild-type osteoblasts and further experiments showed that *Per* gene deficiency in osteoblasts results in elevated *G1 Cyclin* expression that leads to shortening of the cell cycle and increased cell proliferation [80]. While BMAL1 and CLOCK do not affect *Cyclin D1* promoter activity, they downregulate the expression of *c-myc*, a critical regulator of *Cyclin D1* activity [80]. Clock genes also decrease the expression of multiple AP-1 genes causing a further decrease in c-myc activation of *G1 Cyclin* expression. This second arm of regulation in also under the control of the sympathetic tone since in absence of clock genes or of their activity β-adrenergic signaling can induce AP-1 transcription factors and promote osteoblast proliferation [80]. Altogether, these results established that the molecular clock acts downstream of leptin and the sympathetic nervous system in osteoblasts to inhibit their proliferation via inhibition of the c-myc-mediated activation of *Cyclin* gene expression (Fig. 12.3).

Several reports have proposed that leptin directly affects osteoblast differentiation and/or proliferation in vitro [41, 81–83]. In contextualizing these studies it is important to note that most of these reports use leptin concentrations that are supraphysiologic and therefore provide results from which it is difficult to draw meaningful conclusions. Even when more physiologically relevant concentrations of leptin are used [12, 41, 83] in vitro studies have led to different and sometimes opposite results. This could be due to the distinct impact the presence of different concentrations of serum, and therefore of leptin, could have on the cells before or during treatment or to their differentiation status [39]. For instance, deletion of the long-form of the leptin receptor from bone marrow stromal cells in culture delays mineralization by increasing adipogenesis but osteoblasts derived from *db/db* mice behave normally [12, 84]. It remains that analyses involving in vivo tracking of osteoblast lineages through the use of a *LepR* promoter-YFP reporter gene showed that osteoblasts do not express leptin receptors [42] (Fig. 12.2) and that the conditional inactivation of leptin receptor in osteoblasts using α1(I)Collagen-Cre, a transgenic strain that induces recombination early in the osteoblast lineage [85], does not affect trabecular bone mass [30].

Leptin Regulates Bone Resorption Through Adrβ2 Signaling in Osteoblasts

Studies in *Adrβ2*-deficient mice showed that in addition to an increase in bone formation, lack of sympathetic signaling results in a decrease in bone resorption even more pronounced than the one existing in *ob/ob* mice [58, 70]. These observations indicated a neuronal control of bone resorption and posed the question whether leptin-activated SNS signaling impinges on osteoclastogenesis.

Although Adrβ2 is expressed in osteoclasts, attempts to demonstrate a direct effect of sympathetic tone on osteoclasts or on osteoclast precursor cells have failed thus far. For example, while cAMP induction by isoproterenol in primary osteoblast cultures is blocked by the absence of *Adrb2*, deletion of *Adrb2* has no effect on cultured osteoclasts [70]. Instead, a decrease of osteoclast surface and activity can be observed in mice *Adrβ2*-deficient globally or in osteoblasts only, and a decrease in bone resorption can be observed in wild type mice transplanted with *Adrβ2*-deficient osteoblasts [58, 70]. These observations all concur to suggest that osteoblasts mediate the leptin-activated sympathetic signal on osteoclasts. Consistent with this notion leptin-activated sympathetic tone acts on osteoblasts to increase the expression of *RankL*, a most powerful osteoclastogenic cytokine [86], and thus favors bone resorption [58, 70]. This sympathetic function is mediated by the cAMP-dependent activation of protein kinase A (PKA) and subsequent phosphorylation on Ser254 (by PKA) and increase in the transactivation function of ATF4, the cell-specific CREB-related transcription factor essential for osteoblast differentiation and function [70, 87] As a result, ATF4 is recruited and directly binds to a CRE-binding site in the promoter of *Rankl*, thus upregulating the expression of this osteoclastogenic factor [70]. However, sympathetic regulation of *Rankl* expression by ATF4 is independent of its phosphorylation on Ser251 by RSK2, another kinase known to regulate ATF4 functions on osteoblast differentiation [88]. This regulation is also independent of CREB, the downstream mediator of sympathetic signaling in osteoblasts, since leptin icv infusion in mice deficient in *Creb* in osteoblasts can affect bone resorption [58].

Leptin Regulation of Bone Resorption Through CART

The second pathway by which leptin regulates bone mass accrual also affects bone resorption although in contrast to the sympathetic tone it inhibits this process [70]. The mediator of this inhibitory action is CART, a neuropeptide whose expression is increased by leptin and whose levels are in *ob/ob* mice but normal in *Adrb2–/–* mice [70]. *Cart–/–* mice show a low bone mass phenotype which is solely attributed to increases in osteoclast formation and function [26, 70]. CART is not expressed in osteoblasts or osteoclasts, *Cart–/–* bone cells show no cell-autonomous defects and exogenous CART administration does not affect osteoclast formation [70]. In contrast, *Rankl* expression is increased in *Cart–/–* bones suggesting that CART exerts its function by modulating the production of this cytokine by osteoblasts. Thus, leptin controls bone resorption through, at least, two distinct and antagonistic pathways. On the one hand, sympathetic signaling via Adrβ2 promotes osteoclast differentiation; on the other hand, CART inhibits it. The transcriptional mechanisms by which CART regulates bone resorption remain unknown in absence of a specific CART receptor.

Leptin Actions on Bone Remodeling and Human Bone Biology

The most straightforward indications that leptin's effect on bone mass accrual is conserved from rodents to humans were obtained from a patient with a mutation in the *ob* gene, who displayed a high bone mass phenotype, and the observation that human patients with lipodystrophy display advanced the bone age, an indirect indicator of bone formation [70]. More generally, however, the situation is more complex. Indeed, positive, negative or no associations between serum leptin levels and bone mineral density have been reported, which confounds the interpretation of leptin's effect on bone mass and the correlation with rodent studies [89–93]. Moreover, in obese individuals body weight can be positively correlated with increased bone mass [7]. Considering that leptin levels are proportional to fat mass this observation can be viewed as a direct contradiction with the negative role defined in animal studies. Obesity, however, is also associated with the development of leptin resistance, which could explain this discrepancy as it explains the persistence of appetite despite high levels of leptin [37, 38, 94, 95].

Only a few human studies have examined the direct effect of leptin administration on bone-mineral density. One study reported an increase in bone mass and decrease in bodyweight after long-term leptin therapy in an obese 9-year-old girl with congenital leptin deficiency [96]. In view of the patient's age, however, it is difficult to make any firm conclusions because of the effects of ongoing skeletal growth on bone mass. More recently, subcutaneous administration of leptin was found to have no significant effect on bone-mineral density in two women with lipodystrophy [97]. Larger clinical studies are therefore necessary to clarify leptin's role in human vivo and to assess the contribution of the central and peripheral role of leptin to the overall maintenance of bone turnover in human beings.

The donwstream effectors of leptin's regulation of bone remodeling are also conserved betwwen rodents and mice. Indeed, patients heterozygous for inactivating mutations in *MC4R* develop a late onset increase in bone mass associated with a decrease in bone resorption [26, 98]. As it is the case in *Mc4r*-deficient mice these patients have significantly increased serum levels or CART [26]. The mouse studies have also indicated that β-adrenergic antagonists, commonly used to control blood pressure and cardiovascular disease, induce bone formation and increase osteoblast numbers. They also showed that such treatment can overcome hypogonadism-induced loss of bone mass [33] suggesting that β-blockers may overcome the loss of bone mass in postmenopausal women. Many epidemiological studies have reported beneficial effects of β-blockers on BMD and/or fracture risk [99–102]. More generally, a meta-analysis of eight studies demonstrated that β-blockers reduce hip fracture risk (pooled relative risk 0.72) and any fracture risk (pooled relative risk 0.86) [103]. Similarly, reflex sympathetic dystrophy, a disease characterized by local sympathetic activation and bone loss, is most often treated with β-blockers [104, 105]. However, most studies are observational and prospective randomized clinical trials that take the specificity and dosage of β-blockers into consideration are needed.

References

1. Kronenberg HM. Developmental regulation of the growth plate. Nature. 2003;423(6937):332–6.
2. Karsenty G, Wagner EF. Reaching a genetic and molecular understanding of skeletal development. Dev Cell. 2002;2(4):389–406.
3. Ducy P, Schinke T, Karsenty G. The osteoblast: a sophisticated fibroblast under central surveillance. Science. 2000;289:1501–4.
4. Teitelbaum SL. Bone resorption by osteoclasts. Science. 2000;289:1504–8.
5. Karsenty G, Ferron M. The contribution of bone to whole-organism physiology. Nature. 2012;481(7381):314–20.
6. Denver RJ, Bonett RM, Boorse GC. Evolution of leptin structure and function. Neuroendocrinology. 2011;94(1):21–38.
7. Holbrook TL, Barrett-Connor E. The association of lifetime weight and weight control patterns with bone mineral density in an adult community. Bone Miner. 1993;20(2):141–9. Epub 1993/02/01.
8. Legroux-Gerot I, Vignau J, Collier F, Cortet B. Bone loss associated with anorexia nervosa. Joint Bone Spine. 2005;72(6):489–95. Epub 2005/10/26.
9. Legroux-Gerot I, Vignau J, D'Herbomez M, Collier F, Marchandise X, Duquesnoy B, et al. Evaluation of bone loss and its mechanisms in anorexia nervosa. Calcif Tissue Int. 2007;81(3):174–82. Epub 2007/08/02.
10. Misra M, Klibanski A. Bone health in anorexia nervosa. Curr Opin Endocrinol Diabetes Obes. 2011;18(6):376–82. doi:10.1097/MED.0b013e32834b4bdc.
11. Riggs BL, Khosla S, Melton 3rd LJ. A unitary model for involutional osteoporosis: estrogen deficiency causes both type I and type II osteoporosis in postmenopausal women and contributes to bone loss in aging men. J Bone Miner Res. 1998;13(5):763–73.
12. Ducy P, Amling M, Takeda S, Priemel M, Schilling AF, Beil FT, et al. Leptin inhibits bone formation through a hypothalamic relay: a central control of bone mass. Cell. 2000;100(2):197–207.
13. Friedman JM. Obesity in the new millennium. Nature. 2000;404:632–4.
14. Friedman JM, Halaas JL. Leptin and the regulation of body weight in mammals. Nature. 1998;395(6704):763–70.
15. Spiegelman BM, Flier JS. Adipogenesis and obesity: rounding out the big picture. Cell. 1996;87(3):377–89.
16. Tartaglia LA, Dembski M, Weng X, Deng N, Culpepper J, Devos R, et al. Identification and expression cloning of a leptin receptor OB-R. Cell. 1995;83(7):1263–71.
17. Zhang Y, Proenca R, Maffei M, Barone M, Leopold L, Friedman JM. Positional cloning of the mouse obese gene and its human homologue. Nature. 1994;372:425–32.
18. Ahima RS. Body fat, leptin, and hypothalamic amenorrhea. N Engl J Med. 2004;351(10):959–62.
19. Baldock PA, Sainsbury A, Allison S, Lin EJ, Couzens M, Boey D, et al. Hypothalamic control of bone formation: distinct actions of leptin and y2 receptor pathways. J Bone Miner Res. 2005;20(10):1851–7.
20. Vaira S, Yang C, McCoy A, Keys K, Xue S, Weinstein EJ, et al. Creation and preliminary characterization of a leptin knockout rat. Endocrinology. 2012;153(11):5622–8. Epub 2012/09/06.
21. Solomon G, Atkins A, Shahar R, Gertler A, Monsonego-Ornan E. Effect of peripherally administered leptin antagonist on whole body metabolism and bone microarchitecture and biomechanical properties in the mouse. Am J Physiol Endocrinol Metab. 2014;306(1):E14–27. Epub 2013/10/31.
22. Ahima RS, Kelly J, Elmquist JK, Flier JS. Distinct physiologic and neuronal responses to decreased leptin and mild hyperleptinemia. Endocrinology. 1999;140(11):4923–31. Epub 1999/10/28.
23. Reid IR. Glucocorticoid osteoporosis–mechanisms and management. Eur J Endocrinol. 1997;137(3):209–17. Epub 1997/10/23.
24. Reid IR. Steroid-induced osteoporosis. Osteoporos Int. 1997;7 Suppl 3:S213–6. Epub 1997/01/01.
25. Suva LJ, Gaddy D, Perrien DS, Thomas RL, Findlay DM. Regulation of bone mass by mechanical loading: microarchitecture and genetics. Curr Osteoporos Rep. 2005;3(2):46–51. Epub 2005/07/23.
26. Ahn JD, Dubern B, Lubrano-Berthelier C, Clement K, Karsenty G. Cart overexpression is the only identifiable cause of high bone mass in melanocortin 4

receptor deficiency. Endocrinology. 2006;147(7): 3196–202.

27. Moitra J, Mason MM, Olive M, Krylov D, Gavrilova O, Marcus-Samuels B, et al. Life without white fat: a transgenic mouse. Genes Dev. 1998;12(20):3168–81. Epub 1998/10/24.
28. Elefteriou F, Takeda S, Ebihara K, Magre J, Patano N, Kim CA, et al. Serum leptin level is a regulator of bone mass. Proc Natl Acad Sci U S A. 2004; 101(9):3258–63.
29. Chehab FF, Lim ME, Lu R. Correction of the sterility defect in homozygous obese female mice by treatment with the human recombinant leptin. Nat Genet. 1996;12(3):318–20.
30. Shi Y, Yadav VK, Suda N, Liu XS, Guo XE, Myers Jr MG, et al. Dissociation of the neuronal regulation of bone mass and energy metabolism by leptin in vivo. Proc Natl Acad Sci U S A. 2008;105:20529.
31. Iwaniec UT, Boghossian S, Lapke PD, Turner RT, Kalra SP. Central leptin gene therapy corrects skeletal abnormalities in leptin-deficient ob/ob mice. Peptides. 2007;28(5):1012–9. Epub 2007/03/10.
32. Pogoda P, Egermann M, Schnell JC, Priemel M, Schilling AF, Alini M, et al. Leptin inhibits bone formation not only in rodents, but also in sheep. J Bone Miner Res. 2006;21(10):1591–9.
33. Takeda S, Elefteriou F, Levasseur R, Liu X, Zhao L, Parker KL, et al. Leptin regulates bone formation via the sympathetic nervous system. Cell. 2002;111(3): 305–17.
34. Sato S, Hanada R, Kimura A, Abe T, Matsumoto T, Iwasaki M, et al. Central control of bone remodeling by neuromedin U. Nat Med. 2007;13:1234.
35. Bjorbak C, Lavery HJ, Bates SH, Olson RK, Davis SM, Flier JS, et al. SOCS3 mediates feedback inhibition of the leptin receptor via Tyr985. J Biol Chem. 2000;275(51):40649–57.
36. Bjornholm M, Munzberg H, Leshan RL, Villanueva EC, Bates SH, Louis GW, et al. Mice lacking inhibitory leptin receptor signals are lean with normal endocrine function. J Clin Invest. 2007;117(5):1354–60.
37. Könner AC, Brüning Jens C. Selective insulin and leptin resistance in metabolic disorders. Cell Metab. 2012;16(2):144–52.
38. Mark AL. Selective leptin resistance revisited. Am J Physiol Regul Integr Comp Physiol. 2013;305(6): R566–81.
39. Motyl KJ, Rosen CJ. Understanding leptin-dependent regulation of skeletal homeostasis. Biochimie. 2012;94(10):2089–96.
40. Steppan CM, Crawford DT, Chidsey-Frink KL, Ke H, Swick AG. Leptin is a potent stimulator of bone growth in ob/ob mice. Regul Pept. 2000;92(1–3): 73–8.
41. Cornish J, Callon KE, Bava U, Lin C, Naot D, Hill BL, et al. Leptin directly regulates bone cell function in vitro and reduces bone fragility in vivo. J Endocrinol. 2002;175(2):405–15.
42. Ding L, Saunders TL, Enikolopov G, Morrison SJ. Endothelial and perivascular cells maintain haematopoietic stem cells. Nature. 2012;481(7382): 457–62.
43. Yadav VK, Oury F, Suda N, Liu ZW, Gao XB, Confavreux C, et al. A serotonin-dependent mechanism explains the leptin regulation of bone mass, appetite, and energy expenditure. Cell. 2009;138(5): 976–89.
44. Balthasar N, Coppari R, McMinn J, Liu SM, Lee CE, Tang V, et al. Leptin receptor signaling in POMC neurons is required for normal body weight homeostasis. Neuron. 2004;42(6):983–91.
45. Oury F, Karsenty G. Towards a serotonin-dependent leptin roadmap in the brain. Trends Endocrinol Metab. 2011;22(9):382–7. Epub 2011/05/24.
46. Ducy P, Karsenty G. The two faces of serotonin in bone biology. J Cell Biol. 2010;191(1):7–13. Epub 2010/10/06.
47. Hay-Schmidt A, Helboe L, Larsen PJ. Leptin receptor immunoreactivity is present in ascending serotonergic and catecholaminergic neurons of the rat. Neuroendocrinology. 2001;73(4):215–26. Epub 2001/05/08.
48. Scott MM, Lachey JL, Sternson SM, Lee CE, Elias CF, Friedman JM, et al. Leptin targets in the mouse brain. J Comp Neurol. 2009;514(5):518–32. Epub 2009/04/08.
49. Collin M, Håkansson-Ovesjö M-L, Misane I, Ögren SO, Meister B. Decreased 5-HT transporter mRNA in neurons of the dorsal raphe nucleus and behavioral depression in the obese leptin-deficient ob/ob mouse. Mol Brain Res. 2000;81(1–2):51–61.
50. Heath MJ, Hen R. Serotonin receptors. Genetic insights into serotonin function. Curr Biol. 1995;5(9):997–9. Epub 1995/09/01.
51. Berger M, Gray JA, Roth BL. The expanded biology of serotonin. Annu Rev Med. 2009;60:355–66. Epub 2009/07/28.
52. Flomen R, Knight J, Sham P, Kerwin R, Makoff A. Evidence that RNA editing modulates splice site selection in the 5-HT2C receptor gene. Nucleic Acids Res. 2004;32(7):2113–22.
53. Drago A, Serretti A. Focus on HTR2C: a possible suggestion for genetic studies of complex disorders. Am J Med Genet B Neuropsychiatr Genet. 2009; 150B(5):601–37.
54. Burns CM, Chu H, Rueter SM, Hutchinson LK, Canton H, Sanders-Bush E, et al. Regulation of serotonin-2C receptor G-protein coupling by RNA editing. Nature. 1997;387(6630):303–8.
55. Oury F, Yadav VK, Wang Y, Zhou B, Liu XS, Guo XE, et al. CREB mediates brain serotonin regulation of bone mass through its expression in ventromedial hypothalamic neurons. Genes Dev. 2010;24(20): 2330–42. Epub 2010/10/19.
56. Coleman DL. Effects of parabiosis of obese with diabetes and normal mice. Diabetologia. 1973;9(4): 294–8.
57. Bray GA, York DA. The MONA LISA hypothesis in the time of leptin. Recent Prog Horm Res. 1998; 53:95–117.

58. Kajimura D, Hinoi E, Ferron M, Kode A, Riley KJ, Zhou B, et al. Genetic determination of the cellular basis of the sympathetic regulation of bone mass accrual. J Exp Med. 2011;208(4):841–51. Epub 2011/03/30.
59. Bonnet N, Benhamou CL, Beaupied H, Laroche N, Vico L, Dolleans E, et al. Doping dose of salbutamol and exercise: deleterious effect on cancellous and cortical bones in adult rats. J Appl Physiol. 2007; 102(4):1502–9.
60. Bonnet N, Benhamou CL, Brunet-Imbault B, Arlettaz A, Horcajada MN, Richard O, et al. Severe bone alterations under β2 agonist treatments: bone mass, microarchitecture and strength analyses in female rats. Bone. 2005;37(5):622–33.
61. Kondo H, Togari A. Continuous treatment with a low-dose β-agonist reduces bone mass by increasing bone resorption without suppressing bone formation. Calcif Tissue Int. 2011;88(1):23–32.
62. Bonnet N, Laroche N, Vico L, Dolleans E, Benhamou CL, Courteix D. Dose effects of propranolol on cancellous and cortical bone in ovariectomized adult rats. J Pharmacol Exp Ther. 2006;318(3):1118–27.
63. Bonnet N, Benhamou CL, Malaval L, Goncalves C, Vico L, Eder V, et al. Low dose beta-blocker prevents ovariectomy-induced bone loss in rats without affecting heart functions. J Cell Physiol. 2008; 217(3):819–27.
64. Thim L, Kristensen P, Larsen PJ, Wulff BS. CART, a new anorectic peptide. Int J Biochem Cell Biol. 1998;30(12):1281–4.
65. Thim L, Kristensen P, Nielsen PF, Wulff BS, Clausen JT. Tissue-specific processing of cocaine- and amphetamine-regulated transcript peptides in the rat. Proc Natl Acad Sci. 1999;96(6):2722–7.
66. Wierup N, Kuhar M, Nilsson BO, Mulder H, Ekblad E, Sundler F. Cocaine- and amphetamine-regulated transcript (CART) is expressed in several islet cell types during rat development. J Histochem Cytochem. 2004;52(2):169–77.
67. Vrang N, Kristensen P, Tang-Christensen M, Larsen PJ. Effects of leptin on arcuate pro-opiomelanocortin and cocaine-amphetamine-regulated transcript expression are independent of circulating levels of corticosterone. J Neuroendocrinol. 2002;14(11):880–6.
68. Kristensen P, Judge ME, Thim L, Ribel U, Christjansen KN, Wulff BS, et al. Hypothalamic CART is a new anorectic peptide regulated by leptin. Nature. 1998;393(6680):72–6.
69. Elias CF, Lee C, Kelly J, Aschkenasi C, Ahima RS, Couceyro PR, et al. Leptin activates hypothalamic CART neurons projecting to the spinal cord. Neuron. 1998;21(6):1375–85.
70. Elefteriou F, Ahn JD, Takeda S, Starbuck M, Yang X, Liu X, et al. Leptin regulation of bone resorption by the sympathetic nervous system and CART. Nature. 2005;434(7032):514–20.
71. Mounzih K, Lu R, Chehab FF. Leptin treatment rescues the sterility of genetically obese ob/ob males. Endocrinology. 1997;138(3):1190–3.
72. Pierroz D, Baldock PA, Bouxsein ML, Ferrari S. Low cortical bone mass in mice lacking beta 1 and beta 2 adrenergic recptors is associated with low bone formation and circulating IGF-1. J Bone Miner Res. 2006;21 Suppl 1:S26 (Abstract no 1091).
73. Dhillon H, Zigman JM, Ye C, Lee CE, McGovern RA, Tang V, et al. Leptin directly activates SF1 neurons in the VMH, and this action by leptin is required for normal body-weight homeostasis. Neuron. 2006; 49(2):191–203.
74. Benovic JL, Bouvier M, Caron MG, Lefkowitz RJ. Regulation of adenylyl cyclase-coupled beta-adrenergic receptors. Annu Rev Cell Biol. 1988;4: 405–28.
75. Yadav VK, Ryu JH, Suda N, Tanaka KF, Gingrich JA, Schutz G, et al. Lrp5 controls bone formation by inhibiting serotonin synthesis in the duodenum. Cell. 2008;135(5):825–37.
76. Kode A, Mosialou I, Silva BC, Rached MT, Zhou B, Wang J, et al. FOXO1 orchestrates the bone-suppressing function of gut-derived serotonin. J Clin Invest. 2012;122(10):3490–503. Epub 2012/09/05.
77. Russell JE, Simmons DJ, Huber B, Roos BA. Meal timing as a zeitgeber for skeletal deoxyribonucleic acid and collagen synthesis rhythms. Endocrinology. 1983;113(6):2035–42.
78. Nielsen HK. Circadian and circatrigintan changes in osteoblastic activity assessed by serum osteocalcin. Physiological and methodological aspects. Dan Med Bull. 1994;41(2):216–27. Epub 1994/04/01.
79. Szulc P, Seeman E, Delmas PD. Biochemical measurements of bone turnover in children and adolescents. Osteoporos Int. 2000;11(4):281–94. Epub 2000/08/06.
80. Fu L, Patel MS, Bradley A, Wagner EF, Karsenty G. The molecular clock mediates leptin-regulated bone formation. Cell. 2005;122(5):803–15.
81. Thomas T, Gori F, Khosla S, Jensen MD, Burguera B, Riggs BL. Leptin acts on human marrow stromal cells to enhance differentiation to osteoblasts and to inhibit differentiation to adipocytes. Endocrinology. 1999;140(4):1630–8.
82. Gordeladze JO, Drevon CA, Syversen U, Reseland JE. Leptin stimulates human osteoblastic cell proliferation, de novo collagen synthesis, and mineralization: impact on differentiation markers, apoptosis, and osteoclastic signaling. J Cell Biochem. 2002;85(4):825–36.
83. Kim GS, Hong JS, Kim SW, Koh JM, An CS, Choi JY, et al. Leptin induces apoptosis via ERK/cPLA2/cytochrome c pathway in human bone marrow stromal cells. J Biol Chem. 2003;278(24):21920–9.
84. Scheller EL, Leinninger GM, Hankenson KD, Myers JMG, Krebsbach PH. Ectopic expression of Col2.3 and Col3.6 promoters in the brain and association with leptin signaling. Cells Tissues Organs. 2011; 194(2–4):268–73.
85. Dacquin R, Starbuck M, Schinke T, Karsenty G. Mouse alpha1(I)-collagen promoter is the best known promoter to drive efficient Cre recombinase

expression in osteoblast. Dev Dyn. 2002;224(2):245–51.

86. Teitelbaum SL, Ross FP. Genetic regulation of osteoclast development and function. Nat Rev Genet. 2003;4(8):638–49.
87. Yang X, Matsuda K, Bialek P, Jacquot S, Masuoka HC, Schinke T, et al. ATF4 is a substrate of RSK2 and an essential regulator of osteoblast biology; implication for Coffin-Lowry Syndrome. Cell. 2004;117(3):387–98.
88. Elefteriou F, Benson MD, Sowa H, Starbuck M, Liu X, Ron D, et al. ATF4 mediation of NF1 functions in osteoblast reveals a nutritional basis for congenital skeletal dysplasiae. Cell Metab. 2006;4(6):441–51.
89. Iwamoto I, Douchi T, Kosha S, Murakami M, Fujino T, Nagata Y. Relationships between serum leptin level and regional bone mineral density, bone metabolic markers in healthy women. Acta Obstet Gynecol Scand. 2000;79(12):1060–4.
90. Sato M, Takeda N, Sarui H, Takami R, Takami K, Hayashi M, et al. Association between serum leptin concentrations and bone mineral density, and biochemical markers of bone turnover in adult men. J Clin Endocrinol Metab. 2001;86(11):5273–6.
91. Blum M, Harris SS, Must A, Naumova EN, Phillips SM, Rand WM, et al. Leptin, body composition and bone mineral density in premenopausal women. Calcif Tissue Int. 2003;73(1):27–32. Epub 2003/09/26.
92. Rauch F, Blum WF, Klein K, Allolio B, Schonau E. Does leptin have an effect on bone in adult women? Calcif Tissue Int. 1998;63(6):453–5. Epub 1998/11/18.
93. Martini G, Valenti R, Giovani S, Franci B, Campagna S, Nuti R. Influence of insulin-like growth factor-1 and leptin on bone mass in healthy postmenopausal women. Bone. 2001;28(1):113–7.
94. Caro JF, Kolaczynski JW, Nyce MR, Ohannesian JP, Opentanova I, Goldman WH, et al. Decreased cerebrospinal-fluid/serum leptin ratio in obesity: a possible mechanism for leptin resistance. Lancet. 1996;348(9021):159–61.
95. Schwartz MW, Peskind E, Raskind M, Boyko EJ, Porte Jr D. Cerebrospinal fluid leptin levels: relationship to plasma levels and to adiposity in humans. Nat Med. 1996;2(5):589–93. Epub 1996/05/01.
96. Farooqi IS, Jebb SA, Langmack G, Lawrence E, Cheetham CH, Prentice AM, et al. Effects of recombinant leptin therapy in a child with congenital leptin deficiency. N Engl J Med. 1999;341(12):879–84. Epub 1999/09/16.
97. Simha V, Zerwekh JE, Sakhaee K, Garg A. Effect of subcutaneous leptin replacement therapy on bone metabolism in patients with generalized lipodystrophy. J Clin Endocrinol Metabol. 2002;87(11):4942–5.
98. Yeo GS, Farooqi IS, Aminian S, Halsall DJ, Stanhope RG, O'Rahilly S. A frameshift mutation in MC4R associated with dominantly inherited human obesity. Nat Genet. 1998;20(2):111–2.
99. Schlienger RG, Kraenzlin ME, Jick SS, Meier CR. Use of beta-blockers and risk of fractures. JAMA. 2004;292(11):1326–32.
100. Bonnet N, Gadois C, McCloskey E, Lemineur G, Lespessailles E, Courteix D, et al. Protective effect of beta blockers in postmenopausal women: influence on fractures, bone density, micro and macroarchitecture. Bone. 2007;40(5):1209–16.
101. Pasco JA, Henry MJ, Nicholson GC, Schneider HG, Kotowicz MA. Beta-blockers reduce bone resorption marker in early postmenopausal women. Ann Hum Biol. 2005;32(6):738–45.
102. Turker S, Karatosun V, Gunal I. Beta-blockers increase bone mineral density. Clin Orthop Relat Res. 2006;443:73–4.
103. Wiens M, Etminan M, Gill SS, Takkouche B. Effects of antihypertensive drug treatments on fracture outcomes: a meta-analysis of observational studies. J Intern Med. 2006;260(4):350–62.
104. Kurvers HA. Reflex sympathetic dystrophy: facts and hypotheses. Vasc Med. 1998;3(3):207–14.
105. Patel MS, Elefteriou F. The new field of neuroskeletal biology. Calcif Tissue Int. 2007;80(5):337–47.

Leptin, Cell Cycle, and Cancer

13

Olorunseun O. Ogunwobi

Introduction

Leptin is one of the best known adipocytokines. Successful cloning of the leptin gene was first reported in 1994 [1]. Since then it has become an important target of study by researchers interested in understanding the biological basis for the strong association between obesity and many cancers. Some of the cancers associated with obesity include colon cancer [2–5], breast cancer [6], endometrial cancer [7, 8], esophageal adenocarcinoma [9–12], kidney cancer [13–17], leukemia [18], melanoma [19–23], multiple myeloma [24], non-Hodgkin's lymphoma [25–28], pancreatic cancer [29–32], prostate cancer [33, 34] rectal cancer [35, 36] and thyroid cancer [37–40]. The most strongly associated cancers with obesity in men are esophageal adenocarcinoma, thyroid cancer, colon cancer, and kidney cancer [41]. In women, the cancers most strongly associated with obesity are endometrial cancer, esophageal adenocarcinoma, and kidney cancer [41]. There is increasing evidence indicating that high circulating leptin levels characteristic of obesity may be promoting the development and progression of many of these obesity-associated cancers. Some of the observational and laboratory-based mechanistic data will be discussed in later sections of this chapter. The discussion will be particularly focused on the role of leptin in the development and progression of esophageal adenocarcinoma and colon cancer, although Table 13.1 summarizes the main cancer types where increased leptin and leptin receptor expression have been reported. The current state of scientific knowledge regarding how leptin regulates signal transduction and the cell cycle to promote carcinogenesis will be described. The main molecular mechanisms underlying the role of leptin in carcinogenesis are listed in Table 13.2. For completion, it must be mentioned that there are other adipocytokines that may regulate carcinogenesis. These include adiponectin, resistin, chemerin, collagenous repeat-containing sequence of 26 kDa protein (CORS-26), omentin, and visfatin [42–44].

Leptin and Esophageal Adenocarcinoma

Esophageal adenocarcinoma is one of two types of esophageal cancer. The more common type of esophageal cancer is esophageal squamous cell carcinoma. However, the incidence of esophageal squamous cell carcinoma has been decreasing whereas the incidence of esophageal adenocarcinoma (EAC) has been rapidly increasing worldwide [45]. This has especially been the case in the western world [45]. In fact, some researchers feel that

O.O. Ogunwobi, M.D., Ph.D. (✉)
Department of Biological Sciences, Hunter College of The City University of New York, 695 Park Avenue, New York, NY, 10065, USA
e-mail: ogunwobi@genectr.hunter.cuny.edu

S. Dagogo-Jack (ed.), *Leptin: Regulation and Clinical Applications*,
DOI 10.1007/978-3-319-09915-6_13, © Springer International Publishing Switzerland 2015

Table 13.1 Cancers associated with increased leptin and leptin receptor expression

Cancer type discussed	Leptin expression	Leptin receptor expression
Esophageal adenocarcinoma	Yes	Yes
Colon cancer	Yes	Yes
Breast cancer	Yes	Yes
Endometrial cancer	Yes	Yes
Kidney cancer	Yes	Yes
Leukemia	Yes	Yes
Melanoma	Yes	Yes
Multiple Myeloma	Yes	Yes
Non-Hodgkin's Lymphoma	Yes	Yes
Pancreatic cancer	No	No
Prostate cancer	Yes	Yes
Thyroid cancer	Yes	Yes
Ovarian	Yes	Yes

Table 13.2 Mechanisms of leptin action in cancer

Mechanism	Cancer type discussed
Cell proliferation	Esophageal adenocarcinoma (EAC), colon cancer, ovarian cancer, thyroid cancer
Inhibition of apoptosis	EAC, colon cancer, thyroid cancer
Motility	Colon cancer
Migration	EAC
Invasiveness	Colon cancer
Extracellular signal-regulated kinase (ERK)	EAC
p38 mitogen-activated protein kinase (p38 MAPK)	EAC
c-Jun NH_2-terminal kinase (JNK)	EAC
Akt	EAC
Janus kinase 2 (JAK2)	EAC
Signal transducer and activation of transcription 3 (STAT3)	EAC
Cyclooxygenase-2 (COX-2)	EAC
Prostaglandin E-2 (PGE2)	EAC
Epidermal growth factor receptor (EGFR)	EAC
Increased cell population in the S phase of the cell cycle	Ovarian cancer, endometrial cancer
Increased cell population in the G2/M phase of the cell cycle	Ovarian cancer
Decreased cell population in the G0/G1 phase of the cell cycle	Endometrial cancer
Cyclin D1-dependent cell cycle progression	Thyroid cancer
Downregulation of p21	Thyroid cancer
Upregulation of cyclin D, cyclin G, cyclin-dependent kinase 2, p27, p21, and p16	Breast cancer
Downregulation of transforming growth factor beta (TGFβ)	Breast cancer

the incidence of EAC worldwide is rising faster than that of any other solid cancer.

As mentioned above, there is a very strong association between obesity and esophageal adenocarcinoma. One of the earlier well-performed studies in this area was done in Sweden. The study showed that the odds ratio between obese persons (those with body mass index (BMI) greater than 30 kg/m^2) as compared to the leanest persons (individuals with BMI less than 22 kg/m^2) was 16.2 [46]. Around the same time, a group of researchers in the USA conducted a population-based case–control study of 589 patients of esophageal and gastric adenocarcinoma and 695 healthy control volunteers. After adjusting for age, sex, race, and cigarette smoking, they found that the odds ratio for esophageal adenocarcinoma for men in the highest quartile of BMI as compared to those in the lowest quartile was 3.0 (95 % confidence interval was 1.7–5.0) while the odds ratio for women in the highest quartile as compared to those in the lowest quartile was 2.6 (95 % confidence interval was 0.8–8.5) [47]. Many other studies performed since then have consistently showed that obesity is strongly associated with EAC [9, 10, 12, 45, 48]. Some have suggested that the reason for this association is the increased incidence of gastro-esophageal reflux disease (GERD) among obese people and that increased GERD leads to increased Barrett's esophagus (BE) and consequently increased EAC. It should be noted, however, that the association between obesity and EAC is stronger than that between GERD and EAC [46, 49]. Obesity is, therefore, a direct risk factor for EAC independent of GERD [50]. Consequently, it is very likely that there is a more direct link between obesity and EAC.

Adipocytokines are dysregulated in obesity and are known to exert effects on a wide variety of peripheral tissues [51–53]. Therefore, any or a combination of adipocytokines may provide a direct biological link between obesity and EAC. Leptin is a very strong candidate for this role because serum leptin concentrations correlate with percentage body mass and BMI [51, 54]. Consequently, many researchers have specifically investigated the direct role of leptin in the development and progression of many cancers. Although only few studies have specifically investigated EAC, their results have been clear and consistent.

In 2003, Somasundar et al. reported that leptin stimulated the proliferation of two different EAC cell lines but they were not able to detect an anti-apoptotic effect using their experimental approach [55]. However, 3 years later and working with a different EAC cell line, Ogunwobi et al. showed very clearly that leptin stimulated proliferation of an EAC cell line in a dose-dependent manner [56]. They were also able to detect an anti-apoptotic effect for leptin on the EAC cells. More importantly, they elucidated a cascade of intracellular signaling mechanisms via which leptin stimulates proliferation and inhibits apoptosis of EAC cells. Their studies showed that leptin stimulation resulted in the activation of cyclooxygenase-2 (COX-2) and prostaglandin E2 (PGE2) production in a manner dependent upon activation of extracellular signal-regulated kinase (ERK), p38 mitogen-activated protein kinase (MAPK), phosphatidylinositol 3′-kinase (PI3K)/Akt, and janus kinase (JAK) 2. They also showed that the PGE2 produced was subsequently involved in the transactivation of the epidermal growth factor receptor and c-Jun amino terminal kinase (JNK) [56]. It is noteworthy that all of the signaling pathways activated by leptin in the Ogunwobi et al. study have been shown by multiple studies and research groups to be important in the development and progression of EAC [57–59]. Furthermore, the leptin receptor is expressed in the OE33 EAC cell line used in the Ogunwobi et al. study. Moreover, leptin receptor expression has been demonstrated throughout the mouse gastrointestinal epithelium including the esophagus [60]. More importantly, leptin receptor expression has been demonstrated in the epithelium of the human lower esophagus [61] and it has been shown to increase as the lower esophagus changes from normal to Barrett's esophagus and finally to development of EAC [62].

Mention should also be made of data that suggest that hyperleptinemia in obesity likely cooperates with GERD in contributing to the development and progression of EAC. Beales et al. investigated the combined effects of acid and leptin exposure on EAC cells [63]. They found that there was a positive synergistic effect on proliferation and inhibition of apoptosis [63]. Additionally, these effects were via synergistic activation of the epidermal growth factor receptor (EGFR) and ERK [63].

Taken together, these studies provide a strong basis for concluding that increased circulating leptin in obese people may play a direct role in the increased incidence and progression of EAC in obesity.

Leptin and Colon Cancer

The role of leptin as a direct promoter of colon cancer is also clear. Expression of the leptin receptor in the epithelium of the human colon was described by Hardwick et al. in their 2001 publication [64]. In that paper, they also demonstrated that treatment of mice with leptin resulted in significant increase in colonic epithelial cell proliferation [64]. More recently, Koda and colleagues reported that leptin is overexpressed in human colon cancer [65]. Multiple research groups have independently demonstrated that leptin is able to promote proliferation, motility, invasiveness, and inhibit apoptosis of colonic epithelial cells by activation of a complex cascade of intracellular signaling mechanisms that have all been implicated in the development of human colon cancer [64, 66–69]. It is noteworthy that many of the intracellular signaling mechanisms activated by leptin in esophageal epithelial cells are also activated by leptin in colonic epithelial cells. However, one striking difference is that whereas leptin-induced proliferation is dependent on activation of the COX-2 pathway in esophageal epithelial cells [56], in colonic epithelial cells leptin is able to potently induce proliferation and inhibit apoptosis independent of activation of COX-2 [67].

The epidemiologic data supporting leptin's role in the promotion of colon cancer is also compelling. In Stattin et al's 2003 Sweden-based case–control study, they measured the prediagnostic plasma leptin levels of 75 men, 93 women, and 327 control volunteers. They performed statistical analysis using logistic regression and found that plasma leptin was associated with increased risk of colon cancer in men. The odds ratio (OR) between the highest and lowest quartiles was 1.96 (95 % confidence interval (CI) was 0.72–5.29) [70]. Subsequently, in 2005 Tamakoshi and colleagues performed a separate case–control study in Japan where they found an association between plasma leptin and colon cancer risk in women. Their study assessed 58 colon cancer patients and 145 colon cancer-free volunteers matched for study area and age. They also used logistic regression for their statistical analysis. In addition, however, they also accounted for BMI, life-style factors, reproductive factors, and insulin-like growth factor and its binding protein. Their analysis revealed that the ORs of female colorectal cancer risk for the second and third quintiles combined and the fourth and fifth quintiles combined relative to the first quintile were 1.40 (95 % CI was 0.41–4.78) and 4.84 (95 % CI was 1.29–18.1) respectively [71]. Around the same time, Stattin and colleagues reported a case–control study they performed in Norway wherein they analyzed serum levels of leptin in cryopreserved prediagnostic sera of 235 men with colon cancer and 378 control volunteers matched for age and date of blood collection. This time they performed logistic regression analysis and their data showed about a threefold increase in the risk of colon cancer associated with increasing concentrations of leptin. The odds ratio between the lowest and highest quartiles was up to 2.72 (95 % CI was 1.44–5.12); *p* (trend) was 0.008 [72].

Consequently, there is compelling evidence that circulating leptin concentrations correlate with colon cancer risk and that leptin directly promotes colon cancer.

Leptin and Cell Cycle in Cancer

Dysregulation of the cell cycle is undoubtedly a fundamental factor in the development and progression of cancer. This is especially the case with the uncontrolled proliferation and the genetic alterations that are characteristic of cancer cells (reviewed in [73]). It is, therefore, not surprising that the role of leptin in promoting many cancers often involves dysregulation of the cell cycle.

Consider a few examples. In an ovarian cancer study that used leptin receptor-expressing OVCAR-3 ovarian cancer cells, leptin was found to stimulate proliferation by upregulating cell cycle progression genes and suppressing cell cycle inhibitor genes. The authors also reported that leptin promoted cell cycle progression, as demonstrated by an increased cell population in both the S and G2/M phases [74]. In a separate study that used a mouse model of spontaneous thyroid cancer, consumption of a high-fat diet resulted in the development of obesity and elevated serum leptin levels. This in turn resulted in increased speed of tumor growth and reduced survival. Interestingly, thyroid tumor cell proliferation was increased via cyclin D1-dependent cell cycle progression [38]. Also, in an endometrial cancer model, leptin exposure reduced the number of cells in the G0/G1 phase while increasing the number of cells in the S-phase of the cell cycle. These regulatory effects on the cell cycle were also associated with differential regulation of cyclin D1 and the cyclin-dependent kinase inhibitor, p21: there was upregulation of cyclin D1 and downregulation of p21 [75]. Furthermore, in a separate study using the MCF-7 human breast cancer cell line, leptin treatment led to upregulation of the cell cycle genes cyclin D, cyclin G, cyclin-dependent kinase 2, p27, p21, and p16 as well as downregulation of the cell cycle suppressor, transforming growth factor beta [76].

The authors of the study further demonstrated that leptin down-regulates apoptosis-inducing genes and inhibits apoptosis. And they concluded that these tumorigenic effects of leptin in the MCF-7 human breast cancer model are mediated in part via regulation of the cell cycle [76].

The above examples clearly show that leptin is able to dysregulate the cell cycle to promote the development and progression of cancer.

Leptin and Adiponectin Cross-Talk to Regulate Carcinogenesis

As mentioned above, obesity is an established risk factor for many cancers. And it is characterized by hyperleptinemia and hypoadiponectinemia. It is, therefore, possible that either elevated serum leptin levels or reduced serum adiponectin levels may independently contribute to the development of obesity-associated cancers. In the previous sections of this chapter, compelling evidence indicating that leptin directly promotes development and progression of obesity-related cancers has been presented. It should be noted that there is also independent evidence that reduced circulating levels of adiponectin may contribute to the development of obesity-associated cancers [77–80]. Nevertheless, it is most likely that a variety of molecular factors inter-play to regulate the development and progression of cancers. Consequently, it is not surprising that there is increasing experimental evidence that leptin and adiponectin cross-talk to regulate the development and progression of obesity-associated cancers.

For example, using multiple cellular models of esophageal adenocarcinoma (EAC), Ogunwobi and Beales demonstrated that the globular form of adiponectin inhibited leptin-induced proliferation of EAC cells in a manner dependent on the adipoR1 receptor isoform and 5′-AMP-activated protein kinase [81]. In a more recent study of the OE33 esophageal adenocarcinoma model, Beales et al. further reported that the globular form of adiponectin inhibited leptin-induced proliferation, migration, and anti-apoptosis via protein tyrosine phosphatase 1B-mediated downregulation of signal transducer and activator of transcription 3 (STAT3) transcriptional activity [82]. Similar findings have been reported in other cancer types. A recent case–control study of 516 Chinese women specifically evaluated potential correlation between serum leptin and adiponectin levels with the presence of endometrial carcinoma. The study found that patients with endometrial carcinoma had higher serum leptin and lower serum adiponectin concentrations than normal healthy volunteers. After adjusting for cholesterol, triglycerides, fasting insulin, serum glucose, BMI, and age, logistic regression analysis of their data revealed that high serum leptin concentration and low serum adiponectin concentration are both significantly associated with endometrial carcinoma [83]. Data from the study by Jardé and colleagues published in 2009 are also very interesting [84]. They found that leptin mRNA expression in the MCF-7 breast cancer model was 34.7 times higher than adiponectin mRNA expression [84]. Furthermore, they found that adiponectin treatment resulted in loss of expression of leptin and its receptors whereas leptin treatment resulted in loss of expression of the adiponectin receptor, adipoR1 [84]. They also found that adiponectin treatment inhibited the proliferation of the MCF-7 breast cancer cells whereas leptin treatment stimulated their proliferation [84]. In addition, adiponectin inhibited leptin-induced proliferation of the MCF-7 breast cancer cells [84].

Consequently, there is epidemiological as well as experimental evidence suggesting that leptin likely is not the only adipocytokine regulating tumor development and progression. The role of leptin in cancer development and progression is probably dependent in ways not yet fully understood on adiponectin activity.

Potential Clinical Impact of Understanding the Role of Leptin in Carcinogenesis

Understanding the pathophysiological role of leptin in cancer development and progression is undoubtedly important. It is especially important that we understand the molecular signaling mechanisms mediating leptin activity as it relates to cancer. This may reveal novel insights into cancer development and progression in general. More importantly, it is possible that some of these mechanisms may be exploitable for screening, diagnostic, therapeutic, or monitoring purposes.

The good news is that there is already indication that knowledge gained so far from researching the role of leptin in cancer may be useful clinically. For example, a retrospective analysis of leptin and leptin receptor expression in normal lung tissue in comparison to non-small cell lung cancer tissue revealed that leptin expression significantly affected survival time and that leptin expression is an independent prognostic factor in non-small cell lung cancer [85]. Also, a study of 71 consecutive colon cancer patients that examined serum leptin and leptin receptor levels found that serum leptin and leptin receptor levels correlate with advanced tumor stage [86], thus indicating that information regarding serum leptin and tissue leptin receptor expression may be clinically useful in this setting. Data from breast cancer studies also suggest potential clinical usefulness in that setting. Several research groups have reported that leptin and leptin receptor expression may be useful as prognostic factors in breast cancer [87, 88]. Interestingly, there are even data suggesting that leptin levels may predict response or resistance to anti-estrogen therapy during breast cancer treatment [89]. Also, in gastric cancer, there is evidence that leptin expression may be useful clinically as a prognostic factor [90].

Therefore, there is real potential for the use of leptin or its receptor as clinical biomarkers. And our understanding of its pathophysiologic signaling mechanisms in cancer may also lead to clinical applications. Figure 13.1 summarizes the key signaling pathways that may be important in the role of leptin in carcinogenesis. These are also potential molecular targets that can be exploited for clinical applications.

Contrarian Reports

There is, of course, some data (though fewer) that may suggest that leptin does not play a role or that it plays an anti-tumorigenic role in certain cancers. For example, a 2013 report of a case–control study and meta-analysis of the association between leptin and colorectal adenoma or colon cancer mentioned that there was a positive association of serum leptin with colorectal adenoma, but not colorectal cancer [91]. It should be noted, though, that even the authors of the report explicitly mentioned that there was significant heterogeneity between the studies they analyzed and that there may have been multiple effect modifiers [91]. Another 2013 report partly focused on the association between leptin and prostate cancer [92]. The authors used nested case–control methodology and utilized both conditional and unconditional logistic regression for their analyses [92]. And they reported that there was no compelling evidence of an association between leptin and prostate cancer stage [92]. An earlier study that examined breast, esophageal, prostate, and pancreatic cancer cell lines found that the effects of leptin may be cell line specific. They found that whereas leptin had a proliferative effect on the breast, esophageal, and prostate cancer cell lines, it had an anti-proliferative effect on the pancreatic cancer cell lines [93]. More recently, it was reported that leptin exerted significant anti-tumor effects in hepatocellular carcinoma [94]. In athymic nude mice implanted with Hep3B human hepatocellular carcinoma cells, leptin significantly reduced tumor size and improved animal survival [94]. Furthermore, it was reported that leptin exerted anti-proliferative effects on the MDA-MB-231 breast cancer cell line via downregulation of protein kinase A [95].

These reports, although not exhaustive, certainly indicate that in some organs or cell types leptin may not have a pro-carcinogenic role.

Conclusion

There is much more that can be said about the role of leptin in the cell cycle and cancer development and progression. This chapter has, somewhat narrowly, focused on only some of the peer-reviewed scientific evidence that leptin does indeed play a role in cancer development and progression. As discussed in the previous section of this chapter, there is some data that may

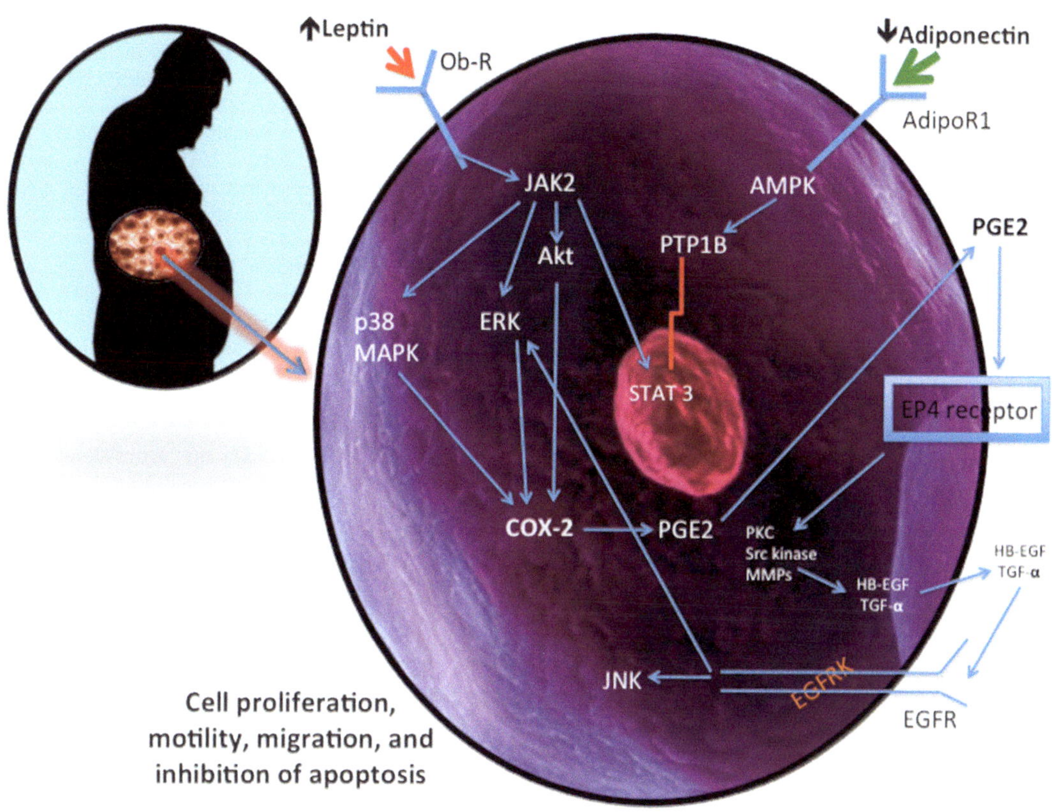

Fig. 13.1 Summary of key signaling pathways that may be important in the role of leptin in carcinogenesis

suggest that leptin does not play a role in certain cancers. Nevertheless, the evidence that leptin is an important player in carcinogenesis is compelling and is very likely to continue to grow.

Acknowledgements Thanks to Pascal DuBois for helping with literature search, preparation of Fig. 13.1, and proofreading of the manuscript. Thanks too to Dr. Ian Beales for his outstanding supervision of Dr. Ogunwobi's initial work on the role of leptin in cancer. Work in Dr. Ogunwobi's laboratory at Hunter College of The City University of New York is currently supported by a NIH RCMI grant to Hunter College, and Pilot Project and Innovation Seed Funding awards from the NIMHD-funded Center for Translational and Basic Research at Hunter College.

References

1. Zhang YY, Proenca R, Maffei M, Barone M, Leopold L, Friedman JM. Positional cloning of the mouse obese gene and its human homolog. Nature. 1994; 372(6505):425–32.
2. Ma YL, Yang YZ, Wang F, Zhang P, Shi CZ, Zou Y, et al. Obesity and risk of colorectal cancer: a systematic review of prospective studies. PLoS One. 2013; 8(1):16.
3. Campbell PT, Jacobs ET, Ulrich CM, Figueiredo JC, Poynter JN, McLaughlin JR, et al. Case-control study of overweight, obesity, and colorectal cancer risk, overall and by tumor microsatellite instability status. J Natl Cancer Inst. 2010;102(6):391–400.
4. Moghaddam AA, Woodward M, Huxley R. Obesity and risk of colorectal cancer: a meta-analysis of 31 studies with 70,000 events. Cancer Epidemiol Biomarkers Prev. 2007;16(12):2533–47.
5. LeMarchand L, Wilkens LR, Kolonel LN, Hankin JH, Lyu LC. Associations of sedentary lifestyle, obesity, smoking, alcohol use, and diabetes with the risk of colorectal cancer. Cancer Res. 1997;57(21):4787–94.
6. Nichols HB, Trentham-Dietz A, Egan KM, Titus-Ernstoff L, Holmes MD, Bersch AJ, et al. Body mass index before and after breast cancer diagnosis: associations with all-cause, breast cancer, and cardiovascular disease mortality. Cancer Epidemiol Biomarkers Prev. 2009;18(5):1403–9.
7. Reeves KW, Carter GC, Rodabough RJ, Lane D, McNeeley SG, Stefanick ML, et al. Obesity in relation to endometrial cancer risk and disease characteristics

in the Women's Health Initiative. Gynecol Oncol. 2011;121(2):376–82.

8. Meredith I, Sarfati D, Ikeda T, Atkinson J, Blakely T. High rates of endometrial cancer among Pacific women in New Zealand: the role of diabetes, physical inactivity, and obesity. Cancer Causes Control. 2012; 23(6):875–85.
9. Duggan C, Onstad L, Hardikar S, Blount PL, Reid BJ, Vaughan TL. Association between markers of obesity and progression from Barrett's esophagus to esophageal adenocarcinoma. Clin Gastroenterol Hepatol. 2013;11(8):934–43.
10. Ryan AM, Duong M, Healy L, Ryan SA, Parekh N, Reynolds JV, et al. Obesity, metabolic syndrome and esophageal adenocarcinoma: epidemiology, etiology and new targets. Cancer Epidemiol. 2011;35(4): 309–19.
11. Lofdahl HE, Lane A, Lu YX, Lagergren P, Harvey RF, Blazeby JM, et al. Increased population prevalence of reflux and obesity in the United Kingdom compared with Sweden: a potential explanation for the difference in incidence of esophageal adenocarcinoma. Eur J Gastroenterol Hepatol. 2011;23(2):128–32.
12. Veugelers PJ, Porter GA, Guernsey DL, Casson AG. Obesity and lifestyle risk factors for gastroesophageal reflux disease, Barrett esophagus and esophageal adenocarcinoma. Dis Esophagus. 2006;19(5):321–8.
13. Ildaphonse G, George PS, Mathew A. Obesity and kidney cancer risk in men - a meta-analysis (1992-2008). Asian Pac J Cancer Prev. 2009;10(2):279–86.
14. Mathew A, George PS, Ildaphonse G. Obesity and kidney cancer risk in women - a meta-analysis (1992-2008). Asian Pac J Cancer Prev. 2009;10(3):471–8.
15. Pan SY, DesMeules M, Morrison H, Wen SW, Canadian Canc Registries E. Obesity, high energy intake, lack of physical activity, and the risk of kidney cancer. Cancer Epidemiol Biomarkers Prev. 2006; 15(12):2453–60.
16. Chow WH, Gridley G, Fraumeni JF, Jarvholm B. Obesity, hypertension, and the risk of kidney cancer in men. N Engl J Med. 2000;343(18):1305–11.
17. McCredie M, Stewart JH. Risk-factors for kidney cancer in New South Wales, Australia. 2. Urologic disease, hypertension, obesity, and hormonal factors. Cancer Causes Control. 1992;3(4):323–31.
18. Castillo JJ, Reagan JL, Ingham RR, Furman M, Dalia S, Merhi B, et al. Obesity but not overweight increases the incidence and mortality of leukemia in adults: a meta-analysis of prospective cohort studies. Leuk Res. 2012;36(7):868–75.
19. Brandon EL, Gu J-W, Cantwell L, He Z, Wallace G, Hall JE. Obesity promotes melanoma tumor growth Role of leptin. Cancer Biol Ther. 2009;8(19):1871–9.
20. Dennis LK, Lowe JB, Lynch CF, Alavanja MCR. Cutaneous melanoma and obesity in the Agricultural Health Study. Ann Epidemiol. 2008; 18(3):214–21.
21. Jung J, Her S, Park J. High-fat diet-induced obesity increases solid tumor growth and metastasis of melanoma cells in C57BL/6 mice. Mol Biol Cell. 2011;22.
22. Pandey V, Vijayakumar MV, Ajay AK, Malvi P, Bhat MK. Diet-induced obesity increases melanoma progression: involvement of Cav-1 and FASN. Int J Cancer. 2012;130(3):497–508.
23. Sergentanis TN, Antoniadis AG, Gogas HJ, Antonopoulos CN, Adami H-O, Ekbom A, et al. Obesity and risk of malignant melanoma: a meta-analysis of cohort and case-control studies. Eur J Cancer. 2013;49(3):642–57.
24. Friedman GD, Herrinton LJ. Obesity and multiple myeloma. Cancer Causes Control. 1994;5(5):479–83.
25. Chu D-M, Wahlqvist ML, Lee M-S, Chang H-Y. Central obesity predicts non-Hodgkin's lymphoma mortality and overall obesity predicts leukemia mortality in adult Taiwanese. J Am Coll Nutr. 2011;30(5):310–9.
26. Larsson SC, Wolk A. Obesity and risk of non-Hodgkin's lymphoma: a meta-analysis. Int J Cancer. 2007;121(7):1564–70.
27. Maskarinec G, Erber E, Gill J, Cozen W, Kolonel LN. Overweight and obesity at different times in life as risk factors for non-Hodgkin's lymphoma: the multiethnic cohort. Cancer Epidemiol Biomarkers Prev. 2008;17(1):196–203.
28. Pan SY, Mao Y, Ugnat AM, Canadian Canc R. Physical activity, obesity, energy intake, and the risk of non-Hodgkin's lymphoma: a population-based case-control study. Am J Epidemiol. 2005;162(12):1162–73.
29. Bracci PM. Obesity and pancreatic cancer: overview of epidemiologic evidence and biologic mechanisms. Mol Carcinog. 2012;51(1):53–63.
30. Gong Z, Holly EA, Bracci PM. Obesity and survival in population-based patients with pancreatic cancer in the San Francisco Bay Area. Cancer Causes Control. 2012;23(12):1929–37.
31. Gukovsky I, Li N, Todoric J, Gukovskaya A, Karin M. Inflammation, autophagy, and obesity: common features in the pathogenesis of pancreatitis and pancreatic cancer. Gastroenterology. 2013;144(6):1199.
32. White PB, Ziegler KM, Swartz-Basile DA, Wang SS, Lillemoe KD, Pitt HA, et al. Obesity, but not high-fat diet, promotes murine pancreatic cancer growth. J Gastrointest Surg. 2012;16(9):1680–5.
33. Golabek T, Bukowczan J, Chlosta P, Powroznik J, Dobruch J, Borowka A. Obesity and prostate cancer incidence and mortality: a systematic review of prospective cohort studies. Urol Int. 2014;92(1):7–14.
34. De Nunzio C, Albisinni S, Freedland SJ, Miano L, Cindolo L, Agro EF, et al. Abdominal obesity as risk factor for prostate cancer diagnosis and high grade disease: a prospective multicenter Italian cohort study. Urol Oncol Semi Orig Investig. 2013;31(7):997–1002.
35. Mao Y, Pan SY, Wen SW, Johnson KC. Candian Canc Epidemiology Res G. Physical inactivity, energy intake, obesity and the risk of rectal cancer in Canada. Int J Cancer. 2003;105(6):831–7.
36. Larsson SC, Wolk A. Obesity and colon and rectal cancer risk: a meta-analysis of prospective studies. Am J Clin Nutr. 2007;86(3):556–65.

37. Han JM, Kim TY, Jeon MJ, Yim JH, Kim WG, Song DE, et al. Obesity is a risk factor for thyroid cancer in a large, ultrasonographically screened population. Eur J Endocrinol. 2013;168(6):879–86.
38. Kim WG, Park JW, Willingham MC, Cheng S-y. Diet-induced obesity increases tumor growth and promotes anaplastic change in thyroid cancer in a mouse model. Endocrinology. 2013;154(8):2936–47.
39. Marcello MA, Sampaio AC, Geloneze B, Vasques ACJ, Assumpcao LVM, Ward LS. Obesity and excess protein and carbohydrate consumption are risk factors for thyroid cancer. Nutr Cancer. 2012;64(8):1190–5.
40. Zhao ZG, Guo XG, Ba CX, Wang W, Yang YY, Wang J, et al. Overweight, obesity and thyroid cancer risk: a meta-analysis of cohort studies. J Int Med Res. 2012;40(6):2041–50.
41. Khandekar MJ, Cohen P, Spiegelman BM. Molecular mechanisms of cancer development in obesity. Nat Rev Cancer. 2011;11(12):886–95.
42. Garcia JM, Splenser AE, Kramer J, Alsarraj A, Fitzgerald S, Ramsey D, et al. Circulating inflammatory cytokines and adipokines are associated with increased risk of Barrett's esophagus: a case-control study. Clin Gastroenterol Hepatol. 2014;12(2):229.
43. Ntikoudi E, Kiagia M, Boura P, Syrigos KN. Hormones of adipose tissue and their biologic role in lung cancer. Cancer Treat Rev. 2014;40(1):22–30.
44. Wurm S, Neumeier M, Weigert J, Schaeffler A, Buechler C. Plasma levels of leptin, omentin, collagenous repeat-containing sequence of 26-kDa protein (CORS-26) and adiponectin before and after oral glucose uptake in slim adults. Cardiovasc Diabetol. 2007;6:7.
45. Dubecz A, Solymosi N, Stadlhuber RJ, Schweigert M, Stein HJ, Peters JH. Does the incidence of adenocarcinoma of the esophagus and gastric cardia continue to rise in the twenty-first century?-a SEER database analysis. J Gastrointest Surg. 2014;18(1):124–9.
46. Lagergren J, Bergstrom R, Nyren O. Association between body mass and adenocarcinoma of the esophagus and gastric cardia. Ann Intern Med. 1999; 130(11):883.
47. Chow WH, Blot WJ, Vaughn TL, Risch HA, Gammon MD, Stanford JL, et al. Body mass index and risk of adenocarcinomas of the esophagus and gastric cardia. J Natl Cancer Inst. 1998;90(2):150–5.
48. Merry AHH, Schouten LJ, Goldbohm RA, van den Brandt PA. Body mass index, height and risk of adenocarcinoma of the oesophagus and gastric cardia: a prospective cohort study. Gut. 2007;56(11):1503–11.
49. Lagergren J, Bergstrom R, Lindgren A, Nyren O. Symptomatic gastroesophageal reflux as a risk factor for esophageal adenocarcinoma. N Engl J Med. 1999;340(11):825–31.
50. Lagergren J. Adenocarcinoma of oesophagus: what exactly is the size of the problem and who is at risk? Gut. 2005;54:I1–5.
51. Considine RV, Sinha MK, Heiman ML, Kriauciunas A, Stephens TW, Nyce MR, et al. Serum immunoreactive leptin concentrations in normal-weight and obese humans. N Engl J Med. 1996;334(5):292–5.
52. Heinonen MV, Purhonen AK, Miettinen P, Paakkonen M, Pirinen E, Alhava E, et al. Apelin, orexin-A and leptin plasma levels in morbid obesity and effect of gastric banding. Regul Pept. 2005;130(1–2):7–13.
53. Baratta M. Leptin–from a signal of adiposity to a hormonal mediator in peripheral tissues. Med Sci Monit. 2002;8(12):RA282–92.
54. Maffei M, Halaas J, Ravussin E, Pratley RE, Lee GH, Zhang Y, et al. Leptin levels in human and rodent - measurement of plasma leptin and ob RNA in obese and weight-reduced subjects. Nat Med. 1995;1(11): 1155–61.
55. Somasundar P, Riggs D, Jackson B, Vona-Davis L, McFadden DW. Leptin stimulates esophageal adenocarcinoma growth by nonapoptotic mechanisms. Am J Surg. 2003;186(5):575–8.
56. Ogunwobi O, Mutungi G, Beales I. Leptin stimulates proliferation and inhibits apoptosis in Barrett's esophageal adenocarcinoma cells by cyclooxygenase-2-dependent, prostaglandin-E2-mediated transactivation of the epidermal growth factor receptor and c-Jun NH2-terminal kinase activation. Endocrinology. 2006;147(9):4505–16.
57. Abdalla SI, Sanderson IR, Fitzgerald RC. Effect of inflammation on cyclooxygenase (COX)-2 expression in benign and malignant oesophageal cells. Carcinogenesis. 2005;26(9):1627–33.
58. Moons LMG, Kuipers EJ, Rygiel AM, Groothuismink AZM, Geldof H, Bode WA, et al. COX-2 CA-haplotype is a risk factor for the development of esophageal adenocarcinoma. Am J Gastroenterol. 2007;102(11):2373–9.
59. Tuynman JB, Buskens CJ, Kemper K, ten Kate FJW, Offerhaus GJA, Richel DJ, et al. Neoadjuvant selective COX-2 inhibition down-regulates important oncogenic pathways in patients with esophageal adenocarcinoma. Ann Surg. 2005;242(6):840–50.
60. Dal Farra C, Zsurger N, Vincent JP, Cupo A. Binding of a pure I-125-monoiodoleptin analog to mouse tissues: a developmental study. Peptides. 2000;21(4):577–87.
61. Francois F, Roper J, Goodman AJ, Pei Z, Ghumman M, Mourad M, et al. The association of gastric leptin with oesophageal inflammation and metaplasia. Gut. 2008;57(1):16–24.
62. Ahmed S, Khan AL, Pazmany L, Bogder K. Epithelial cells over-express the leptin receptor during malignant progression in Barrett's oesophagus. Gastroenterology. 2006;130(4):A564.
63. Beales ILP, Ogunwobi OO. Lept in synergistically enhances the anti-apoptotic and growth-promoting effects of acid in OE33 oesophageal adenocarcinoma cells in culture. Mol Cell Endocrinol. 2007;274(1–2): 60–8.
64. Hardwick JCH, Van den Brink GR, Offerhaus GJ, Van Deventer SJH, Peppelenbosch MP. Leptin is a growth factor for colonic epithelial cells. Gastroenterology. 2001;121(1):79–90.

65. Koda M, Sulkowska M, Kanczuga-Koda L, Surmacz E, Sulkowski S. Overexpression of the obesity hormone leptin in human colorectal cancer. J Clin Pathol. 2007;60(8):902–6.
66. Jaffe T, Schwartz B. Leptin promotes motility and invasiveness in human colon cancer cells by activating multiple signal-transduction pathways. Int J Cancer. 2008;123(11):2543–56.
67. Ogunwobi O, Beales I. Cyclo-oxygenase-independent inhibition of apoptosis and stimulation of proliferation by leptin in human colon cancer cells. Dig Dis Sci. 2007;52(8):1934–45.
68. Ogunwobi OO, Beales ILP. The anti-apoptotic and growth stimulatory actions of leptin in human colon cancer cells involves activation of JNK mitogen activated protein kinase, JAK2 and PI3 kinase/Akt. Int J Colorectal Dis. 2007;22(4):401–9.
69. Rouet- Benzineb P, Aparicio T, Guilmeau S, Pouzet C, Descatoire V, Buyse M, et al. Leptin counteracts sodium butyrate-induced apoptosis in human colon cancer HT-29 cells via NF-kappaB signaling. J Biol Chem. 2004;279(16):16495–502.
70. Stattin P, Palmqvist R, Soderberg S, Biessy C, Ardnor B, Hallmans G, et al. Plasma leptin and colorectal cancer risk: a prospective study in Northern Sweden. Oncol Rep. 2003;10(6):2015–21.
71. Tamakoshi K, Toyoshima H, Wakai K, Kojima M, Suzuki K, Watanabe Y, et al. Leptin is associated with an increased female colorectal cancer risk: a nested case-control study in Japan. Oncology. 2005;68(4–6): 454–61.
72. Stattin P, Lukanova A, Biessy C, Soderberg S, Palmqvist R, Kaaks R, et al. Obesity and colon cancer: does leptin provide a link? Int J Cancer. 2004; 109(1):149–52.
73. Williams GH, Stoeber K. The cell cycle and cancer. J Pathol. 2012;226(2):352–64.
74. Ptak A, Kolaczkowska E, Gregoraszczuk EL. Leptin stimulation of cell cycle and inhibition of apoptosis gene and protein expression in OVCAR-3 ovarian cancer cells. Endocrine. 2013;43(2):394–403.
75. Catalano S, Giordano C, Rizza P, Gu G, Barone I, Bonofiglio D, et al. Evidence that leptin through STAT and CREB signaling enhances cyclin D1 expression and promotes human endometrial cancer proliferation. J Cell Physiol. 2009;218(3):490–500.
76. Perera CN, Chin HG, Duru N, Camarillo IG. Leptin-regulated gene expression in MCF-7 breast cancer cells: mechanistic insights into leptin-regulated mammary tumor growth and progression. J Endocrinol. 2008;199(2):221–33.
77. Aleksandrova K, Boeing H, Jenab M, Bueno-de-Mesquita HB, Jansen E, van Duijnhoven FJB, et al. Total and high-molecular weight adiponectin and risk of colorectal cancer: the European Prospective Investigation into Cancer and Nutrition Study. Carcinogenesis. 2012;33(6):1211–8.
78. Pinthus J, Hopmans S, Paschos A, Austin R, Duivenvoorden W. ERP46 mediates prostate cancer tumorigenesis *in vitro* by inhibiting adiponectin-induced tumor-suppressive effects - linking obesity to prostate cancer. J Urol. 2013;189(4):E128.
79. Chung SJ, Saxena N, Sharma D. Adiponectin induces autophagic cell death in breast cancer cells through SIRT1 mediated deacetylation of LKB1 leading to ATG1 activation. Cancer Res. 2013;73(8, Suppl 1): 1673.
80. Erdogan S, Sezer S, Baser E, Eryilmaz OG, Gungor T, Uysal S, et al. Low serum adiponectin and vaspin levels as novel risk factors for postmenopausal endometrial cancer. Int J Gynecol Cancer. 2013;23(8).
81. Ogunwobi OO, Beales ILP. Globular adiponectin, acting via adiponectin receptor-1, inhibits leptin-stimulated oesophageal adenocarcinoma cell proliferation. Mol Cell Endocrinol. 2008;285(1–2):43–50.
82. Beales ILP, Garcia-Morales C, Ogunwobi OO, Mutungi G. Adiponectin inhibits leptin-induced oncogenic signalling in oesophageal cancer cells by activation of PTP1B. Mol Cell Endocrinol. 2014; 382(1):150–8.
83. Ma Y, Liu Z, Zhang Y, Lu B. Serum leptin, adiponectin and endometrial cancer risk in Chinese women. J Gynecol Oncol. 2013;24(4):336–41.
84. Jarde T, Caldefie-Chezet F, Goncalves-Mendes N, Mishellany F, Buechler C, Penault-Llorca F, et al. Involvement of adiponectin and leptin in breast cancer: clinical and in vitro studies. Endocr Relat Cancer. 2009;16(4):1197–210.
85. Xu Y-J, Shao Y-F, Zhao X, Geng Y-T, Wang K, Yin Y-M. Expression and clinical significance of leptin, the functional receptor of leptin (OB-Rb) and HER-2 in non-small-cell lung cancer: a retrospective analysis. J Cancer Res Clin Oncol. 2011;137(12):1841–8.
86. Tutino V, Notarnicola M, Guerra V, Lorusso D, Caruso MG. Increased soluble leptin receptor levels are associated with advanced tumor stage in colorectal cancer patients. Anticancer Res. 2011;31(10):3381–3.
87. Miyoshi Y, Funahashi T, Tanaka S, Taguchi T, Tamaki Y, Shimomura I, et al. High expression of leptin receptor mRNA in breast cancer tissue predicts poor prognosis for patients with high, but not low, serum leptin levels. Int J Cancer. 2006;118(6):1414–9.
88. Ishikawa M, Kitayama J, Nagawa H. Enhanced expression of leptin and leptin receptor (OB-R) in human breast cancer. Clin Cancer Res. 2004;10(13):4325–31.
89. Maccio A, Madeddu C, Gramignano G, Mulas C, Floris C, Massa D, et al. Correlation of body mass index and leptin with tumor size and stage of disease in hormone-dependent postmenopausal breast cancer: preliminary results and therapeutic implications. J Mol Med. 2010;88(7):677–86.
90. Zhao X, Huang K, Zhu Z, Chen S, Hu R. Correlation between expression of leptin and clinicopathological features and prognosis in patients with gastric cancer. J Gastroenterol Hepatol. 2007;22(8):1317–21.
91. Gialamas SP, Sergentanis TN, Antonopoulos CN, Dessypris N, Chrousos GP, Petridou ET. Circulating leptin levels and risk of colorectal cancer and adenoma:

a case-control study and meta-analysis. Cancer Causes Control. 2013;24(12):2129–41.

92. Burton A, Martin RM, Holly J, Lane JA, Donovan JL, Hamdy FC, et al. Associations of adiponectin and leptin with stage and grade of PSA-detected prostate cancer: the ProtecT study. Cancer Causes Control. 2013;24(2):323–34.
93. Somasundar P, Yu AK, Vona-Davis L, McFadden DW. Differential effects of leptin on cancer *in vitro*. J Surg Res. 2003;113(1):50–5.
94. Elinav E, Abd-Elnabi A, Pappo O, Bernstein I, Klein A, Engelhardt D, Rabbani E, Ilan Y. Suppression of hepatocellular carcinoma growth in mice via leptin, is associated with inhibition of tumor cell growth and natural killer cell activation. J Hepatol. 2006;44(3):529–36.
95. Naviglio S, Di Gesto D, Illiano F, Chiosi E, Giordano A, Illiano G, Spina A. Leptin potentiates antiproliferative action of cAMP elevation via protein kinase A down-regulation in breast cancer cells. J Cell Physiol. 2010;225(3):801–9.

Leptin, the Autonomic Nervous System, and Hypertension

14

Alexandre A. da Silva, Jussara M. do Carmo, Zhen Wang, and John E. Hall

Introduction

The worldwide prevalence of obesity and its associated cardiometabolic diseases has increased dramatically in the past 2–3 decades, rapidly becoming a major health care challenge in the United States as well as in most industrialized and developing countries. Current estimates indicate that more than one *billion* people in the world are overweight or obese [1]. In the United States, at least 65 % of adults are overweight and approximately one-third of adults are obese with a body mass index (BMI), defined as kg weight/m^2 height, greater than 30 [2].

Epidemiological studies show that obesity affects 17 % of children and adolescents in the United States, a number that has tripled from one generation ago, indicating that the prevalence of childhood obesity has also risen rapidly, in parallel with increasing obesity in adults. A recent report indicates that 18.4 % of 4-year-old children in the United States are obese, with significantly higher rates in Hispanic, Black, and Native American children [3].

These numbers are alarming since excess weight gain enhances the risk for developing many chronic diseases including diabetes, cancer, kidney disease, hypertension, and cardiovascular diseases (CVD). In this chapter we discuss the role of leptin as a major link between obesity, sympathetic nervous system (SNS) activity and hypertension.

Role of SNS Activity and Renal Nerves in Obesity-Hypertension

Although the multiple mechanisms by which obesity elevates BP are still not fully understood, all forms of hypertension studied thus far, including obesity-induced hypertension, are accompanied by impaired renal pressure natriuresis [4–6]. In obesity-hypertension, impaired pressure natriuresis is due mainly to increased renal sodium reabsorption caused by at least three major mechanisms (Fig. 14.1): (1) physical compression of the kidneys by surrounding visceral and retroperitoneal fat as well as renal sinus fat, (2) mild activation of the renin-angiotensin-aldosterone system (RAAS), and (3) mild SNS overactivity [5, 7, 8]. In this chapter we focus on the role of leptin in promoting increased SNS activity and contributing to elevated BP in obesity.

Clinical and experimental studies have demonstrated that excess weight gain, especially when

A.A. da Silva, Ph.D. (✉)
Department of Physiology and Biophysics, University of Mississippi Medical Center, Jackson, MS, USA
e-mail: asilva@umc.edu

J.M. do Carmo, Ph.D. • Z. Wang, Ph.D.
J.E. Hall, Ph.D.
Department of Physiology and Biophysics, Mississippi Center for Obesity Research, Cardiovascular-Renal Research Center, University of Mississippi Medical Center, 2500 North State St, Jackson, MS 39216, USA

S. Dagogo-Jack (ed.), *Leptin: Regulation and Clinical Applications*,
DOI 10.1007/978-3-319-09915-6_14,

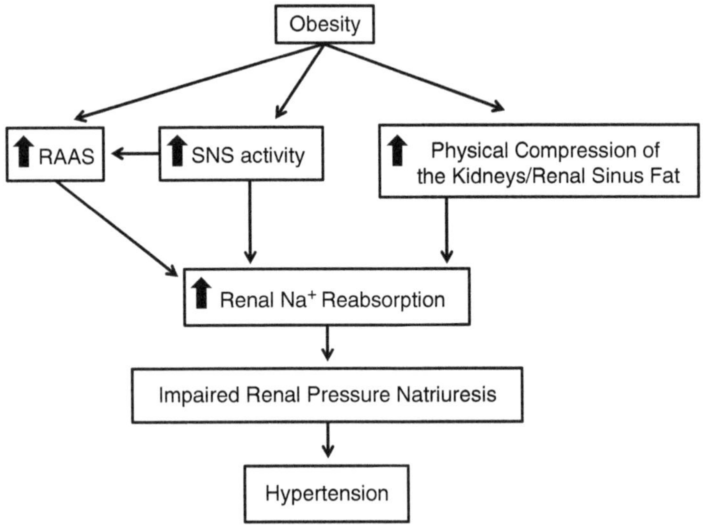

Fig. 14.1 Schematic representation of potential mechanisms linking obesity with hypertension. Na^+ = sodium; RAAS = renin-angiotensin-aldosterone system; SNS = sympathetic nervous system

excess visceral adiposity is present, is accompanied by increased SNS activation to several organs and tissues [8, 9]. The rise in SNS activity can occur as early as 1 week after exposure to high fat diets in experimental animals and even with modest weight gain in nonobese subjects [8, 10, 11]. There is evidence that excess weight gain is associated with selective, mild increases in SNS to a few organs and tissues, including the kidneys and skeletal muscle, rather than widespread SNS activation [8, 12]. For example, cardiac SNS activity is normal or reduced in obese compared to lean subjects and increased heart rate is due mainly to decreased parasympathetic activity rather than increased SNS activity [13]. Also, the rise in SNS activity to key organs such as the kidneys is modest and insufficient to cause vasoconstriction, albeit enough to promote sodium retention and to activate the RAAS [5, 7].

Evidence for an important role of increased renal SNS activity in obesity-hypertension derives from studies showing that chronic pharmacological blockade of adrenergic receptors elicits greater reductions in BP in obese versus lean hypertensive subjects [14] and that bilateral renal denervation markedly attenuates sodium retention and elevated BP in obese dogs fed a high fat diet [15]. Also, renal denervation substantially reduces BP in patients with resistant hypertension who, in most cases, are overweight or obese [16].

The degree of SNS activation in obesity appears to vary according to body fat distribution with visceral obesity being associated with greater increases in SNS activity compared to the effects of subcutaneous obesity [8, 9]. Unfortunately, due to technical challenges, in most human studies only muscle SNS activity has been evaluated rather than renal SNS activity which mediates most of the SNS effects to increase BP in obesity [8, 9, 12]. However, renal norepinephrine spillover, an index of renal sympathetic activity, is increased in obese subjects with increased visceral adiposity [13, 17].

Role of Leptin in Obesity-Induced SNS Activation and Hypertension

Several factors have been suggested to contribute to increased SNS activity in obesity including impaired baroreflex sensitivity, angiotensin II, hyperinsulinemia, chemoreceptor-mediated reflexes associated with sleep apnea, hypoghrelinemia, and hypoadiponectemia, to name a few [7, 14, 18, 19]. However, considerable evidence suggests that hyperleptinemia may be a critical factor linking excess weight gain with increased SNS activity and hypertension.

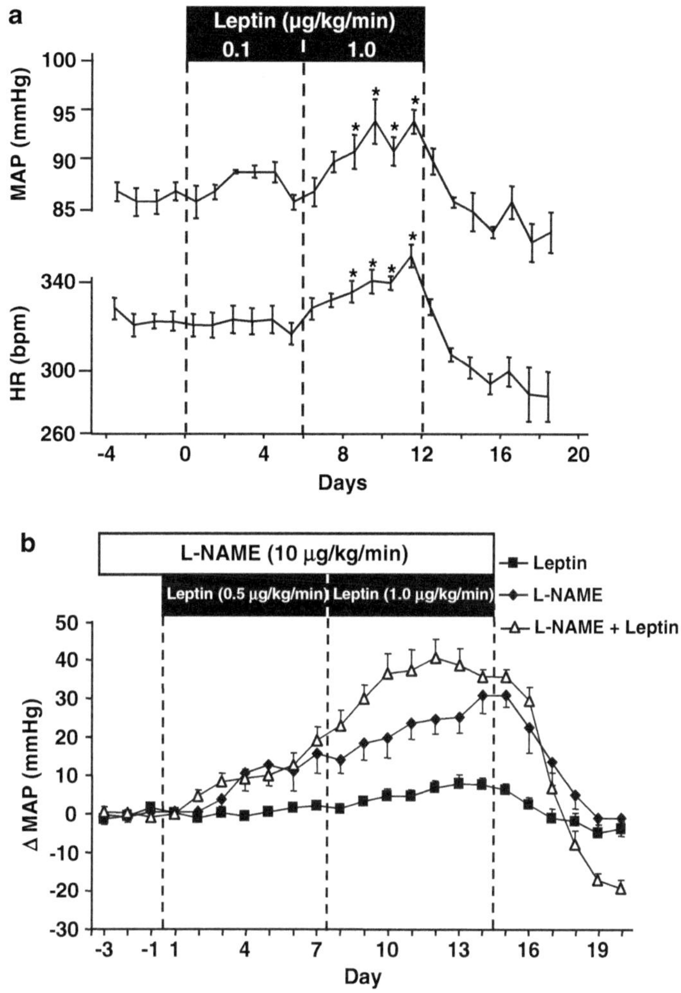

Fig. 14.2 Compilation of data demonstrating the pressor effects of chronic leptin infusion at doses that raise plasma leptin levels to those found in severe obesity (**a**) and the exacerbation of these effects in the presence of the nitric oxide synthase inhibitor L-NAME (**b**). HR = heart rate; L-NAME = L-NG-nitroarginine methyl ester; MAP = mean arterial pressure. * indicates $p < 0.05$ versus baseline values (Modified from [25] and [36])

Acute and Chronic Effects of Leptin on SNS Activity and BP

Shortly after its discovery in 1994, investigators noticed a positive relationship between circulating leptin levels and muscle SNS activity [20]. Haynes et al. [21] and Dunbar et al. [22] also demonstrated that acute intravenous or intracerebroventricular (ICV) administration of leptin in lean rats increased SNS to brown adipose tissue, kidneys, and adrenal gland, suggesting a possible role for leptin in controlling sympathetic activity and thermogenesis. Recent studies in humans confirmed that acute hyperleptinemia increases muscle SNS activity, as assessed by microneurography [23]. Despite increasing SNS activity, acute injections of leptin have little effect on BP perhaps due, in part, to counterbalancing vasodilator effects of nitric oxide (NO) which is also stimulated by leptin [18, 24]. Also, leptin-mediated increases in SNS activity are mild and do not appear to be sufficient to directly cause peripheral vasoconstriction or acute increases in BP.

In 1998 we first demonstrated that chronic infusions of leptin to produce increases in circulating leptin levels comparable to those found in severe obesity-evoked sustained increases in BP [25] (Fig. 14.2a). In 2000, Aizawa-Abe et al. [26] found that transgenic mice with ectopic liver overexpression of leptin also exhibited increased BP. Leptin-mediated increases in BP are gradual and occur over several days, indicating a slow-acting mechanism consistent with the modest increases in renal SNS activity and increased renal tubular sodium reabsorption [25]. Although the chronic hypertensive effects of leptin in lean animals are modest, they are more impressive if one considers the accompanying marked decreases in food intake and weight loss which would normally tend to lower SNS activity and BP.

To test the role of increased SNS activity in mediating the rise in BP with chronic hyperleptinemia, we blocked α and β adrenergic receptors and showed that adrenergic blockade completely abolished leptin's ability to raise BP over several days [27]. Chronic adrenergic receptor antagonism also reversed the increased BP observed in transgenic mice overexpressing leptin [26].

Some studies, however, have reported no changes in BP during chronic leptin administration in humans. For example, Zelissen et al. [28] reported that recombinant leptin administration subcutaneously for 12 weeks at three different doses did not raise BP in 284 overweight or obese subjects during a randomized, double-blind, placebo-controlled multicenter study. However, these investigators also reported no significant changes in body weight compared to placebo treated subjects. Brooke et al. [29] also reported that acute leptin administration in lean human subjects did not raise BP a finding that is not surprising in view of previous studies showing that leptin's effects on BP are slow to develop and often require several days to manifest [25].

The importance of endogenous leptin in contributing to increased BP is supported by the studies of Lim and colleagues who showed that increases in BP and renal SNS activity in obese rabbits fed a high fat diet were attenuated by acute (90 min) ICV administration of a specific leptin receptor antagonist [30]. Although acute administration of the leptin antagonist did not restore BP to normal in obese rabbits, this is perhaps not surprising since the chronic hypertensive effects of leptin are slow to develop and would likely require several days of blockade to fully reverse its chronic BP effects. Thus, blockade of the actions of endogenous leptin lowers BP in obese animals, further supporting the concept that leptin, at physiological concentrations, can cause chronic increases in BP, at least in experimental animals. It should be noted, however, that currently there are no studies showing that chronic leptin administration raises BP in humans, although acute studies indicate important effects to stimulate SNS activity.

Sympathetic Activity and BP in Obese, Leptin-Deficient Subjects

Mice with leptin deficiency (ob/ob mice) are extremely obese and have many metabolic abnormalities, including insulin resistance, hyperinsulinemia, and dyslipidemia which have been suggested to raise BP. However, mice with leptin deficiency are not hypertensive and tend to have lower BP and reduced SNS activity compared to lean control mice [31, 32]. Moreover, leptin infusion in ob/ob mice increased BP despite reducing body weight [26].

Humans with leptin deficiency also exhibit early-onset morbid obesity and many characteristics of the metabolic syndrome [33, 34]. Although BP and SNS activity have been assessed in only a few human subjects with leptin deficiency, these individuals generally are not hypertensive and do not have evidence of increased SNS activity [34]. In fact, humans with leptin gene mutation show postural hypotension and attenuated RAAS responses to upright posture [34].

Collectively, these clinical and experimental observations support a role for leptin as a link between obesity, increased SNS activity and elevated BP although data on the chronic BP effects of leptin in humans are still limited.

Role of Changes in Body Weight and Endothelial Function in Modulating Chronic BP Effects of Leptin

A difficulty in evaluating the chronic effects of leptin on BP regulation is that leptin also has effects that tend to counterbalance its actions to increase SNS activity. As discussed previously, leptin decreases appetite and increases energy expenditure which both tend to reduce adiposity and cause rapid weight loss, at least in lean subjects who are sensitive to the metabolic effects of leptin. These effects would normally tend to reduce BP. The fact that chronic administration leptin often increases renal SNS activity and BP, despite marked weight loss and decreased adiposity, suggests that leptin may have even more potent effects on BP in the setting of obesity where there is resistance to the metabolic effects of leptin and preservation of the effects on renal SNS activity [35].

A second effect of leptin that partially counterbalances the effects of SNS activation on BP is stimulation of endothelial-derived nitric oxide (NO) formation, at least in subjects with normal endothelial function. Fruhbeck et al. [24] showed, for example, that acute infusion of leptin increased serum NO concentrations and that after inhibition of NO synthesis leptin significantly raised BP. After SNS blockade, however, acute leptin infusion reduced BP [24]. We demonstrated that blockade of NO synthesis greatly exacerbated the chronic effects of leptin to raise BP (Fig. 14.2b) and heart rate [36].

Thus, a major reason for modest effects of leptin to raise BP in lean subjects with normal endothelial function is the offsetting BP lowering effects of increased NO formation. To the extent that obesity causes endothelial dysfunction and impaired NO formation, one might expect greater leptin-mediated increases in BP than in lean subjects, especially if obesity does not induce resistance to the SNS responses to leptin. Moreover, if obesity is associated with resistance to the anorexic effects of leptin with preserved effects on SNS activity, as has been previous suggested [35], this would also amplify the hypertensive effects of leptin since the effects of leptin to cause weight loss and associated decreases in BP would be attenuated.

CNS Sites of Leptin Action on SNS Activity and BP Regulation

Deletion of the long-form of the leptin receptor (LR) in the entire brain recapitulates most of the known metabolic phenotypes of leptin-deficient mice, including obesity, hyperphagia, decreased thermogenesis, and impaired glucose homeostasis, indicating that the CNS actions of leptin play a dominant role in mediating its metabolic actions [37]. As mentioned above, ICV administration of leptin at doses that do not raise circulating leptin levels also evokes increases in SNS activity in metabolic and cardiovascular relevant organs and tissues that can be blocked by ICV infusion of LR antagonists [22, 30], indicating that most, if not all, of the effects of leptin on SNS activity are mediated by leptin's action in the CNS.

High levels of leptin receptor mRNA and protein are expressed in the forebrain, especially in the ventromedial hypothalamus, arcuate nucleus (ARC), and dorsomedial areas of the hypothalamus, as well as in vasomotor centers of the brainstem and intermediolateral medulla (IML) [35, 38]. Although the brain centers that mediate leptin's action on SNS activity and cardiovascular function have not been precisely mapped, hypothalamic centers as well as certain extra-hypothalamic regions (e.g. brainstem, subfornical organ (SFO)) appear to be important in mediating the effects of leptin on SNS activity and BP [35]. For example, acute microinjections of leptin into the ARC increase SNS activity to the kidneys and to brown adipose tissue (BAT) [39]. Also ARC lesions prevent leptin's ability to increase BAT SNS activity when infused intravenously [35], and site specific ARC deletion of LR markedly attenuates the rise in renal and BAT SNS activity evoked by leptin [40]. This is consistent with previous studies showing that neurons of the ARC send projections to sympathetic preganglionic neurons in the IML [41, 42] and suggest that the ARC is an important site for leptin-mediated modulation of SNS activity to several tissues. In fact, deletion of LR only in proopiomelanocortin (POMC) neurons which comprise an important portion of the neuronal types within the ARC prevents the rise in BP evoked by chronic hyperleptinemia [43].

Other nuclei in the hypothalamus have also been implicated in the effects of leptin on SNS activity. The ventromedial and dorsomedial hypothalamus, for example, appear to contribute to leptin-mediated increases in SNS activity

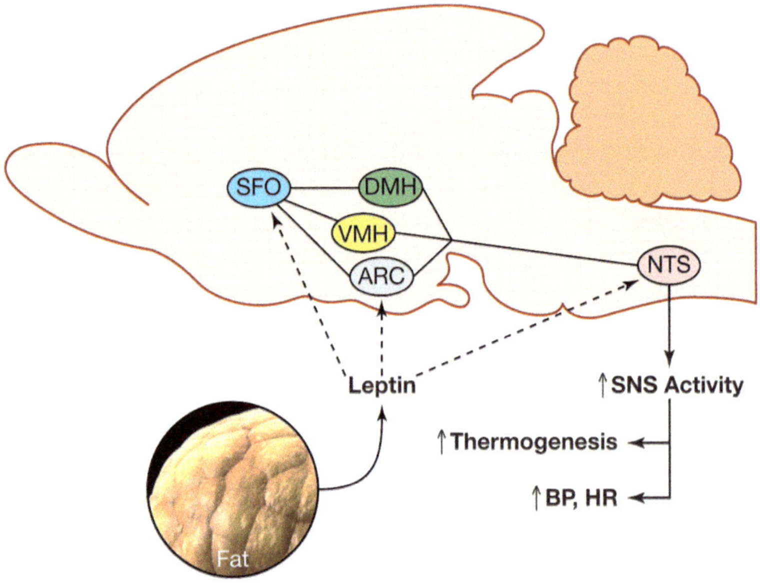

Fig. 14.3 Schematic representation of the potential brain regions that mediate the effects of leptin on sympathetic nervous system (SNS) activity. ARC = arcuate nucleus of the hypothalamus; DMH = dorsomedial hypothalamic nucleus; NTS = nucleus of the tractus solitarius; SFO = subfornical organ; VMH = ventromedial hypothalamic nucleus

to the kidneys, skeletal muscle, and BAT [35]. These nuclei seem to be particularly important in modulation of BAT thermogenesis and peripheral vasoconstriction as acute injections of leptin into the dorsomedial hypothalamus increase HR and BP but do not alter renal SNS activity, a key sympathetic target for long-term BP regulation.

Extra-hypothalamic regions may also play an important role in mediating leptin's effect on SNS activity. Microinjection of leptin into the nucleus of the tractus solitarius (NTS) of the brainstem, especially in the caudal portion of the NTS, increases renal SNS activity and acutely raised BP while SNS activity to BAT remained unchanged [44]. Conversely, leptin microinjection into the SFO, located in the forebrain, caused rapid acute decreases in BP in lean rats, an effect that was absent in diet-induced obese rats [45]. Young and colleagues [46], however, showed that mice with specific deletion of LR in SFO neurons had normal BAT SNS activity responses to systemic or ICV administration of leptin but did not exhibit the expected increase in renal SNS activity. Taken together, these studies suggest that several brain regions may work in concert to regulate SNS activity in response to leptin (Fig. 14.3) and that leptin's effects on SNS activity in various organs and tissues can be differentially controlled by activation of leptin receptors in these multiple brain regions.

Obesity and "Selective" Leptin Resistance

The fact that most obese humans have markedly elevated circulating leptin levels and still continue to ingest excess calories suggests that obesity may be associated with resistance to leptin's anorexic effects, in much the same way that subjects with type 2 diabetes are resistant to the metabolic effects of insulin. Experimental studies have also shown that leptin is much less effective in suppressing appetite in obese than in lean animals [35, 47]. There is evidence, however, that if leptin is administered ICV, bypassing the blood–brain barrier, appetite is substantially suppressed in obese rodents fed a high fat diet [48]. These observations, as well as other studies, suggest that at least part of the resistance to exogenously administered leptin in obese subjects may be attributed to defective transport, or saturation of transport, of leptin across the blood–brain barrier [49, 50]. However, obese subjects have higher cerebrospinal fluid (CSF) leptin levels compared to lean subjects [50] suggesting that there is also resistance to leptin signaling, likely related to a post-receptor defect [51]. As discussed later, there has been substantial progress in identifying some of the signaling pathways that modulate/attenuate CNS leptin signaling in obesity.

To the extent that excess weight gain causes global leptin resistance, including resistance to leptin's effects on SNS activity, one might expect that leptin's effects to increase SNS activity and BP would also be attenuated in obese subjects. However, obesity has been suggested to induce "selective" leptin resistance, whereby the effects of leptin to increase renal SNS activity are preserved while appetite suppression is attenuated [35]. Acute experimental studies support this concept [52–56]. In obese mice the leptin mediated reductions in food intake over a 24-h period were attenuated whereas the acute effects to increase renal SNS activity were preserved [54, 55]. However, there have been few studies that have tested whether the chronic effects of hyperleptinemia on BP and SNS activity are attenuated in obese compared to lean subjects. Also, the CNS pathways and cell signaling mechanisms that may underlie selective leptin resistance in obesity are only beginning to be elucidated and represent an important area for investigation.

Intracellular Signaling and Specific CNS Areas That May Mediate Differential Control of Cardiovascular and Metabolic Functions by Leptin

The LR is a cytokine receptor that activates janus tyrosine kinases (JAK), especially JAK2 [57]. In the CNS, upon binding to its receptor, leptin increases activity of intracellular janus activating kinase (JAK2) leading to subsequent activation of three major intracellular pathways: (1) phosphorylation of tyrosine (Tyr) residue 1138 to recruit latent signal transducers and activators of transcription 3 (STAT3) to the LR-JAK2 complex, resulting in phosphorylation and nuclear translocation of STAT3 to regulate transcription; (2) insulin receptor substrate (IRS2) phosphorylation which activates phosphatidylinositol 3-kinase (PI3K) which appears to be involved in regulating rapid nongenomic events affecting neuronal activity and neuropeptide release; and (3) Tyr985 phosphorylation which recruits the tyrosine phosphatase (SHP2) to activate the ERK (MAPK).

Deletion of each of these signaling pathways in the CNS results in varying degrees of obesity, but only neuron-specific deletion of STAT3 appears to mimic the obese phenotype found in ob/ob mice [58]. In addition to its well-known importance in regulating body weight homeostasis, STAT3 signaling may also contribute to leptin's chronic effects on BP. Dubinion et al. showed that deletion of STAT3 specifically in POMC neurons attenuated leptin's ability to raise BP but had only minor effects on leptin's actions on food intake and energy expenditure [59]. These observations suggest that leptin-mediated activation of STAT3 in POMC neurons is important for BP regulation whereas STAT3 activation in other neuronal types is more important in mediating the effects of leptin on appetite and energy expenditure.

Previous acute studies also indicate that the IRS2-PI3K pathway may contribute to leptin's effect on SNS activity and BP. For instance, pharmacological blockade of PI3K abolished the acute effects of leptin to increase renal SNS activity [60]. To our knowledge, however, no long-term studies have been published on whether chronic blockade of the IRS2-PI3K pathway abolishes or attenuates the long-term effects of sustained hyperleptinemia to increase SNS activity and BP. Deletion of IRS2 in the entire CNS causes only moderate obesity and slight hyperphagia associated with normal anorexic and weight loss responses to leptin [61–63]. These observations suggest that IRS2-PI3K signaling contributes modestly to body weight regulation and that it may also mediate, at least in part, the action of leptin on SNS activity. Further studies are needed, however, to assess the role of

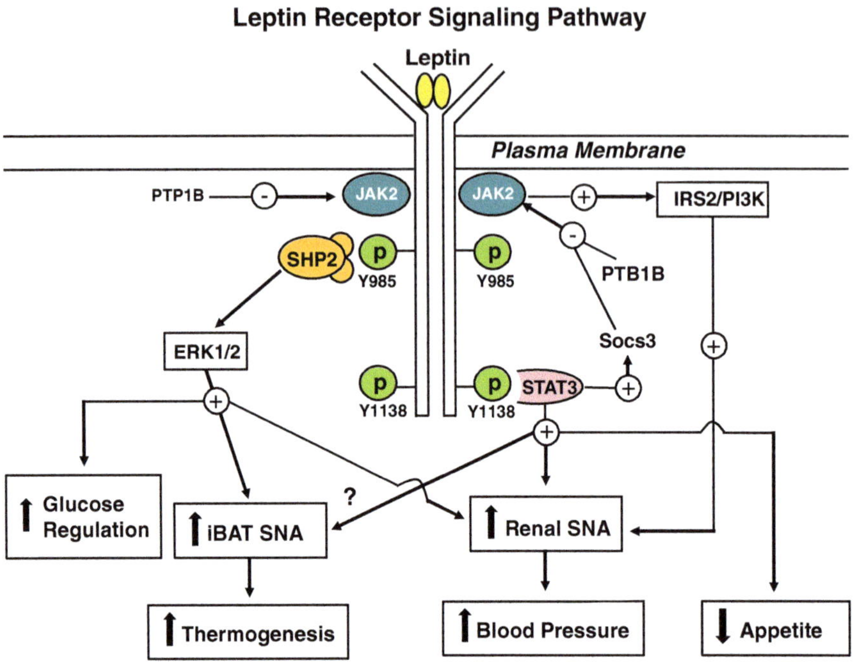

Fig. 14.4 Schematic representation of the leptin receptor signaling events that may contribute to differential of appetite, metabolic and cardiovascular function by leptin and that represent potential mechanisms leading to selective leptin resistance in obesity. ERK = extracellular signal-regulated kinases; JAK = janus tyrosine kinases; STAT3 = signal transducers and activators of transcription 3; iBAT = interscapular brown adipose tissue; IRS2 = insulin receptor substrate 2; PI3K = phosphatidylinositol 3-kinase; PTP1B = protein tyrosine phosphatase-1B; Shp2 = src homology protein 2; SNA = sympathetic nerve activity; SOCS3 = suppressor of cytokines signaling-3

this pathway in mediating the chronic effects of leptin on renal SNS activity and BP in obesity.

The SHP2-MAPK pathway has been shown to participate in energy balance and metabolism as neuronal deletion of SHP2 causes obesity associated with hyperphagia and diabetes [64]. Deletion of SHP2 specifically in forebrain neurons of mice, however, appears to cause early-onset obesity and metabolic syndrome mainly by reducing energy expenditure rather than promoting increased food intake [65], although we observed hyperphagia at a young age in this model [66]. We and others have also found an important role for SHP2 signaling in regulation of glucose homeostasis [64, 66]. Moreover, we found that the chronic effects of hyperleptinemia to increase BP was attenuated in mice with forebrain deletion of SHP2 [66] suggesting that SHP2 signaling may also be important in mediating the effects of leptin on SNS activity and BP.

Collectively, these observations are consistent with the possibility that differential activation of these three intracellular signaling pathways by the LR may mediate divergent control of appetite, energy balance, glucose homeostasis, and cardiovascular function (Fig. 14.4). To the extent that these signaling pathways are differentially regulated in obesity, this may help explain the development of selective leptin resistance. Leptin receptor activation in different regions of the CNS may also contribute to development of selective leptin resistance in obesity. Thus, depending on its site of action leptin may control appetite independently of its effect to increase SNS activity and BP.

Vong and Colleagues [67] showed that leptin receptor deletion in gabaergic neurons mimics most of the obese phenotype observed in ob/ob mice. Although the authors suggest that leptin's action on presynaptic gabaergic neurons decreases

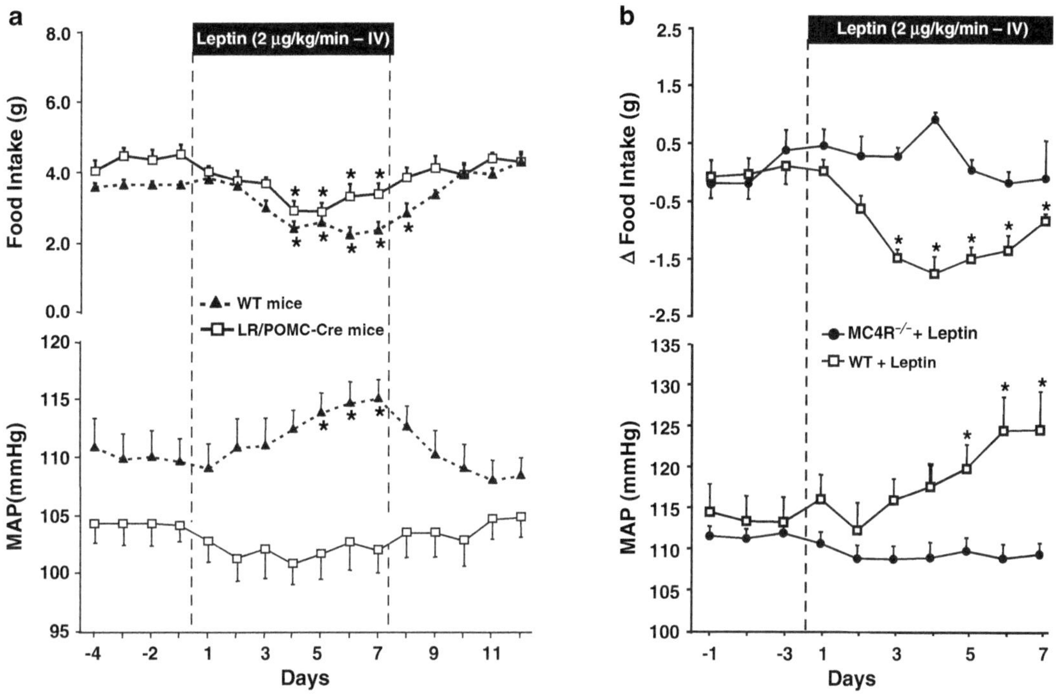

Fig. 14.5 Compilation of data demonstrating the selective importance of POMC neurons for leptin's ability to increase blood pressure but not to reduce appetite (**a**), and the necessity of functional MC4R for leptin to be able to raise blood pressure (**b**). Δ food intake = indicates average change in food intake; LR/POMC-Cre mice = mice with leptin receptor deletion specifically in POMC neurons; MAP = mean arterial pressure; $MC4R^{-/-}$ = melanocortin-4 receptor knockout; POMC = proopiomelanocortin; WT = wild-type. * indicates $p < 0.05$ versus baseline values (Modified from [43] and [74])

inhibitory tone to postsynaptic POMC neurons, the mechanism responsible for the obesity in these mice are still unclear. In addition, gabaergic neurons are widely distributed in the CNS and further studies are still needed to examine which neuronal types and brain sites are most important in mediating the effects of leptin on appetite and body weight regulation as well as on SNS activity. As discussed previously, deletion of leptin receptors in the ARC markedly reduced the acute effects of leptin to increase renal SNS activity and attenuated the rise in BP induced by high fat feeding [40]; and we have shown that leptin receptor activation in POMC neurons, which are present in the ARC and brainstem, is critical for leptin's ability to increase BP (Fig. 14.5a) and improve glucose homeostasis but not for leptin's effect to reduce appetite [43]. These findings suggest that POMC neurons are an important component of the chronic effects of leptin on SNS activity, BP regulation, and glucose regulation, whereas leptin receptor activation in other neurons may play a more important role in mediating the effects of leptin on appetite and energy expenditure.

Negative Regulators of Leptin's Actions on SNS Activity and BP May Contribute to Selective Leptin Resistance

Another potential mechanism that may contribute to selective leptin resistance in obesity is differential control of LR signaling by negative regulators such as protein tyrosine phosphatase-1B (PTP1B) and suppressor of cytokine signaling-3 (SOCS3). PTP1B regulates the janus kinase/signal transducer and activator of transcription (JAK/STAT3) signaling pathway by dephosphorylation of JAK2 [68], whereas Socs3 negatively regulates leptin receptor signaling by inhibiting JAK activity [69]. Deletion of PTP1B enhances leptin sensitivity and confers resistance to high-fat diet induced obesity and type II diabetes [70]. Mice with whole body PTP1B deficiency also exhibit higher baseline BP and amplified BP response to leptin compared to wild-type controls [70]. Although specific deletion of PTP1B in POMC neurons increases energy expenditure [71], it does not alter food intake, suggesting that alterations in PTP1B levels in certain areas of the brain or in specific neuronal types (e.g. POMC neurons) may modulate SNS activity and BP with minimal impact on the anorexic action of leptin.

SOCS-3 expression is regulated by the STAT3 pathway and, like PTP1B, is a negative regulator of leptin receptor signaling that may contribute to leptin resistance. For instance, SOCS3 deficiency increases leptin sensitivity and attenuates development of obesity caused by a high fat diet [72]. The importance of SOCS3 signaling in regulating SNS activity, however, is still unclear. Together, PTP1B and SOCS3 could play an important role in modulating the appetite, metabolic and cardiovascular actions of leptin and contribute to the development of selective leptin resistance in obesity. However, additional studies are needed to explore how obesity alters PTP1B and SOCS3 expression and whether these negative regulators of leptin receptor signaling may be potential targets for novel therapies to treat obesity and its metabolic and cardiovascular abnormalities.

As discussed previously, other factors associated with obesity, such as endothelial dysfunction and impaired NO release, may also selectively amplify the effects of leptin on SNS activity and BP. Thus, obesity induces a complex set of pathophysiological events that not only modulate LR signaling but also elicit changes in renal, vascular, and SNS function that contribute to unaltered, or even augmented, effects of leptin on SNS activity and BP whereas leptin's action on appetite, energy expenditure, and glucose homeostasis are attenuated.

The CNS Melanocortin System Mediates Most of the Effects of Leptin on SNS Activity and BP Regulation

Although the precise intracellular events and brain regions by which leptin regulates body weight homeostasis and cardiovascular function are not completely understood, strong evidence shows that leptin requires activation of the brain melanocortin system, including activation of POMC neurons and melanocortin 4 receptors (MC4R) to exert most of its effects on renal SNS activity and BP regulation [19, 73, 74]. We already discussed the importance of leptin receptors in POMC neurons for leptin's ability to increase SNS activity and BP [43], but multiple acute and chronic studies further support a key role for the brain melanocortin system in mediating the cardiovascular effects of leptin. For example, activation of MC4R using synthetic agonists increases renal SNS activity, BP, and HR in experimental animal models as well as in humans [19, 75–78], and mice with whole body MC4R deficiency are hyperphagic and obese, and have many characteristics of metabolic syndrome including hyperglycemia, hyperinsulinemia, visceral adiposity, and dislypidemia despite markedly elevated blood leptin levels [73]; and importantly, mice with MC4R deficiency are also completely unresponsive to the effects of leptin to increase renal SNS activity raise BP [74, 79] (Fig. 14.5b). In addition, mutations in POMC or MC4R genes lead to severe early-onset obesity and dysregulation of appetite in humans who, despite pronounced obesity, exhibit reduced BP, HR and 24-h urinary catecholamine excretion, lower prevalence of hypertension, and reduced SNS activity in response to acute stress [76–78]. Taken together, these studies strongly suggest that a functional MC4R is necessary for obesity and hyperleptinemia to increase SNS activity and cause hypertension.

Differential control of appetite, metabolic and cardiovascular function by MC4R activation in various regions of the brain may also contribute to selective leptin resistance in obesity. For example,

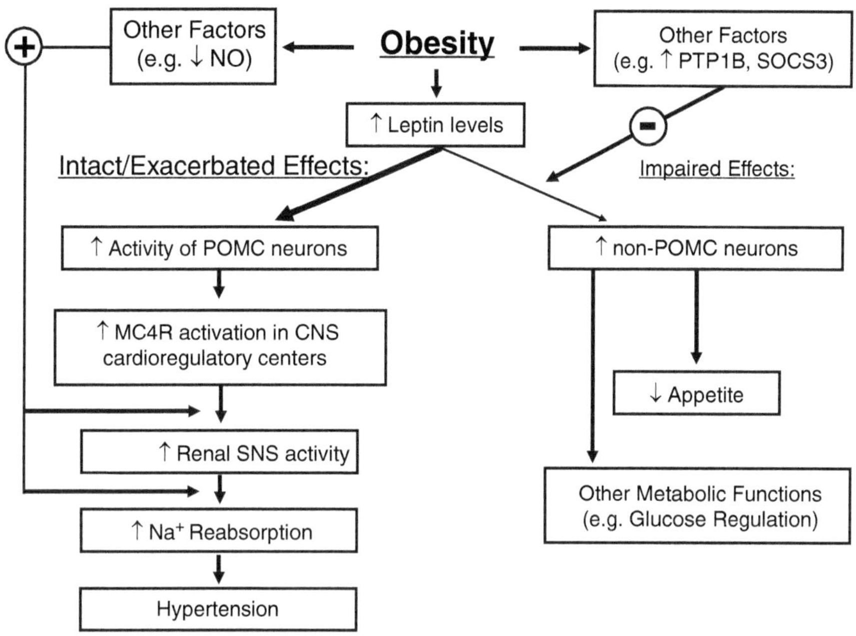

Fig. 14.6 Schematic representation of the complex set of events associated with obesity that results in augmented renal, vascular, and SNS responses to hyperletinemia that contribute to increased sympathetic activity and hypertension, whereas leptin's action on appetite and other metabolic functions are attenuated. CNS = central nervous system; MC4R = melanocortin-4 receptor; Na^+ = sodium; NO = nitric oxide; POMC = proopiomelanocortin; PTP1B = protein tyrosine phosphatase-1B; SNS = sympathetic nervous system; SOCS3 = suppressor of cytokines signaling-3

MC4R located in PVN neurons appear to be more important in regulating appetite while exerting minimal role in the control of thermogenesis, whereas MC4R located in POMC neurons seem to play a more prominent role in regulating thermogenesis and energy expenditure [80, 81]. Although previous studies suggest that MC4R in the PVN and preganglionic sympathetic neurons in the brainstem modulate SNS activity and BP [82, 83], additional long-term studies are needed to examine the brain regions where MC4R regulate SNS activity and cardiovascular function.

Conclusions

Obesity is a major cause of human essential hypertension. Excess weight gain leads to activation of the SNS which plays a key role in increasing renal sodium reabsorption, impairing pressure natriuresis, and raising BP in obese subjects. SNS activation in obesity is mediated, in part, by increased leptin, stimulation of POMC neurons, and subsequent activation of MC4R in the CNS. Other factors associated with obesity, such as endothelial dysfunction and impaired NO release, enhanced negative LR feedback mechanisms (e.g. PTP1B and SOCS3), and altered activation of LR and/or MC4R in distinct regions of the brain may also selectively amplify the effects of leptin on SNS activity and BP. Thus, obesity induces a complex set of events that may ultimately result in augmented renal, vascular, and SNS responses to hyperletinemia that contribute to increased SNS activity and hypertension, whereas leptin's action on appetite, energy expenditure, and glucose homeostasis are attenuated (Fig. 14.6). The molecular pathways by which the CNS leptin-melanocortin system differentially regulates energy balance, SNS activity, and BP in obesity, however, is still unclear and remains an important area for further investigation.

Sources of Funding The authors' research was supported by grants from the National Heart, Lung and Blood Institute (PO1 HL51971), the National Institute of General Medical Sciences (P20 GM104357), and by an American Heart Association Scientist Development Grant to Jussara M. do Carmo.

References

1. Yach D, Stuckler D, Brownell KD. Epidemiologic and economic consequences of the global epidemics of obesity and diabetes. Nat Med. 2006;12:62–6.
2. Ogden CL, Carroll MD, Curtin LR, McDowell MA, Tabak CJ, Flegal KM. Prevalence of overweight and obesity in the United States, 1999-2004. JAMA. 2006;295:1549–55.
3. Anderson SE, Whitaker RC. Prevalence of obesity among US preschool children in different racial and ethnic groups. Arch Pediatr Adolesc Med. 2009;163: 344–8.
4. Guyton AC. The surprising kidney-fluid mechanism for pressure control: its infinite gain! Hypertension. 1990;16:425–30.
5. Hall JE, Crook ED, Jones DW, Wofford MR, Dubbert PM. Mechanisms of obesity-associated cardiovascular and renal disease. Am J Med Sci. 2002;324: 127–37.
6. Hall JE. The kidney, hypertension, and obesity. Hypertension. 2003;41:625–33.
7. Davy KP, Hall JE. Obesity and hypertension: two epidemics or one? Am J Physiol Regul Integr Comp Physiol. 2004;286:R803–13.
8. Davy KP, Orr JS. Sympathetic nervous system behavior in human obesity. Neurosci Biobehav Rev. 2009;33: 116–24.
9. Vaz M, Jennings G, Turner A, Cox H, Lambert G, Esler M. Regional sympathetic nervous activity and oxygen consumption in obese normotensive subjects. Circulation. 1997;18:3423–9.
10. Armitage JA, Burke SL, Prior LJ, Barzel B, Eikelis N, Lim K, Head GA. Rapid onset of renal sympathetic nerve activation in rabbits fed a high-fat diet. Hypertension. 2012;60:163–71.
11. Hall JE, da Silva AA, do Carmo JM, Dubinion J, Hamza S, Munusamy S, Smith G, Stec DE. Obesity-induced hypertension: role of sympathetic nervous system, leptin, and melanocortins. J Biol Chem. 2010;285:17271–6.
12. Straznicky NE, Eikelis N, Lambert EA, Esler MD. Mediators of sympathetic activation in metabolic syndrome obesity. Curr Hypertens Rep. 2008;10: 440–7.
13. Esler M, Straznicky N, Eikelis N, Masuo K, Lambert G, Lambert E. Mechanisms of sympathetic activation in obesity-related hypertension. Hypertension. 2006;48:787–96.
14. Wofford MR, Anderson DC, Brown CA, Jones DW, Miller ME, Hall JE. Antihypertensive effect of alpha and beta adrenergic blockade in obese and lean hypertensive subjects. Am J Hypertens. 2001;14:694–8.
15. Kassab S, Kato T, Wilkins FC, Chen R, Hall JE, Granger JP. Renal denervation attenuates the sodium retention and hypertension associated with obesity. Hypertension. 1995;25:893–7.
16. Hering D, Marusic P, Walton AS, Lambert EA, Krum H, Narkiewicz K, Lambert GW, Esler MD, Schlaich MP. Sustained sympathetic and blood pressure reduction 1 year after renal denervation in patients with resistant hypertension. Hypertension 2014;64:118–24.
17. Rumantir MS, Vaz M, Jennings GL, Collier G, Kaye DM, Seals DR, Wiesner GH, Brunner-La Rocca HP, Esler MD. Neural mechanisms in human obesity-related hypertension. J Hypertens. 1999;17:1125–33.
18. da Silva AA, do Carmo JM, Dubinion J, Hall JE. The role of the sympathetic nervous system in obesity-related hypertension. Curr Hypertens Rep. 2009;11: 206–11.
19. da Silva AA, do Carmo JM, Wang Z, Hall JE. The brain melanocortin system, sympathetic control, and obesity hypertension. Physiology (Bethesda). 2014;29: 196–202.
20. Snitker S, Pratley RE, Nicolson M, Tataranni PA, Ravussin E. Relationship between muscle sympathetic nerve activity and plasma leptin concentration. Obes Res. 1997;5:338–40.
21. Haynes WG, Morgan DA, Walsh SA, Mark AL, Sivitz WI. Receptor-mediated regional sympathetic nerve activation by leptin. J Clin Invest. 1997;100:270–8.
22. Dunbar JC, Hu Y, Lu H. Intracerebroventricular leptin increases lumbar and renal sympathetic nerve activity and blood pressure in normal rats. Diabetes. 1997;46: 2040–3.
23. Machleidt F, Simon P, Krapalis AF, Hallschmid M, Lehnert H, Sayk F. Experimental hyperleptinemia acutely increases vasoconstrictory sympathetic nerve activity in healthy humans. J Clin Endocrinol Metab. 2013;98:E491–6.
24. Frühbeck G. 460. Pivotal role of nitric oxide in the control of blood pressure after leptin administration. Diabetes. 1999;48:903–8.
25. Shek EW, Brands MW, Hall JE. Chronic leptin infusion increases arterial pressure. Hypertension. 1998;31:409–14.
26. Aizawa-Abe M, Ogawa Y, Masuzaki H, Ebihara K, Satoh N, Iwai H, Matsuoka N, Hayashi T, Hosoda K, Inoue G, Yoshimasa Y, Nakao K. Pathophysiological role of leptin in obesity-related hypertension. J Clin Invest. 2000;105:1243–52.
27. Carlyle M, Jones OB, Kuo JJ, Hall JE. Chronic cardiovascular and renal actions of leptin-role of adrenergic activity. Hypertension. 2002;39:496–501.
28. Zelissen PM, Stenlof K, Lean ME, Fogteloo J, Keulen ET, Wilding J, Finer N, Rössner S, Lawrence E, Fletcher C, McCamish M. Effect of three treatment schedules of recombinant methionyl human leptin on body weight in obese adults: a randomized, placebo-controlled trial. Diabetes Obes Metab. 2005;7:755–61.
29. Brook RD, Bard RL, Bodary PF, Eitzman DT, Rajagopalan S, Sun Y, Depaoli AM. Blood pressure and vascular effects of leptin in humans. Metab Syndr Relat Disord. 2007;5:270–4.
30. Lim K, Burke SL, Head GA. Obesity-related hypertension and the role of insulin and leptin in high-fat-fed rabbits. Hypertension. 2013;61:628–34.
31. Mark AL, Shafer RA, Correia ML, Morgan DA, Sigmund CD, Haynes WG. Contrasting blood pressure

effects of obesity in leptin deficient ob/ob mice and agouti yellow obese mice. J Hypertens. 1999;17: 1949–53.
32. do Carmo JM, Bassi M, da Silva AA, Hall JE. Control of cardiovascular, metabolic and respiratory functions during prolonged obesity in leptin-deficient and diet-induced obese mice. Hypertension. 2008;15:109.
33. Farooqi S, O'Rahilly S. Genetics of obesity in humans. Endocr Rev. 2006;27:710–8.
34. Ozata M, Ozdemir IC, Licinio J. Human leptin deficiency caused by a missense mutation: multiple endocrine defects, decreased sympathetic tone, and immune system dysfunction indicate new targets for leptin action, greater central than peripheral resistance to the effects of leptin, and spontaneous correction of leptin-mediated defects. J Clin Endocrinol Metab. 1999;10:3686–95.
35. Mark AL. Selective leptin resistance revisited. Am J Physiol Regul Integr Comp Physiol. 2013;305: R566–81.
36. Kuo JJ, Jones OB, Hall JE. Inhibition of NO synthesis enhances chronic cardiovascular and renal actions of leptin. Hypertension. 2001;37:670–6.
37. Cohen P, Connie Z, Cai X, Montez JM, Rohani SC, Feinstein P, Mombaerts P, Friedman JM. Selective deletion of leptin receptor in neurons leads to obesity. J Clin Invest. 2001;108:1113–21.
38. Schwartz MW, Woods SC, Porte Jr D, Seeley RJ, Baskin DG. Central nervous system control of food intake. Nature. 2000;404:661–71.
39. Rahmouni K, Morgan DA. Hypothalamic arcuate nucleus mediates the sympathetic and arterial pressure responses to leptin. Hypertension. 2007;49: 647–52.
40. Harlan SM, Morgan DA, Agassandian K, Guo DF, Cassell MD, Sigmund CD, Mark AL, Rahmouni K. Ablation of the leptin receptor in the hypothalamic arcuate nucleus abrogates leptin-induced sympathetic activation. Circ Res. 2011;108:808–12.
41. Elias CF, Lee C, Kelly J, Aschkenasi C, Ahima RS, Couceyro PR, Kuhar MJ, Saper CB, Elmquist JK. Leptin activates hypothalamic CART neurons projecting to the spinal cord. Neuron. 1998;21:1375–85.
42. Elmquist JK. Hypothalamic pathways underlying the endocrine, autonomic, and behavioral effects of leptin. Physiol Behav. 2001;74:703–8.
43. do Carmo JM, da Silva AA, Cai Z, Lin S, Dubinion JH, Hall JE. Control of blood pressure, appetite, and glucose by leptin in mice lacking leptin receptors in proopiomelanocortin neurons. Hypertension. 2011;57: 918–26.
44. Mark AL, Agassandian K, Morgan DA, Liu X, Cassell MD, Rahmouni K. Leptin signaling in the nucleus tractus solitarii increases sympathetic nerve activity to the kidney. Hypertension. 2009;53:375–80.
45. Smith PM, Ferguson AV. Cardiovascular actions of leptin in the subfornical organ are abolished by diet-induced obesity. J Neuroendocrinol. 2012;24:504–10.
46. Young CN, Morgan DA, Butler SD, Mark AL, Davisson RL. The brain subfornical organ mediates leptin-induced increases in renal sympathetic activity but not its metabolic effects. Hypertension. 2013;61: 737–44.
47. Mark AL, Correia ML, Rahmouni K, Haynes WG. Selective leptin resistance: a new concept in leptin physiology with cardiovascular implications. J Hypertens. 2002;20:1245–50.
48. Dubinion JH, da Silva AA, Hall JE. Chronic blood pressure and appetite responses to central leptin infusion in rats fed a high fat diet. J Hypertens. 2011;29:758–62.
49. Banks WA, Kastin AJ, Huang W, Jaspan JB, Maness LM. Leptin enters the brain by a saturable system independent of insulin. Peptides. 1996;17:305–11.
50. Caro JF, Kolaczynski JW, Nyce MR, Ohannesian JP, Opentanova I, Goldman WH, Lynn RB, Zhang PL, Sinha MK, Considine RV. Decreased cerebrospinal-fluid/serum leptin ratio in obesity: a possible mechanism for leptin resistance. Lancet. 1996;348:159–61.
51. Münzberg H, Myers Jr MG. Molecular and anatomical determinants of central leptin resistance. Nat Neurosci. 2005;8:566–70.
52. Kalil GZ, Haynes WG. Sympathetic nervous system in obesity-related hypertension: mechanisms and clinical implications. Hypertens Res. 2012;35:4–16.
53. Correia ML, Haynes WG, Rahmouni K, Morgan DA, Sivitz WI, Mark AL. The concept of selective leptin resistance: evidence from agouti yellow obese mice. Diabetes. 2002;51:439–42.
54. Rahmouni K, Fath MA, Seo S, Thedens DR, Berry CJ, Weiss R, Nishimura DY, Sheffield VC. Leptin resistance contributes to obesity and hypertension in mouse models of Bardet-Biedl syndrome. J Clin Invest. 2008;118:1458–67.
55. Rahmouni K, Morgan DA, Morgan GM, Mark AL, Haynes WG. Role of selective leptin resistance in diet-induced obesity hypertension. Diabetes. 2005;54:2012–8.
56. Prior LJ, Eikelis N, Armitage JA, Davern PJ, Burke SL, Montani JP, Barzel B, Head GA. Exposure to a high-fat diet alters leptin sensitivity and elevates renal sympathetic nerve activity and arterial pressure in rabbits. Hypertension. 2010;55:862–8.
57. Ghilardi N, Skoda RC. The leptin receptor activates janus kinase 2 and signals for proliferation in a factor-dependent cell line. Mol Endocrinol. 1997;11:393–9.
58. Gao Q, Wolfgang MJ, Neschen S. Disruption of neural signal transducer and activator of transcription 3 causes obesity, diabetes, infertility, and thermal dysregulation. Proc Natl Acad Sci U S A. 2004;101: 4661–6.
59. Dubinion JH, do Carmo JM, Adi A, Hamza S, da Silva AA, Hall JE. Role of signal transducer and activator of transcription 3 in proopiomelanocortin neurons in cardiovascular and metabolic actions of leptin. Hypertension. 2013;61:1066–74.
60. Rahmouni K, Haynes WG, Morgan DA, Mark AL. Intracellular mechanisms involved in leptin regulation of sympathetic outflow. Hypertension. 2002;41: 763–7.

61. Choudhury AI, Heffron H, Smith MA, Al-Qassab H, Xu AW, Selman C, Simmgen M, Clements M, Claret M, Maccoll G, Bedford DC, Hisadome K, Diakonov I, Moosajee V, Bell JD, Speakman JR, Batterham RL, Barsh GS, Ashford ML, Withers DJ. The role of insulin receptor substrate 2 in hypothalamic and beta cell function. J Clin Invest. 2005;15:940–50.
62. Lin X, Taguchi A, Park S, Kushner JA, Li F, Li Y, White MF. Dysregulation of insulin receptor substrate 2 in beta cells and brain causes obesity and diabetes. J Clin Invest. 2004;114:908–16.
63. Burks D, de Mora JF, Schubert M, Withers DJ, Myers MG, Towery HH, Altamuro SL, Flint CL, White MF. IRS-2 pathways integrate female reproduction and energy homeostasis. Nature. 2000;407:377–82.
64. Krajewska M, Banares S, Zhang EE, Huang X, Scadeng M, Jhala US, Feng GS, Krajewski S. Development of diabesity in mice with neuronal deletion of Shp2 tyrosine phosphatase. Am J Pathol. 2008;172:1312–24.
65. Zhang EE, Chapeau E, Hagihara K, Feng GS. Neuronal Shp2 tyrosine phosphatase controls energy balance and metabolism. Proc Natl Acad Sci U S A. 2004;9:16064–9.
66. do Carmo JM, da Silva AA, Sessums PO, Ebaady SH, Pace BR, Rushing JS, Davis MT, Hall JE. Role of Shp2 in forebrain neurons in regulating metabolic and cardiovascular functions and responses to leptin. Int J Obes (Lond). 2014;38:775.
67. Vong L, Ye C, Yang Z, Choi B, Chua Jr S, Lowell BB. Leptin action on GABAergic neurons prevents obesity and reduces inhibitory tone to POMC neurons. Neuron. 2011;71:142–54.
68. Myers MP, Anderson JN, Cheng A, Tremblay ML, Horvath CM, Parisien JP, Salmeen A, Barford D, Tonks NK. TYK2 and JAK2 are substrates of protein-tyrosine phosphatase 1B. J Biol Chem. 2001;276: 47771–4.
69. Bjorbaek C, El-Haschimi K, Frantz JD, Flier JS. The role of SOCS3 in leptin signaling and leptin resistance. J Biol Chem. 1999;274:30059–65.
70. Belin de Chantemele EJ, Muta K, Mintz J, Tremblay ML, Marrero MB, Fulton DJ, Stepp DW. Protein tyrosine phosphatase 1B, a major regulator of leptin-mediated control of cardiovascular function. Circulation. 2009;120:753–63.
71. Banno R, Zimmer D, De Jonghe BC, Atienza M, Rak K, Yang W, Bence KK. PTP1B and SHP2 in POMC neurons reciprocally regulate energy balance in mice. J Clin Invest. 2010;120:720–34.
72. Mori H, Hanada R, Hanada T, Aki D, Mashima R, Nishinakamura H, Torisu T, Chien KR, Yasukawa H, Yoshimura A. Socs3 deficiency in the brain elevates leptin sensitivity and confers resistance to diet-induced obesity. Nat Med. 2004;10:739–43.
73. Tallam LS, Stec DE, Willis MA, da Silva AA, Hall JE. Melanocortin-4 receptor-deficient mice are not hypertensive or salt-sensitive despite obesity, hyperinsulinemia, and hyperleptinemia. Hypertension. 2005; 46:326–32.
74. Tallam LS, da Silva AA, Hall JE. Melanocortin-4 receptor mediates chronic cardiovascular and metabolic actions of leptin. Hypertension. 2006;48:58–64.
75. Kievit P, Halem H, Marks DL, Dong JZ, Glavas MM, Sinnayah P, Pranger L, Cowley MA, Grove KL, Culler MD. Chronic treatment with a melanocortin 4 receptor agonist causes weight loss, reduces insulin resistance, and improves cardiovascular function in diet-induced obese Rhesus Macaques. Diabetes. 2013;62:490–7.
76. Greenfield JR. Melanocortin signaling and the regulation of blood pressure in human obesity. J Neuroendocrinol. 2011;23:186–93.
77. Sayk F, Heutling D, Dodt C, Iwen KA, Wellhoner JP, Scherag S, Hinney A, Hebebrand J, Lehnert H. Sympathetic function in human carriers of melanocortin-4 receptor gene mutations. J Clin Endocrinol Metab. 2010;95:1998–2002.
78. Greenfield JR, Miller JW, Keogh JM, Henning E, Satterwhite JH, Cameron GS, Astruc B, Mayer JP, Brage S, See TC, Lomas DJ, O'Rahilly S, Farooqi IS. Modulation of blood pressure by central melanocortinergic pathways. N Engl J Med. 2009;360: 44–52.
79. Rahmouni K, Haynes WG, Morgan DA, Mark AL. Role of melanocortin-4 receptors in mediating renal sympathoactivation to leptin and insulin. J Neurosci. 2003;23:5998–6004.
80. Balthasar N, Dalgaard LT, Lee CE, Yu J, Funahashi H, Williams T, Ferreira M, Tang V, McGovern RA, Kenny CD, Christiansen LM, Edelstein E, Choi B, Boss O, Aschkenasi C, Zhang CY, Mountjoy K, Kishi T, Elmquist JK, Lowell BB. Divergence control of melanocortin pathways in the control of food intake and energy expenditure. Cell. 2005;123:493–505.
81. do Carmo JM, da Silva AA, Rushing JS, Pace B, Hall JE. Differential control of appetite and cardiovascular function after selective rescue of melanocortin-4 receptor in proopiomelanocortin neurons. Am J Physiol Regul Integr Comp Physiol. 2013;305: R359–68.
82. Li P, Cui BP, Zhang LL, Sun HJ, Liu TY, Zhu GQ. Melanocortin 3/4 receptors in paraventricular nucleus modulate sympathetic outflow and blood pressure. Exp Physiol. 2013;98:435–43.
83. Sohn JW, Harris LE, Berglund ED, Liu T, Vong L, Lowell BB, Balthasar N, Williams KW, Elmquist JK. Melanocortin 4 receptors reciprocally regulate sympathetic and parasympathetic preganglionic neuron. Cell. 2013;152:612–9.

Dynamic Leptin Secretion in Obesity and Diabetes

15

Sam Dagogo-Jack

Glucocorticoid-Induced Leptin Secretion

The hypothalamic-pituitary-adrenal axis plays a clinically recognized role in the regulation of appetite and body weight [1–4]. Patients with glucocorticoid deficiency or excess, such as Addison's disease or Cushing's syndrome, manifest alterations in appetite resulting in weight loss or obesity, respectively [4, 5] . On the other hand, obesity per se results in perturbation of the hypothalamic-pituitary-adrenal axis, such as false-positive screening tests for Cushing's syndrome [6]. Several lines of evidence confirm that glucocorticoids are potent stimuli for leptin production at the mRNA and secreted protein levels in humans [7–14]. Pathological hypercortisolemia, as occurs in patients with Cushing's syndrome, is associated with hyperleptinemia [12, 15, 16]. The glucocorticoid effect on leptin production occurs after a lag period of several hours (consistent with a transcriptional mechanism), and the proportionate increase in plasma leptin levels is similar in men and women [10, 17].

Administration of recombinant leptin inhibits the secretion of insulin by the pancreatic islet beta-cells [18] and glucocorticoid secretion in *ob*/*ob* mice in vitro as well as in vivo [19, 20]. These findings together with the aforementioned well-documented stimulatory effects of glucocorticoids on leptin secretion suggest the existence of a feedback loop between leptin and glucocorticoids. Besides their effects on adipocytes [21, 22], glucocorticoids also have central effects (including interaction with glucocorticoid receptors in the hypothalamus [23] and modulation of neuropeptide Y expression [19, 24, 25]) that alter food intake. A putative feedback loop between leptin and glucocorticoid secretion could subserve an important physiological function by coordinately modulating hunger and ingestive behavior and glucocorticoid availability under various metabolic and stressful conditions.

Physiological Response or Pharmacological Epiphenomenon?

Evidence that the glucocorticoid effect on leptin production might be of physiological significance include (1) demonstration of a linear relationship between serum dexamethasone concentration and leptin levels [10], (2) the potency of physiological doses and a dose–response relationship between glucocorticoid and plasma leptin response [26]; (3) the demonstration that fasting abolished the

S. Dagogo-Jack, M.D., M.B.B.S. (✉)
Division of Endocrinology, Diabetes and Metabolism, The University of Tennessee Health Science Center, 920 Madison Avenue, Suite 300A, Memphis, TN 38163, USA
e-mail: sdj@uthsc.edu

S. Dagogo-Jack (ed.), *Leptin: Regulation and Clinical Applications*,
DOI 10.1007/978-3-319-09915-6_15, © Springer International Publishing Switzerland 2015

expected leptin response to glucocorticoids [26, 27]; (4) the finding that inhibition of endogenous steroidogenesis with metyrapone decreases plasma leptin levels) [28, 29]; and (5) modulation of ad libitum food intake by glucocorticoid-induced hyperleptinemia in humans [30]. Moreover, unlike the sexual dimorphism observed in basal leptin levels, the leptin response to glucocorticoids (as a percentage of baseline leptin) does not differ by gender [10]. These observations underscore the probable physiological relevance of glucocorticoid–leptin interactions.

Effects of Fasting and Feeding

To provide further physiological insight, the glucocorticoid effect on leptin secretion was studied under fasting or fed conditions in healthy volunteers (mean age 35 yr, BMI 27.1 ± 2.1 kg/m^2) [26]. The study subjects received, in random order, i.v. infusion of hydrocortisone (300 mg/24 h) in the fed state or hydrocortisone (300 mg/24 h) with total caloric deprivation, with saline infusion serving as the control arm. The peak/baseline plasma leptin levels (ng/ml) were 32.5 ± 12.5/12.0 ± 8.4 (+171 %, $P<0.001$) during hydrocortisone infusion in the fed state and 14.6 ± 6.0/12.5 ± 6.5(+17 %) during hydrocortisone infusion in the fasting state, compared with 16.1 ± 5.8/12.8 ± 5.9 (+26 %) during saline infusion in the fed state. Thus, fasting completely abolished the leptin response to glucocorticoid (Fig. 15.1). Similar findings were reported by Laferrere et al. [27]. These findings suggest that a behavioral input (feeding) is required for glucocorticoids to stimulate leptin production. Because feeding increases circulating levels of insulin and cortisol [31–33], two known leptin secretagogues, the marked attenuation of glucocorticoid-induced leptin secretion may be due, at least in part, to the lack of insulin augmentation in fasting subjects. Recognize, however, that glucocorticoids directly stimulate leptin mRNA synthesis in adipocytes [11, 21, 34], and that the reported effect of co-incubation with insulin in cultured human adipocytes seems antagonistic rather than additive or synergistic [35]. Thus, it is not fully clear by what exact mechanism fasting exerts such a profoundly negative effect on leptin secretory responses to glucocorticoids [26, 27]. In this regard, the potential role of gastrointestinal hormones (besides insulin), whose expression can be altered by fasting, has not

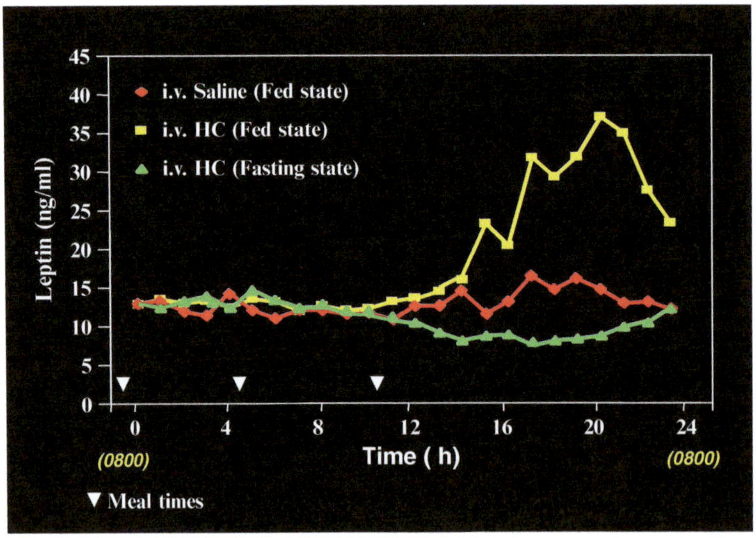

Fig. 15.1 Plasma leptin levels during continuous infusion of hydrocortisone (300 mg/24 h) in the fasting or fed state compared with saline (placebo) infusion in the fed state. The peak/baseline plasma leptin levels (ng/ml) were 32.5 ± 12.5/12.0 ± 8.4 (+171 %, $P<0.001$) during hydrocortisone infusion in the fed state and 14.6 ± 6.0/12.5 ± 6.5 (+17 %) during hydrocortisone infusion in the fasting state, compared with 16.1 ± 5.8/12.8 ± 5.9 (+26 %) during saline infusion in the fed state. Adapted from Dagogo-Jack S, Umamaheswaran I, Askari H, Tykodi G [26]

been fully explored. Thus, what can be concluded from the available data is that feeding is required for glucocorticoids to stimulate leptin secretion in vivo in humans.

Endogenous Hyperleptinemia and Caloric Intake

Despite being hyperleptinemic relative to lean persons, obese persons who were treated with subcutaneous doses of exogenous recombinant leptin experienced a mean weight loss of ~7 kg [36]. Although there was marked individual variation in the magnitude of the effect of leptin therapy, the demonstration of significant weight loss indicates that augmentation of the already elevated leptin levels in obese persons exerts an anti-ingestive effect that could result in weight loss. Whether manipulation of endogenous native leptin levels (without recourse to injection of recombinant leptin) could impact feeding behavior in humans is an important question. Answering that question requires the deployment of a potent leptin secretagogue. Insulin, estrogens, and glucocorticoids have potent stimulatory effects on leptin production [37]. However, each of these hormones has metabolic and systemic effects as well as safety concerns, if deployed as a long-term leptin secretagogue. Thus, there is currently no pure leptin secretagogue that is devoid of intrinsic metabolic effects. Of the three hormonal options for increasing leptin production, glucocorticoids seem the most appealing, because of convenience, avoidance of hypoglycemia, acceptability to both genders, and demonstrated greater potency on leptin production compared to insulin [34].

As a proof-of-concept study, our group assessed energy consumption during administration of hydrocortisone in healthy adults. Study participants were admitted overnight on two occasions, separated by a 2-week wash-out period, were randomly assigned to receive either hydrocortisone (12.5 mg/h IV) or saline infusion for 24 h (0800–0800) in a crossover design [30]. During each admission, participants had ad libitum access to meals and snacks. The subjects were given a printed menu from the hospital kitchen from which they were to order three meals and snacks on day 1 and breakfast on day 2. The study participants marked their food choices from the same menu during each entry. All meals and snacks were served on a tray and delivered by a research dietitian, who checked the food trays before and after meal/snack consumption. At the end of each mealtime, the uneaten items were recorded. The total energy and amounts of protein, fat, and carbohydrates consumed were analyzed. Hydrocortisone infusion increased plasma leptin level within ~5 h from initiation, and the increase was sustained throughout the study period (Fig. 15.2). The total energy consumed was ~500 kcal lower during hydrocortisone-induced hyperleptinemia compared to saline infusion (Fig. 15.2) [30]. Decreases in the intake of carbohydrates and fat accounted for most of the caloric reduction observed during glucocorticoid-induced hyperleptinemia [30].

These results indicate that stimulation of native leptin secretion decreases energy consumption, similar to the effect observed with exogenous leptin therapy. The challenge is that the secretagogue utilized in this acute study would not be appropriate for longer term use, owing to the numerous adverse systemic effects of corticosteroids. Nonetheless, this proof-of-concept study does provide a sound rationale for searching for safer nonsteroidal or steroidomimetic leptin secretagogues for antiobesity drug development. The clinical significance of the finding that endogenous hyperleptinemia induced by glucocorticoid suppressed food intake needs to be interpreted carefully. Experiments of nature, such as Cushing's syndrome, in which chronic hypercortisolemia results in chronic hyperleptinemia, are associated with obesity rather than anorexia and weight loss, as would have been predicted from our model. A similar experience applies to patients treated chronically with pharmacological doses of glucocorticoids. In contrast, patients with Addison's disease do not develop obesity during lifelong replacement therapy with physiological doses of glucocorticoids. Thus, the physiological effects of glucocorticoids on ingestive behavior may be different from the effects of chronic therapy with pharmacological

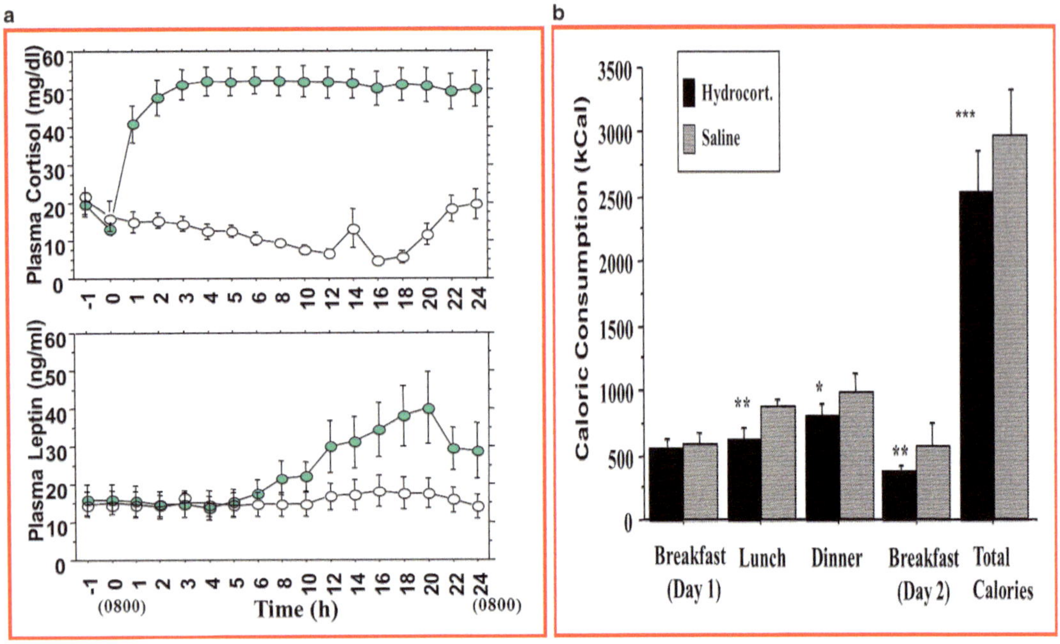

Fig. 15.2 (**a**) Plasma cortisol (*upper panel*) and leptin (*lower panel*) levels during infusion of hydrocortisone (*closed circles*) or saline (*open circles*) in healthy subjects; (**b**) Caloric intake during induced hyperleptinemia (*closed rectangles*) or saline infusion (*hatched rectangles*) in healthy subjects. *$P=0.04$, **$P=0.02$, ***$P=0.005$. Reproduced from Askari H, Liu J, Dagogo-Jack S [30]

doses or pathological hypercortisolemia. Chronic exposure to high concentrations of glucocorticoids appears to override the anti-ingestive effects of the resultant hyperleptinemia, presumably by activating central glucocorticoid receptors [38] and stimulating hypothalamic orexigenic pathways [39–41].

Integrated Physiology of Glucocorticoid–Leptin Interaction

Postprandial increases in plasma insulin and free cortisol [31–33] levels represent a physiological response to meal ingestion. The subsequent release of leptin, triggered by the combined effects of insulin and cortisol, is theorized to induce satiety and prevent hunger between meals. Indeed, the ability of an individual to observe fasting periods of several hours between the three main meals might be related to interprandial leptin levels. Glucocorticoids exert orexigenic effects that are mediated, at least in part, by augmentation of neuropeptide Y (NPY) [25], an effect that is inhibited by leptin [19, 24]. The metabolic effects of leptin result from coordinate activation of anorexigenic pathways and inhibition of orexigenic pathways via leptin-responsive neurons in the hypothalamus [42]. The possibility that increased leptin secretion represents a compensatory response to glucocorticoid-induced insulin resistance cannot be dismissed, as leptin is a potent endogenous insulin sensitizer in hyperglycemic ob/ob mice [43, 44]. Additionally, leptin secretion could be a response to glucocorticoid activation of central orexigenic signals, such as NPY-secreting neurons [25], since leptin suppresses the expression of NPY [19, 24]. Finally, to complete the feedback loop, leptin suppresses glucocorticoid release by the adrenal cortex [20], thus restraining hypercortisolemia and maintaining homeostasis. The interactions among adipocyte leptin secretion, islet cell insulin secretion, adrenocortical output of glucocorticoids, and central orexigenic/anorexogenic responses are schematized in Fig. 15.3.

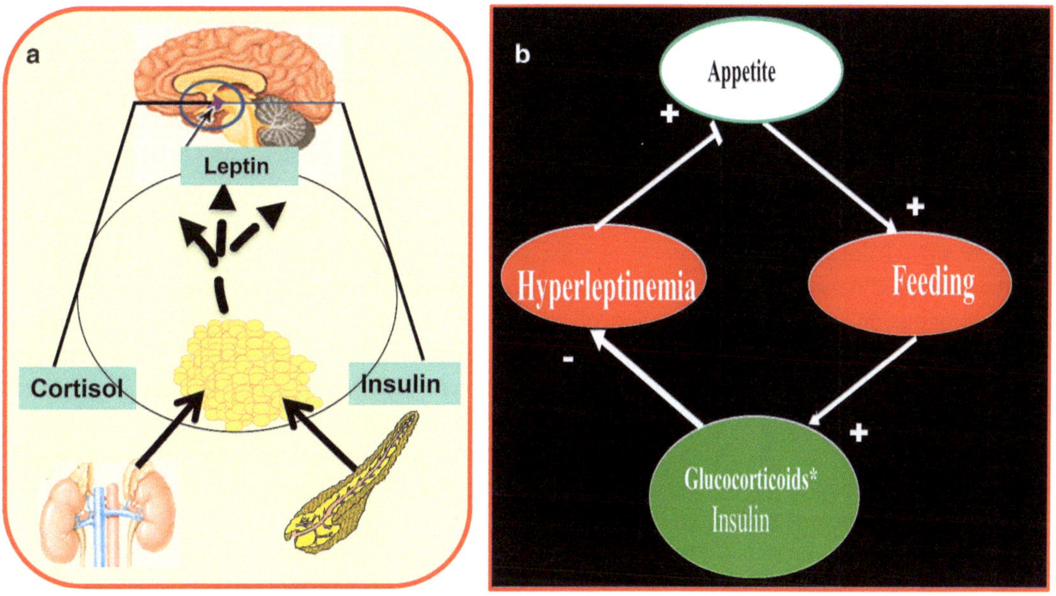

Fig. 15.3 The adrenoinsular-adipocyte axis. (**a**) Increased plasma insulin and cortisol levels in the postprandial period stimulate leptin secretion by adipocytes, which can induce satiety and prevent hunger between meals and during sleep. Leptin, glucocorticoids, and insulin have central effects on brain nuclei that modulate hunger, meal size, and satiety nuclei (*small circle*), in part, by altering neuropeptide Y expression. A peripheral feedback loop (*wider circle*) involves direct suppression of glucocorticoid and insulin secretion by leptin, thus ensuring homeostasis. (**b**) Model of diabetic dysleptinemia: Impaired insulin- and glucocorticoid-stimulated leptin secretion in patients with diabetes would be permissive of increased caloric intake, weight gain, insulin resistance, and worsening hyperglycemia. *Postprandial increase in free cortisol levels is well-documented [31–33]

The interaction between glucocorticoids and leptin can be conceptualized as having a direct short-loop and an indirect long-loop component. The short loop involves direct transcriptional activation of leptin gene, demonstrable in vitro, following glucocorticoid interaction with glucocorticoid receptors and glucocorticoid response element in adipocytes [34, 35, 45, 46]. No prior orexigenic signals or energy flux are required for activation of the short-loop pathway. On the other hand, the putative long loop operates indirectly by requires prior ingestive behavior (presumably driven by upregulation of hypothalamic NPY signal) before secretion of leptin can be triggered. Consistent with the preceding notion, the long-loop pathway to leptin secretion cannot be activated by glucocorticoids (even at pharmacological doses) under fasting conditions (Fig. 15.1) [26, 27].

Dynamic Leptin Secretion in Obesity

Common forms of acquired obesity in rodents and humans are characterized by hyperleptinemia, resulting from increased leptin synthesis and secretion by the abundant fat cell mass [47–51]. Notably, obesity is also associated with insulin resistance, hyperinsulinemia, and high risk for type 2 diabetes. There are parallels between the finding of hyperleptinemia in obese persons and the hyperinsulinemia of insulin resistance and early type 2 diabetes mellitus. Both conditions are characterized by the overexpression of a hormone that fails to regulate the desired physiological process—normoglycemia in diabetes and appetite and weight regulation in obesity. Because leptin has weight-reducing effects, the coexistence of hyperleptinemia and obesity is a physiological paradox that has generally been attributed to "leptin resistance" [52]. The mechanisms of leptin resistance are not fully understood, but factors such as mutations in post-receptor signaling [53] have been proposed. States of hormone resistance usually elicit hypersecretion of the index hormone, in a physiological attempt at compensation for the decreased hormone action. In the case of glucose regulation, most overweight and obese subjects with insulin resistance do not develop the sequela of diabetes, because they are able to maintain euglycemia through compensatory hyperinsulinemia. Those who progress to type 2 diabetes show a blunted insulin secretory response to a glucose challenge, even though their fasting insulin may be normal or elevated [54, 55].

Analogous to insulin resistance and progression to diabetes, many overweight or obese individuals maintain their body weight for long periods without progressing to higher degrees of obesity, whereas some progress to massive obesity. The factors that regulate progression from normal weight to obesity, and thence to massive or extreme obesity, are not fully understood. We, therefore, explored dynamic leptin secretion in 79 nondiabetic adults, of whom 27 were lean (BMI ≤25 kg/m^2), 28 were obese (BMI 30–40 kg/m^2), and 26 were massively obese (BMI >40 kg/m^2) [56]. For these experiments, we utilized two different leptin secretagogues: a single oral dose of dexamethasone [7, 8, 10] and insulin [34, 57].

During separate outpatient visits to the GCRC, each subjects received oral dexamethasone (4 mg), with blood sampling before, and after 8 and 16 h post-ingestion. For insulin as leptin secretagogue, subjects underwent a two-step hyperinsulinemic (1.0 mU kg^{-1}/min for 3 h, followed by 2.0 mU kg^{-1}/min), euglycemic (~100 mg/dl) clamp for 3 h. Blood samples were obtained at baseline and every 20 min during the clamp. The basal and peak leptin levels during dexamethasone or insulin treatment were higher in women than men, but the percentage increases from baseline were similar [56]. For both sexes, the peak leptin levels (% baseline) following dexamethasone ingestion were 178 ± 13.9 % in lean, 166 ± 10.5 % in obese, and 145 ± 10.4 % in massively obese subjects (P = 0.02 vs. lean and 0.05 vs. obese). Peak insulin-stimulated leptin levels were 152 ± 7.6 % in lean, 141 ± 5.9 % in obese, and 128 ± 3.7 % in massively obese subjects (P = 0.007 vs. lean and 0.035 vs. obese) [56]. Thus, despite being hyperleptinemic at baseline, obese and massively obese men and women were able to augment leptin levels in response to two separate secretagogues. However, the fold-increase over baseline leptin values is diminished among massively obese subjects compared with lean subjects (Fig. 15.4). These findings suggest that impaired dynamic leptin secretion might be one of the factors associated with transition to higher degrees of obesity.

Diabetic Dysleptinemia

Early suspicions that the hyperphagia of diabetes might be due to leptin deficiency were not borne out by subsequent studies that showed no gross leptin deficiency in patients with diabetes [58–60]. In our study [60], fasting blood specimens for measurement of leptin and other hormones were obtained at baseline from 65 healthy subjects and 54 diabetic patients (classified by C-peptide status: "negative" if <0.1 ng/ml or "positive" if >0.3 ng/ml, in fasting plasma). The results showed that basal plasma leptin levels were 13.4 ± 1.5 ng/ml in C-peptide negative patients and 26.1 ± 3.7 ng/ml in C-peptide positive patients, compared with 19.7 ± 2.3 ng/ml in nondiabetic subjects. Although the C-peptide negative patients had lower leptin levels (P = 0.001) than healthy subjects and C-peptide positive diabetic patients, the basal leptin levels reflected the BMI of subjects in the three groups, and the regression of leptin vs. BMI showed a similar relationship in healthy and diabetic subjects (Fig. 15.5a). Thus, fasting leptin levels are within the normal or expected range for BMI in persons with type 1 (C-peptide negative) or type 2 (C-peptide positive) diabetes. Our findings are in accord with other observations that plasma leptin levels generally lie within the expected range for BMI in patients with type 1(51) or type 2 diabetes [58, 59, 61], compared to gender-matched nondiabetic subjects.

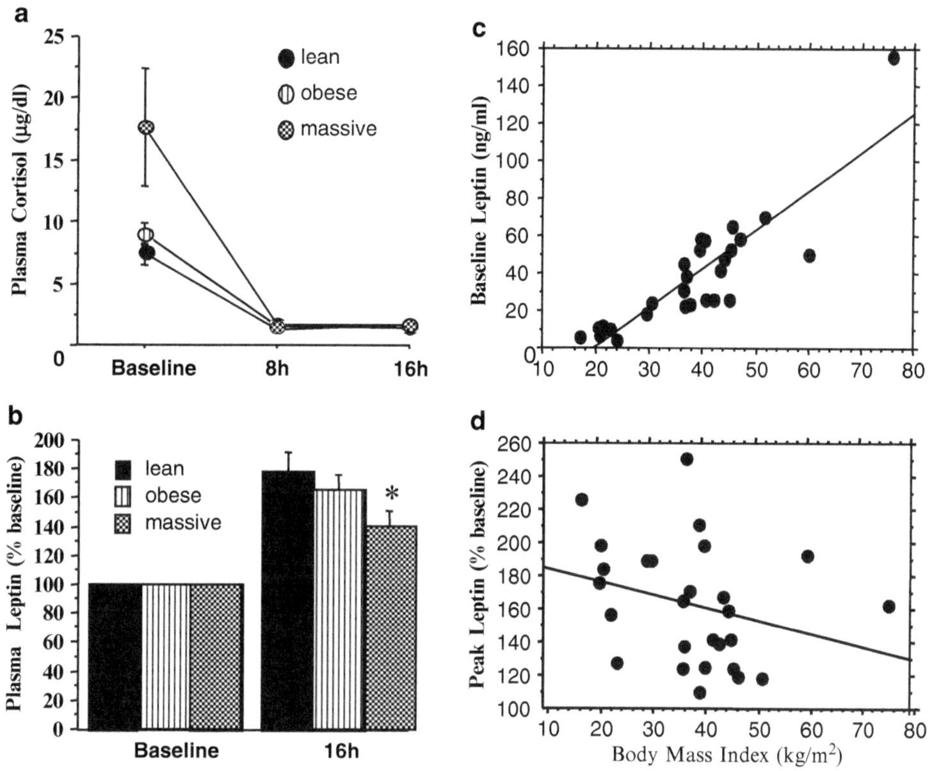

Fig. 15.4 Changes in plasma cortisol (**a**) and leptin (**b**) following dexamethasone ingestion in lean, obese, and massively obese subjects, and the relationship between body mass index (BMI) and baseline (fasting) plasma leptin (**c**) or post-dexamethasone leptin levels (**d**). Baseline (fasting) leptin levels were positively correlated with BMI ($R^2=0.76$) but peak dexamethasone-stimulated leptin levels showed a trend toward an inverse correlation. *$P=0.02$ vs. lean and 0.05 vs. obese. Adapted from Dagogo-Jack S, Askari H, Tykodi G, Liu J, Umamaheswaran I [56]

As is well-known, patients with type 2 diabetes have normal or elevated plasma insulin levels in the basal (fasting) state, but show defective dynamic insulin secretion in response to iv or oral glucose [54, 55, 62, 63]. To determine whether an analogous situation exists with regard to leptin regulation, we obtained blood specimens before and 8, 16, and 40 h following ingestion of a single dose (4 mg) of dexamethasone in healthy and diabetic subjects, classified by C-peptide status [60]. The peak plasma leptin level (as a percentage of basal values) following dexamethasone challenge was 224±18 % in healthy subjects, 126±23 % in C-peptide negative diabetic patients, and 144±16 % in C-peptide positive diabetic patients [60] (Fig. 15.5b). Compared to nondiabetic subjects, the peak glucocorticoid-stimulated leptin responses were lower in C-peptide positive diabetic patients ($P=0.011$) and C-peptide negative patients ($P=0.003$) (Fig. 15.5b). These results indicate that diabetes is associated with normal basal leptin levels, but markedly attenuated dynamic leptin secretion following glucocorticoid stimulation. We have proposed the term, "diabetic dysleptinemia," to describe the defective dynamic leptin secretion in diabetes.

Cause or Consequence

With the known postprandial increases in plasma insulin and cortisol [31–33], the resultant increase in plasma leptin, driven by the two hormones, could serve a physiological role of restraining appetite between meals and during sleep. Based

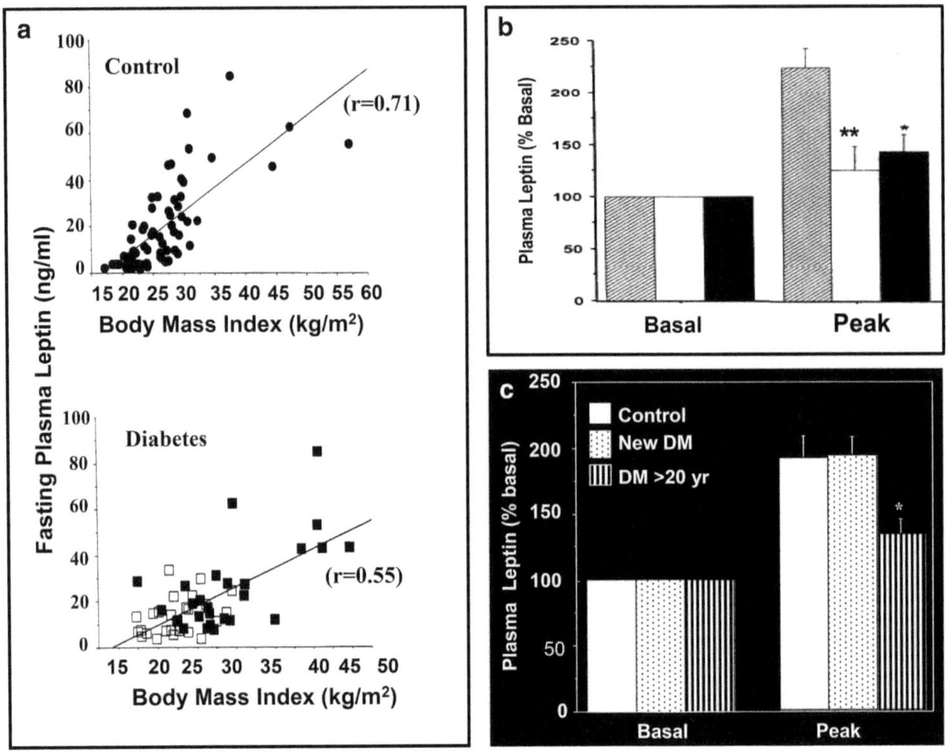

Fig. 15.5 Basal and stimulated plasma leptin levels in healthy and diabetic subjects: (**a**) regression of fasting leptin vs. BMI in nondiabetic subjects (*upper panel*), C-peptide negative diabetic patients (*lower panel*, *open squares*) and C-peptide diabetic positive patients (*lower panel*, *closed squares*); (**b**) Plasma leptin responses to a single oral dose (4 mg) of dexamethasone in nondiabetic subjects (*hatched bars*), C-peptide negative diabetic patients (*open bars*) and C-peptide diabetic positive patients (*closed bars*). The peak leptin response (% baseline) was 224 ± 18 % in healthy subjects, 126 ± 23 % in C-peptide negative diabetic patients, and 144 ± 16 % in C-peptide positive diabetic patients; (**c**) Dexamethasone-stimulated plasma leptin responses among healthy controls (white bars), newly diagnosed type 2 diabetes patients (*stippled bars*), and patients with type 2diabetes of >20 years duration (*striped bars*). $*P=0.01$, $**P=0.003$ vs. nondiabetic controls. Adapted from Liu J, Askari H, Dagogo-Jack S [60] and Dagogo-Jack S, Liu J, Askari H, Tykodi G, Umamaheswaran I [66]

on the physiological understanding of leptin as an endogenous satiety factor with anti-obesity and insulin-sensitizing properties [43, 44, 64, 65], impaired dynamic leptin secretory secretion could be a risk factor for hyperphagia, obesity, and insulin resistance. To determine whether such a secretory defect precedes or follows the diagnosis of diabetes, we studied 37 adults: 11 with type 2 DM diagnosed within 6 months prior to study, 16 with chronic (≥20 yr) type 2 DM, and 10 healthy controls [66]. After baseline measurements, study subjects ingested a single dose (4 mg) of dexamethasone, followed by blood sampling for assay of leptin and other hormones and metabolites. The peak dexamethasone stimulated plasma leptin responses (% baseline) were 188 ± 18.7 % among healthy controls, 180 ± 13.8 % among newly diagnosed type 2 DM patients, and 127 ± 10.5 % ($P<0.01$) in chronic DM patients [66] (Fig. 15.5c). Following dexamethasone ingestion, plasma insulin increased significantly in control subjects and newly diagnosed type 2 diabetes patients, but not in patients with chronic DM [66]. These results indicate that plasma leptin responses to glucocorticoid challenge are preserved in patients with newly diagnosed type 2 DM but markedly attenuated in patients with long-standing diabetes, who also were unable to augment insulin secretion during glucocorticoid treatment.

Data from Insulin as Leptin Secretagogue

To extend the findings from the preceding studies, we tested the effects of insulin as a leptin secretagogue. Previous studies have established that insulin is a weaker leptin secretagogue than glucocorticoids (peak effect ~50 % above baseline vs. ~100 % above baseline) [34, 57]. With that in mind, we investigated whether leptin secretory responses to insulin would show evidence of dysleptinemia along the lines observed with glucocorticoid. Using oral glucose tolerance tests, we screened 64 subjects with previously unknown glycemic status, and enrolled three groups of subjects matched for age, gender, and BMI: Group I: subjects with normal glucose tolerance (NGT) (age 43.6±4.80 yr, BMI 36.6±4.93 kg/m^2, N=6); Group II: subjects with impaired glucose tolerance (IGT) (age 40.2±4.95 yr, BMI 36.2±5.10 kg/m^2, N=6); Group III: subjects with newly diagnosed T2DM (age 42.5±5.0 yr, BMI 33.4±3.37 kg/m^2, N=6) [67]. The subjects were not taking any diabetes medications or drugs known to affect leptin or glucoregulatory metabolism. The study subjects underwent a two-step hyperinsulinemic (1.0 mU kg^{-1}/min for 3 h, followed by 2.0 mU kg^{-1}/min for 3 h), euglycemic (~100 mg/dl). Blood samples were obtained at baseline and every 20 min during the clamp. The peak insulin-stimulated leptin levels (% baseline) were 145±2.67 %% in NGT control subjects, 151±6.74 % in IGT subjects, and 125±1.30 % in newly diagnosed T2DM patients (P=0.005 vs. NGT and IGT groups) (Fig. 15.6). Thus, plasma leptin responses during hyperinsulinemic clamp were similar in NGT and IGT subjects, but were decreased significantly in patients with newly diagnosed T2DM. Malmstrom et al. [68] measured plasma leptin concentrations during an 8.5-h hyperinsulinemic clamp or saline infusion in eight healthy subjects (age 51±3 yr, BMI 26.3±0.6 kg/m^2) and seven patients with T2DM (age 54±2 yr, BMI 27.0±0.9 kg/m^2, fasting plasma glucose 11.1±0.8 mmol/L). Plasma leptin levels decreased significantly during 8.5 h of saline infusion. During insulin infusion, plasma leptin concentrations (% above saline control) were 32±13 %, 53±14 %, 106±15 %, and

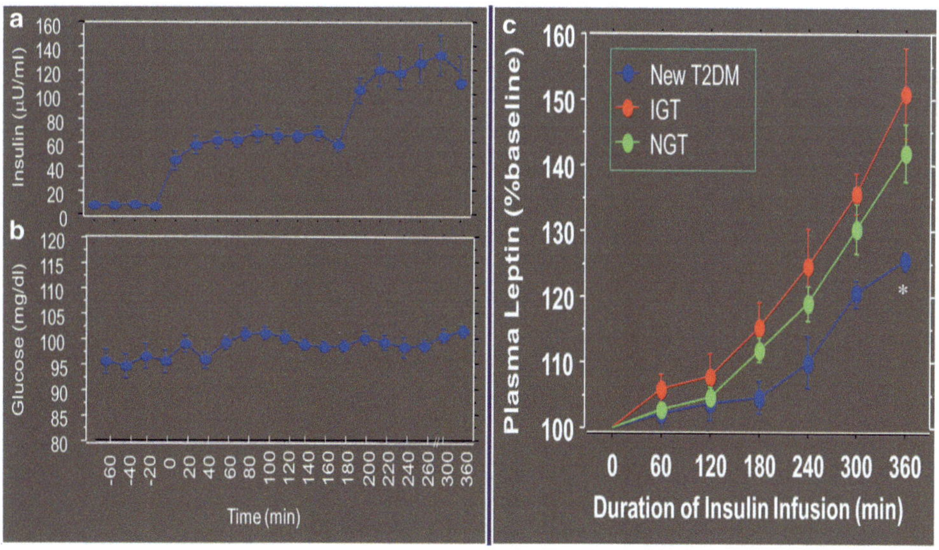

Fig. 15.6 Plasma levels of insulin (**a**) and glucose (**b**) during two-step hyperinsulinemic (1.0 mU kg^{-1}/min for 3 h, followed by 2.0 mU kg^{-1}/min for 3 h), euglycemic (~100 mg/dl) clamp; (**c**) plasma leptin responses during two-step hyperinsulinemic in subjects with normal glucose tolerance (NGT), impaired glucose tolerance (IGT), and type 2 diabetes (T2DM). *P=0.005 vs. NGT and IGT groups

165 ± 21 % at 2 h, 4 h, 6 h and 8.5 h in the healthy subjects, and 11 ± 9 %, 27 ± 10 %, 58 ± 7 %, and 106 ± 13 % in the patients with T2DM, respectively [68]. The plasma leptin response to insulin infusion at every time point was numerically lower in the diabetic patients, and there was a nominal 59 % reduction in the peak leptin secretory response to prolonged insulin infusion in the diabetic patients, compared to healthy controls [68]. Other workers have reported impaired leptin secretion in patients with poorly controlled diabetes [69], as well as defective postprandial leptin secretion in patients with type 1 diabetes, which was improved by preprandial injections of rapid acting insulin [70].

Although diabetic dysleptinemia was first demonstrated, using glucocorticoid as the leptin secretagogue in patients with long-standing diabetes [60, 66], the defect can also be demonstrated with insulin. Furthermore, the leptin response to insulin was found to be impaired in patients with newly diagnosed, but not subjects with prediabetes (IGT) [67]. Taken together, these observations indicate that diabetic dysleptinemia is most probably an acquired defect, rather than a causal factor in the etiology of diabetes. The exact pathogenesis of dysleptinemia remains to be elucidated; however, current evidence suggests that insulin deficiency, insulin resistance, glucotoxicity, and the duration as well as state of metabolic control of diabetes may all be contributory factors. Even with the notion of dysleptinemia as a consequence rather than a causal factor in diabetes, the persistence of diabetic dysleptinemia could, theoretically, be permissive of hyperphagia, progressive weight gain, insulin resistance, and worsening dysglycemia.

Apart from the lone report of the effect of preprandial rapid acting insulin [70], no formal studies have been undertaken to test interventions for the reversal or amelioration diabetic dysleptinemia. The role of β-cell function (insulin secretion) in orchestrating the leptin responsiveness to glucocorticoid is strongly suggested by several lines of evidence [26, 27, 66, 70]. Impaired flux through the nutrient-sensing hexosamine pathway during states of insulin deficiency, insulin resistance, or glucotoxicity would decrease the abundance of intracellular UDP-N-acetylglucosamine, a mediator of adipocyte leptin secretion [71–74]. Also, perturbations along the inositol pathway [75] might be involved in the mechanism of diabetic dysleptinemia. Two families of inositol phosphoglycans (IPG-A and IPG-B) serve as second messengers in the insulin signaling cascade. The ratio of IPG-A/IPG-B is elevated in obesity and type 2 diabetes; IPG-A inhibits leptin secretion from adipocytes [75]. Thus, in addition to limitation of glucose metabolism and nutrient sensing along the hexosamine pathway [71–74], the elevated IPG-A levels in diabetic subjects [75] could contribute to impaired leptin secretion.

The rational deployment of exogenous leptin therapy requires careful selection of individuals who are most likely to benefit from such therapy. Persons with congenital leptin deficiency [64, 65] and lipodystrophy [76, 77] are prime examples. Outside the latter groups, one approach would be to target patients who manifest evidence of relative leptin deficiency. In this regard, the demonstration of impaired dynamic leptin secretion among subsets of obese and diabetic subjects [56, 60, 66–70] suggests a possible screening strategy for the selection of subjects for an intervention trial. Notably, current experience from nontargeted human trials of recombinant leptin therapy indicates modest and markedly variable efficacy on weight and metabolic parameters [36, 78]. With the recent approval of Metreleptin for clinical use, it should become feasible to design studies to test the metabolic effects of targeted leptin augmentation therapy in carefully selected patients with evidence of dysleptinemia.

Acknowledgements The author gratefully acknowledges the sacrifice of research volunteers and the research grants from the National Institutes of Health and the American Diabetes Association that enabled his studies on the metabolic significance of leptin in humans.

References

1. Guyenet SJ, Schwartz MW. Clinical review: regulation of food intake, energy balance, and body fat mass: implications for the pathogenesis and treatment of obesity. J Clin Endocrinol Metab. 2012;97:745–55.

2. Bray GA, York DA. Hypothalamic and genetic obesity in experimental animals: an autonomic and endocrine hypothesis. Physiol Rev. 1979;59:719–809.
3. Kopelman PG. Neuroendocrine function in obesity. Clin Endocrinol. 1988;28:675–98.
4. Lamberts SW, Birkenhager JC. Body composition in Cushing's syndrome. J Clin Endocrinol Metab. 1976; 42:864–8.
5. Ross IL, Levitt NS. Addison's disease symptoms—a cross sectional study in urban South Africa. PLoS One. 2013. doi:10.1371/journal.pone.0053526. Epub 2013 Jan 7.
6. Baid SK, Rubino D, Sinaii N, Ramsey S, Frank A, Nieman LK. Specificity of screening tests for Cushing's syndrome in an overweight and obese population. J Clin Endocrinol Metab. 2009;94:3857–64.
7. Larsson H, Ahren B. Short-term dexamethasone increases plasma leptin independently of changes in insulin sensitivity in healthy women. J Clin Endocrinol Metab. 1996;81:4428–32.
8. Miell JP, Englaro P, Blum WF. Dexamethasone induces an acute and sustained rise in circulating leptin levels in normal human subjects. Horm Metab Res. 1996;28:704–7.
9. Kolaczynski JW, Goldstein BJ, Considine RV. Dexamethasone, OB gene, and leptin in humans; effect of exogenous hyperinsulinemia. J Clin Endocrinol Metab. 1997;82:3895–7.
10. Dagogo-Jack S, Selke G, Melson AK, Newcomer JW. Robust leptin secretory responses to dexamethasone in obese subjects. J Clin Endocrinol Metab. 1997;82:3230–3.
11. Papaspyrou-Rao S, Schneider SH, Petersen RN, Fried SK. Dexamathasone increases leptin expression in humans in vivo. J Clin Endocrinol Metab. 1997;82: 1635–7.
12. Masuzaki H, Ogawa Y, Hosoda K, et al. Glucocorticoid regulation of leptin synthesis and secretion in humans: elevated plasma leptin levels in Cushing's syndrome. J Clin Endocrinol Metab. 1997;82:2542–7.
13. Berneis K, Vosmeer S, Keller U. Effects of glucocorticoids and of growth hormone on serum leptin concentration in man. Eur J Endocrinol. 1996;135: 663–5.
14. Bornstein SR, Licinio J, Tauchnitz R, et al. Plasma leptin levels are increased in survivors of acute sepsis: associated loss of diurnal rhythm in cortisol and leptin secretion. J Clin Endocrinol Metab. 1997;83:280–3.
15. Widjaja A, Schurmeyer TH, Von Zur Muhlenh A, Brabant G. Determinants of serum leptin levels in Cushing's syndrome. J Clin Endocrinol Metab. 1998; 83:600–3.
16. Cizza G, Lotsikas AJ, Licinio J, Gold PW, Chrousos GP. Plasma leptin levels do not change in patients with Cushing's disease after correction of hypercortisolism. J Clin Endocrinol Metab. 1997;82:2747–50.
17. Newcomer JW, Selke G, Melson AK, Gross J, Volger GP, Dagogo-Jack S. Dose-dependent cortisol-induced increases in plasma leptin concentration in healthy humans. Arch Gen Psychiatry. 1998;55:995–1000.
18. Kieffer TJ, Heller RS, Leech CA, Holz GG, Habener JF. Leptin suppression of insulin secretion by activation of ATP-sensitive K+ channels in pancreatic beta-cells. Diabetes. 1997;46:1087–93.
19. Stephens TW, Basinski M, Bristow PK, et al. The role of neuropeptide Y in the antiobesity action of the obese gene product. Nature. 1995;377:530–2.
20. Pralong FP, Roduit R, Waeber G, et al. Leptin inhibits directly glucocorticoid secretion by normal human and rat adrenal gland. Endocrinology. 1998;139:4264–8.
21. De Vos P, Saladin R, Auwerx J, Staels B. Induction of ob gene expression by corticosteroids is accompanied by body weight loss and reduced food intake. J Biol Chem. 1995;270:15958–61.
22. Wolf G. The molecular mechanism of the stimulation of adipocyte differentiation by a glucocorticoid. Nutr Rev. 1999;57:324–6.
23. Stevens W, Grosser GI, Reed DJ. Corticosterone-binding moleculess in rat brain cytosols. Regional distribution. Brain Res. 1971;35:602–7.
24. Schwartz MW, Baskin DG, Bukowski TR, et al. Specificity of leptin action on elevated blood glucose levels and hypothalamic neuropeptide Y gene expression in *ob/ob* mice. Diabetes. 1996;45:531–5.
25. Wilding JPH, Gilbey SG, Lambert PD, Ghatei MA, Bloom SR. Increases in neuropeptide Y content and gene expression in the hypothalamus of rats treated with dexamethasone are prevented by insulin. Neuroendocrinology. 1993;57:581–7.
26. Dagogo-Jack S, Umamaheswaran I, Askari H, Tykodi G. Leptin response to glucocorticoid occurs at physiological doses and is abolished by fasting. Obes Res. 2003;11:232–7.
27. Laferrère B, Fried SK, Hough K, Campbell SA, Thornton J, Pi-Sunyer FX. Synergistic effects of feeding and dexamethasone on serum leptin levels. J Clin Endocrinol Metab. 1998;83:3742–5.
28. Dagogo-Jack S, Tykodi G, Umamaheswaran I. Inhibition of cortisol biosynthesis decreases circulating leptin levels in obese humans. J Clin Endocrinol Metab. 2005;90:5333–5.
29. Laferrère B, Abraham C, Awad M, et al. Inhibiting endogenous cortisol blunts the meal-entrained rise in serum leptin. J Clin Endocrinol Metab. 2006;91: 2232–8.
30. Askari H, Liu J, Dagogo-Jack S. Energy adaptation to glucocorticoid-induced hyperleptinemia in human beings. Metabolism. 2005;54:876–80.
31. Kirschbaum C, Bono EG, Rohleder N, et al. Effects of fasting and glucose load on free cortisol responses to stress and nicotine. J Clin Endocrinol Metab. 1997; 82:1101–5.
32. Rosmond R, Chagnon YC, Holm G, et al. A glucocorticoid receptor gene marker is associated with abdominal obesity, leptin, and dysregulation of the hypothalamic-pituitary-adrenal axis. Obes Res. 2000; 8:211–8.
33. Stimson RH, Mohd-Shukri NA, Bolton JL, Andrew R, Reynolds RM, Walker BR. The postprandial rise in plasma cortisol in men is mediated by macronutrient-

specific stimulation of adrenal and extra-adrenal cortisol production. J Clin Endocrinol Metab. 2014; 99:160–8.
34. Askari H, Liu J, Dagogo-Jack S. Hormonal regulation of human leptin in vivo: effects of hydrocortisone and insulin. Int J Obes Relat Metab Disord. 2000;24: 1254–9.
35. Considine RV, Nyce MR, Kolaczynski JW, et al. Dexamethasone stimulates leptin release from human adipocytes: unexpected inhibition by insulin. J Cell Biochem. 1997;65:254–8.
36. Heymsfield SB, Greenberg AS, Fujioka K, et al. Recombinant leptin for weight loss in obese and lean adults: a randomized, controlled, dose escalation trial. JAMA. 1999;282:1568–75.
37. Dagogo-Jack S. Human leptin regulation and promise in pharmacotherapy. Curr Drug Targets. 2001;2: 181–95.
38. Spencer RL, Young EA, Choo PH, McEwen BS. Adrenal steroid type I and type II receptor binding: estimates of in vivo receptor number, occupancy, and activation with varying levels of steroid. Brain Res. 1990;514:37–48.
39. Zarjevski N, Cusin I, Vettor A, Rohner-Jeanrenaud F, Jeanrenaud B. Chronic intracerebroventricular neuropeptide-Y administration to normal rats mimics hormonal and metabolic changes of obesity. Endocrinology. 1993;133:1753–8.
40. Schwartz MW, Woods SC, Porte D, Seeley RJ, Baskin DG. Central nervous system control of food intake. Nature. 2000;404:661–71.
41. Kalra SP, Dube MG, Pu S, Xu B, Horvath TL, Kalra PS. Interacting appetite-regulating pathways in the hypothalmic regulation of body weight. Endocr Rev. 1999;20:68–100.
42. List JF, Habener JF. Defective melanocortin 4 receptors in hyperphagia and morbid obesity. N Engl J Med. 2003;348:1160–6.
43. Halaas JL, Gajiwala KS, Maffei M, et al. Weight-reducing effects of the plasma protein encoded by the obese gene. Science. 1995;269:543–6.
44. Pelleymounter MA, Cullen MJ, Baker MB, et al. Effects of the obese gene product on body weight regulation in ob/ob mice. Science. 1995;269: 540–3.
45. Kronfeld-Schor N, Zhao J, Silva BA, et al. Steroid-dependent upregulation of adipose tissue leptin secretion in vitro during pregnancy in mice. Biol Reprod. 2000;63:274–80.
46. Feldman D, Loose D. Glucocorticoid receptors in adipose tissue. Endocrinology. 1977;100:398–405.
47. Lonnqvist F, Aener P, Nordfors L, Schalling M. Overexpression of the obese (ob) gene in adipose tissue of obese subjects. Nat Med. 1995;1:950–3.
48. Hamilton BS, Paglia D, Kwan AYM, Deitel M. Increased obese mRNA expression in omental fat cells from massively obese humans. Nat Med. 1995; 1:953–6.
49. Considine RV, Sinha MK, Heiman ML, et al. Serum immunoreactive-leptin concentrations in normal-weight and obese humans. N Engl J Med. 1996; 334:292–5.
50. Dagogo-Jack S, Fanelli C, Paramore D, Brothers J, Landt M. Plasma leptin and insulin relationships in obese and nonobese humans. Diabetes. 1996;45: 695–8.
51. Schwartz MW, Peskind E, Boyko EJ, Porte Jr D. Cerebrospinal fluid leptin levels: relationship to plasma levels and to adiposity in humans. Nat Med. 1996;2:589–93.
52. Caro JF, Kolaczynski JW, Nyce MR, et al. Decreased cerebrospinal-fluid/serum leptin ratio in obesity: a possible mechanism for leptin resistance. Lancet. 1996;348:159–61.
53. Yang Z, Hulver M, McMillan RP, et al. Regulation of insulin and leptin signaling by muscle suppressor of cytokine signaling 3 (SOCS3). PLoS One. 2012. doi:10.1371/journal.pone.0047493.
54. Porte D. Banting lecture 1990: beta-cells in type II diabetes mellitus. Diabetes. 1991;40:166–80.
55. Defronzo RA. Banting lecture. From the triumvirate to the ominous octet: a new paradigm for the treatment of type 2 diabetes mellitus. Diabetes. 2009; 58:773–95.
56. Dagogo-Jack S, Askari H, Tykodi G, Liu J, Umamaheswaran I. Dynamic responses to leptin secretagogues in lean, obese, and massively obese men and women. Horm Res. 2008;70:174–81.
57. Saad MF, Khan A, Sharma A, et al. Physiological insulinemia acutely modulates plasma leptin. Diabetes. 1998;47:544–9.
58. Haffner SM, Stern MP, Miettinen H, Wei M, Gingerich RL. Leptin concentrations in diabetic and nondiabetic Mexican-Americans. Diabetes. 1996;45:822–4.
59. Widjaja A, Stratton IM, Horn R, Holman RR, Turner R, Brabant G. UKPDS 20: plasma leptin, obesity, and plasma insulin in type 2 diabetic subjects. J Clin Endocrinol Metab. 1997;82:654–7.
60. Liu J, Askari H, Dagogo-Jack S. Basal and stimulated plasma leptin in diabetic subjects. Obes Res. 1999; 7:537–44.
61. Sinha MK, Ohannesian JP, Heiman ML, et al. Nocturnal rise of leptin in lean, obese, and non-insulin-dependent diabetes mellitus subjects. J Clin Invest. 1996;97:1344–7.
62. Pfeifer MA, Halter JB, Porte Jr D. Insulin secretion in diabetes mellitus. Am J Med. 1981;70:578–88.
63. Weyer C, Bogardus C, Mott DM, Pratley RE. The natural history of insulin secretory dysfunction and insulin resistance in the pathogenesis of type 2 diabetes. J Clin Invest. 1999;104:787–94.
64. Farooqi IS, Matarese G, Lord GM, et al. Beneficial effects of leptin on obesity, T cell hyporesponsiveness, and neuroendocrine/metabolic dysfunction of human congenital leptin deficiency. J Clin Invest. 2002;110:1093–103.
65. Licinio J, Caglayan S, Ozata M. Phenotypic effects of leptin replacement on morbid obesity, diabetes mellitus, hypogonadism, and behavior in leptin-deficient adults. Proc Natl Acad Sci U S A. 2004;101:4531–6.

66. Dagogo-Jack S, Liu J, Askari H, Tykodi G, Umamaheswaran I. Impaired leptin response to glucocorticoid as a chronic complication of diabetes. J Diabetes Complications. 2000;14:1–6.
67. Tykodi G, Askari H. Dagogo-Jack S. Impaired leptin response to insulin in newly diagnosed type 2 diabetes. Endocrine Society. 87th Annual Scientific Meetings, San Diego, CA, June 2005. Abstract # P2-701.
68. Malmstrom R, Taskinen MR, Karonen SL, Yki-Jarvinen H. Insulin increases plasma leptin concentrations in normal subjects and patients with NIDDM. Diabetologia. 1996;39:993–6.
69. Clement K, Lahlou N, Ruiz J, et al. Association of poorly controlled diabetes with low serum leptin in morbid obesity. Int J Obes. 1997;21:556–61.
70. Griffen SC, Oostema K, Stanhope KL, et al. Administration of Lispro insulin with meals improves glycemic control, increases circulating leptin, and suppresses ghrelin, compared with regular/NPH insulin in female patients with type 1 diabetes. J Clin Endocrinol Metab. 2006;91:485–91.
71. Mueller WM, Gregoire F, Stanhope KL, et al. Evidence that glucose metabolism regulates leptin secretion from cultured adipocytes. Endocrinology. 1998;139:551–8.
72. Patel BK, Koenig JI, Kaplan LM, Hooi SC. Increase in plasma leptin and Lep mRNA concentrations by food intake is dependent on insulin. Metabolism. 1998;47:603–7.
73. Rossetti L. Perspective: hexosamines and nutrient sensing. Endocrinology. 2000;141:1922–5.
74. Wellhoener P, Fruehwald-Schultes B, Kern W, et al. Glucose metabolism rather than insulin is a main determinant of leptin secretion in humans. J Clin Endocrinol Metab. 2000;85:1267–71.
75. Kunjara S, Wang DY, Mclean P, Greenbaum AL, Rademacher TW. Inositol phosphoglycans and the regulation of the secretion of leptin: in vitro effects on leptin release from adipocytes and the relationship to obesity. Mol Genet Metab. 2000;70:61–8.
76. Oral EA, Simha V, Ruiz E, et al. Leptin-replacement therapy for lipodystrophy. N Engl J Med. 2002; 346:570–8.
77. Javor ED, Cochran EK, Musso C, Young JR, Depaoli AM, Gorden P. Long-term efficacy of leptin replacement in patients with generalized lipodystrophy. Diabetes. 2005;54:1994–2002.
78. Moon HS, Dalamaga M, Kim SY, et al. Leptin's role in lipodystrophic and nonlipodystrophic insulin-resistant and diabetic individuals. Endocr Rev. 2013; 34:377–412.

Leptin Therapy in People with Congenital Leptin Deficiency

16

Gilberto Paz-Filho and Julio Licinio

Introduction

Adipose tissue is not just a store of fat, but it is also an endocrine organ, where adipokines are synthesized [1]. Although excess fat (obesity) leads to complications such as diabetes [2], cardiovascular disease [3] and cancer [4], its absence can also cause disease, due to low levels of adipokines.

Leptin is one of the most abundant adipokines, and in its absence, severe and potentially lethal disruptions in body homeostasis occur [5]. Leptin has crucial roles in regulating body weight and energy balance, reproduction, glucose homeostasis, tissue remodeling, and inflammation, as well as in other elements of the endocrine and immune systems [5]. Leptin is an indicator of the size of somatic energy stores (fat mass), and is a major contributor to the regulation of energy balance [6]. Leptin deficiency is a cause of several diseases, such as lipodystrophy syndromes, functional hypothalamic amenorrhea, and congenital leptin deficiency due to mutations in the leptin gene [7].

Congenital leptin deficiency (CLD) is a rare condition, caused by mutations in the leptin gene that result in the synthesis of biologically inactive truncated proteins. The phenotype of patients with mutations in the leptin gene is diverse, and include manifestations such as diabetes, dyslipidaemia, hormonal deficiencies, impaired cognitive development, and potentially lethal T-cell hyporesponsiveness [7–13].

Leptin replacement therapy (LRT) with recombinant human leptin is the only available treatment for CLD. The study of the effects of LRT represent an unparalleled human experimental model of endocrine-based obesity, and has promoted a better understanding of leptin's physiology, providing the basis for the development of novel potential therapies for obesity, diabetes, and neurodegenerative disorders.

Forms of Partial Leptin Deficiency

The complete absence of leptin is seen in cases of CLD, but relative leptin deficiency is also observed in cases of lipodystrophy and functional hypothalamic amenorrhea. In lipodystrophy, fat mass is decreased due to molecular defects in genes that regulate adipocyte differentiation, lipid metabolism, and lipid droplet morphology [5], or to the use of highly active antiretroviral therapy (HAART).

G. Paz-Filho, M.D. (✉)
The John Curtin School of Medical Research, Australian National University, Garran Rd, Building 131, Canberra, ACT 0200, Australia
e-mail: gilbertjpf@hotmail.com

J. Licinio, M.D.
Mind and Brain Theme, South Australian Health and Medical Research Institute, Adelaide, SA, Australia

Department of Psychiatry, Flinders University, Adelaide, SA, Australia
e-mail: Julio.licinio@sahmri.com

S. Dagogo-Jack (ed.), *Leptin: Regulation and Clinical Applications*,
DOI 10.1007/978-3-319-09915-6_16, © Springer International Publishing Switzerland 2015

Functional hypothalamic amenorrhea is a state of energy deprivation, usually associated with exercise, in the absence of organic disease or ovarian failure, where reduced leptin levels lead to impaired secretion of gonadotropin-releasing hormone and reproductive dysfunction. These features are similar to those of individuals with anorexia nervosa, where fat mass is reduced due to energy deprivation. In all conditions (including non-athletic forms of hypothalamic amenorrhea), fat mass is decreased, which determine substantial reductions in serum leptin levels [14].

Congenital Leptin Deficiency Pretreatment Phenotype

Cases of CLD caused by mutation in the leptin gene are rare. To date, mutations leading to the leptin-deficient phenotype have been reported in children of Pakistani [15–20], Egyptian [21], Austrian [22], and Turkish origins [10, 23, 24]. Worldwide, a total of 34 patients with CLD have been described in the literature, harboring eight different mutations (Table 16.1).

For over 15 years, our group has been evaluating the phenotypic findings and effects of leptin replacement in four unique leptin-deficient adults from a consanguineous extended Turkish family [7]. These individuals have a Mendelian recessive mutation in the leptin gene, consisting of a C→T substitution in codon 105 of this gene (the same that is observed in the leptin-deficient *ob/ob* mouse), resulting in an Arg→Trp replacement in the mature protein.

Initially, a 22-year-old male, and two females (34 and 6 years old), from the same highly consanguineous Turkish family, were identified with a homozygous mutation in the leptin gene [24]. The male patient had a body mass index (BMI) of 55.8 kg/m^2, and very low leptin levels (0.9 ng/ml). The female adult had a BMI of 46.9 kg/m^2, and equally low serum leptin levels (1.6 ng/ml). The girl had a BMI of 32.6 kg/m^2, and low leptin levels of 1.1 ng/ml. Both adult patients had hypogonadotropic hypogonadism, and the three patients were hyperinsulinemic. The girl had subclinical hypothyroidism, and the female was diagnosed with type 2 diabetes.

Further investigation in the same family led to the diagnosis of CLD in two additional family members who harbored the same mutation in homozygosity: a 30-year-old female [23] and a 5-year-old male [10], who had a similar phenotype, with extremely high BMI (54.8 kg/m^2 and 39.6 kg/m^2, respectively), hyperphagia, and low leptin levels (0.6 ng/ml in the female, undetectable in the child). The female patient also had hypogonadotropic hypogonadism, and all patients had sympathetic system dysfunction (assessed by cold pressor response test, orthostatic hypotension test, and sympathetic skin response test).

Leptin Replacement Therapy

In the leptin-deficient *ob/ob* mouse model, the obese phenotype is prevented or reversed by the administration of exogenous leptin [25]. Physiological doses of recombinant methionyl human leptin (metreleptin, Myalept®, Amylin Pharmaceuticals, USA; now owned by AstraZeneca) were initiated on these leptin-deficient individuals at ages 5 (boy), 27 (male), 30 and 40 (females). The girl that had been initially described died before treatment could be initiated. Treatment led to significant improvements in weight, endocrine function, and behavior [8]. Leptin replacement was lifesaving, as eight members of this family with severe early-onset obesity, whom we presume to have been leptin-deficient, died during childhood due to infections and sepsis. In the Turkish cohort of patients with CLD, treatment was initiated with metreleptin 0.02–0.04 mg/kg/day, administered once a day subcutaneously, at 6 p.m. That time in the evening was chosen to mimic leptin's normal circadian rhythm, which peak occurs at early in the morning around 2 a.m. [26]. In adults, this dose increases serum leptin to levels that are observed in healthy adult males with 20 % body fat, or in healthy adult females with 30 % body fat. The child's initial dose was calculated to increase the peak serum leptin to 70 ng/ml. Patients were evaluated regularly and doses were then recalculated, avoiding excessively rapid weight loss.

Table 16.1 List of individuals with congenital leptin deficiency and their respective mutations

Article where patients were first reported (first author, year)	Number of patients	Ethnicity	Mutation
Montague, 1997 Farooqi, 2002 Gibson, 2004	4 (2 M, 2 F)	Pakistani	Homozygous frame-shift mutation consisting of a deletion of a G nucleotide in codon 133 (delta133G)
Farooqi, 2008[a]	4	Pakistani	Homozygous frame-shift mutation consisting of a deletion of a G nucleotide in codon 133 (delta133G)
Strobel, 1998 Ozata, 1999 Paz-Filho, 2008	5[b] (2 M, 3 F)	Turkish	Homozygous missense mutation consisting of a C to T substitution in codon 105 (R105W)
Fischer-Posovzky, 2010	1 F	Austrian	Homozygous missense mutation consisting of a T to C substitution in codon 72 (L72S)
Mazen, 2009	1 M	Egyptian	Homozygous missense mutation consisting of a C to A substitution in codon 103 (N103K)
Fatima, 2011	7 (4 M, 3 F)	Pakistani	Homozygous frame-shift mutation consisting of a deletion of a G nucleotide in codon 133 (delta133G)
Fatima, 2011	1 M	Pakistani	Homozygous frame-shift mutation consisting of deletions of CT nucleotides in codon 161 (delta161CT)
Fatima, 2011	1 F	Pakistani	Homozygous frame-shift mutation consisting of deletions of TC nucleotides in codons 35 and 36 (delta36TC)
Saeed, 2012	9 (5 M, 4 F)	Pakistani	Homozygous frame-shift mutation consisting of a deletion of a G nucleotide in codon 398
Saeed, 2012	1 F	Pakistani	Homozygous mutation involving deletion of three base pairs involving codons 35 and 36

M male, *F* female
[a]The author has not provided clinical data from those patients in the article
[b]The youngest female patient died of sepsis before being treated with leptin

The adults' initial mean dose was 4.1 ± 1.2 mg/day: 2.8 mg for oldest male, 4.2 mg for youngest female, and 5.3 mg for oldest female [8]. After 13 years of treatment, the most current dose is 1.95 ± 2.05 mg/day: 0.6 mg for the oldest male, 1.0 mg for the youngest female, and 5.0 mg for the oldest female. The child's initial dose was 1.36 mg/day [10], and the current dose is 1.2 mg/day. The oldest female is under a considerably higher dose, for whom dose decreases led to significant weight gain. That patient had type 2 diabetes before treatment, which reversed after metreleptin initiation [8, 10]. No leptin antibodies have been detected in that patient (nor the others), and it is very likely that her higher dose requirements are attributed to increased leptin resistance, in the context of common obesity combined with leptin deficiency. For the additional cases of CLD described by other investigators, the dose of metreleptin is calculated in the same manner, but some investigators prefer to divide the dose into two daily injections, or to administer a single injection in the morning. Efficacy does not seem to be different when a single injection is administered per day, but we have observed increased adherence with that regimen.

Myalept® is a recombinant human leptin analog for that binds to and activates the leptin receptor. It is a 147-amino acid, nonglycosylated, polypeptide with one disulfide bond between Cys-97 and Cys-147 and a molecular weight of approximately 16.15 kDa, produced in *E. coli*, and differs from native human leptin by the addition of a methionine residue at its amino terminus [27].

The initial dose physiological dose (0.02–0.04 mg/kg/day) is calculated to achieve 10 % predicted serum leptin concentration based on gender, age, and percentage of body fat (calculations based on pharmacodynamic and pharmacokinetic data from AMGEN Inc., Thousand Oaks, California, USA). The dose administered remains the same if weight reduces or stabilizes. If weight increases over two consecutive 2-month periods, the dose is increased to achieve 20 %, and subsequently 50, 100, and 150 % predicted serum leptin concentrations.

After subcutaneous administration of single doses of Myalept® ranging from 0.1 to 0.3 mg/kg in healthy subjects, peak serum leptin concentration (Cmax) occurred approximately 4.0–4.3 h after. The median Tmax of metreleptin was 4 h (range: 2–8 h; $N=5$ lipodystrophy patients) following single-dose administration of metreleptin. In studies of healthy adult subjects, leptin volume of distribution was approximately 4–5 times plasma volume after intravenous administration of metreleptin. No formal metabolism studies have been conducted with metreleptin, but data indicate that renal clearance is the major route of metreleptin elimination, with no apparent contribution of systemic metabolism or degradation. The half-life was 3.8–4.7 h following single administration of subcutaneous doses of 0.01–0.3 mg/ml in healthy subjects. In the presence of leptin antibodies, the clearance of metreleptin is expected to be delayed [27].

Myalept® has been recently approved by the FDA for the treatment of congenital or acquired generalized lipodystrophy (non-HIV-related), but not for the partial forms of the disease, for which safety and effectiveness have not been established yet. For lipodystrophy, the recommended starting dose is 0.06 mg/kg/day (if body weight 40 kg or less), increasing or decreasing by 0.02 mg/kg to a maximum daily dose of 0.13 mg/kg. For males with body weight >40 kg, the recommended starting dose is 2.5 mg/day, increasing or decreasing by 1.25 mg to 2.5 mg/day, to a maximum dose of 10 mg/day. For females with body weight >40 kg, the recommended starting dose is 5 mg/day, increasing or decreasing by 1.25 mg to 2.5 mg/day, to a maximum dose of 10 mg/day. Myalept is administered once daily at the same time every day, subcutaneously [27].

The most common reported adverse reactions ($\geq$10 %) are headache, hypoglycemia, decreased weight, and abdominal pain. T-cell lymphoma has also been reported in patients with acquired generalized lipodystrophy being treated with Myalept®. However, a causal relationship between Myalept® and the development and/or progression of lymphoma has not been established, since lymphoproliferative disorders, including lymphomas, have been reported in patients with acquired generalized lipodystrophy not treated with the drug. Therefore, doctors should consider the benefits and risks of treatment with Myalept® in patients with significant hematologic abnormalities and/or acquired generalized lipodystrophy. Due to the risk of hypoglycemia, dose adjustment of insulin or insulin secretagogues may be necessary, if in use, and blood glucose levels should be closely monitored in those patients. Since autoimmune disorder progression has been observed in patients treated with Myalept® (autoimmune hepatitis and membranoproliferative glomerulonephritis), risks and benefits and risks of Myalept® treatment should be weighed in patients with autoimmune disease. Hypersensitivity reactions (e.g., urticaria or generalized rash) have also been reported [27].

Anti-metreleptin antibodies with neutralizing activity have been identified in 84 % of patients treated with Myalept®, which titers ranged from 1:5 to 1:1,935,125, and which consequences have not been well characterized yet. Although these antibodies could inhibit endogenous leptin action and cause loss of drug efficacy, neutralizing activity was observed in 2 out of 33 patients tested. In addition, clinical trials have reported loss of metabolic control and/or severe infections in the presence of antibodies against metreleptin. In the package insert, the company recommends testing for anti-metreleptin antibodies with neutralizing activity in patients with severe infections or loss of efficacy during Myalept® treatment. The contraindications listed by the package insert are general obesity not associated with congenital leptin deficiency, and hypersensitivity to metreleptin. It is uncertain whether

Myalept® can be used during pregnancy no adequate and well-controlled studies have been conducted with the drug in pregnant women. If case of nursing women, Myalept® or nursing should be discontinued. No clinically meaningful differences have been observed in the efficacy and safety of Myalept® between pediatric and adult patients. In case of the geriatric population, existing clinical trials have not included sufficient numbers of participants >65 years old. However, due to decreased hepatic, renal and/or cardiac function, dose selection should be cautious and start at the low end of the dosing range [27].

No formal drug interaction studies have been performed to evaluate drug interactions. However, leptin is a cytokine that has the potential to alter the formation of cytochrome P450 (CYP450) enzymes. Therefore, caution is warranted when prescribing concomitant drugs metabolized by CYP450, such as oral contraceptives and drugs with a narrow therapeutic index [27].

Effects of Leptin Replacement Therapy in Patients with CLD

Body Composition, Food Intake, and Energy Expenditure

Leptin replacement therapy leads to significant decreases in body weight, BMI, and fat mass. Our Turkish adult patients' mean BMI was 51.2±2.5 kg/m^2 before treatment. After 18 months of treatment, the patients reached a mean BMI of 26.9±2.1 kg/m^2, which remained fairly stable since then. The youngest male also lost a significant amount of weight, from a BMI of 39.6 kg/m^2 before treatment at age 5, to 26.5 kg/m^2 at age 11. Most of the decrease in BMI was attributed to fat mass loss, as measured by Dual-energy X-ray absorptiometry (DXA) [8]. In 2001, the adults' mean initial total body fat percentage was 46.4±3.2 %, which decreased to 35.9±17.7 % after 10 years of therapy. The child's fat percentage was 27.9 % at age 11.

Patients were not instructed to changes their diets or physical activity, and their weight loss was attributed to voluntary decrease in energy intake.

Table 16.2 Behavioral and anthropometric effects of leptin replacement

Decrease in total body weight
Decrease in total fat mass
Decrease in food intake
Decrease in hunger and in desire to eat
Greater fullness after eating
Voluntary increase in physical activity
Attenuated decrease in weight loss-associated reduction of energy expenditure

While on leptin, patients reported less hunger, less desire to eat, and greater fullness, both before and after the meals. Also, the patients found different foods equally appealing in taste, texture, aroma, and with similar filling qualities [28]. In addition, activity levels were measured in the adults by actigraphy, which showed progressive and linear increases [8]. Leptin replacement changed the macronutrient content of the patients' diets, with an increase in carbohydrate and a decrease in fat consumption [29].

Before treatment, energy expenditure and fat oxidation were comparable to those of age-, sex-, and weight-matched controls. Leptin therapy did not increase energy expenditure, but it prevented the reduction in metabolic rate that is associated with weight loss [30]. Farooqi et al. have also reported that leptin therapy did not increase energy expenditure [15, 31]. Table 16.2 summarizes the behavioral and anthropometric effects of leptin replacement.

Lipids and Glucose Metabolism

Before treatment, all patients had low HDL-cholesterol and normal or high triglycerides and insulin. The older female was also diagnosed with type 2 diabetes [23]. Leptin replacement normalized blood lipids (reducing triglycerides and increasing HDL), insulin levels, and glucose (in the patient that had type 2 diabetes). Also, glucose levels in the oldest patient decreased to normal levels, outside the diabetes range [8]. Similar effects on triglycerides, HDL, and insulin have been observed in the other patients as well [15, 18].

Glucose, insulin, and C-peptide were measured during meal tolerance tests in the oldest male patient. Leptin replacement increased insulin sensitivity by at least 5.7-fold, increased insulin hepatic extraction, and decreased insulin secretion [32]. The adult patients were also submitted to euglycemic hyperinsulinemic clamps during the 4th, 5th, and 6th years of treatment, while on treatment and 6 weeks after therapy was briefly interrupted. Leptin withdrawal led to substantial weight gain, up to 10.0 kg, which determined an acute and transient increase in insulin sensitivity while off leptin, as the newly acquired adipose tissue absorbed glucose in excess [10]. Oral glucose tolerance tests (OGTT) were also performed, showing substantial decrease in insulin resistance in two patients after leptin replacement was interrupted and weight gain occurred. In the male adult, the increase in insulin sensitivity, associated with a decreased hepatic extraction of insulin, resulted in a hypoglycemic episode during the off-leptin OGTT [10]. Regarding insulin secretion, we observed that it was increased in the absence of leptin in two of our adult patients. In those patients, insulin hepatic extraction was also decreased, resulting in an increase in post-hepatic insulin delivery, in the absence of leptin [10]. By evaluating the dynamics of plasma proteome during acute and chronic leptin therapy, we observed that leptin treatment was associated with the upregulation of pathways and processes involved in glycolysis and gluconeogenesis, and also cell adhesion, cytoskeleton remodeling, cell cycle, blood coagulation [33].

Hypothalamic-Pituitary-Gonadal Axis

Before treatment, the adults had signs of hypogonadism. The adult male was prepuberal; the youngest female had normal pubic and axillary hair, small ovaries and borderline uterus, and diminished mammary tissue; the oldest female had sparse pubic and axillary hair, small uterus and ovaries, and no mammary tissue. Both females had delayed spontaneous menarche between ages 29 and 35, with irregular menses. Gonadotropins responses to GnRH stimulation were normal, compatible with hypogonadotropic hypogonadism [8].

After treatment, the most remarkable effect was the full development of secondary sexual characteristics [8]. In addition, menstrual periods became regular in the females, with serial midluteal phase progesterone measurements >10 ng/ml, indicative of ovulation. In the adult male, testosterone and free testosterone levels reached normal values for adults. The youngest male is now 12 years 6 months, and has now begun entering puberty, with testicular enlargement and pubarche. The effects of leptin therapy on raising basal and stimulated LH and FSH levels to pubertal values, and on the initiation of nocturnal pulsatility have been also described in the Austrian patient, whose menarche occurred at age 16.3 years, 76 weeks after leptin was initiated [34].

Hypothalamic-Pituitary-Adrenal Axis and Biomarkers of Cardiovascular Disease

Our patients had normal levels serum and urinary cortisol, differently to the hypercorticosteronemia that is observed in the *ob/ob* mice [8]. Serum cortisol levels were fully suppressed with 1 mg of dexamethasone [23]. During a 24-h frequent blood sampling, leptin replacement increased the mean 24-h levels of serum cortisol, from 4.04 ± 0.22 to 5.97 ± 0.30 μg/dl, and altered its circadian rhythm, by decreasing the number of pulses from 25 to 19, increasing their amplitude, increasing the morning peak, and increasing regularity [8]. In the patients of Pakistani origin, urinary and serum cortisol levels were within normal ranges as well, before and during leptin therapy [15].

Levels of biomarkers of inflammation, coagulation, fibrinolysis, and platelet aggregation were heterogeneous in the three adult Turkish patients. Leptin replacement led to changes in most of those biomarkers, but a pattern could not be established. However, leptin withdrawal tended to determine changes towards a decreased state of thrombogenesis and increased fibrinolysis [12], suggesting that the absence of leptin may protect against cardiovascular disease, even in a morbidly obese state, and that leptin excess leads to a proinflammatory state [35].

Hypothalamic-Pituitary Somatotropic Axis

In the adults, all of the IGF-related parameters were within the normal range, except for a low postprandial IGFBP-1 [8]. At baseline, and 2 and 18 months after treatment initiation, we observed no significant changes in IGF-I (141 ± 14, 137 ± 15, 154 ± 16 respectively, reference range 120–140 ng/ml), IGF-II (484 ± 17, 480 ± 16, 487 ± 17 respectively, reference range 290–730 ng/ml), IGFBP-3 (1,606 ± 96, 1,588 ± 78, 1,633 ± 821 respectively, reference range 500–3,600 ng/ml) and IGFBP-6 (299 ± 12, 288 ± 10, 282 ± 12 respectively, reference range 100–340 ng/ml). We observed significant increases in IGFBP-1 levels at the 18th month, both while fasting (21.1 ± 1.3 at baseline, 30.8 ± 7.1 at the 2nd month, 140 ± 42 at the 18th month; reference range 13–120 ng/ml; $p = 0.02$), and postprandial (3.7 ± 0.5 at baseline, 8.6 ± 1.9 at the 2nd month, 18.1 ± 2.6 at the 18th month; reference range 10–30 ng/ml; $p = 0.0001$). Mean IGFBP-2 also increased from 571 ± 32 to 936 ± 53 ng/ml ($p < 0.001$), possibly attributed to the decrease in insulin levels [36]. In three leptin-deficient patients of Pakistani origin, baseline mean IGFBP-2 levels were lower than those observed by us (71 ng/ml), which increased in two of the patients 6 months after leptin therapy (to 88 and 132 ng/ml). Those levels were considerably lower than those we have observed, and no statistical significance between baseline and post-therapy IGFBP-2 levels was reported [37].

The adult patients' heights were within the family mean heights, with no history of delayed or impaired growth. Growth hormone levels were undetectable, and responses to insulin-induced hypoglycemia and exercise tests were absent in the male (nadir glucose level, 37 mg/dl; GH of 0.1 ng/ml in both tests) and in the younger adult female (nadir glucose level, 35 mg/dl; GH, 0.1 ng/ml in the hypoglycemia test and 0.3 ng/ml in the exercise tests). These results are probably attributed to obesity, given the absence of clinical features of growth hormone deficiency [23].

Before treatment, the youngest male's height was at the 50th percentile in the growth chart, with growth deceleration after treatment was initiated (from the 50th to the 10th percentile), possibly due to weight gain and inadequate dose adjustments. Doses were adjusted, and now the patient is between the 10th and the 25th percentile, within the targeted height. In patients of Pakistani origin, growth was normal before and during leptin therapy, with normal levels of IGF-1 [15].

Hypothalamic-Pituitary-Thyroid Axis

Leptin has a highly organized circadian rhythm [38], with a pattern similar to that of TSH: a nadir in late morning and peak in the early morning [39]. Thyroid function tests were normal for all our patients [11], but the leptin-deficient adult male had dysregulated patterns of TSH pulsatile and circadian rhythms [39]. Also, the girl that died before receiving treatment had subclinical hypothyroidism. Leptin has a role in regulating TSH secretion, and its absence may lead to thyroid dysfunction [40]. Leptin replacement did not increase free T4 or T3 [11], as previously observed [15]. Subclinical hypothyroidism has been reported in the other patients as well, which subsided upon leptin therapy initiation [18].

Immunity

The youngest male had had normal blood cells count; after 6 weeks of therapy, leptin replacement led to a decrease in the absolute lymphocyte count, from 3.5×10^3 to $2.9 \times 10^3/\mu l$. His immunoglobulin levels were normal, except for elevated IgE, indicating atopy. By flow cytometry, we determined that the decrease in lymphocytes corresponded to decreases in CD3, CD4, and CD19 cells. Lymphocyte proliferative responses to the mitogens phytohemaglutinin, concanavalin A, pokeweed, and tetanus and candida antigens were normal at baseline (except for tetanus). Two and 6 weeks after treatment, leptin enhanced T cell responsiveness, as shown by significant increases of responses to antigens, except for tetanus [12]. Farooqi et al. reported T cell hyporesposiveness before leptin therapy in two patients, which increased to normal levels during treatment [15].

No changes in immune blood counts were observed in the Turkish adults after leptin therapy was initiated. Also, neither hypersensitivity reactions nor autoimmune diseases were detected. No hematologic abnormalities suggesting the development of lymphoma have been observed in nearly 14 years of leptin therapy.

Gibson et al. have reported that, in a Pakistani girl, white blood cell count doubled within the 1st month of therapy and remained elevated for the first 3 months, without any evidence of infection. Interestingly, the patient was asthmatic before therapy, and did not require hospital visits for asthma in the 12 months following therapy initiation [18]. Farooqi et al. reported that another child of Pakistani origin had a normal total lymphocyte number and a normal number of CD3 cells, with reduced CD4 cell number and increased CD8 and B cells, which normalized during leptin therapy [15].

Brain Structure and Function

Eighteen months of leptin therapy increased grey matter concentration in three brain regions of the adults: anterior cingulate gyrus, parietal lobe, and medial cerebellum [41]. Annual withholding of replacement for several weeks reversed this effect in the anterior cingulate gyrus and medial cerebellum, and treatment reinitiation did not significantly restore grey matter concentration in the short-term (11–22 days), but led to an unexpected increase in grey matter concentration in the posterior half of the left thalamus, particularly the pulvinar nucleus [42]. Those areas are implicated in neural circuits regulating hunger and satiation, and shows leptin's effect on neuroplasticity.

In functional studies, leptin replacement reduced activation of regions linked to hunger (insula, parietal, and temporal cortex) and enhanced activation of regions linked to inhibition and satiety (prefrontal cortex), as well as the posterior lobe of the cerebellum, the brain region with the highest concentration of leptin receptors [43]. These results show that leptin has extra-hypothalamic effects in the regulation of food intake, reversibly altering neural structure and function, and modulating plasticity-dependent brain physiology in response to food cues [44]. In the Austrian patient, acute leptin therapy elicited activation in reward- and food-related areas (ventral striatum and the orbitofrontal cortex), when comparing high- and low-calorie pictures. Moreover, acute and long-term effects were observed in the hypothamalus, striatum, amygdala, orbitofrontal cortex, and substantia nigra/ventral tegmental area, when comparing food and nonfood pictures, and high- vs. low-caloric pictures [45]. Those results were sustained in the amygdala and in the orbitofrontal cortex, 1 and 2 years after leptin therapy, with a reduction of the frontopolar cortex activity [46]. In that patient, leptin therapy did not reduce activity in hunger-related regions, as we have previously reported [44]. This might be attributed to the fact that the Austrian patient had high cognitive control over her food choices, and voluntarily chose a low-calorie diet. Differently to what is observed in *ob/ob* mice, leptin therapy did not increase striatal dopamine receptor availability in the adult Turkish patients [47]. However, it is uncertain whether D2/D3 receptor availability and other dopamine system parameters are abnormal before the initiation of leptin replacement in patients with CLD, and leptin therapy fails to produce any effect.

The procognitive effects of leptin were observed in the youngest male patient, who showed improvements of several subtests of the Differential Ability Scale (DAS), a measure of general verbal and nonverbal functioning, and of several subtests from the NEPSY, a measure of neuropsychological functioning in children [10].

The adult patients were evaluated for anxiety and depression, by employing the Hamilton Anxiety Rating Scale and the Hamilton Depression Rating Scale. Their scores were normal at baseline, and did not change during treatment.

However, it was noted that the patients' behavior changed from very infantile and docile, to assertive and adult-like [8].

Our results demonstrated that leptin therapy is associated with structural and functional changes in the brain, providing further evidence to the hypothesis that leptin plays an important role in brain development and cognition [48]. Furthermore, low leptin levels or leptin resistance may be involved in the pathogenesis of neurodegenerative diseases such as Alzheimer's disease [49, 50], as previously demonstrated in a study from the Framingham cohort [51].

Liver Steatosis

In the Turkish cohort, liver enzymes and other biomarkers of liver function were normal before and after leptin replacement was initiated. In the Austrian patient, severe hepatic steatosis was reported before treatment. After 23 weeks of leptin replacement, liver fat content was reduced from 49.7 to 9.4 %, with concomitant normalization of serum transaminases [52]. This is in concordance with previous animal [53] and human studies on the effects of leptin on the improvement of liver steatosis in lipodystrophy patients [54], providing the basis for clinical trials evaluating leptin as a potential therapeutic agent for nonalcoholic fatty liver disease [55].

Table 16.3 Metabolic and endocrine changes following leptin replacement

Metabolic changes	Decrease in triglycerides
	Increase in HDL-cholesterol
	Decrease in insulin
	Decrease in plasma glucose, with resolution of type 2 diabetes in one patient
	Increase in insulin sensitivity
	Decrease in insulin secretion
	Increase in insulin hepatic extraction
	Decrease in liver fat content and in serum transaminases
Endocrine changes	Reversal of hypogonadotropic hypogonadism
	Increase in basal and stimulated LH and FSH levels to pubertal values
	Initiation of nocturnal pulsatility of LH and FSH
	Establishment of ovulatory menstrual cycles
	Establishment of normal adult levels of testosterone and estrogens
	Increase in mean 24-h serum cortisol
	Changes in cortisol circadian rhythm: decrease in total number of pulses, increase in amplitude, increase in morning peak, increase in regularity
	Increase in IGFBP-1 and in IGFBP-2
	Resolution of subclinical hypothyroidism

Conclusions

Currently, very few cases of congenital leptin deficiency caused by mutations in the leptin gene have been reported so far. However, as demonstrated by Fatima et al. [17] and Saeed et al. [20], screening of severe early-onset cases of obesity may lead to the diagnosis of new cases of CLD.

Nevertheless, the study of leptin replacement therapy on these patients has provided insightful information on the roles of leptin, not only on the regulation of food intake, energy expenditure, and body weight (Table 16.2), but also of its extra-hypothalamic effects. It has been shown that leptin regulates hypothalamic-pituitary axes (thyroid, adrenal, somatotropic, and gonadotropic), lipid metabolism, glucose/insulin homeostasis, and hepatic steatosis (Table 16.3). Moreover, leptin therapy is associated with changes in immunological parameters, and determines structural and functional changes in the brain (Table 16.4).

Continued studies on the effects of leptin replacement therapy on these patients with CLD, as well as novel studies on the effects of leptin in patients with lipodystrophy, will generate new knowledge on leptin's physiology, providing the foundation for evaluating leptin in other disorders, such as diabetes, fatty liver disease, and neurodegenerative diseases.

Table 16.4 Immunological and neuroimaging findings following leptin replacement

Immunological changes	Decrease in the absolute lymphocyte count
	Decreases in CD3, CD4, and CD19 cells
	Increase in T cell responsiveness
	Switch from the secretion of predominantly Th2 to Th1 cytokines
	Increase in total white blood cell count
	Normalization of CD4 cells count (from reduced numbers), and of CD8 and B cells counts (from increased numbers)
Neuroimaging changes	Increase in grey matter concentration in the anterior cingulate gyrus, parietal lobe, and medial cerebellum
	Increase in grey matter concentration in the posterior half of the left thalamus (particularly the pulvinar nucleus), following treatment withholding/re-initiation
	Decrease in activation of regions linked to hunger (insula, parietal, and temporal cortex)
	Increase in activation of regions linked to inhibition and satiety (prefrontal cortex)
	Increase in activation of posterior lobe of the cerebellum

References

1. Ahima RS. Adipose tissue as an endocrine organ. Obesity (Silver Spring). 2006;14 Suppl 5:242S–9.
2. Chen GC, Qin LQ, Ye JK. Leptin levels and risk of type 2 diabetes: gender-specific meta-analysis. Obes Rev. 2014;15:134–42.
3. Chai SB, Sun F, Nie XL, Wang J. Leptin and coronary heart disease: a systematic review and meta-analysis. Atherosclerosis. 2014;233:3–10.
4. Paz-Filho G, Lim EL, Wong ML, Licinio J. Associations between adipokines and obesity-related cancer. Front Biosci. 2011;16:1634–50.
5. Mantzoros CS, Magkos F, Brinkoetter M, et al. Leptin in human physiology and pathophysiology. Am J Physiol Endocrinol Metab. 2011;301:E567–84.
6. Boguszewski CL, Paz-Filho G, Velloso LA. Neuroendocrine body weight regulation: integration between fat tissue, gastrointestinal tract, and the brain. Endokrynol Pol. 2010;61:194–206.
7. Paz-Filho G, Wong ML, Licinio J. Ten years of leptin replacement therapy. Obes Rev. 2011;12:e315–23.
8. Licinio J, Caglayan S, Ozata M, et al. Phenotypic effects of leptin replacement on morbid obesity, diabetes mellitus, hypogonadism, and behavior in leptin-deficient adults. Proc Natl Acad Sci U S A. 2004;101:4531–6.
9. Paz-Filho GJ, Ayala A, Esposito K, et al. Effects of leptin on lipid metabolism. Horm Metab Res. 2008;40:572–4.
10. Paz-Filho GJ, Babikian T, Asarnow R, et al. Leptin replacement improves cognitive development. PLoS One. 2008;3:e3098.
11. Paz-Filho GJ, Andrews D, Esposito K, et al. Effects of leptin replacement on risk factors for cardiovascular disease in genetically leptin-deficient subjects. Horm Metab Res. 2009;41:164–7.
12. Paz-Filho GJ, Delibasi T, Erol HK, Wong ML, Licinio J. Cellular immunity before and after leptin replacement therapy. J Pediatr Endocrinol Metab JPEM. 2009;22:1069–74.
13. Paz-Filho G, Mastronardi C, Wong ML, Licinio J. Leptin therapy, insulin sensitivity, and glucose homeostasis. Indian J Endocrinol Metab. 2012;16: S549–55.
14. Chan JL, Mantzoros CS. Role of leptin in energy-deprivation states: normal human physiology and clinical implications for hypothalamic amenorrhoea and anorexia nervosa. Lancet. 2005;366:74–85.
15. Farooqi IS, Matarese G, Lord GM, et al. Beneficial effects of leptin on obesity, T cell hyporesponsiveness, and neuroendocrine/metabolic dysfunction of human congenital leptin deficiency. J Clin Invest. 2002;110:1093–103.
16. Farooqi IS, O'Rahilly S. Leptin: a pivotal regulator of human energy homeostasis. Am J Clin Nutr. 2009;89: 980S–4.
17. Fatima W, Shahid A, Imran M, et al. Leptin deficiency and leptin gene mutations in obese children from Pakistan. Int J Pediatr Obes. 2011;6:419–27.
18. Gibson WT, Farooqi IS, Moreau M, et al. Congenital leptin deficiency due to homozygosity for the Delta133G mutation: report of another case and evaluation of response to four years of leptin therapy. J Clin Endocrinol Metab. 2004;89:4821–6.
19. Montague CT, Farooqi IS, Whitehead JP, et al. Congenital leptin deficiency is associated with severe early-onset obesity in humans. Nature. 1997;387: 903–8.
20. Saeed S, Butt TA, Anwer M, Arslan M, Froguel P. High prevalence of leptin and melanocortin-4 receptor gene mutations in children with severe obesity from Pakistani consanguineous families. Mol Genet Metab. 2012;106:121–6.
21. Mazen I, El-Gammal M, Abdel-Hamid M, Amr K. A novel homozygous missense mutation of the leptin gene (N103K) in an obese Egyptian patient. Mol Genet Metab. 2009;97:305–8.
22. Fischer-Posovszky P, von Schnurbein J, Moepps B, et al. A new missense mutation in the leptin gene

causes mild obesity and hypogonadism without affecting T cell responsiveness. J Clin Endocrinol Metab. 2010;95:2836–40.
23. Ozata M, Ozdemir IC, Licinio J. Human leptin deficiency caused by a missense mutation: multiple endocrine defects, decreased sympathetic tone, and immune system dysfunction indicate new targets for leptin action, greater central than peripheral resistance to the effects of leptin, and spontaneous correction of leptin-mediated defects. J Clin Endocrinol Metab. 1999;84:3686–95.
24. Strobel A, Issad T, Camoin L, Ozata M, Strosberg AD. A leptin missense mutation associated with hypogonadism and morbid obesity. Nat Genet. 1998;18:213–5.
25. Pelleymounter MA, Cullen MJ, Baker MB, et al. Effects of the obese gene product on body weight regulation in ob/ob mice. Science. 1995;269:540–3.
26. Licinio J, Negrao AB, Mantzoros C, et al. Synchronicity of frequently sampled, 24-h concentrations of circulating leptin, luteinizing hormone, and estradiol in healthy women. Proc Natl Acad Sci U S A. 1998;95:2541–6.
27. Company B-MS. Myalept Package Insert. 2014.
28. Williamson DA, Ravussin E, Wong ML, et al. Microanalysis of eating behavior of three leptin deficient adults treated with leptin therapy. Appetite. 2005;45:75–80.
29. Licinio J, Milane M, Thakur S, et al. Effects of leptin on intake of specific micro- and macronutrients in a woman with leptin gene deficiency studied off and on leptin at stable body weight. Appetite. 2007;49: 594–9.
30. Galgani JE, Greenway FL, Caglayan S, Wong ML, Licinio J, Ravussin E. Leptin replacement prevents weight loss-induced metabolic adaptation in congenital leptin-deficient patients. J Clin Endocrinol Metab. 2010;95:851–5.
31. Farooqi IS, Jebb SA, Langmack G, et al. Effects of recombinant leptin therapy in a child with congenital leptin deficiency. N Engl J Med. 1999;341:879–84.
32. Andreev VP, Paz-Filho G, Wong ML, Licinio J. Deconvolution of insulin secretion, insulin hepatic extraction post-hepatic delivery rates and sensitivity during 24-hour standardized meals: time course of glucose homeostasis in leptin replacement treatment. Horm Metab Res. 2009;41:142–51.
33. Andreev VP, Dwivedi RC, Paz-Filho G, et al. Dynamics of plasma proteome during leptin-replacement therapy in genetically based leptin deficiency. Pharmacogenomics J. 2011;11:174–90.
34. von Schnurbein J, Moss A, Nagel SA, et al. Leptin substitution results in the induction of menstrual cycles in an adolescent with leptin deficiency and hypogonadotropic hypogonadism. Horm Res Paediatr. 2012;77:127–33.
35. Paz-Filho G, Mastronardi C, Franco CB, Wang KB, Wong ML, Licinio J. Leptin: molecular mechanisms, systemic pro-inflammatory effects, and clinical implications. Arq Bras Endocrinol Metabol. 2012;56:597–607.
36. Wheatcroft SB, Kearney MT. IGF-dependent and IGF-independent actions of IGF-binding protein-1 and -2: implications for metabolic homeostasis. Trends Endocrinol Metab. 2009;20:153–62.
37. Hedbacker K, Birsoy K, Wysocki RW, et al. Antidiabetic effects of IGFBP2, a leptin-regulated gene. Cell Metab. 2010;11:11–22.
38. Licinio J, Mantzoros C, Negrao AB, et al. Human leptin levels are pulsatile and inversely related to pituitary- adrenal function. Nat Med. 1997;3:575–9.
39. Mantzoros CS, Ozata M, Negrao AB, et al. Synchronicity of frequently sampled TSH and leptin concentrations in healthy adults and leptin deficient subjects: evidence for possible partial TSH regulation by leptin in humans. J Clin Endocrinol Metab. 2001;86:3284–91.
40. Moura EG, Moura CC. regulation of thyrotropin synthesis and secretion. Arq Bras Endocrinol Metabol. 2004;48:40–52.
41. Matochik JA, London ED, Yildiz BO, et al. Effect of leptin replacement on brain structure in genetically leptin-deficient adults. J Clin Endocrinol Metab. 2005;90:2851–4.
42. London ED, Berman SM, Chakrapani S, et al. Short-term plasticity of gray matter associated with leptin deficiency and replacement. J Clin Endocrinol Metab. 2011;96:E1212–20.
43. Berman SM, Paz-Filho G, Wong ML, Kohno M, Licinio J, London ED. Effects of leptin deficiency and replacement on cerebellar response to food-related cues. Cerebellum. 2013;12:59–67.
44. Baicy K, London ED, Monterosso J, et al. Leptin replacement alters brain response to food cues in genetically leptin-deficient adults. Proc Natl Acad Sci U S A. 2007;104:18276–9.
45. Frank S, Heni M, Moss A, et al. Leptin therapy in a congenital leptin-deficient patient leads to acute and long-term changes in homeostatic, reward, and food-related brain areas. J Clin Endocr Metab. 2011;96: E1283–7.
46. Frank S, Heni M, Moss A, et al. Long-term stabilization effects of leptin on brain functions in a leptin-deficient patient. PLoS One. 2013;8.
47. Ishibashi K, Berman SM, Paz-Filho G, et al. Dopamine D2/D3 receptor availability in genetically leptin-deficient patients after long-term leptin replacement. Mol Psychiatry. 2012;17:352–3.
48. Paz-Filho G, Wong ML, Licinio J. The procognitive effects of leptin in the brain and their clinical implications. Int J Clin Pract. 2010;64:1808–12.
49. Clark I, Atwood C, Bowen R, Paz-Filho G, Vissel B. Tumor necrosis factor-induced cerebral insulin resistance in Alzheimer's disease links numerous treatment rationales. Pharmacol Rev. 2012;64:1004–26.
50. Paz-Filho G, Wong ML, Licinio J. Leptin levels and Alzheimer disease. JAMA J Am Med Assoc. 2010;303:1478. author reply 9.

51. Lieb W, Beiser AS, Vasan RS, et al. Association of plasma leptin levels with incident Alzheimer disease and MRI measures of brain aging. JAMA. 2009;302: 2565–72.
52. von Schnurbein J, Heni M, Moss A, et al. Rapid improvement of hepatic steatosis after initiation of leptin substitution in a leptin-deficient girl. Horm Res Paediatr. 2013;79:310–7.
53. Paz-Filho G, Mastronardi CA, Parker BJ, et al. Molecular pathways involved in the improvement of non-alcoholic fatty liver disease. J Mol Endocrinol. 2013;51:167–79.
54. Javor ED, Ghany MG, Cochran EK, et al. Leptin reverses nonalcoholic steatohepatitis in patients with severe lipodystrophy. Hepatology. 2005;41: 753–60.
55. NIH. Research Portfolio Online Reporting Tools (RePORT) 2014. Available from http://projectreporter.nih.gov/project_info_description.cfm?aid=8600674

Leptin Therapy in People with a Normal Leptin Gene

17

Steven B. Heymsfield and Heike Münzberg

Abbreviations

BMI	Body mass index
CSF	Cerebrospinal fluid levels
C_{max}	Peak concentrations
IGF	Insulin-like growth factor
OB-R	Leptin receptor
PEG	Polyethylene glycol
PEG-OB protein	Pegylated recombinant native human leptin
REE	Resting energy expenditure
r-metHu-Leptin and metreleptin	Recombinant methionyl leptin
RQ	Respiratory quotient
SC	Subcutaneous
VLED	Very-low energy diet

Introduction

Late in 1994 Zhang et al. first reported that a mutation in the mouse *obese* (*ob*, aka *lep*) gene results in severe obesity and type II diabetes as part of a syndrome resembling morbid obesity in humans [1]. Zhang and her colleagues proposed that the *ob* gene product is part of the now-classic signaling pathway from adipose tissue that works to regulate fat depot stores and energy balance. Less than 1 year later, in 1995, Halaas et al. reported that the 167-amino acid protein *ob* gene product was present in mouse and human plasma but was absent from the plasma of obese (*ob/ob*) mice and greatly increased in the plasma of diabetic (*db/db*) mice [2]. Intraperitoneal injection of recombinant OB protein, now referred to as leptin, had no effect in *db/db* mice but reduced food intake, increased energy expenditure, and reduced body fat stores and weight in *ob/ob* mice. On the 1 year anniversary of Zhang's report, Tartaglia and his colleagues identified and cloned the leptin receptor [3].

These three publications within one year not only revolutionized energy balance and body weight regulation concepts, but signaled pharmacologic possibilities with the discovery of a receptor target and its natural ligand. The promise of therapeutic potential was further advanced 3 years later in 1997 with the first report of two severely obese children with a homozygous frame-shift mutation leading to deletion of a single guanine nucleotide in codon 133 of the leptin gene [4]. Both children had very low leptin levels in the presence of a greatly expanded adipose tissue compartment. Two years later, in 1999, the group reported treatment of the older child with subcutaneously administered recombinant methionyl leptin (r-metHu-Leptin) [5]. The administered dose was calculated to achieve a peak serum

S.B. Heymsfield, M.D. (✉) • H. Münzberg, Ph.D.
Pennington Biomedical Research Center,
LSU System, 6400 Perkins Road, Baton Rouge,
LA 70808, USA
e-mail: Steven.Heymsfield@pbrc.edu

S. Dagogo-Jack (ed.), *Leptin: Regulation and Clinical Applications*,
DOI 10.1007/978-3-319-09915-6_17, © Springer International Publishing Switzerland 2015

concentration 10 % of that predicted for the child's sex, age, and body composition. Treatment led to a sustained weight loss, primarily body fat, over the following year.

However, not all of these early studies supported the likelihood of leptin's therapeutic potential in people without *ob* mutations. Two years following leptin's discovery, Considine et al. in 1996 [6] used a newly developed radioimmunoassay to measure serum leptin levels in normal weight and obese subjects. Serum leptin levels were significantly positively correlated with percent body fat and adipocyte ob mRNA was also substantially elevated in obese subjects. Considine and colleagues concluded in their 1996 report that most obese subjects are insensitive to endogenous leptin production [6]. The question then remained if obese humans without leptin mutations would respond with weight loss to pharmacologic levels of exogenously administered leptin.

The first proof-of concept study in human subjects without mutations in the *ob* receptor was started in 1997 and reported in 1999 [7]. This report was based on treatment with recombinant methionyl leptin, now referred to as metreleptin. A second series of reports first appeared in 2000 with treatment by pegylated recombinant native human leptin, now referred to as PEG-OB protein [8]. Our focus in the following sections is on the pharmacokinetics and weight-loss efficacy of these two leptin preparations. Pivotal studies often included secondary endpoints and we also provide a summary of these observations in the broad context of leptin biology.

Weight-Loss Effects

Metreleptin

Pharmokinetics

Metreleptin is produced by *Escherichia coli* as a 147 amino acid-16.2 kDa protein. Peak concentrations (C_{max}) are observed after subcutaneous (SC) administration 3–4 h post dose (0.1–0.3 mg/kg) with a 1–3.5 h terminal half-life and 90 % bioavailability [9–11]. Metreleptin is mainly eliminated through the kidneys by glomerular filtration and no losses are recognized via degradation or systemic metabolism.

Fujioka et al. in 1999 [12] administered either SC metreleptin ($n=4$, 1 mg/kg) or placebo ($n=2$) to obese adults over a 1-week period and observed increased cerebrospinal fluid levels (CSF, 0.36–2.15 ng/mL vs. 0.18–0.24 ng/mL) with a significant ($P=0.003$) correlation observed between CSF and serum levels.

Clinical Trials

The first human proof-of-concept study reported in 1999 [7] aimed to test the hypothesis that increasing administered doses of leptin will lead to dose-dependent weight loss. The study was designed as a double-blind, placebo-controlled escalating dose cohort trial in lean and obese adults with body weight and composition as endpoints (Table 17.1).

The study consisted of two parts with lean and obese subjects treated for 4 weeks in Part A and obese subjects continuing on for 20 additional weeks in Part B. The lean subjects were prescribed a weight maintenance diet while the obese subjects were prescribed an energy deficit diet of 500 kcal/day. Metreleptin was administered SC to subjects stratified by body mass index (BMI) into four cohorts at doses of 0.01, 0.03, 0.10, or 0.30 mg/kg. Eight subjects were treated for 2 weeks at the specified dose and the safety monitoring board allowed activation of the next dose cohort if no adverse event signals were present. Six subjects (four active and two placebo) were evaluated for weight loss in each BMI strata. Subject enrollment was discontinued if the active-placebo weight-loss difference over 2 weeks was >1.5 kg or <0.5 kg.

The 4-week Part A protocol was completed by 87 subjects in the metreleptin group and 36 subjects in the placebo group. The corresponding samples were 35 and 12 subjects in Part B. The range of weight loss averaged between −0.4 and −1.9 kg over the 4 weeks of Part A. The range of weight loss observed over 20 weeks across the groups in Part B averaged −0.7 to −7.1 kg. Dose–response relationships were statistically significant for weight loss at 4 weeks

Table 17.1 Weight-loss effects observed in leptin clinical trials in subjects without leptin gene mutations

Reference	Agent/dose	Subjects	Protocol	Results
Metreleptin				
Heymsfield et al. 1999 [7]	Escalating SC doses of metreleptin up to 0.30 mg/kg or placebo	54 lean and 73 obese adults	A. 4 weeks (lean and obese) B. 20 weeks (obese). Obese subjects prescribed a 500 kcal/day deficit diet in Parts A and B	Dose–response for weight and fat loss in both lean and obese subjects
Zelissen et al. 2005 [13]	SC metreleptin; randomized double-blind trial	284 obese adults	12 weeks with 6 groups: 20 mg/day with 10 mg am and 10 mg pm; 10 mg/day morning; 10 mg/day evening; matching placebo groups; 500 kcal/day deficit diet	No significant weight loss vs. placebo
PEG-OB protein				
Hukshorn et al. 2000 [8]	PEG-OB protein 20 mg/week	30 obese men	12 weeks + 500 kcal/day energy restriction	No differences in delta or % weight loss
Lejeune et al. 2003 [16] Hukshorn et al. 2003 [14]	PEG-OB protein 80 mg/week	24 overweight men	46 days + 500 kcal/day VLED.	With PEG-OB protein treatment and diet, additional weight loss (X ± SEM; 14.6 ± 0.8 vs. placebo 11.8 ± 0.9 kg; $p < 0.03$) was observed; during 8 weeks follow-up weight increase was larger in the PEG-OB protein group ($p < 0.05$).

PEG-OB protein Pegylated recombinant native human leptin, *r-metHu-Leptin and metreleptin* Recombinant methionyl leptin, *SC* subcutaneous, *VLED* very-low energy diet

($p = 0.02$) and 24 weeks of treatment ($p = 0.01$). The difference in weight loss across doses was statistically significant between lean and obese subjects in Part A ($p = 0.03$). Over 95 % of weight loss was accounted for by fat mass in the two highest dose cohorts. The pattern of weight change observed in the metreleptin-treated obese subjects over the 24 weeks of Parts A and B is shown in Fig. 17.1.

Almost three-fourths of the metreleptin-treated obese subjects tested positive for anti-leptin antibodies, although antibody status did not influence weight loss or adverse events. Injection site reactions were the most common adverse event and these reactions (e.g., ecchymoses, erythema, pruritus, etc.) showed a dose–response relation.

This first proof-of-concept study established that a dose–response relationship is present after 4 weeks of metreleptin treatment in lean and obese subjects and after 24 weeks of treatment in obese subjects. Weight loss was dose-related and consisted mainly of body fat.

As shown by Fujioka et al. [12], exogenous peripheral metreleptin infusion leads to elevated CSF leptin concentrations in humans. Direct cerebrospinal fluid administration of leptin in rodent models leads to weight loss [7], thus suggesting that leptin's weight-loss effects are centrally mediated.

The highest metreleptin dose of 0.3 mg/kg administered in the study of Heymsfield et al. [7] translates to a volume of about 6 ml/day. This level of metreleptin administration was not well

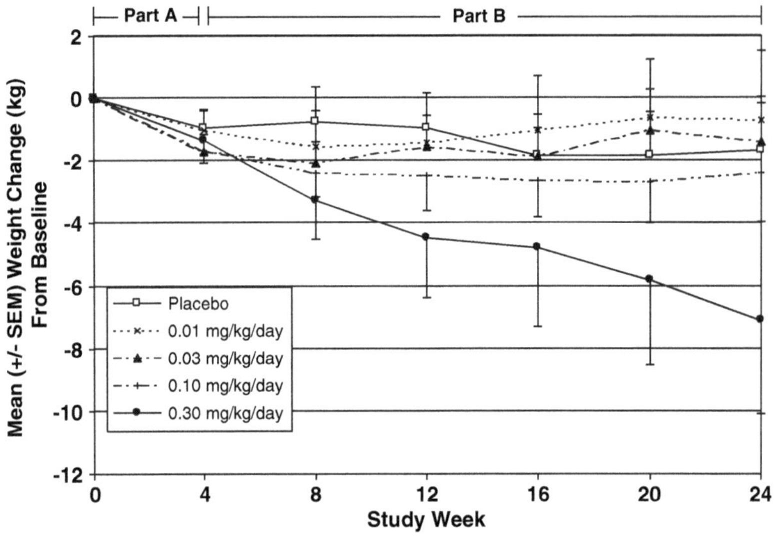

Fig. 17.1 Pattern of weight change from baseline to week 24 in obese subjects who received recombinant metreleptin (methionyl human leptin). From Heymsfield et al. with permission [7]. *Error bars* indicate SEM; *gray line* indicates baseline. The number of subjects is not constant over the course of the study

tolerated, a problem that was addressed in the 2005 study of Zelissen et al. in 2005 [13]. The authors examined if lower doses of metreleptin improve tolerance and promote weight loss if hormone is administered at night in a paradigm that resembles leptin's normal diurnal rhythm. The Zelissen study was a randomized, double-blind, placebo-controlled, investigation of 284 overweight or obese subjects that began with a 3-week dietary lead-in which was then followed by a 12-week metreleptin or placebo treatment period. Subjects were allocated to three metreleptin treatment groups or matching placebo groups. Metreleptin was given SC as 10 mg/morning, 10 mg/evening, or 10 mg twice daily. As with the study of Heymsfield et al. [7], patients were counseled to lower dietary intake by 500 kcal/day.

Upon completion of the 12-week protocol there were no significant changes in body weight with metreleptin treatment versus placebo ($p = 0.68$). As with the study of Heymsfield et al. [7], there were no important adverse effects other than an increase in injection-site reactions in patients with metreleptin treatment (83 %) compared to placebo (36 %). Over 80 % of metreleptin-treated subjects developed antibodies, although immunogenicity did not appear to be clinically significant during the 12-week protocol.

The Zelissen study [13] confirms the findings of Heymsfield et al. [7] that metreleptin treatment of overweight or obese subjects is not effective as a means of promoting substantial weight loss at the selected doses. The study results do not support the author's hypothesis that nocturnal administration of metreleptin will lead to specific weight-loss effects.

Pegylated OB-Protein

Pharmokinetics

The serum half-life of many proteins can be increased by covalent linkage to polyethylene glycol (PEG) polymers. Native human leptin can be expressed from *Escherichia coli* and chemically conjugated to a species of branched PEGs [8]. The resulting PEG-native human leptin polymer (PEG-OB protein) has an increased molecular mass of 42 kDa compared to native leptin (16 kDa). PEG-OB protein has an extended half-life of >48 h with peak serum levels reached 72 h post SC dose and sustained increased blood levels following weekly injections.

Clinical Trials

The first PEG-OB protein study was reported by Hukshorn and colleagues in 2000 [8]. Thirty obese men were randomized to double-blind treatment with weekly SC injections of 20 mg PEG-OB protein or placebo for 12 weeks, in addition to a hypocaloric diet (deficit, ~500 kcal/day). The study was powered to detect a 4 kg difference in weight loss between active and placebo groups at 12 weeks following randomization.

Weekly SC PEG-OB protein injections at a dose of 20 mg/week led to sustained serum PEG-OB protein and leptin concentrations throughout treatment. By contrast, leptin levels decreased with weight loss in the placebo-treated subjects. No significant differences in the absolute weight change (active, −4.3 kg vs. placebo, −6.4 kg) were observed between the PEG-OB protein and placebo groups.

The sponsor prematurely stopped the study after a planned interim analysis indicated the 20 mg PEG-OB dose lacked weight-loss efficacy. Additional doses beyond the 20 mg PEG-OB protein dose were therefore not evaluated in this study.

The authors concluded that weekly SC injection of PEG-OB protein leads to sustained serum concentrations of PEG-OB protein and leptin throughout the 12-week treatment period and that the drug is generally well tolerated.

The next series of studies with PEG-OB protein involved a higher dose with publications distributed across several reports that included secondary endpoints. In the primary study, Hukshorn and colleagues reported a randomized double-blind trial of PEG-OB protein at a SC dose of 80 mg/week versus placebo in 24 overweight men in 2003 [14]. Hukshorn et al. and Lejeune et al. reported additional details of this study in 2003 [15, 16], Hukshorn et al. in 2004 [17], and Lejeune et al. in 2007 [18]. The six-week treatment protocol included a 500 kcal/day very-low energy-diet (VLED) that promoted rapid weight loss. Following the 6-week treatment phase PEG-OB protein treatments were stopped and subjects were followed for several additional weeks as they transitioned from the VLED to regular foods.

Weight loss at the end of the 6-week phase was (X ± SEM) 14.6 ± 0.80 kg in the 12 completing PEG-OB-treated subjects and 11.8 ± 0.9 kg in the ten completing placebo-treated subjects ($p = 0.03$) (Fig. 17.2). Both groups regained weight during the 8 weeks of follow up, increasing by 2.7 kg in the active treatment group and by 1.8 kg in the placebo group ($p < 0.05$).

Secondary Endpoints

While weight loss is the primary endpoint of clinical interest, several metreleptin and PEG-OB protein studies also evaluated secondary endpoints that are of clinical or basic science interest. These studies are summarized in Table 17.2. As most of these studies are based on post-hoc analyses and were not powered to test secondary effects, caution should be used in their interpretation and replication of the findings of interest in future studies is encouraged.

Appetitive Effects

Metreleptin

In a 1999 report, O'Neil et al. [19] examined eating behaviors and mood in obese subjects before and after a 4-week open label course of metreleptin at a twice-daily SC dose of 10 mg. The metreleptin treatment phase was proceeded by a 3-week diet phase with a 500-kcal/day-deficit diet that was continued during the subsequent 4-week protocol. Analysis of behavioral questionnaires supported the hypothesis that metreleptin treatment promotes improvements in weight-loss management strategies, notably less negative emotional eating. Causal pathways could not be established as the study did not include a placebo group.

PEG-OB Protein

Active treatment with PEG-OB protein at a SC dose of 20 mg/week led to reduction in appetite ($P < 0.05$) after 12 weeks even though weight loss did not differ significantly from the placebo group [20].

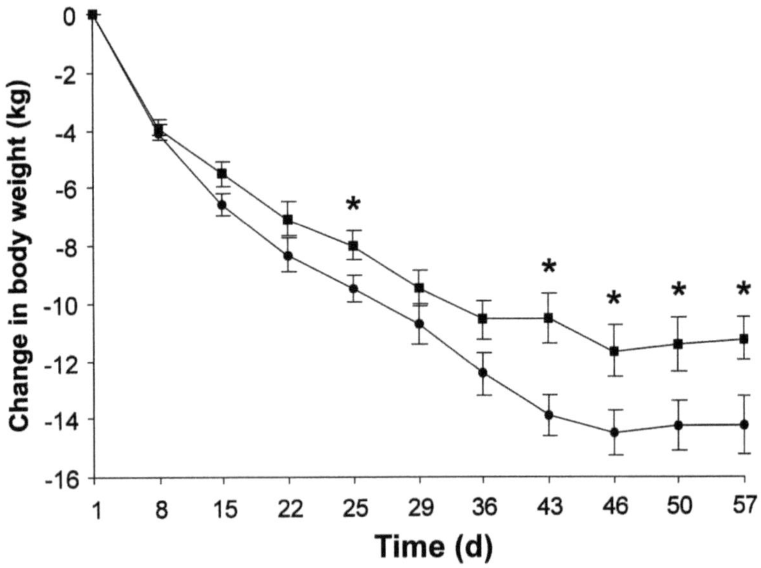

Fig. 17.2 Effect of 80 mg pegylated human recombinant leptin [polyethylene glycol–OB protein (PEG-OB)] (*filled circle*; $n=12$) or matching placebo (*filled square*; $n=10$) administered weekly and of severe energy restriction (500 kcal/day) on mean (±SEM) weight loss from the start of the treatment (day 1), through the diet period (day 46), to the end of the 2-weeks follow-up period (day 57). (*asterisk*)Significantly different from the PEG-OB protein group, $P<0.05$ (interaction of time and treatment; two-factor repeated-measures ANOVA with Scheffe's F procedure). From Hukshorn et al. [14] with permission

Lejeune et al. [16] examined dietary restraint during and following 6 weeks of a VLED (500 kcal/day) combined with SC PEG-OB protein (80 mg/week) or placebo treatment in a cohort of overweight men. Dietary restraint was measured by the Three-Factor Eating Questionnaire. Weight loss during active treatment was significantly greater than the placebo group ($p<0.03$) while dietary restraint increased to the same extent in both groups. By contrast, the weight increase following cessation of the VLED and PEG-OB protein/placebo treatments was significantly larger ($p<0.05$) in the PEG-OB protein group compared to placebo.

The regain in weight was inversely correlated with the increase in dietary restraint during treatment. The authors concluded that PEG-OB protein treatment led to greater weight loss compared to placebo, but that weight maintenance thereafter was likely accomplished by dietary restraint that was more effective in the placebo-treated group. Lejeune et al. [16] speculated that leptin treatment might limit the lifestyle changes needed for long-term weight maintenance. The authors suggest that PEG-OB protein treatment, albeit at a reduced dosage, might have to be continued in order to achieve long-term weight maintenance.

Neuroendocrine Response

Metreleptin

Shetty et al. in 2011 [21] examined leptin and neuroendocrine changes in obese subjects during long-term (6-months) weight loss. The authors evaluated a small cohort ($n=24$) of overweight and obese adults with comorbidities who were placed on a 500-kcal/day-deficit diet and randomly assigned to either SC metreleptin (10 mg/day in two divided doses) or placebo. These subjects were retrospectively selected from a larger pool of 208 subjects based on their moderate weight loss (≥8 % of initial weight) over the 6-month active treatment phase. Weight loss at the end of 6 months did not differ significantly between metreleptin (X ± SEM, 12.7 ± 1.2 %) and placebo groups (10.2 ± 1.7 %) even though active treatment increased serum leptin levels six- to

Table 17.2 Secondary outcome effects observed in leptin clinical trials in subjects without leptin mutations

Reference	Dose	Subjects	Results
Metreleptin			
O'Neil et al. 1999 [19]	SC metreleptin 10 mg 2×/day × 4 weeks; 500 kcal/day deficit diet beginning at 3-week lead-in	16 obese adults	Significant improvement in Emotional Eating Factor of DIET and Disinhibition Scale of the Three Factor Eating Questionnaire. No significant mood changes. There was no placebo group in this open-label trial
Chan et al. 2005 [23]	SC metreleptin 10 mg 2×/day or placebo; 500 kcal/day deficit diet × 16 weeks	Initial short-term studies of lean and obese men; 117 obese subjects with diet-controlled type 2 diabetes mellitus	Increasing leptin from low to high physiologic levels in lean men and from high physiologic to low pharmacologic levels in obese men over a 3 day period did not alter serum interferon-γ, IL-10, TNF-α, monocyte chemoattractant protein-1, or soluble intercellular adhesion molecule-1. Metreleptin treatment for 4 or 16 weeks in subjects with diabetes did not activate the TNF-α system or increase cytokines or inflammatory markers. These observations do not support a role for leptin in hyperleptinemic proinflammatory states
Shetty et al. 2011 [21]	SC metreleptin 10-20 mg/day or placebo; 500 kcal/day deficit diet × 24 weeks	Post-hoc analysis of larger trial; 24 overweight and obese adults	Changes in thyroid and IGF axes at 12 and 24 weeks did not differ significantly between placebo- and metreleptin-treated groups; leptin does not appear to mediate neuroendocrine changes in response to weight loss associated with a hypocaloric diet
Pegylated OB protein			
Hukshorn et al. 2003 [14] Lejeune et al. 2003 [16]	SC PEG-OB protein 80 mg/week + 500 kcal/day VLED × 46 days	Overweight men	Between-group differences in percentage fat, fat-free mass, or fat mass reductions nonsignificant; lowering of REE, sleeping metabolic rate, or RQ did not differ between active and placebo groups
Hukshorn et al. 2003 [14]			Dietary restraint increased and hunger, REE, and RQ decreased similarly in PEG-OB protein and the placebo groups
Hukshorn et al. 2004 [17]			No significant between-group differences in thyroid, corticotropic, somatotropic axes, and sympathetic nervous system activity; fasting-induced reduction in luteinizing hormone levels attenuated after weight loss adjustment in the PEG-OB protein group
Lejeune et al. 2007 [18]			The findings did not support leptin's proinflammatory role in obese subjects with a normal leptin gene
			No significant PEG-OB protein treatment effects observed over treatment course for changes in insulin, glucose, and adiponectin. No correlation observed between plasma levels of ghrelin and leptin

PEG-OB protein Pegylated recombinant native human leptin, *REE* Resting energy expenditure, *r-metHu-Leptin and metreleptin* Recombinant methionyl leptin, *RQ* Respiratory quotient, *SC* subcutaneous, *VLED* Very-low energy diet

eightfold ($p<0.001$). As in the previous metreleptin studies, anti-leptin antibodies were present and were observed in 56 % of subjects at 3 and 6 months of treatment. Although serum levels of free leptin were increased, thyroid and IGF axis hormones did not differ significantly between the active and placebo treatment. The authors conclude that leptin is not a likely mediator of the neuroendocrine changes observed in response to the weight loss observed when overweight and obese subjects without leptin mutations are placed on a hypocaloric diet.

PEG-OB Protein

Leptin levels decrease during a fast and the drop in hormone levels is thought to act as a feedback signal that promotes food intake and reduces energy expenditure as means of restoring energy equilibrium. Hukshorn et al. [15] examined this hypothesis by evaluating neuroendocrine signals in overweight men prescribed a 500 kcal/day VLED that induced a semi-starvation state for 46 days. Subjects during this period were randomized to receive either 80 mg/week of PEG OB protein or placebo. Although subjects in the active treatment group lost more weight than in the placebo group (Δ2.8 kg. $p=0.027$), there were no significant between-group differences in semi-starvation induced changes in thyroid, corticotropic, somatotropic axes, and sympathetic nervous system activity. Compared to the placebo group, the fasting-induced reduction in luteinizing hormone levels was attenuated after weight loss adjustment in the PEG-OB protein group. Hukshorn et al. [15] conclude that reduced leptin levels accompanying semi-starvation in humans with a normal leptin gene might be a component of fasting-induced neuroendocrine inhibition of the reproductive axis.

Lejeune et al. [18] examined plasma levels of ghrelin, adiponectin, insulin, and glucose during semi-starvation (VLED, 500 kcal/day for up to 46 days) in overweight/obese men who also received either leptin treatment (SC PEG-OB protein, 80 mg/week) or placebo. Weight loss at the end of treatment was significantly greater in the PEG-OB protein group compared to the placebo group (X±SD, 14.6±0.8 kg vs. 11.8±0.9 kg, $p=0.03$). No significant PEG-OB protein treatment effects were observed over the treatment course for changes in insulin, glucose, and adiponectin. Although ghrelin levels are reduced in the presence of high leptin levels [22], no correlation was observed in this study between plasma levels of ghrelin and leptin, a finding leading the authors to conclude that over the 46 days treatment period the weight-loss effects on plasma ghrelin levels was dominant over the high plasma leptin levels.

Inflammatory Marker Response

Metreleptin

Chan et al. in 2005 [23] examined the response of inflammatory markers and other cytokines that are important in the T helper cell to metreleptin in lean, obese, and obese diabetic men. Short-term (3 days) dose-ranging metreleptin treatments did not alter serum interferon-γ, IL-10, TNF-α, monocyte chemoattractant protein-1, or soluble intercellular adhesion molecule-1 levels in lean and obese men. Metreleptin administration to the obese men with type 2 diabetes for up to 16 weeks failed to activate the TNF-α system or increase cytokines or inflammatory markers. The authors conclude that their observations do not support a pathophysiologic role for leptin in proinflammatory states such as is present in people who are obese and who do not have mutations in the leptin gene.

PEG-OB Protein

To examine the suggestion that elevated leptin levels are the basis of the low grade proinflammatory state observed in human obesity, Hukshorn et al. [17] determined if SC PEG-OB protein at a dose of 80 mg/week for 46 days prevents the reduction in cellular and humoral inflammation mediators during VLED treatment in overweight men. The study rationale was that exogenous leptin treatment during rapid weight loss could potentially counteract the beneficial weight-loss effects on the proinflammatory obese state. Treatment with PEG-OB protein failed to influence the decrease in the total leukocyte count and mononuclear subfractions during the VLED diet period. C-reactive protein levels increased ($P<0.05$) and was the only indication of a humoral proinflammatory leptin action. These findings did not support leptin's proinflammatory role in nonsyndromic human obesity and are complementary to those of the metreleptin studies of Chan et al. [23].

Metabolic Responses

PEG-OB Protein

At the 20 mg/day dose there were no between-group differences in fat loss, sleeping metabolic rate, or RQ [8]. Percent change in serum triglycerides from baseline was significantly correlated with body weight loss in the PEG-OB protein group ($p<0.01$), but not in the placebo group. Although larger reductions in serum triglycerides were observed in the PEG-OB protein group compared with the placebo group, these differences were not statistically significant. The trends observed in serum triglycerides suggest that a weekly 20-mg SC treatment with PEG-OB protein may have biological effects in obese men. However, there were no notable plasma triglyceride effects reported in the 80 mg/week PEG-OB dose studies [17], thus suggesting these observations have limited clinical value.

At the 80 mg dose [14, 16] there were no between-group differences in percentage fat, fat-free mass, or fat mass reductions. The lowering of resting energy expenditure, sleeping metabolic rate, or respiratory quotient typically seen with weight loss did not differ between active treatment and placebo groups.

Conclusions

There are two main groups of studies evaluating leptin therapy in subjects without mutations in the leptin gene, one based on metreleptin and the other on PEG-OB protein. While their half-lives differ substantially, both preparations raise blood leptin and with limited data, CNS leptin levels. Thus, the available publications provide a good foundation for testing proof-of-concept that exogenous leptin treatment in subjects without leptin gene mutations promotes weight loss. Indeed, statistically significant weight-loss effects were observed with both hormone preparations, but the effect sizes were relatively small and were detected only at high exogenous leptin doses that were accompanied by prohibitive injection site reactions. Moreover, a scattering of secondary outcomes proved statistically significant in these trials, but these findings were usually found through post-hoc analyses and the reported studies were typically not powered with these endpoints as primary outcomes. Any such findings, should they be of clinical or scientific interest, will thus require replication in appropriately designed future trials. Our review thus suggests that exogenous administration of leptin to subjects without leptin gene mutations meets with substantial hormone resistance and thus a future strategy to overcome this limitation is needed in order for leptin to prove clinically useful as weight-loss treatment.

References

1. Zhang Y, Proenca R, Maffei M, Barone M, Leopold L, Friedman JM. Positional cloning of the mouse obese gene and its human homologue. Nature. 1994;372(6505):425–32. PubMed PMID: 7984236, Epub 1994/12/01. eng.
2. Halaas JL, Gajiwala KS, Maffei M, Cohen SL, Chait BT, Rabinowitz D, et al. Weight-reducing effects of the plasma protein encoded by the obese gene. Science. 1995;269(5223):543–6. PubMed PMID: 7624777, Epub 1995/07/28. eng.
3. Tartaglia LA, Dembski M, Weng X, Deng N, Culpepper J, Devos R, et al. Identification and expression cloning of a leptin receptor OB-R. Cell. 1995;83(7):1263–71. PubMed PMID: 8548812, Epub 1995/12/29. eng.
4. Montague CT, Farooqi IS, Whitehead JP, Soos MA, Rau H, Wareham NJ, et al. Congenital leptin deficiency is associated with severe early-onset obesity in humans. Nature. 1997;387(6636):903–8. PubMed PMID: 9202122, Epub 1997/06/26. eng.
5. Farooqi IS, Jebb SA, Langmack G, Lawrence E, Cheetham CH, Prentice AM, et al. Effects of recombinant leptin therapy in a child with congenital leptin deficiency. N Engl J Med. 1999;341(12):879–84. PubMed PMID: 10486419, Epub 1999/09/16. eng.

6. Considine RV, Sinha MK, Heiman ML, Kriauciunas A, Stephens TW, Nyce MR, et al. Serum immunoreactive-leptin concentrations in normal-weight and obese humans. N Engl J Med. 1996; 334(5):292–5. PubMed PMID: 8532024, Epub 1996/02/01. eng.
7. Heymsfield SB, Greenberg AS, Fujioka K, Dixon RM, Kushner R, Hunt T, et al. Recombinant leptin for weight loss in obese and lean adults: a randomized, controlled, dose-escalation trial. JAMA. 1999;282(16):1568–75. PubMed PMID: 10546697, Epub 1999/11/05. eng.
8. Hukshorn CJSW, Westerterp-Plantenga MS, Farid AR, Smith FJ, Campfield LA. Weekly subcutaneous pegylated recombinant native human leptin (PEG-OB) administration in obese men. J Clin Endocrinol Metab. 2000;85(11):4003–9.
9. Varnerin JP, Smith T, Rosenblum CI, Vongs A, Murphy BA, Nunes C, et al. Production of leptin in Escherichia coli: a comparison of methods. Protein Expr Purif. 1998;14(3):335–42. PubMed PMID: 9882567, Epub 1999/01/12. eng.
10. Chan JL, Wong SL, Orlova C, Raciti P, Mantzoros CS. Pharmacokinetics of recombinant methionyl human leptin after subcutaneous administration: variation of concentration-dependent parameters according to assay. J Clin Endocrinol Metab. 2007;92(6):2307–11. PubMed PMID: 17405837, Epub 2007/04/05. eng.
11. Chan JL, Wong SL, Mantzoros CS. Pharmacokinetics of subcutaneous recombinant methionyl human leptin administration in healthy subjects in the fed and fasting states: regulation by gender and adiposity. Clin Pharmacokinet. 2008;47(11):753–64. PubMed PMID: 18840030, Pubmed Central PMCID: 2737404, Epub 2008/10/09. eng.
12. Fujioka K, Patane J, Lubina J, Lau D. CSF leptin levels after exogenous administration of recombinant methionyl human leptin. JAMA. 1999;282(16):1517–8. PubMed PMID: 10546689, Epub 1999/11/05. eng.
13. Zelissen PM, Stenlof K, Lean ME, Fogteloo J, Keulen ET, Wilding J, et al. Effect of three treatment schedules of recombinant methionyl human leptin on body weight in obese adults: a randomized, placebo-controlled trial. Diabetes Obes Metab. 2005;7(6):755–61. PubMed PMID: 16219020, Epub 2005/10/13. eng.
14. Hukshorn CJ, Westerterp-Plantenga MS, Saris WH. Pegylated human recombinant leptin (PEG-OB) causes additional weight loss in severely energy-restricted, overweight men. Am J Clin Nutr. 2003; 77(4):771–6. PubMed PMID: 12663271, Epub 2003/03/29. eng.
15. Hukshorn CJ, Menheere PP, Westerterp-Plantenga MS, Saris WH. The effect of pegylated human recombinant leptin (PEG-OB) on neuroendocrine adaptations to semi-starvation in overweight men. Eur J Endocrinol. 2003;148(6):649–55. PubMed PMID: 12773137, Epub 2003/05/30. eng.
16. Lejeune MP, Hukshorn CJ, Saris WH, Westerterp-Plantenga MS. Effect of dietary restraint during and following pegylated recombinant leptin (PEG-OB) treatment of overweight men. Int J Obes Relat Metab Disord. 2003;27(12):1494–9. PubMed PMID: 14634680, Epub 2003/11/25. eng.
17. Hukshorn CJ, Lindeman JH, Toet KH, Saris WH, Eilers PH, Westerterp-Plantenga MS, et al. Leptin and the proinflammatory state associated with human obesity. J Clin Endocrinol Metab. 2004; 89(4):1773–8. PubMed PMID: 15070944, Epub 2004/04/09. eng.
18. Lejeune MP, Hukshorn CJ, Saris WH, Westerterp-Plantenga MS. Effects of very low calorie diet induced body weight loss with or without human pegylated recombinant leptin treatment on changes in ghrelin and adiponectin concentrations. Physiol Behav. 2007;91(2–3):274–80. PubMed PMID: 17434547, Epub 2007/04/17. eng.
19. O'Neil P, Rogers R, Malcolm R, Shaub R, Patane J, McCamish M. Assessment of behavioral and mood changes among obese persons receiving exogenous leptin. Obes Res. 1999;7(S1):92S.
20. Westerterp-Plantenga MS, Saris WH, Hukshorn CJ, Campfield LA. Effects of weekly administration of pegylated recombinant human OB protein on appetite profile and energy metabolism in obese men. Am J Clin Nutr. 2001;74(4):426–34. PubMed PMID: 11566639, Epub 2001/09/22. eng.
21. Shetty GK, Matarese G, Magkos F, Moon HS, Liu X, Brennan AM, et al. Leptin administration to overweight and obese subjects for 6 months increases free leptin concentrations but does not alter circulating hormones of the thyroid and IGF axes during weight loss induced by a mild hypocaloric diet. Eur J Endocrinol. 2011;165(2):249–54. PubMed PMID: 21602313, Pubmed Central PMCID: 3159386, Epub 2011/05/24.eng.
22. Barazzoni R, Zanetti M, Stebel M, Biolo G, Cattin L, Guarnieri G. Hyperleptinemia prevents increased plasma ghrelin concentration during short-term moderate caloric restriction in rats. Gastroenterology. 2003;124(5):1188–92. PubMed PMID: 12730858, Epub 2003/05/06. eng.
23. Chan JL, Bullen J, Stoyneva V, Depaoli AM, Addy C, Mantzoros CS. Recombinant methionyl human leptin administration to achieve high physiologic or pharmacologic leptin levels does not alter circulating inflammatory marker levels in humans with leptin sufficiency or excess. J Clin Endocrinol Metab. 2005;90(3):1618–24. PubMed PMID: 15613407, Epub 2004/12/23. eng.

Leptin Therapy in Patients with Lipodystrophy and Syndromic Insulin Resistance

18

Rebecca J. Brown and Phillip Gorden

Abbreviations

ACTH	Adrenocorticotropic hormone
AGL	Acquired generalized lipodystrophy
APL	Acquired partial lipodystrophy
BMI	Body mass index
CGL	Congenital generalized lipodystrophy
CRH	Corticotropin releasing hormone
FDA	Food and Drug Administration
fMRI	Functional magnetic resonance imaging
FPL	Familial partial lipodystrophy
GnRH	Gonadotropin releasing hormone
HIV	Human immunodeficiency
HAART	Highly active antiretroviral therapy
IGF-1	Insulin-like growth factor-1
LH	Luteinizing hormone
NAFLD	Nonalcoholic fatty liver disease
NAS	NAFLD activity score
NASH	Nonalcoholic steatohepatitis
NIH	National Institutes of Health
PCOS	Polycystic ovary syndrome
PI3K	Phosphoinositide 3-kinase
TRH	Thyrotropin releasing hormone
TSH	Thyroid stimulating hormone

The discovery of the adipocyte-derived hormone leptin by Jeffrey Friedman's laboratory in 1994 was a seminal event in the history of science and medicine. Leptin acts as a signal of total body energy sufficiency. Leptin deficiency, either in the physiologic state of starvation or the pathophysiologic states of congenital leptin deficiency and lipodystrophy, leads to hyperphagia and impaired reproduction. Pharmacologic treatment with leptin reverses the hyperphagia of leptin-deficient states, but has little clinical effect in states of endogenous leptin sufficiency or excess, such as obesity. The greatest success of leptin as a pharmaceutical agent has been in patients with lipodystrophy, who have leptin deficiency as a result of deficient adipose mass. Based on the dramatic improvements in metabolic disease seen with leptin replacement, the FDA approved recombinant human methionyl leptin (metreleptin) for patients with generalized lipodystrophy in February, 2014, 20 years after the hormone was first described. Leptin remains an experimental drug for all other conditions, including partial forms of lipodystrophy. The clinical effects of leptin pharmacotherapy in both generalized and partial forms of lipodystrophy are discussed in this chapter.

Lipodystrophy Syndromes

The lipodystrophy syndromes are a heterogeneous group of disorders that are characterized by selective deficiency of subcutaneous adipose

R.J. Brown, M.D. (✉) • P. Gorden, M.D., M.H.Sc.
National Institute of Diabetes and Digestive and Kidney Diseases, National Institutes of Health, Building 10, Room 6-5940, 10 Center Drive, Bethesda, MD 20892, USA
e-mail: brownrebecca@mail.nih.gov; PhillipG@intra.niddk.nih.gov

S. Dagogo-Jack (ed.), *Leptin: Regulation and Clinical Applications*,
DOI 10.1007/978-3-319-09915-6_18, © Springer International Publishing Switzerland 2015

tissue. This deficiency of subcutaneous fat may involve the entire body (generalized lipodystrophy) or selected fat depots, most commonly the limbs and buttocks (partial lipodystrophy) (Fig. 18.1). Lipodystrophies, either generalized or partial, may be genetic or acquired in origin (Fig. 18.2). All known inherited generalized lipodystrophies are autosomal recessive, whereas the majority of inherited partial lipodystrophies are autosomal dominant [1]. Inherited forms of lipodystrophy can also be associated with other syndromic conditions, such as progeria, and may be associated with variable extent of adipose deficiency. The most common form of acquired lipodystrophy is associated with infection with the human immunodeficiency virus (HIV) combined with use of highly active antiretroviral therapy (HAART). Acquired lipodystrophies that are not due to HIV/HAART are thought to be due to autoimmune destruction of adipocytes, because they are commonly associated with other systemic or organ-specific autoimmune diseases [2].

Metabolic Disease in Lipodystrophy

The metabolic complications of lipodystrophy are shown in Table 18.1. The primary physiologic abnormality in lipodystrophy is deficient subcutaneous adipose tissue. This deficiency in adipocytes leads to low levels of adipocyte-derived hormones, including leptin, adiponectin, and others. The low leptin is sensed by the brain as a starvation signal, leading to hyperphagia. Unlike obese patients, those with lipodystrophy cannot store excess caloric intake in subcutaneous fat, and hence these excess calories are stored as triglyceride in ectopic locations, including the muscle and the liver. Ectopic lipid in the liver leads to nonalcoholic fatty liver disease, and ectopic lipid in both the liver and the muscle contributes to insulin resistance. This insulin resistance may be extreme, and frequently results in diabetes as beta-cell function declines. Despite the presence of insulin resistance, lipodystrophy patients (just like those with the obesity-associated metabolic syndrome) retain selective sensitivity to insulin at certain tissues. In the liver, although insulin fails to suppress to glucose production, insulin continues to stimulate lipogenesis, further exacerbating fatty liver disease and leading to hypertriglyceridemia. The ovary similarly maintains sensitivity to insulin, and the extreme hyperinsulinemia of lipodystrophy can lead to ovarian enlargement and hyperandrogenism, analogous to the common polycystic ovary syndrome (PCOS). In addition to subfertility from PCOS, patients with generalized lipodystrophy also have significantly reduced fertility resulting from abnormal secretion of the gonadotropin hormones, luteinizing hormone, and follicle stimulating hormone; this is a direct result of leptin deficiency.

Overall, the metabolic disease of lipodystrophy is a result of the combination of both leptin deficiency (as well as deficiency of other adipokines) plus ectopic lipid deposition. This combination results in more severe metabolic disease than that observed in patients with isolated congenital leptin or leptin receptor deficiency, who have normal adipose tissue storage capacity [3, 4]. Likewise, patients with lipodystrophy have metabolic disease that is analogous to, but more severe than that seen patients with the common, obesity-associated metabolic syndrome [5]. Patients with the obesity-associated metabolic syndrome are thought to have ectopic lipid deposition as a result of exceeding the storage capacity of their subcutaneous adipose tissue; the mechanism of ectopic lipid storage in lipodystrophy is the same, but adipose tissue stores are exhausted much sooner in lipodystrophy than in obesity.

Clinical Effects of Metreleptin in Lipodystrophy

Treatment of lipodystrophy with conventional metabolic therapies, such as insulin, oral hypoglycemic agents, and lipid lowering agents, is extremely challenging. Some patients require thousands of units of insulin per day [6], and many have severe hypertriglyceridemia leading to pancreatitis despite maximal therapy with drugs such as fibrates, statins, or even plasmapheresis [7]. Since 2000, over 100 patients with lipodystrophy have been treated with leptin, most at the National Institutes

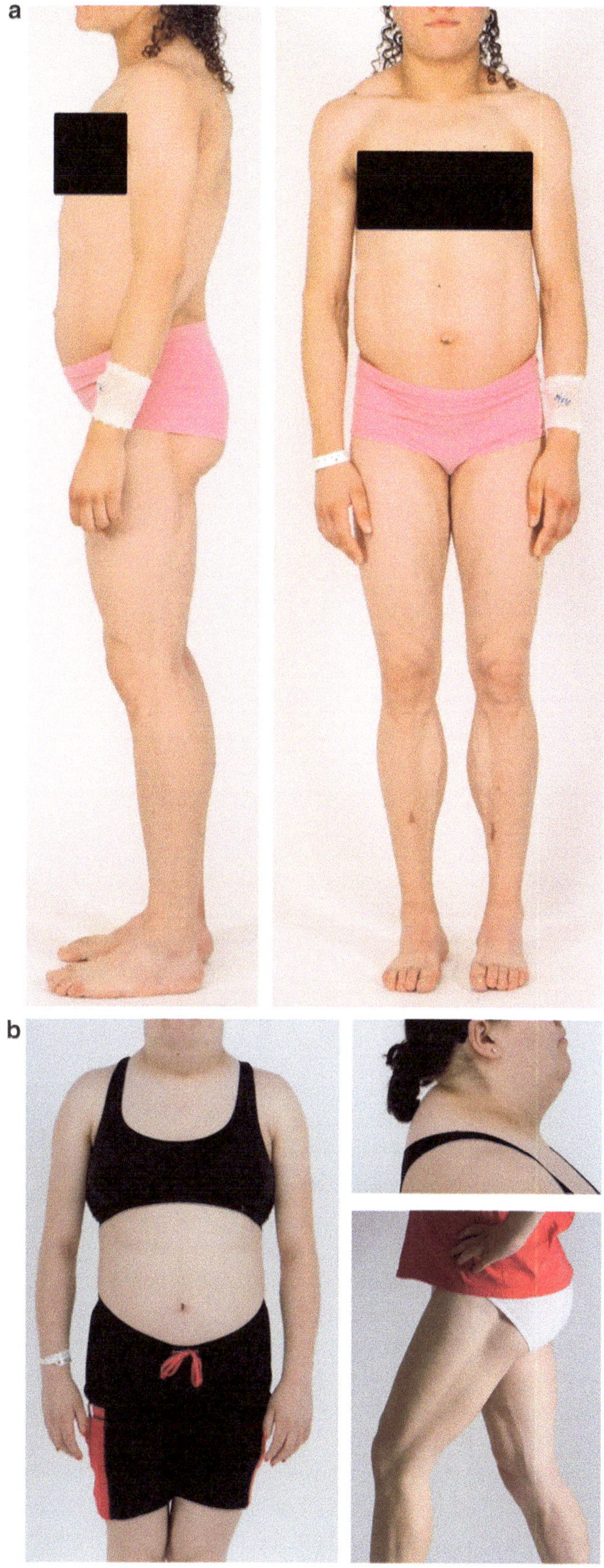

Fig. 18.1 Physical phenotype of generalized versus partial lipodystrophy. (**a**) A young woman with congenital generalized lipodystrophy due to recessive mutation in AGPAT2. She exhibits generalized deficiency of subcutaneous adipose tissue, leading to a muscular appearance with prominent veins. The increase in abdominal girth is secondary to organomegaly. (**b**) An adolescent girl with familial partial lipodystrophy due to dominant mutation in LMNA. She has absent subcutaneous adipose tissue in the legs and gluteal region, resulting in a muscular appearance with prominent veins, similar to the patient with generalized lipodystrophy. Subcutaneous fat is greatly diminished, but not absent, in the arms. There is increased fat present in the head, neck, and trunk, resulting in a Cushingoid appearance

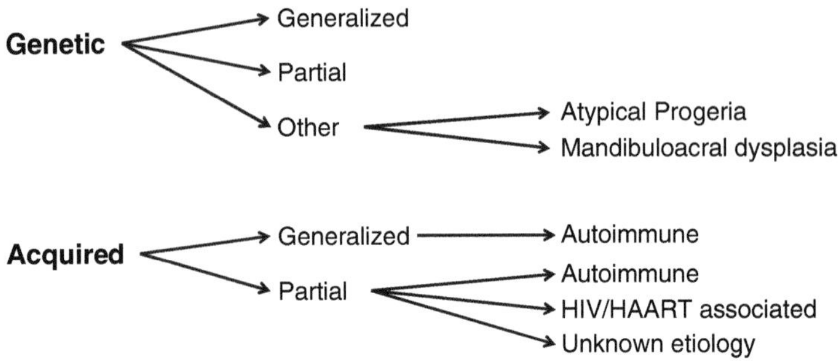

Fig. 18.2 Classification scheme for lipodystrophies. Lipodystrophies are classified according to their origin (genetic or acquired), and the distribution of body fat deficiency (generalized or partial). Lipodystrophy may also occur in patients with progeroid (premature aging) disorders, including atypical progeria and mandibuloacral dysplasia. These disorders are classified separately, as they may lead to either partial or generalized lipodystrophy. The most common form of acquired lipodystrophy arises in individuals treated with highly active antitretroviral therapy (HAART) for the human immunodeficiency virus (HIV). Most other acquired lipodystrophies are thought to be secondary to autoimmune destruction of adipocytes, as they are associated with systemic or organ-specific autoimmune conditions

Table 18.1 Metabolic complications of lipodystrophy

Glucose metabolism:
Insulin resistance
Diabetes
Acanthosis nigricans
Lipid metabolism:
High triglycerides
Eruptive xanthomata
Pancreatitis
Nonalcoholic fatty liver disease (NAFLD)
Steatosis → Nonalcoholic steatohepatitis (NASH) → Cirrhosis
Reproductive:
Polycystic ovary syndrome (PCOS)
Abnormal gonadotropin secretion

Table 18.2 Types of lipodystrophy treated with leptin at the National Institutes of Health

	Inheritance (genes)	Endogenous leptin level mean ± SD (range) (ng/mL)
Congenital generalized lipodystrophy (CGL)	Autosomal recessive (AGPAT2, BSCL2)	1.17 ± 0.8 (0.25–3.3)
Familial partial lipodystrophy (FPL)	Usually autosomal dominant (LMNA, PPARγ, unknown)	5.9 ± 3.0 (0.95–12.3)
Atypical progeria	Autosomal recessive (LMNA, ZMPSTE24, unknown)	1.08 ± 0.5 (0.33–1.8)
Acquired generalized lipodystrophy (AGL)	_	1.05 ± 0.7 (0.25–3.3)
Acquired partial lipodystrophy (APL)	_	7.5 ± 6.8 (0.61–16.9)

of Health (NIH) in Bethesda, MD. The types of lipodystrophy treated with leptin at the NIH are shown in Table 18.2. The initial investigation of leptin in lipodystrophy was designed as a proof of principle study to determine if leptin replacement in this hypoleptinemic state could act as a targeted therapy for the metabolic diseases of lipodystrophy. This uncontrolled study of nine patients with severe hypoleptinemia (leptin <4 ng/mL) showed such dramatic improvements in triglycerides and diabetes control that it was subsequently considered unethical to conduct placebo-controlled trials of leptin in this population [8]. Further studies have shown that leptin replacement in lipodystrophy leads to improvements in ectopic lipid, insulin resistance and diabetes, hypertriglyceridemia and its complications, fatty liver disease, and subfertility. While many of these effects may be mediated via reductions in hyperphagia, rodent data suggest that leptin likely has direct effects to improve metabolic disease independent of central nervous system mediated changes in food intake [9, 10].

Appetite, Weight, and Body Composition

In lipodystrophy, as in other models of leptin deficiency, leptin replacement causes a reduction in spontaneous food intake by approximately 50 % [11, 12]. The neural pathways involved in appetite regulation with leptin replacement in lipodystrophy were investigated by Aotani et al. using functional magnetic resonance imaging (fMRI) [13]. They demonstrated that leptin is most important for postprandial satiety via suppression of neural activity in brain regions including the amygdala, insulin, nucleus accumbens, caudate, putamen, and globus pallidus.

Despite the substantial reduction in food intake, lipodystrophy patients experience only modest weight loss with leptin replacement, averaging approximately 7.5 kg after 1 year, with most of the weight loss occurring during the first 4–6 months of treatment [11]. Some of this weight loss may be attributed to reduction in liver size (from 3,055 to 2,204 cm^3 after 1 year) [11]. Reductions in lean body mass occurred as well, but were not statistically significant. Some patients with generalized lipodystrophy appear to be particularly sensitive to the appetite suppressing effects of leptin, with weight loss of 20 kg or more, and the dose may need to be reduced to prevent excessive weight loss in these patients (unpublished data).

Lipid Metabolism

The most dramatic clinical effect of leptin treatment in lipodystrophy is improvement in hypertriglyceridemia. The first lipodystrophy patient treated with leptin, an adolescent with acquired, generalized lipodystrophy, had extreme hypertriglyceridemia, with serum triglyceride levels consistently greater than 10,000 mg/dL, resulting in painful xanthomata and recurrent pancreatitis. Prior to leptin treatment, this patient required weekly plasmapheresis to maintain triglycerides at ~5,000 mg/dL. After initiating leptin treatment, the patient's triglyceride level fell to ~1,000 mg/dL, plasmapheresis was discontinued, and xanthomata resolved; triglycerides improved further to ~200 mg/dL with inpatient administration of a high mono-unsaturated fat diet. This patient was one of nine patients who participated in the first study of leptin in lipodystrophy, which included eight patients with generalized lipodystrophy and one with partial lipodystrophy, all with endogenous leptin less than 4 ng/mL (mean leptin 1.3±0.3 ng/mL). Thish study showed a 60 % reduction in serum triglycerides after 4 months of treatment [8]. Similar findings have been observed in subsequent, larger and more heterogeneous cohorts. In 55 patients (36 with generalized lipodystrophy and 19 with partial lipodystrophy) with endogenous leptin less than 12 ng/mL (mean leptin 2.8±2.8 ng/mL), leptin treatment decreased triglycerides from 479±80 mg/dL (geometric mean±SEM) to 254±40 after 4 months, and 164±26 after 3 years. Among the subgroup of 41 patients who had hypertriglyceridemia (>200 mg/dL) at baseline, the change was even more dramatic, with triglyceride levels falling from 743±123 mg/dL at baseline to 326±59 after 4 months and 197±35 after 3 years.

Ectopic Lipid

Leptin replacement in lipodystrophy leads to substantial reductions in ectopic lipid, both in the liver and in the muscle. In patients with generalized lipodystrophy, magnetic resonance spectroscopy demonstrated ~80 % reduction in hepatic triglyceride and ~40 % reduction in intramyocellular triglyceride with 2–10 months of leptin treatment [12, 14].

Nonalcoholic Fatty Liver Disease

Patients with lipodystrophy typically have a form of liver disease that most resembles the nonalcoholic fatty liver disease (NAFLD) seen in obesity. However, lipodystrophy patients appear to have a much greater prevalence of the later stages of NAFLD (nonalcoholic steatohepatitis [NASH] and cirrhosis) compared to patients with obesity-associated NAFLD (Table 18.3).

Table 18.3 Prevalence of the stages of nonalcoholic fatty liver disease in lipodystrophy versus obesity

	Obesity [49]	Lipodystrophy [15]
Nonalcoholic fatty liver disease (NAFLD)	40–90 %	90 %
Nonalcoholic steatohepatitis (NASH)	10–20 % of NAFLD	70–90 %
Cirrhosis	0–4 % of NAFLD (over 10–20 years)	17 %
Hepatocellular carcinoma	2–5 % per year in patients with cirrhosis	Not reported

Patients with congenital generalized lipodystrophy due to mutations in the BSCL2 gene (encoding the protein seipin) appear to be at particularly high risk for advanced liver disease at an early age, with 9 of 10 patients, all under 18 years of age, having bridging fibrosis or cirrhosis at the time of pre-leptin liver biopsy.

Leptin treatment reduces liver volume in lipodystrophy by 28 % after 4 months of treatment, presumably secondary to reduction in hepatic triglyceride content [8]. In 27 patients (15 generalized, 12 partial), liver biopsies were performed before and 26±4 months (median 15 months) after leptin treatment [15]. Although 86 % of patients met histologic criteria for definite or borderline NASH prior to leptin, only 33 % had NASH on biopsy after leptin. Mean NAFLD activity scores (NAS) decreased from 4.3 (out of a maximum of 8) to 2.4. This improvement in NAS was attributable to improvements in steatosis and inflammation; no changes in fibrosis were observed. Three of four patients with advanced cirrhosis at baseline remained clinically stable over 2–6 years of follow-up, and the fourth died of liver failure after 17 months of leptin treatment.

Glucose Metabolism

The original study of leptin in lipodystrophy showed a 1.9 % reduction in A1c after 4 months of treatment [8]. This effect has been reconfirmed as numbers of patients treated has grown, including not only the international NIH cohort, but also a cohort in Japan [16]. In generalized lipodystrophy patients, reductions in fasting glucose are seen rapidly after introduction of leptin treatment, with statistically significant declines (from 172 to 120 mg/dL) by day 7 of treatment [16]. Moreover, the beneficial effects on glycemia have been sustained over time [17–19]. The most recent publication based on the NIH cohort showed a 4 month reduction in A1c of 1.2 % ($n=40$), and a 2.1 % reduction after 3 years of treatment ($n=18$) [18]. Reductions were most dramatic in patients with worse glycemia control at baseline; among patients with an initial A1c>7 %, A1c decreased from 9.4 % at baseline, to 7.7 % after 4 months ($n=31$), and to 6.3 % after 3 years ($n=14$). These improvements in A1c were observed despite reductions in concomitant diabetes medications. In 32 patients with various forms of lipodystrophy, the percent taking insulin decreased from 40 to 22, and the percent using oral hypoglycemic agents decreased from 72 to 59 after 12 months of leptin treatment [6].

The beneficial effects of leptin on glycemia in patients with partial lipodystrophy are a bit more ambiguous. Park et al. reported significant improvement in fasting glucose (from 190 to 151 mg/dL) but nonsignificant change in A1c (from 8.4 to 8 %) in six patients with familial parital lipodystrophy of the Dunnigan type [20]. In two of these patients, leptin withdrawal for 3 months resulted in substantial worsening of A1c, suggesting it did have efficacy in these patients. Simha et al. did not observe improvements in fasting glucose, insulin, glucose tolerance, or A1c in 24 patients with familial partial lipodystrophy of the Dunnigan type, although some improvement in insulin sensitivity was observed in the subgroup with more severe hypoleptinemia. In a single patient with familial partial lipodystrophy due to mutation in the PPARγ gene, leptin treatment for 18 months led to a 2.7 % reduction in A1c.

The mechanisms responsible for improvements in clinical glycemic endpoints with leptin treatment in lipodystrophy have not been well explored. Reduction in food intake is likely to play an important role, and a study to determine if leptin has effects independent of changes in food intake is ongoing (NCT01778556). In generalized lipodystrophy, leptin improves total body insulin sensitivity as measured by the hyperinsulinemic–euglycemic clamp [12, 16]. In three subjects, improvements in hepatic insulin sensitivity have been demonstrated as well [12].

Reproduction

Leptin is known to have a permissive role in pubertal GnRH secretion. Leptin replacement in patients with congenital leptin deficiency normalizes GnRH pulsatility [21] and allows normal pubertal development [22]. Lipodystrophic patients, even those with generalized lipodystrophy and very low leptin levels, appear to have sufficient leptin secretion to permit normal pubertal development in the leptin-deficient state. However, there remains some impairment of normal hypothalamic-pituitary-gonadal axis function in lipodystrophy. In the leptin-deficient state, five lipodystrophic women with severe leptin deficiency (<4 ng/mL) had attenuated LH responses to LHRH stimulation, which improved after 4 months of leptin replacement [23], but this finding was not reproduced in a larger cohort of ten women [24]. Despite the uncertain changes in gonadotropin regulation, leptin therapy clearly normalizes menstrual cyclicity in women with lipodystrophy. Eighty percent of post-pubertal women with generalized lipodystrophy are amenorrheic or have menstrual irregularity in the leptin-deficient state, and normal cycles are restored with leptin treatment [16, 23, 24]. Moreover, leptin replacement tends to increase estradiol levels in women [23, 24] and testosterone levels in men [24].

Abnormal menstrual cycles in women with lipodystrophy are not solely attributable to impaired gonadotropin secretion. The hyperinsulinemia that results from insulin resistance in these patients increases ovarian volume and androgen production, analogous to the common polycystic ovarian syndrome (PCOS) [25]. Leptin reduced free testosterone levels in ten lipodystrophic women from 40 ± 11 ng/dL to 19 ± 4 ng/dL after 1 year, although significant reductions in ovarian volume were not observed.

The combination of abnormal gonadotropin secretion and PCOS significantly impairs fertility in women with generalized lipodystrophy. In the NIH cohort, only 1 of 12 women over age 20 years became pregnant in the leptin-deficient state (unpublished data). During experimental leptin treatment, despite strong recommendations to use birth control, three additional women with generalized lipodystrophy had spontaneous pregnancies, with two live births. By contrast, fertility appears to be relatively normal in women with partial lipodystrophy, with a mean of 1.25 children (median, 1) in women over 20 years of age prior to leptin treatment. This finding is, of course, consistent with the autosomal dominant pattern of inheritance of almost all forms of familial partial lipodystrophy. Very little is known about fertility in men with congenital generalized lipodystrophy, although there have been no cases of known or suspected paternity in the NIH cohort, either before or after leptin therapy.

Thyroid

In rodent and in vitro model systems, leptin regulates the expression of thyrotropin releasing hormone (TRH), and leptin-deficient ob/ob mice have central hypothyroidism that is corrected with leptin replacement [26]. Humans with congenital leptin deficiency have a milder phenotype, with disorganized TSH pulsatility and circadian rhythm [27], but the majority do not have overt hypothyroidism [28]. Lipodystrophy patients do not appear to have an overt thyroid phenotype, although TSH pulsatility has not been studied. The initial studies of leptin on the thyroid axis in lipodystrophy patients ($N = 7$) demonstrated statistically significant (but not clinically significant) declines in TSH (from 2.2 ± 1.1 to 1.2 ± 0.2 μU/mL, $P < 0.001$) and total thyroxine (from 126 ± 27 to 92 ± 19 nmol/L, $P < 0.001$), with no change in TSH response to TRH stimulation testing after 4 months of leptin therapy [23]. However, these findings were not reproduced in a larger cohort

($N = 14$) after 8–12 months of leptin treatment [24], suggesting that leptin replacement is unlikely to have clinically important effects on thyroid function in lipodystrophy.

Adrenal

Animal and in vitro models suggest multiple (and sometimes opposing) roles of leptin in regulation of the hypothalamic-pituitary-adrenal axis [26]. However, neither humans with congenital leptin deficiency nor lipodystrophy have any measurable perturbation of adrenal function. In lipodystrophy patients, 4–12 months of leptin replacement did not result in any change in spontaneous adrenocorticotropic hormone (ACTH) or cortisol secretion, or in ACTH and cortisol responses to corticotropin releasing hormone (CRH) stimulation [23, 24].

Growth Hormone and Insulin-Like Growth Factor-1 (IGF-1)

In rodents and in vitro studies, leptin stimulates growth hormone secretion, and leptin deficiency results in impaired linear growth [26]. This does not hold true in humans. However, human models of leptin deficiency including congenital leptin deficiency, leptin receptor mutation, and starvation support the hypothesis that leptin may regulate the ability of growth hormone to stimulate secretion of IGF-1 and its binding proteins [26]. Data from lipodystrophy patients is consistent with other human conditions: leptin replacement in lipodystrophy had no effect on fasting (unstimulated) growth hormone levels, but increased IGF-1 levels by 30–53 % [24, 25]. This increase in IGF-1 may simply be a consequence of improved insulin sensitivity, as IGF-1 is lower in insulin resistant states.

Bone

Rodent models have shown that leptin impacts bone metabolism via two distinct and opposing mechanisms. Leptin increases bone mass via direct stimulation of osteoblast differentiation and proliferation, and decreases bone mass via indirect neural circuitry involving the sympathetic nervous system [29]. The phenotype of leptin deficiency in the rodent skeleton is increased trabecular bone in the vertebrae [30], and decreased cortical bone in the vertebrae and limbs [31, 32], with overall decreased total body bone mass, due to the predominance of cortical bone in the skeleton . This phenotype is reversed by leptin replacement [32, 33]. In contrast, we have found that patients with congenital generalized lipodystrophy have *increased* total body bone mass in the leptin-deficient state, and bone mass is unchanged by leptin replacement in these patients [34]. This finding suggests that pathways linking leptin to bone metabolism in rodents may not be relevant for humans.

Kidney

Kidney disease is a common manifestation of lipodystrophy, particularly among patients with generalized lipodystrophy, and typically manifests as proteinuria and hyperfiltration. Among 15 leptin-treated patients with generalized lipodystrophy, 11 (73 %) had reduction in urine protein excretion after leptin treatment [35]. This occurred in conjunction with a decrease in creatinine clearance (from over 200 to ~120 mL/min), suggesting that improvements in protein excretion may be secondary to reduced hyperfiltration.

Immune System

The leptin deficiency of lipodystrophy is not associated with overt immunodeficiency. Certain T lymphocyte subsets were lower in ten patients with generalized lipodystrophy compared to healthy control subjects, but were within the normal range [36]. Leptin replacement in these lipodystrophy patients normalized both absolute and relative T cell subsets as well as normalizing peripheral blood mononuclear cell responsiveness to stimulation [36].

Leptin Treatment in Patients with HIV/HAART-Associated Lipodystrophy

Four small studies of leptin replacement in men with HIV/HAART-associated lipodystrophy and hypoleptinemia (endogenous leptin <3 or 4 ng/dL) have been conducted, studying a total of 41 patients [37–40]. Three of the studies showed modest improvements in insulin resistance and lipids, while the fourth showed improvements in glycemia, but minimal change in fasting lipids or lipid turnover. Two of the studies also showed reductions in truncal or visceral fat.

Leptin Treatment in Patients with Insulin Receptor Mutations

Patients with mutations of the insulin receptor suffer from extreme insulin resistance and dysglycemia, and patients are at high risk for early morbidity and mortality due to microvascular complications of diabetes [41, 42]. In contrast to lipodystrophy, insulin receptor mutations do not cause NAFLD or hypertriglyceridemia, as intact insulin signaling through its receptor is required for de novo lipogenesis in the liver [43]. Hyperglycemia in these patients is very difficult to treat [44], and glucose-lowering therapies are needed that do not require signaling through the insulin receptor. The idea of treating patients with mutations of the insulin receptor with leptin arose from the discovery that the signal transduction cascades downstream of the insulin and leptin receptors overlap at the level of phosphoinositide 3-kinase (PI3K). We hypothesized that pharmacologic treatment with leptin could increase PI3K levels in patients with insulin receptors, thereby increasing post-receptor insulin signaling while bypassing the defective receptor.

The initial pilot study of leptin treatment in this population included two siblings with the Rabson Mendenhall syndrome due to homozygous mutation of the insulin receptor [45]. Leptin therapy at doses of up to 0.06–0.09 mg/kg/day for 10 months resulted in declines in fasting glucose of 62 and 139 mg/dL, and declines in A1c of 0.9 and 1.3 % in the two patients. After leptin withdrawal for 3 months, glycemia returned to the pre-leptin baseline. These two patients were subsequently followed for 10 years, and treated with escalating doses of leptin (up to 0.22 mg/kg/day), and underwent three cycles of leptin withdrawal and reinitiation. With each withdrawal, A1c rose, and it declined again with each reinitiation, suggesting a lasting effect on glycemia [46]. A total of five patients (including the original two) with this extremely rare condition were treated with leptin at doses of 0.22 mg/kg/day for 1 year, resulting in a decrease in A1c from 11.4 ± 1.1 % at baseline, to 9.3 ± 1.9 % after 6 months, and 9.7 ± 1.6 % after 12 months. This dose of leptin resulted in significant weight loss (presumably due to appetite suppression), with declines in BMI z-score from −1.4 ± 1.8 at baseline to −2.6 ± 1.6 after 12 months. The presumed reduction in food intake likely accounted, at least in part, for the reduction in A1c. Although the 1.8 % reduction in A1c with leptin still left patients considerably above glucose targets, this reduction would be anticipated to substantially reduce the risk of microvascular complications of diabetes.

Adverse Effects of Leptin Treatment

The most common adverse effects of leptin across all treatment studies (including those conducted in obese, lipodystrophic, congenital leptin-deficient, and other populations) include hypoglycemia (in insulin treated patients), weight loss, headache, and abdominal pain (http://packageinserts.bms.com/pi/pi_myalept.pdf). Two adverse events of particular concern are listed as black box warnings in the package insert: neutralizing antibodies to leptin and T cell lymphoma. Neutralizing antibodies were observed in three lipodystrophy patients in the NIH cohort. The clinical consequences of these antibodies remain uncertain, but may include loss of efficacy of the drug, as well as severe infection. T cell lymphoma has been observed in three patients in the NIH cohort, all with a diagnosis of acquired generalized lipodystrophy. Two of these patients had preexisting neutropenia prior to initiating leptin, and were diagnosed with peripheral T cell lymphoma within a few months of starting leptin, suggesting that an active malignancy or precursor condition may have been present prior to initiation of leptin. The third patient developed anaplastic large cell lymphoma after approximately 2 years of leptin treatment. Because acquired generalized lipodystrophy is thought to be an autoimmune disorder, and patients with altered immune function are at increased risk for lymphoma, it is likely that the underlying diagnosis placed these patients at risk for lymphoma. In addition, peripheral T cell lymphoma has been reported in patients with acquired generalized lipodystrophy who never received leptin treatment [47, 48]. However, a role for leptin treatment in lymphoma development or growth cannot be entirely excluded.

Conclusions

The discovery of leptin provided a mechanism to explain how the body regulates energy balance. The fact that leptin is a circulating hormone suggested that replacement of the deficient hormone might provide benefit first in rodent models and then in humans in states of leptin deficiency. Lipodystrophy, especially in its generalized form, is a state of severe leptin deficiency and these patients, as a consequence, have severe metabolic derangements. Leptin replacement has a major effect to ameliorate hypertriglyceridemia, insulin resistance and diabetes, nonalcoholic fatty liver disease, and reproductive abnormalities, particularly in the generalized forms of lipodystrophy where metreleptin is now an approved drug. Continued studies are needed in partial forms of lipodystrophy, but at this time it seems clear that patients with more severe metabolic derangements do respond to metreleptin. Other issues remain a work in progress such as the limiting concentration of leptin in blood below which a therapeutic response can be expected, as well as further studies on optimal dosing, antigenicity, and continued safety monitoring.

References

1. Rother KI, Brown RJ. Novel forms of lipodystrophy: why should we care? Diabetes Care. 2013;36(8):2142–5. PubMed PMID: 23881965. Pubmed Central PMCID: 3714480.
2. Garg A. Clinical review#: lipodystrophies: genetic and acquired body fat disorders. J Clin Endocrinol Metab. 2011;96(11):3313–25. PubMed PMID: 21865368. Epub 2011/08/26. eng.
3. Farooqi IS, Matarese G, Lord GM, Keogh JM, Lawrence E, Agwu C, et al. Beneficial effects of leptin on obesity, T cell hyporesponsiveness, and neuroendocrine/metabolic dysfunction of human congenital leptin deficiency. J Clin Invest. 2002;110(8):1093–103. PubMed PMID: 12393845. Pubmed Central PMCID: 150795. Epub 2002/10/24. eng.
4. Farooqi IS, Wangensteen T, Collins S, Kimber W, Matarese G, Keogh JM, et al. Clinical and molecular genetic spectrum of congenital deficiency of the leptin receptor. N Engl J Med. 2007;356(3):237–47. PubMed PMID: 17229951. Pubmed Central PMCID: 2670197. Epub 2007/01/19. eng.
5. Gorden P, Lupsa BC, Chong AY, Lungu AO. Is there a human model for the 'metabolic syndrome' with a defined aetiology? Diabetologia. 2010;53(7):1534–6. PubMed PMID: 20401463. Epub 2010/04/20. eng.
6. Chong AY, Lupsa BC, Cochran EK, Gorden P. Efficacy of leptin therapy in the different forms of human lipodystrophy. Diabetologia. 2010;53(1):27–35. PubMed PMID: 19727665. Epub 2009/09/04. eng.
7. Gorden P, Zadeh ES, Cochran E, Brown RJ. Syndromic insulin resistance: models for the therapeutic basis of the metabolic syndrome and other targets of insulin resistance. Endocr Pract. 2012;18(5):763–71. PubMed PMID: 23047930.
8. Oral EA, Simha V, Ruiz E, Andewelt A, Premkumar A, Snell P, et al. Leptin-replacement therapy for lipodystrophy. N Engl J Med. 2002;346(8):570–8. PubMed PMID: 11856796. Epub 2002/02/22. eng.
9. Shimomura I, Hammer RE, Ikemoto S, Brown MS, Goldstein JL. Leptin reverses insulin resistance and diabetes mellitus in mice with congenital lipodystrophy. Nature. 1999;401(6748):73–6. PubMed PMID: 10485707. Epub 1999/09/15. eng.
10. Hidaka S, Yoshimatsu H, Kondou S, Tsuruta Y, Oka K, Noguchi H, et al. Chronic central leptin infusion restores hyperglycemia independent of food intake and insulin level in streptozotocin-induced diabetic rats. FASEB J. 2002;16(6):509–18. PubMed PMID: 11919153. Epub 2002/03/29. eng.
11. Moran SA, Patten N, Young JR, Cochran E, Sebring N, Reynolds J, et al. Changes in body composition in patients with severe lipodystrophy after leptin replacement therapy. Metabolism. 2004;53(4):513–9. PubMed PMID: 15045701. Epub 2004/03/27. eng.
12. Petersen KF, Oral EA, Dufour S, Befroy D, Ariyan C, Yu C, et al. Leptin reverses insulin resistance and

hepatic steatosis in patients with severe lipodystrophy. J Clin Invest. 2002;109(10):1345–50. PubMed PMID: 12021250. Pubmed Central PMCID: 150981. Epub 2002/05/22. eng.

13. Aotani D, Ebihara K, Sawamoto N, Kusakabe T, Aizawa-Abe M, Kataoka S, et al. Functional magnetic resonance imaging analysis of food-related brain activity in patients with lipodystrophy undergoing leptin replacement therapy. J Clin Endocrinol Metab. 2012;97(10):3663–71. PubMed PMID: 22872692. Pubmed Central PMCID: 3462942.
14. Simha V, Szczepaniak LS, Wagner AJ, DePaoli AM, Garg A. Effect of leptin replacement on intrahepatic and intramyocellular lipid content in patients with generalized lipodystrophy. Diabetes Care. 2003;26(1):30–5. PubMed PMID: 12502655. Epub 2002/12/28. eng.
15. Safar Zadeh E, Lungu AO, Cochran EK, Brown RJ, Ghany MG, Heller T, et al. The liver diseases of lipodystrophy: the long-term effect of leptin treatment. J Hepatol. 2013;59(1):131–7. PubMed PMID: 23439261.
16. Ebihara K, Kusakabe T, Hirata M, Masuzaki H, Miyanaga F, Kobayashi N, et al. Efficacy and safety of leptin-replacement therapy and possible mechanisms of leptin actions in patients with generalized lipodystrophy. J Clin Endocrinol Metab. 2007;92(2):532–41. PubMed PMID: 17118991. Epub 2006/11/23. eng.
17. Ebihara K, Masuzaki H, Nakao K. Long-term leptin-replacement therapy for lipoatrophic diabetes. N Engl J Med. 2004;351(6):615–6. PubMed PMID: 15295061.
18. Chan JL, Lutz K, Cochran E, Huang W, Peters Y, Weyer C, et al. Clinical effects of long-term metreleptin treatment in patients with lipodystrophy. Endocr Pract. 2011;17(6):922–32. PubMed PMID: 22068254. Pubmed Central PMCID: 3498767.
19. Javor ED, Cochran EK, Musso C, Young JR, Depaoli AM, Gorden P. Long-term efficacy of leptin replacement in patients with generalized lipodystrophy. Diabetes. 2005;54(7):1994–2002. PubMed PMID: 15983199. Epub 2005/06/29. eng.
20. Park JY, Javor ED, Cochran EK, DePaoli AM, Gorden P. Long-term efficacy of leptin replacement in patients with Dunnigan-type familial partial lipodystrophy. Metabolism. 2007;56(4):508–16. PubMed PMID: 17379009. Pubmed Central PMCID: 2595136. Epub 2007/03/24. eng.
21. Farooqi IS, Jebb SA, Langmack G, Lawrence E, Cheetham CH, Prentice AM, et al. Effects of recombinant leptin therapy in a child with congenital leptin deficiency. N Engl J Med. 1999;341(12):879–84. PubMed PMID: 10486419. Epub 1999/09/16. eng.
22. Licinio J, Caglayan S, Ozata M, Yildiz BO, de Miranda PB, O'Kirwan F, et al. Phenotypic effects of leptin replacement on morbid obesity, diabetes mellitus, hypogonadism, and behavior in leptin-deficient adults. Proc Natl Acad Sci U S A. 2004;101(13):4531–6. PubMed PMID: 15070752. Pubmed Central PMCID: 384781.
23. Oral EA, Ruiz E, Andewelt A, Sebring N, Wagner AJ, Depaoli AM, et al. Effect of leptin replacement on pituitary hormone regulation in patients with severe lipodystrophy. J Clin Endocrinol Metab. 2002; 87(7):3110–7. PubMed PMID: 12107209. Epub 2002/07/11. eng.
24. Musso C, Cochran E, Javor E, Young J, Depaoli AM, Gorden P. The long-term effect of recombinant methionyl human leptin therapy on hyperandrogenism and menstrual function in female and pituitary function in male and female hypoleptinemic lipodystrophic patients. Metabolism. 2005;54(2):255–63. PubMed PMID: 15690321. Epub 2005/02/04. eng.
25. Lungu AO, Zadeh ES, Goodling A, Cochran E, Gorden P. Insulin resistance is a sufficient basis for hyperandrogenism in lipodystrophic women with polycystic ovarian syndrome. J Clin Endocrinol Metab. 2012;97(2):563–7. PubMed PMID: 22090274. Pubmed Central PMCID: 3275358. Epub 2011/11/18. eng.
26. Mantzoros CS, Magkos F, Brinkoetter M, Sienkiewicz E, Dardeno TA, Kim SY, et al. Leptin in human physiology and pathophysiology. Am J Physiol Endocrinol Metab. 2011;301(4):E567–84. PubMed PMID: 21791620. Pubmed Central PMCID: 3191548.
27. Mantzoros CS, Ozata M, Negrao AB, Suchard MA, Ziotopoulou M, Caglayan S, et al. Synchronicity of frequently sampled thyrotropin (TSH) and leptin concentrations in healthy adults and leptin-deficient subjects: evidence for possible partial TSH regulation by leptin in humans. J Clin Endocrinol Metab. 2001;86(7):3284–91. PubMed PMID: 11443202.
28. Paz-Filho G, Delibasi T, Erol HK, Wong ML, Licinio J. Congenital leptin deficiency and thyroid function. Thyroid Res. 2009;2(1):11. PubMed PMID: 19889232. Pubmed Central PMCID: 2776005.
29. Motyl KJ, Rosen CJ. Understanding leptin-dependent regulation of skeletal homeostasis. Biochimie. 2012;94(10):2089–96. PubMed PMID: 22534195. Pubmed Central PMCID: 3512082.
30. Ducy P, Amling M, Takeda S, Priemel M, Schilling AF, Beil FT, et al. Leptin inhibits bone formation through a hypothalamic relay: a central control of bone mass. Cell. 2000;100(2):197–207. PubMed PMID: 10660043. Epub 2000/02/05. eng.
31. Hamrick MW, Pennington C, Newton D, Xie D, Isales C. Leptin deficiency produces contrasting phenotypes in bones of the limb and spine. Bone. 2004;34(3):376–83. PubMed PMID: 15003785. Epub 2004/03/09. eng.
32. Iwaniec UT, Boghossian S, Lapke PD, Turner RT, Kalra SP. Central leptin gene therapy corrects skeletal abnormalities in leptin-deficient ob/ob mice. Peptides. 2007;28(5):1012–9. PubMed PMID: 17346852. Pubmed Central PMCID: 1986832. Epub 2007/03/10. eng.
33. Hamrick MW, Della-Fera MA, Choi YH, Pennington C, Hartzell D, Baile CA. Leptin treatment induces loss of bone marrow adipocytes and increases bone formation in leptin-deficient ob/ob mice. J Bone Miner Res. 2005;20(6):994–1001. PubMed PMID: 15883640. Epub 2005/05/11. eng.
34. Christensen JD, Lungu AO, Cochran E, Collins MT, Gafni RI, Rother KI, et al. Bone mineral content in patients with congenital generalized lipodystrophy is

unaffected by metreleptin replacement therapy. J Clin Endocrinol Metab. 2014. PubMed PMID: 25070319.
35. Javor ED, Moran SA, Young JR, Cochran EK, DePaoli AM, Oral EA, et al. Proteinuric nephropathy in acquired and congenital generalized lipodystrophy: baseline characteristics and course during recombinant leptin therapy. J Clin Endocrinol Metab. 2004;89(7):3199–207. PubMed PMID: 15240593. Epub 2004/07/09. eng.
36. Oral EA, Javor ED, Ding L, Uzel G, Cochran EK, Young JR, et al. Leptin replacement therapy modulates circulating lymphocyte subsets and cytokine responsiveness in severe lipodystrophy. J Clin Endocrinol Metab. 2006;91(2):621–8. PubMed PMID: 16317060. Epub 2005/12/01. eng.
37. Lee JH, Chan JL, Sourlas E, Raptopoulos V, Mantzoros CS. Recombinant methionyl human leptin therapy in replacement doses improves insulin resistance and metabolic profile in patients with lipoatrophy and metabolic syndrome induced by the highly active antiretroviral therapy. J Clin Endocrinol Metab. 2006;91(7):2605–11. PubMed PMID: 16636130.
38. Magkos F, Brennan A, Sweeney L, Kang ES, Doweiko J, Karchmer AW, et al. Leptin replacement improves postprandial glycemia and insulin sensitivity in human immunodeficiency virus-infected lipoatrophic men treated with pioglitazone: a pilot study. Metabolism. 2011;60(7):1045–9. PubMed PMID: 21081243. Pubmed Central PMCID: 3057303. Epub 2010/11/18. eng.
39. Mulligan K, Khatami H, Schwarz JM, Sakkas GK, DePaoli AM, Tai VW, et al. The effects of recombinant human leptin on visceral fat, dyslipidemia, and insulin resistance in patients with human immunodeficiency virus-associated lipoatrophy and hypoleptinemia. J Clin Endocrinol Metab. 2009;94(4):1137–44. PubMed PMID: 19174500. Pubmed Central PMCID: 2682465.
40. Sekhar RV, Jahoor F, Iyer D, Guthikonda A, Paranilam J, Elhaj F, et al. Leptin replacement therapy does not improve the abnormal lipid kinetics of hypoleptinemic patients with HIV-associated lipodystrophy syndrome. Metabolism. 2012;61(10):1395–403. PubMed PMID: 22542724.
41. Kahn CR, Flier JS, Bar RS, Archer JA, Gorden P, Martin MM, et al. The syndromes of insulin resistance and acanthosis nigricans. Insulin-receptor disorders in man. N Engl J Med. 1976;294(14):739–45. PubMed PMID: 176581.
42. Musso C, Cochran E, Moran SA, Skarulis MC, Oral EA, Taylor S, et al. Clinical course of genetic diseases of the insulin receptor (type A and Rabson-Mendenhall syndromes): a 30-year prospective. Medicine (Baltimore). 2004;83(4):209–22. PubMed PMID: 15232309.
43. Semple RK, Sleigh A, Murgatroyd PR, Adams CA, Bluck L, Jackson S, et al. Postreceptor insulin resistance contributes to human dyslipidemia and hepatic steatosis. J Clin Invest. 2009;119(2):315–22. PubMed PMID: 19164855. Pubmed Central PMCID: 2631303. Epub 2009/01/24. eng.
44. Semple RK, Williams RM, Dunger DB. What is the best management strategy for patients with severe insulin resistance? Clin Endocrinol (Oxf). 2010;73(3):286–90. PubMed PMID: 20455892.
45. Cochran E, Young JR, Sebring N, DePaoli A, Oral EA, Gorden P. Efficacy of recombinant methionyl human leptin therapy for the extreme insulin resistance of the Rabson-Mendenhall syndrome. J Clin Endocrinol Metab. 2004;89(4):1548–54. PubMed PMID: 15070911.
46. Brown RJ, Cochran E, Gorden P. Metreleptin improves blood glucose in patients with insulin receptor mutations. J Clin Endocrinol Metab. 2013;22. PubMed PMID: 23969187.
47. Aslam A, Savage DB, Coulson IH. Acquired generalized lipodystrophy associated with peripheral T cell lymphoma with cutaneous infiltration. Int J Dermatol. 2013;29. PubMed PMID: 24168394.
48. Yiannias JA, DiCaudo DJ, Maskin E. Peripheral T-cell lymphoma presenting as lipoatrophy and nodules. Int J Dermatol. 2006;45(12):1415–9. PubMed PMID: 17184242.
49. LaBreque D. World Gastroenterology Organisation Global Guidelines on Nonalcoholic Fatty Liver Disease and Nonalcoholic Steatohepatitis 2012. 3/13/2014. Available from http://www.worldgastroenterology.org/assets/export/userfiles/2012_NASH%20and%20NAFLD_Final_long.pdf

Leptin Therapy in Women with Hypothalamic Amenorrhea

19

Sharon H. Chou and Christos Mantzoros

Hypothalamic amenorrhea (HA) is characterized by dysfunction of the hypothalamic–pituitary–gonadal (HPG) axis, leading to anovulation and cessation of menstrual cycles in the absence of organic disease. Impaired pulsatile secretion of gonadotropin-releasing hormone (GnRH) with low amplitude and/or frequency leads to low or normal gonadotropin and, subsequently, low estrogen concentrations. This condition is associated with chronic energy deficiency from disproportionately high levels of energy expenditure and/or insufficient nutritional intake. More than 30 % of cases of amenorrhea in reproductive women are attributed to HA [1].

About 6–8 % of high school athletes experience amenorrhea [2, 3], and many more experience more subtle forms of menstrual dysfunction including oligomenorrhea and regular menses with inadequate luteal phase [4]. Training intensity and type of activity are important factors as up to 40–50 % of long-distance runners, gymnasts, and ballet dancers have menstrual irregularities compared to 12 % of swimmers and cyclists [4]. The difference has been attributed to lower body weight and body fat percentage associated with aerobic type activities [5].

Although HA is one of the cardinal features of anorexia nervosa (AN), AN is also associated with severe restriction of food intake, distorted attitudes toward food, and altered body image, resulting in a body weight of less than 85 % of that expected for age and height. Patients with AN also have severe hypothalamic dysfunction, including abnormal responses to heat and cold and bradycardia [6]. HA can also be caused by subclinical nutritional deficiency. Women with HA have been found to score higher on eating disorder questionnaires and tend to have decreased caloric and fat intakes [7–9].

Psychosocial stress may also lead to HA in weight-stable, non-athletic women [10, 11]. These women tend to score higher on depression scales as well as eating disorder questionnaires, compared to eumenorrheic women and amenorrheic women due to an organic cause [12]. Unbalanced nutrient intake in psychogenic HA has been proposed to contribute to the development of associated neuroendocrine and metabolic aberrations [7].

In these conditions of chronic energy deficiency, Frisch had proposed in 1974 that menstrual

S.H. Chou, M.D.
Section of Adult and Pediatric Endocrinology, Diabetes and Metabolism, The University of Chicago, 5841 S. Maryland Avenue, MC 1027, Chicago, IL 60637, USA
e-mail: Sharon.chou@uchospitals.edu

C. Mantzoros, M.D., D.Sc. (✉)
Section of Endocrinology, Boston VA Healthcare System, Jamaica Plain, MA, USA

Department of Medicine, Beth Israel Deaconess Medical Center, Harvard Medical School and Boston Medical Center, Boston, MA 02215, USA
e-mail: cmantzor@bidmc.harvard.edu

S. Dagogo-Jack (ed.), *Leptin: Regulation and Clinical Applications*,
DOI 10.1007/978-3-319-09915-6_19,

function depends on a certain threshold of body fat (about 22 %) that serves as the minimal store of energy necessary for ovulation and menstruation [13]. Leptin, a product of adipose tissue discovered in 1994 [14], eventually emerged as the predominant candidate linking adipose tissue, energy availability, and the reproductive system [15, 16]. Hypoleptinemia, observed in association with acute starvation, weight loss, and HA, indicates a state of energy deficiency and mediates adaptive responses, such as amenorrhea. As discussed in detail below, replacement of leptin in women with HA has been shown not only to improve reproduction function but also to normalize neuroendocrine function [17, 18], increase bone mass [19], and improve immune function parameters [20].

Leptin Levels in HA

Compared to weight-matched [8, 21] and activity-matched [22, 23] eumenorrheic controls, women with HA have lower leptin levels. Miller et al. showed that women with HA have leptin levels of 7.1 ± 3.0 μg/L compared to 10.6 ± 4.9 μg/L in age-, weight-, and body fat-matched eumenorrheic controls [8]. Due to extremely low body weight and fat mass, patients with AN have even lower leptin levels, usually <2 μg/L [24], and may have an even lower free leptin index due to increased concentrations of the soluble leptin receptor [25–28], which is the main binding protein for leptin and may serve as an additional regulator of energy homeostasis [16]. Diurnal rhythm of leptin secretion is lost in female athletes with HA [29, 30] and patients with AN [31], while patients with HA of the psychogenic type are less severely affected [7].

As expected, leptin levels positively correlate with body weight, body mass index (BMI), and body fat percentage in women with HA, but other factors involved in energy balance also play a role. An increase in 1 kg/m^2 in BMI in women with HA corresponds to an increase in leptin levels that is 50 % lower than that observed in control women [21]. Puder et al. found that independent of body fat the extent of physical activity correlates inversely with leptin levels [32]. Serum leptin concentrations are also very sensitive to acute energy deprivation. Complete fasting results in a rapid fall in leptin levels that is out of proportion to changes in fat mass [33–35] and is restored with feeding [36].

Leptin levels also significantly increase with recovery from HA and AN [27, 37, 38]. In a study of woman with HA and restrictive eating disorder undergoing a nutritional rehabilitation program, leptin levels were predictive of menstrual recovery in univariate logistic regression but was no longer significant when analyzed with change in BMI [38]. Interestingly, in another study of women with psychogenic HA, treatment with cognitive behavior therapy increased leptin levels and rate of ovarian recovery compared to observation without changing BMI [39].

Neuroendocrine Axes in HA

In addition to dysfunctional HPG axis resulting in anovulation and estrogen deficiency, all other neuroendocrine axes are affected in women with HA (see Table 19.1). In response to stress, whether metabolic, physical, or psychological, the hypothalamic–pituitary–adrenal (HPA) axis is activated to stimulate lipolysis and glycogenolysis [40]. Increased levels of corticotropin-releasing hormone (CRH), adrenocorticotropic hormone (ACTH), and cortisol have been consistently observed in patients with HA [8, 29, 41–44]; increased adrenal sensitivity to ACTH has been less consistently documented [41, 42, 45, 46]. Hyperactivity of the HPA axis, in turn, suppresses GnRH and LH (luteinizing hormone) release directly as well as indirectly via stimulation of central β-endorphin release [40].

Also contributing to HPG axis dysfunction in HA are abnormalities in the hypothalamic–pituitary–thyroid (HPT) axis. In general, these include low to normal levels of thyrotropin (TSH), decreased levels of thyroid hormone, and increased levels of the inactive reverse triiodothyronine, all of which are consistent with sick euthyroid syndrome seen in chronic illness [9, 22, 23, 40, 44, 47–49]. In HA total triiodothyronine (T3) levels correlate with resting energy

Table 19.1 Neuroendocrine abnormalities in hypothalamic amenorrhea

Axis	Abnormalities	Effect of leptin replacement in hypothalamic amenorrhea
HPG	Low amplitude/frequency of GnRH pulses	Increased LH frequency, mean LH levels
	Low/normal LH, FSH levels	No change in mean FSH levels
	Low estradiol levels	Increased estradiol, progesterone levels
	Anovulation	Increased number of dominant follicles, maximal follicular diameter, and endometrial thickness
	Amenorrhea	Ovulation in 40 %
		Menstruation in 70 %
HPA	Increased CRH levels	No acute change in ACTH pulses
	Increased ACTH levels	
	Increased cortisol levels	Decreased cortisol levels
	Increased adrenal sensitivity to ACTH	
HPT	Low/normal TSH levels	No acute change in TSH levels or pulses
	Low thyroid hormone levels	Increased free T3, free T4 levels
	Increased reverse triiodothyronine levels	
Growth hormone	Increased levels of GH overnight to all day	Borderline increased mean GH levels, no acute change in pulses
	Low IGF-1 levels or IGF-1:IGFBP-1 ratio	Increased IGF-1 levels, IGF-1:IGFBP-3 ratio

HPG hypothalamic–pituitary–gonadal, *HPA* hypothalamic–pituitary–adrenal, *HPT* hypothalamic–pituitary–thyroid

expenditure (REE) corrected for fat free mass [49]. Furthermore, total T3 levels and REE fell across the continuum of menstrual function (from ovulatory to luteal phase deficiency, anovulation, and amenorrhea) in a dose–response relationship [49]. These changes towards lower basal metabolism are consistent with both the proposed role of leptin in regulating thyroid function in states of energy deficiency and the underlying hypothesis that an adaptive response to conserve energy is activated in HA.

Women with HA also have acquired growth hormone (GH) resistance. Abnormalities in GH secretion range from distorted pattern of release with nocturnal elevations in psychogenic HA [7, 47] to elevations throughout the day in amenorrheic athletes [50] and in women with AN [51]. Twelve hour overnight GH pulsatility profiles in women with exercise-induced HA reveal a pattern with less distinct peaks and wider pulses compared to eumenorrheic controls [52]. Despite higher levels of GH, insulin growth factor-1 (IGF-1) activity is lower. In weight-stable psychogenic or exercise-induced HA, basal IGF-1 levels may be lower [52] or similar to controls but with elevated IGF binding protein-1 (IGFBP-1) levels, resulting in reduced IGF-I:IGFBP-1 ratio that reflects lower free IGF-1 concentrations [7, 21, 50]. In women with weight-loss associated amenorrhea, basal IGF-1 levels are significantly lower [53] as they are in women with AN [51].

The mechanism of GH resistance in starvation and chronic energy deficiency is not well understood but has many contributing factors. Tissue GH receptor concentrations may be decreased in women with HA, as reflected by low growth hormone binding protein (GHBP) levels [7, 52, 54]. Undernutrition also directly inhibits IGF-1 production from the liver, thereby increasing GH levels due to lack of negative feedback [51]. Metabolic signals also play a role as GH is positively regulated by ghrelin [55], which simulates appetite and is elevated in women with HA, and IGFBP-1 is negatively regulated by insulin [56], which is low in women with HA [57]. FGF-21, which increases with fasting to induce ketogenesis and decrease metabolic activity, may also play a role as levels are positively correlated with GH levels and negatively with IGF-1 levels in women with AN [58].

Overall, the increase in GH activity may serve to prevent hypoglycemia while the reduction in IGF-1 activity may serve to slow growth-related processes [52] and further suppress GnRH secretion [21].

Leptin in Relation to Neuroendocrine Axes in HA

These changes in neuroendocrine function apparently serve as an adaptive response to conditions of negative energy balance—decreasing reproductive hormones levels to prevent pregnancy, decreasing thyroid hormone levels to slow metabolism, increasing growth hormone levels to mobilize energy stores, and decreasing IGF-1 levels to slow growth [59]. Hypoleptinemia has been found to be a key mediator of these neuroendocrine adaptations [60]. Leptin levels positively correlate with LH, thyroid hormone, and IGF-1 levels and negatively correlate with IGFBP-1 and cortisol levels in women with HA [21–23, 29]. Levels of leptin and these neuroendocrine hormones also correlate with REE [49], further supporting the role of hypoleptinemia in adaptation to chronic energy deficiency. With a goal of correcting hypoleptinemia, physiological doses of recombinant leptin have been shown to restore normal neuroendocrine physiology in clinical trials (see Table 19.1).

In addition to observational studies, the two pivotal clinical trials detailing the effects of leptin in women with HA are reviewed in this chapter—a proof-of-concept, pilot study of 3 month duration [18] and a randomized, placebo-controlled trial of 9 month duration [17]. In the first of these trials, the HPG axis and reproductive function were studied extensively in a 3-month open-label trial that used pelvic ultrasonography to follow dominant follicles and confirm ovulation [18]. Participants were women with HA for a mean (±SD) of 5.1 ± 4.0 years and a normal BMI of 20.5 ± 2.0 kg/m^2 with a stable weight of at least 6 months and within 15 % of ideal body weight. Eight women were started on a leptin dose of 0.08 mg/kg/day given twice a day for the first 2 months and, if ovulation had not yet occurred, an increased dose of 0.2 mg/kg/day for the third month. Leptin levels increased from 3.4 ± 1.5 to 37.4 ± 30.1 ng/mL after 3 months in this study.

In the second study similar participants were randomized to receive leptin or placebo [17]. The ten participants receiving leptin had HA for 5.1 ± 1.3 years and BMI of 20.9 ± 0.6 kg/m^2, while the nine participants receiving placebo had HA for 4.0 ± 1.1 years and BMI of 19.8 ± 0.7 kg/m^2. Starting dose for the treatment arm of this trial was the same at 0.08 mg/kg/day, given once in the evening, and increased to 0.12 mg/kg/day if participants had not begun menstruating by week 12. Over the 9 months leptin levels increase from 4.6 ± 0.6 to 59.3 ± 14.2 ng/mL in the treatment arm, while the placebo arm continued to have low levels (see Table 19.2 for summary of results).

Leptin and the Gonadal Axis

In the open-label trial six women with HA where observed off treatment to serve as controls [18]. These women had similarly low levels of LH, FSH, and estradiol levels compared to the HA participants receiving leptin, and these levels remained low throughout the observational period. No changes in LH pulsatility parameters were noted either. In accordance, the control women with HA were not noted to have any dominant follicles, withdrawal bleeding, or spontaneous menstrual cycles at any time during the study.

In contrast, the eight participants receiving leptin in the open-label trial had significant increases in LH levels and LH pulse frequency but not amplitude; mean follicle-stimulating hormone (FSH) levels did not change. Estradiol levels also increased significantly in these treated women. With these changes in gonadal hormones, ovarian volume during the follicular phase was greater and endometrium was thicker on ultrasound, compared to baseline. Significant increases in the number of dominant follicles and maximal follicular diameter were also observed. Ovulation was confirmed in three out of the eight treated women, occurring 28, 35, and 58 days after the start of treatment. In these three women levels of LH, FSH, estradiol, and inhibin A

Table 19.2 Changes in body composition, neuroendocrine axes, and markers of bone turnover during leptin treatment

Variable		Baseline			Week 12			Week 24			Week 36			Week 52 (follow up)					
		Mean	±	SE	Mean	±	SE	Mean	±	SE	Mean	±	SE	Mean	±	SE	p (trt)[a]	p (trt*time)[b]	p (follow up)[c]
Leptin																			
Leptin (ng/mL)		4.55	±	0.64	44.51	±	8.74	57.26	±	11.36	59.33	±	14.15	8.64	±	3.92	<0.0001	<0.0001	0.05
		4.10	±	0.64	3.65	±	0.61	3.51	±	0.52	3.09	±	0.51	2.64	±	0.57			
Free leptin (ng/mL)		4.75	±	1.24	23.87	±	3.97	47.52	±	11.98	49.04	±	13.78	3.78	±	1.00	<0.0001	<0.0001	0.18
		3.77	±	0.62	3.35	±	0.43	3.25	±	0.41	2.75	±	0.40	2.34	±	0.30			
Body composition																			
Body weight (kg)	Leptin	56.9	±	1.8	55.5	±	1.7	54.6	±	1.9	54.8	±	2.3	56.1	±	2.1	0.86	0.48	0.95
	Placebo	54.9	±	2.1	55.6	±	2.0	54.9	±	2.2	55.0	±	2.2	55.9	±	2.6			
BMI (kg/m²)	Leptin	20.9	±	0.6	20.6		0.5	20.2		0.6	20.8		0.6	21.3		0.5	0.50	0.49	0.07
	Placebo	19.8	±	0.7	20.2		0.6	19.7		0.5	19.6		0.4	19.9		0.5			
Fat Mass by DXA																			
kg	Leptin	13.1	±	1.1	12.5	±	0.9	10.8	±	1.0	10.9	±	1.3	12.2	±	1.6	0.96	0.02	0.49
	Placebo	11.7	±	0.9	10.9	±	0.7	11.3	±	1.0	10.7	±	0.9	10.8	±	1.0			
%	Leptin	22.8	±	1.6	22.2	±	1.4	19.6	±	1.5	19.8	±	2.2	21.4	±	2.6	0.99	0.01	0.27
	Placebo	20.8	±	1.3	19.7	±	1.2	20.0	±	1.5	19.1	±	1.2	19.0	±	1.5			
Neuroendocrine hormones																			
FSH (IU/L)	Leptin	5.3	±	0.5	5.0	±	0.4	4.9	±	0.4	5.0	±	0.6	5.0	±	0.6	0.69	0.70	0.99
	Placebo	4.9	±	0.5	4.9	±	0.4	4.7	±	0.5	4.8	±	0.5	5.0	±	0.7			
LH (IU/L)	Leptin	8.8	±	3.3	11.8	±	4.4	9.7	±	3.5	13.4	±	5.3	8.2	±	3.2	0.86	0.40	0.40
	Placebo	14.3	±	5.0	8.7	±	2.2	12.9	±	3.9	10.0	±	3.6	5.4	±	3.4			
Estradiol (pg/mL)	Leptin	23.0	±	9.0	19.3	±	4.5	27.2	±	8.0	25.4	±	7.8	22.0	±	7.8	0.01	0.52	0.22
	Placebo	14.0	±	1.7	13.9	±	1.8	12.3	±	1.4	11.8	±	1.3	11.6	±	1.8			
Progesterone (ng/mL)	Leptin	4.5	±	0.4	4.9	±	0.3	14.5	±	5.6	7.3	±	3.5	7.8	±	3.9	0.03	0.33	0.30
	Placebo	4.6	±	0.4	4.4	±	0.4	4.4	±	0.3	5.2	±	0.7	3.7	±	0.2			
Cortisol (μg/dl)	Leptin	20.9	±	1.1	18.2	±	1.0	17.1	±	1.1	12.8	±	1.3	14.9	±	1.6	0.02	0.24	0.17
	Placebo	20.0	±	1.3	19.6	±	1.4	20.2	±	1.0	19.7	±	0.9	17.7	±	1.1			
TSH (μIU/mL)	Leptin	1.8	±	0.2	2.1	±	0.3	2.2	±	0.4	1.8	±	0.3	2.0	±	0.3	0.78	0.70	0.97
	Placebo	1.9	±	0.2	2.1	±	0.2	1.9	±	0.2	1.9	±	0.2	2.1	±	0.3			

(continued)

Table 19.2 (continued)

Variable		Baseline			Week 12			Week 24			Week 36			Week 52 (follow up)			p (trt)[a]	p (trt*time)[b]	p (follow up)[c]
		Mean	±	SE	Mean	±	SE	Mean	±	SE	Mean	±	SE	Mean	±	SE			
Free T4 (ng/dl)	Leptin	1.00	±	0.08	1.03	±	0.08	1.07	±	0.08	1.05	±	0.08	1.08	±	0.09	0.43	0.95	0.47
	Placebo	0.91	±	0.08	0.98	±	0.09	0.99	±	0.10	1.00	±	0.10	0.97	±	0.11			
Free T3 (pg/mL)	Leptin	1.90	±	0.17	2.28	±	0.19	2.22	±	0.24	2.05	±	0.21	1.83	±	0.22	0.49	0.02	1.00
	Placebo	2.09	±	0.13	1.87	±	0.07	2.04	±	0.12	1.94	±	0.12	1.83	±	0.06			
IGF-1 (ng/mL)	Leptin	498.1	±	66.7	462.2	±	51.1	543.2	±	49.7	491.0	±	69.8	382.3	±	71.7	0.23	0.08	0.58
	Placebo	422.1	±	41.9	434.3	±	37.2	404.4	±	33.1	388.4	±	40.9	331.6	±	50.6			
IGF1:IGFBP-3	Leptin	5.35	±	0.49	5.14	±	0.37	6.09	±	0.40	5.46	±	0.61	4.58	±	0.72	0.32	0.04	0.48
	Placebo	5.05	±	0.45	5.14	±	0.38	4.82	±	0.33	4.63	±	0.42	3.91	±	0.56			
Bone markers																			
BSAP (U/L)	Leptin	26.6	±	5.7	28.2	±	6.1	29.6	±	7.3	30.7	±	7.5	22.7	±	4.5	0.09	0.29	0.20
	Placebo	16.7	±	4.4	17.2	±	4.3	13.4	±	2.7	13.5	±	2.4	14.2	±	4.2			
Osteocalcin (ng/mL)	Leptin	13.9	±	2.6	20.9	±	3.1	19.8	±	3.1	20.9	±	3.1	12.3	±	2.1	0.0019	0.21	0.17
	Placebo	9.3	±	0.8	8.5	±	1.0	8.1	±	0.9	7.7	±	0.7	8.7	±	1.1			
Urinary NTX:creatinine	Leptin	49.4	±	5.4	72.3	±	9.0	56.1	±	13.6	52.8	±	13.4	45.9	±	20.2	0.03	0.43	0.68
	Placebo	30.8	±	3.1	42.0	±	10.0	56.9	±	21.5	58.1	±	12.0	38.2	±	8.3			
CTX (ng/mL)	Leptin	1.09	±	0.11	1.16	±	0.14	1.02	±	0.15	1.12	±	0.14	0.96	±	0.24	0.13	0.39	0.24
	Placebo	0.97	±	0.14	0.84	±	0.15	0.79	±	0.11	0.82	±	0.10	0.64	±	0.06			

All data are presented as mean± SE. Overall p values were based on repeated measure ANOVA

[a]Effect of metreleptin and placebo treatment

[b]Metreleptin and placebo treatment over time interaction

[c]One-way ANOVA was used to compare the difference between metreleptin and placebo treatment groups at week 52 follow-up

(a protein secreted by granulosa cells of the dominant follicle and corpus luteum) during the ovulatory cycle were within 1 standard deviation of the mean for women with normal cycles; progesterone levels were within 2 standard deviations. An additional two treated participants had dominant follicles that grew to preovulatory size; although these follicles regressed without ovulating, the women did have withdrawal bleeding. One participant had developed a dominant follicle during the third month but did not ovulate or experience withdrawal bleeding. The participant with the lowest level of leptin during treatment (maximum of 12.4 compared to mean of 37.4 ± 30.1 ng/mL) did not have a dominant follicle. The last treated participant withdrew after 1 month for reasons unrelated to the study.

Similar results were observed in the follow-up randomized, placebo-controlled trial of 36 weeks [17]. Although LH and FSH levels did not change significantly with leptin compared to placebo, these were drawn every 12 weeks from trial initiation and were not coordinated with menstrual activity. Estradiol and progesterone levels did increase significantly. Seven of ten participants receiving leptin therapy developed menses, compared to two of nine participants on placebo ($p = 0.0046$). Menstruation occurred 4–32 weeks after initiation of leptin therapy. Menses started out irregularly but became more regular with time. Of the five treated participants who regained menses and completed the study, three continued to have menses 16 weeks after discontinuation of leptin. Four of the menstruating participants on leptin were determined to be ovulating based on elevated serum progesterone levels during the midluteal phase. One of these women became pregnant at 24 weeks. The improvements in reproduction function in these treated women were not due to changes in activity level, weight gain, or increase in fat mass.

The observed abnormalities in LH pulsatile secretion in HA are similar to that during prepuberty or peripuberty [16]. Puberty has been described to be "metabolically gated" as a means to prevent fertility in conditions of energy insufficiency [61]. Administration of leptin has been shown to initiate puberty in individuals with congenital leptin deficiency [62, 63]. Leptin likely plays a permissive role in the onset of puberty, especially in females in whom leptin levels rise prior to pubertal transition [61, 64, 65]. Likewise, leptin may also permit the return of reproductive function in HA. Leptin treatment increases LH pulse frequency, which also occurs with initiation of puberty, and the pattern of follicular growth and regression without ovulation in the treated HA women is also reminiscent of that seen in puberty [18].

As there are no leptin receptors on GnRH neurons [66], the effect of leptin on GnRH regulation is indirect and has been shown to involve a large network of neurons, particularly in the hypothalamus. Leptin directly and/or indirectly activates Kiss1 neurons in the arcuate nucleus (ARC) of the hypothalamus, which then stimulate GnRH neurons [61]. A subpopulation of Kiss1 neurons are also influenced by their own secretion of neurokinin B and dynorphin, which respectively stimulate and inhibit the release of kisspeptins via autocrine and/or paracrine signaling [67]. The effect of kisspeptin on GnRH neurons is further influenced by glutamatergic and GABAergic inputs [67]. Lack of leptin inhibition on another set of neurons in the ARC, the agouti-related peptide (AgRP)/neuropeptide Y (NPY) neurons, results in increased levels of AgRP and NPY, which then inhibit LH release and reproductive function [68, 69]. In women with HA, activation of the HPA axis, including an increase in central β-endorphin levels, and suppression of IGF-1 activity may also contribute to HPG dysfunction [57]. Finally, leptin has also been found to have both direct stimulatory and inhibitory effects at the levels of the pituitary and gonads, and the net effects of leptin on gonadotrophs and gonads may depend on the individual's metabolic status and sensitivity to leptin [70, 71].

Leptin and the Adrenal Axis

Cortisol levels were elevated in the participants of the two clinical trials with a mean of 17.2 ± 3.3 and 20.9 ± 1.1 μg/dL [17, 18]. During the open-label pilot trial, no significant changes were observed in either the level of cortisol or the pulsatility parameters of corticotropin secretion over the 3 months of leptin replacement [18]. However, over 9 months of leptin treatment, there was a significant progressive decline in cortisol levels compared a stable level of cortisol in the placebo-treated women (19.7 ± 0.9 in the placebo group; $p = 0.019$–19.7 ± 0.9 in the placebo group; $p = 0.019$) [17]. Cortisol levels increased after discontinuation of leptin and no longer differed from that of the placebo group. Improvement in cortisol levels may also have implications for bone health, immune function, mental health, and neurocognitive function (discussed below).

It is unclear if leptin directly regulates CRH neurons in the paraventricular nuclei (PVN) or indirectly via ARC neurons [72]. The effect of leptin on the HPA axis also involves several neuropeptides, including neuropeptide Y (NPY) [57, 73] and neuromedian U [74]. The net effect may depend on metabolic status as well as stress level. In ex vivo hypothalamic explants and in rats, leptin has been show to stimulate CRH release [74]. However, in the setting of stress, administration of leptin has been shown to inhibit hypothalamic CRH release and, subsequently, block increases in ACTH and cortisol in mice [75] and in ovariectomized female rhesus monkeys [76].

Leptin and the Thyroidal Axis

In the open-label trial, free T3 and free thyroxine (T4) levels started in the range of normal and increased significantly within the normal range [18]. TSH levels trended up, but pulse frequency and amplitude did not change [18]. The randomized controlled trial confirmed the increase in free T3 with leptin compared to placebo, but no significant changes were seen in free T4 or TSH [17]. The effect of leptin on the HPT axis mirrored that seen in recovery of sick euthyroid syndrome and dissipated after discontinuation.

In vitro and in vivo rodent studies have shown that leptin directly and indirectly, via melanocortins and AgRP, upregulates proTRH gene expression as well as prohormone convertases 1 and 2 to cleave TRH from proTRH in PVN neurons [77]. It may also be possible that leptin directly stimulates T4 release from the thyroid gland and/or increase the bioactivity of TSH since interventional human studies show that leptin increases thyroid hormone levels without changing TSH levels [78].

Leptin and the Growth Hormone Axis

In the open-label trial total and free IGF-1 levels were lower in HA women at baseline compared with eumenorrheic controls [52]. Leptin replacement significantly increased levels of IGF-1, which remained significant after adjustment for estradiol and weight, and tended to increase free IGF-1, which became significant after adjustment for estradiol and weight [18, 52]. In the randomized controlled trial IGF-1 levels trended up with leptin, and the ratio of IGF-1:IGFBP-3, the main circulating carrier protein for IGF-1, was significantly higher in the treatment group compared to the placebo group [17].

The HA women in the open-label trial also had 24 h GH secretion profiled before and after 2 weeks of leptin therapy [52]. Although not directly compared due to procedural differences, the GH pulsatility characteristics were similar in the HA women as the eumenorrheic, euleptinemic controls and the HA women did not have increased mean overnight GH levels. Two weeks of leptin treatment resulted in only borderline increases in mean GH concentration and area under the curve but did not change other GH pulsatility characteristics. During these first 2 weeks of leptin replacement, there were no significant changes in estradiol levels. GH parameters were not studied later.

Leptin has been show to increase GH secretion, particularly in the fasted compared to fed state, and decrease somatostatin secretion in ex vivo and in vivo animal studies [79, 80]. However, minimal changes in GH pulsatility characteristics were observed in response to leptin in women with HA [52]. The effects of leptin on IGF-1 levels may be independent of GH secretion as well as GH receptor expression. GHBP levels, which may reflect that of GH receptor, were low in women with HA at baseline, compared to eumenorrheic controls, and did not change over the 3 months of leptin therapy. This is in contrast to women with AN after weight recuperation, when GHBP levels increase to normal [81]. Leptin may be directly increasing IGF-1 levels, and this occurred in the absence of changes in nutritional status in the clinical trial [52]. Leptin's effect on FGF-21 levels in patients with HA has not been studied. However, in healthy, lean women undergoing 72 h fast, administration of leptin to restore physiological levels did not prevent the fasting-induced increase in FGF-21 levels [82].

Bone Metabolism

A large amount of energy is required for bone remodeling, and leptin may be the key hormone linking the regulation of energy homeostasis with bone metabolism [83]. Osteoporosis is part of the female athlete triad along with amenorrhea and disordered eating, and bone mineral density (BMD) has been found to be lower in amenorrheic athletes than eumenorrheic athletes. In one study 38 % of athletes with amenorrhea had lumbar BMD z-score below −1 compared to 11 % of athletes with eumenorrhea and 11 % of control subjects ($p=0.05$) [84]. Furthermore, 24 % of athletes with amenorrhea reported a history of fractures compared to 5 % of athletes with eumenorrhea, though the difference was not significant [84]. In addition to the lack of the antiresorptive and anabolic effects of gonadal steroids, women with HA have other risk factors for bone loss, including lack of the anabolic effects of IGF-1, high cortisol levels, high thyroid hormone levels, poor nutritional status, lack of sufficient calcium and vitamin D intake, low lean body mass, and low fat mass [85]. In addition, female athletes with HA may not benefit from weight-bearing exercise since estrogen may be required for the positive effects of mechanical loading on bone strength [86].

Leptin, either via normalization of neuroendocrine hormones and/or directly, may help improve bone health. In the 3-month clinical trial leptin replacement increased levels of bone-specific alkaline phosphatase and osteocalcin, both bone formation markers, without significantly changing levels of urinary N-telopeptide, a marker of bone resorption [18]. The 9-month trial confirmed a significant increase in osteocalcin within 4 weeks and stabilization of urinary N-telopeptide compared to placebo, but no significant differences were seen in serum levels of bone-specific alkaline phosphatase, osteoprotegerin, or C-telopeptide [17]. Six participants of the 9-month trial enrolled in an optional open-label extension of leptin treatment for another 12 months; 4 of these participants completed the extension trial [19]. In intention-to-treat analysis lumbar bone mineral content (BMC) increased significantly from baseline. In on-treatment analysis both lumbar BMC and BMD increased significantly from baseline by 6 % and 4 %, respectively. Mean lumbar BMD z-score increased from the osteopenic range to the reference range with both analyses. Adjustments for changes in body weight intensified the significance of leptin's effect since there was a non-significant decrease in body weight. Whole-body, hip, and radial BMC and BMD were not affected by leptin replacement. These results suggest that the skeletal effects of leptin may be primarily on the trabecular bone, which predominates in the lumbar spine. It is also possible that with longer treatment duration, favorable effects at the hip and radius may be observed as vertebral bone has a faster turnover rate and changes are often observed at this location first.

The effect of leptin on BMD appears to be better than that of estrogen therapy, albeit no direct comparison studies are available. The use of estrogen supplementation has been controversial [87]. One of the largest randomized controlled trials studied the effects of oral contraceptives on BMD in oligo/amenorrheic runners over 2 years [88]. Only on-treatment analysis revealed a 1 % gain in spine BMD per year, which was similar to runners who regained periods spontaneously but significantly greater than those for runners who remained oligo/amenorrheic [88]. Estrogen may have limited effects in amenorrheic athletes since estrogen has primarily anti-resorptive effects on bone and these women are often found to have

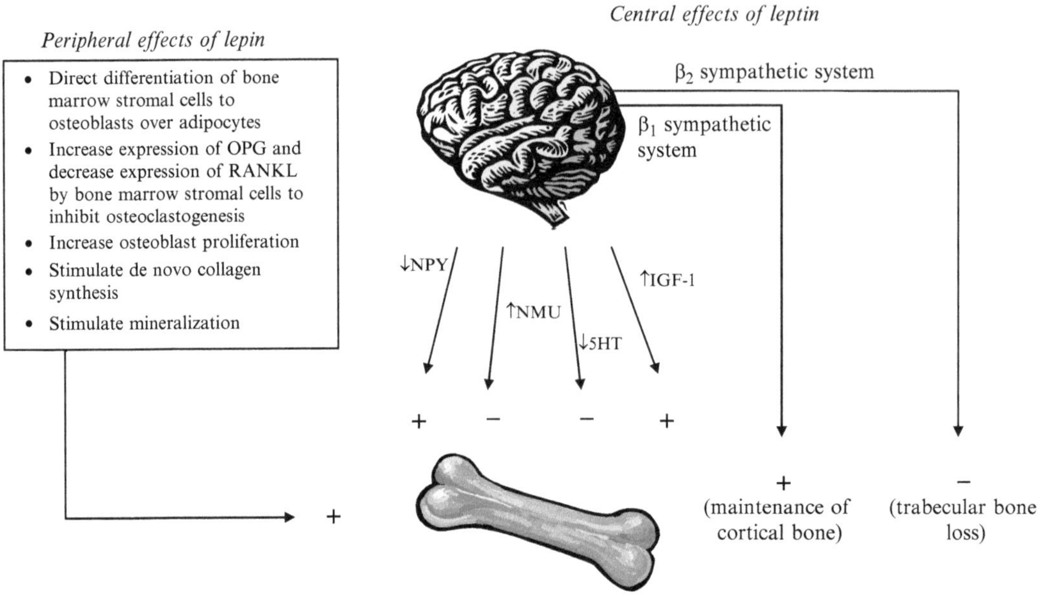

Fig. 19.1 Proposed mechanisms of interaction between leptin and bone metabolism. In in vitro and in vivo mice studies, leptin has been found to regulate bone metabolism through peripheral and central means [77, 92]. The peripheral effects of leptin increase bone formation, while the central effects seem to be more complex involving both stimulatory and inhibitory influences. Overall, leptin treatment increased bone mineral content and density in leptin-deficient *ob/ob* mice, which have otherwise decreased stature [131]. It is unclear though if the data will also apply to humans as patients with congenital leptin deficiency have normal bone mineral content and density [62]. *5HT* serotonin, *IGF-1* insulin growth factor-1, *NMU* neuromedin U, *NPY* neuropeptide Y, *OPG* osteoprotegerin, *RANKL* receptor activator of NF-κB ligand

reduced markers of bone turnover [87]. A decrease in bone turnover is consistent with the need to conserve such high energy requiring processes in women with HA. Estrogen therapy, unlike leptin replacement, also does not address the disturbances in thyroid hormone, IGF-1, and cortisol levels. Likewise, recombinant human IGF-1 [89] and androgens [90] have modest responses in bone metabolism in women with AN; a lesser response may be suspected in women with the less severe condition of HA.

Leptin may also have direct effects on bone (see Fig. 19.1). Centrally, leptin both positively and negatively regulates bone metabolism via hypothalamic expression of several neuropeptides and regulation of sympathetic pathways [91, 92]. Leptin also interacts with bone marrow stromal cells and osteoblasts to increase overall bone mass. In leptin-deficient *ob/ob* mice administration of leptin has been shown to increase expression of osteogenic genes in stromal cells to favor differentiation into osteoblasts over adipocytes [93]. In women with HA, this effect of leptin does not seem to be mediated by preadipocyte factor 1 (pref-1), which has been found to be increased in AN and HA, negatively associated with BMD, and positively associated with bone marrow fat [94, 95]; treatment with leptin did not affect pref-1 levels in women with HA [95]. Overall, the direct effect of leptin on bone is likely less important than the effect of normalizing neuroendocrine hormones in HA women. In patients with congenital leptin deficiency, BMC and BMD are appropriate for age and gender and after treatment increase in line with normal age-related development [62]. In the general population, no correlation between BMD and serum leptin levels has been found in normal-weight children and adolescents [96] or healthy postmenopausal women [97].

Immune Function

As the helical structure of leptin is similar to that of cytokines, leptin has also been proposed to link energy metabolism with the immune response [98–100]. Individuals with congenital leptin deficiency have more frequent childhood infections compared to their wild-type siblings and reduction in $CD4^+$ T cell number, particularly naïve $CD4^+$ T cells [62]. Leptin treatment not only normalized the immune phenotype but also improved the proliferative and functional responses of $CD4^+$ T cells [62]. Studies in women with AN show a reduction of total lymphocyte count and their subpopulations [101–103]. However, the relative proportions of lymphocyte subpopulations were found to be different with one study finding a reduction of naïve $CD4^+$ T cells [101] and another study finding a reduction of $CD8^+$ T cells, particular memory cells [102]; all improved with refeeding. T cell activation and T-cell–B-cell cooperation have also been found to be impaired [101]. Indeed, AN patients are found to have a reduced response to delayed-hypersensitivity skin test, a marker of cell-mediated immune function [103].

The women with HA in the randomized controlled trial were found to have reduced total number of lymphocytes, B cells, and natural killer cells, and the administration of leptin restored their total lymphocyte count with increases in $CD4^+$ and $CD8^+$ T-cells [20]. In the placebo-treated HA subjects, lymphocyte count trended down from a mild degree of lymphopenia to frank lymphopenia over time. Women with HA were also found to have reduced T-cell proliferative capacity, compared to normoleptinemic control women, which was partially restored with leptin. No significant changes in circulating survival cytokines such as IL-1, IL-7, or IL-15 were observed. In this small study these effects of leptin were not associated with significant changes in serum hormone levels of cortisol, ACTH, or insulin; circulating cytokines; or metabolic/inflammatory parameters such as CD40-CD40 ligand, soluble TNF receptors, monocyte chemoattractant protein-1, myeloperoxidase, and C-reactive protein. In peripheral bone marrow cells leptin treatment was found to upregulate genes involved in lymphocyte survival, proliferation, and migration (e.g., IL-7, neurotrophin-3, ADAM-metallopeptidase-23 [ADAM-23], and vascular adhesion molecule-1 [VCAM-1]) and downregulate genes involved in apoptosis (e.g., B-cell chronic lymphocytic leukemia/lymphoma 10 [BCL-10] and TP53-regulator of apoptosis-1 [TRIAP-1]).

Total Energy Expenditure

Women with exercise-induced HA have significantly lower ratio of REE to fat-free mass compared to eumenorrheic women who exercise, and this was predicted more by menstrual status than leptin levels [49, 104]. In accordance, leptin treatment did not affect REE by indirect calorimetric testing in women with HA [17, 18]. Total body expenditure was not studied in the two clinical trials.

Regulation of Appetite

The regulation of food intake involves complex neuronal circuits with input from the brain, gastrointestinal tract, and adipose tissue, converging at the ARC. There, leptin stimulates expression of the anorexigenic neuropeptides pro-opiomelanocortin (POMC) and cocaine- and amphetamine-regulated transcript (CART) and inhibits the expression of orexigenic neuropeptides AgRP and NPY [77]. From the gut, insulin and polypeptide YY has similar affects, while ghrelin has the opposite [105]. Furthermore, leptin and ghrelin together influence the mesolimbic dopamine system in the anticipation and motivation for food [106]. These hormones can also affect the HPG axis and bone metabolism [107].

Gut Neuropeptides

Ghrelin, which is secreted by the stomach, has the opposite metabolic effects of leptin. Levels peak before each meal, fall following food consumption, and increase following exercise

[107]. Ghrelin stimulates food intake, increases gastric motility and acid secretion, enhances the use of carbohydrates over fat, and reduces locomotor activity [105] and administration in rats induces weight gain [108]. Furthermore, ghrelin inhibits gonadotropin secretion, in contrast to leptin [109]. Ghrelin levels are elevated in women with exercise-induced HA [104] and AN [110]. However, ghrelin levels are not consistently associated with disordered eating psychopathology [111]. It has been proposed that these women may be in a state of ghrelin resistance similar to leptin resistance seen in obesity [105]. Although the effect of leptin on ghrelin was not studied in women with HA, it has been studied in healthy lean men undergoing 72-h fasting. In these men neither fasting induced hypoleptinemia nor the replacement of leptin administration had an acute effect on the diurnal pattern of ghrelin secretion [112].

Secreted by the endocrine pancreas, amylin and pancreatic polypeptide are important in energy homeostasis. Both are secreted in response to food and have been proposed to act as short-term satiety signals by decreasing appetite, inhibiting gastric emptying, and reducing gastric acid secretion; weight loss in response to both have been shown in rodents [113]. Levels of amylin and pancreatic peptide are similar in woman with HA compared to weight-matched control subjects and did not change with treatment of leptin [113].

Polypeptide YY is another anorexigenic hormone that is secreted by the intestine in response to food. Levels are elevated in women with AN and exercise-induced HA compared to healthy controls and are positively associated with disordered eating psychopathology independent of BMI [111, 114]. Polypeptide YY in response to leptin has not been studied in HA.

Given the complexity of the control of appetite, it is not surprising that in women with HA food intake was not affected by leptin treatment, although this was only assessed by 3-day food diaries [17]. There were no differences in intake of total calories, fat, protein, or carbohydrate.

Metabolism

Insulin sensitivity increases with the severity of HA conditions [29, 115], and insulin levels are lower in women with HA than weight-matched controls and positively correlate with leptin levels [8, 21, 22]. Insulin may stimulate leptin [116], and low levels of insulin may contribute to the low levels of leptin. Treatment with leptin did not affect insulin levels in women with HA; insulin sensitivity was not studied [19]. In contrast, children with congenital leptin deficiency [62, 63] and patients with lipodystrophy and relative hypoleptinemia [117–121] are insulin resistant, and leptin replacement improves insulin sensitivity. The cause of insulin resistance in these populations may be due to increased triglyceride content in liver and muscle, and administration of leptin has been shown to decrease triglyceride content and improve insulin sensitivity in these organs [119]. Leptin has also been shown to protect pancreatic β-cell from lipotoxicity and apoptosis [122].

Aside from leptin, several other adipokines are involved in insulin sensitivity. Adiponectin is the most abundant hormone secreted from adipocytes, and levels are low in obesity, typically increase with weight loss, and are positively associated with insulin sensitivity [107]. Adiponectin levels are elevated in women with AN but not HA and tend to decline with weight recovery [114, 123–125]. The effect of leptin on adiponectin levels in HA women is unknown. Two other hormones that augment the effects of insulin, vaspin and visfatin, do not seem to play a large role in HA as they are not affected by leptin administration [126].

Psychological Aspects

Adolescents with HA have a higher incidence of subclinical psychosomatic discomfort and mild depressive traits than eumenorrheic controls [44]. Leptin, but not ghrelin, has been found to be inversely associated with scores on depression and anxiety scales, independent of body fat or weight [127]. The effect of leptin administration on mood in women with HA has not been studied yet.

Safety of Leptin

The major limitation of leptin as a therapeutic agent is the anticipated decrease in weight and fat mass. With careful monitoring and dose adjustments, however, weight can be maintained and loss of total body fat mass and percentage can be minimized on leptin therapy [17]. Out of the ten leptin-treated participants who completed more than one follow up visit in the randomized controlled trial, one was removed from the study at week 28 and four required a decrease in leptin dosing due to weight loss. Although BMI did not change in the leptin group (20.8 ± 0.6 kg/m^2 at week 36 compared with 21.1 ± 0.6 kg/m^2 at baseline) compared with the control group (19.6 ± 0.4 kg/m^2 at week 36 compared with 19.8 ± 0.7 kg/m^2 at baseline) ($p = 0.23$), the leptin group did experience a progressive loss of total body fat mass and percentage with a mean loss of 2 kg of fat. The loss of fat was noted from both peripheral and central compartments and reverted 16 weeks after discontinuation of leptin. Lean body mass was not affected [128].

Antileptin antibody levels developed in seven out of eight leptin-treated participants [17]. The antibodies were nonneutralizing; free leptin levels increased significantly and were maintained throughout the study duration. Antileptin antibodies have also been observed transiently after treatment in children with congenital leptin deficiency [62] and adults with obesity [129]. Neutralizing antibodies have been reported by others, however, in response to leptin used in subjects treated for long periods of time for either obesity or lipodystrophy, and this has halted the development of leptin as a therapeutic for those indications [130].

Finally, local injection-site reaction occurred in 1 participant who withdrew from the study [17]. Her symptoms resolved spontaneously within 1 week.

Conclusion

Based on limited but thorough studies, leptin treatment in physiological doses effectively normalizes or improves HA-associated dysfunction of neuroendocrine axes, reproductive system, bone metabolism, and immune system. Leptin, however, does not address the underlying cause of HA—chronic energy deficiency; it circumvents it, so weight loss is an unwanted effect for which careful monitoring is needed. The ideal treatment for HA should focus on lifestyle changes, including cutting back the exercise regimen, eating a balanced diet, gaining weight, and reducing stress. In select patients who find it difficult to make lifestyle changes, those who need a temporizing measure while waiting for lifestyle changes to take effect, or otherwise healthy women with anovulation who wish to become pregnant, leptin may be a potential option in the future. Thus, larger and longer studies are needed to verify the efficacy and safety of leptin in women with HA.

References

1. Reindollar RH, Novak M, Tho SP, McDonough PG. Adult-onset amenorrhea: a study of 262 patients. Am J Obstet Gynecol. 1986;155(3):531–43.
2. Nichols JF, Rauh MJ, Lawson MJ, Ji M, Barkai HS. Prevalence of the female athlete triad syndrome among high school athletes. Arch Pediatr Adolesc Med. 2006;160(2):137–42.
3. Thein-Nissenbaum JM, Rauh MJ, Carr KE, Loud KJ, McGuine TA. Menstrual irregularity and musculoskeletal injury in female high school athletes. J Athl Train. 2012;47(1):74–82.
4. Warren MP. Health issues for women athletes: exercise-induced amenorrhea. J Clin Endocrinol Metab. 1999;84(6):1892–6.
5. Highet R. Athletic amenorrhoea. An update on aetiology, complications and management. Sports Med. 1989;7(2):82–108.
6. Ahima RS. Body fat, leptin, and hypothalamic amenorrhea. N Engl J Med. 2004;351(10):959–62.
7. Laughlin GA, Dominguez CE, Yen SS. Nutritional and endocrine-metabolic aberrations in women with functional hypothalamic amenorrhea. J Clin Endocrinol Metab. 1998;83(1):25–32.
8. Miller KK, Parulekar MS, Schoenfeld E, Anderson E, Hubbard J, Klibanski A, et al. Decreased leptin

levels in normal weight women with hypothalamic amenorrhea: the effects of body composition and nutritional intake. J Clin Endocrinol Metab. 1998;83(7):2309–12.
9. Warren MP, Voussoughian F, Geer EB, Hyle EP, Adberg CL, Ramos RH. Functional hypothalamic amenorrhea: hypoleptinemia and disordered eating. J Clin Endocrinol Metab. 1999;84(3):873–7.
10. Perkins RB, Hall JE, Martin KA. Aetiology, previous menstrual function and patterns of neuro-endocrine disturbance as prognostic indicators in hypothalamic amenorrhoea. Hum Reprod. 2001; 16(10):2198–205.
11. Wiksten-Almstromer M, Hirschberg AL, Hagenfeldt K. Menstrual disorders and associated factors among adolescent girls visiting a youth clinic. Acta Obstet Gynecol Scand. 2007;86(1):65–72.
12. Marcus MD, Loucks TL, Berga SL. Psychological correlates of functional hypothalamic amenorrhea. Fertil Steril. 2001;76(2):310–6.
13. Frisch RE, McArthur JW. Menstrual cycles: fatness as a determinant of minimum weight for height necessary for their maintenance or onset. Science. 1974;185(4155):949–51.
14. Zhang Y, Proenca R, Maffei M, Barone M, Leopold L, Friedman JM. Positional cloning of the mouse obese gene and its human homologue. Nature. 1994;372(6505):425–32.
15. Mantzoros CS, Magkos F, Brinkoetter M, Sienkiewicz E, Dardeno TA, Kim SY, et al. Leptin in human physiology and pathophysiology. Am J Physiol Endocrinol Metab. 2011;301(4):E567–84.
16. Chan JL, Mantzoros CS. Role of leptin in energy-deprivation states: normal human physiology and clinical implications for hypothalamic amenorrhoea and anorexia nervosa. Lancet. 2005;366(9479): 74–85.
17. Chou SH, Chamberland JP, Liu X, Matarese G, Gao C, Stefanakis R, et al. Leptin is an effective treatment for hypothalamic amenorrhea. Proc Natl Acad Sci U S A. 2011;108(16):6585–90.
18. Welt CK, Chan JL, Bullen J, Murphy R, Smith P, DePaoli AM, et al. Recombinant human leptin in women with hypothalamic amenorrhea. N Engl J Med. 2004;351(10):987–97.
19. Sienkiewicz E, Magkos F, Aronis KN, Brinkoetter M, Chamberland JP, Chou S, et al. Long-term metreleptin treatment increases bone mineral density and content at the lumbar spine of lean hypoleptinemic women. Metab Clin Exp. 2011;60(9):1211–21.
20. Matarese G, La Rocca C, Moon HS, Huh JY, Brinkoetter MT, Chou S, et al. Selective capacity of metreleptin administration to reconstitute CD4+ T-cell number in females with acquired hypoleptinemia. Proc Natl Acad Sci U S A. 2013;110(9):E818–27.
21. Andrico S, Gambera A, Specchia C, Pellegrini C, Falsetti L, Sartori E. Leptin in functional hypothalamic amenorrhoea. Hum Reprod. 2002;17(8):2043–8.
22. Thong FS, McLean C, Graham TE. Plasma leptin in female athletes: relationship with body fat, reproductive, nutritional, and endocrine factors. J Appl Physiol. 2000;88(6):2037–44.
23. Corr M, De Souza MJ, Toombs RJ, Williams NI. Circulating leptin concentrations do not distinguish menstrual status in exercising women. Hum Reprod. 2011;26(3):685–94.
24. Hebebrand J, Muller TD, Holtkamp K, Herpertz-Dahlmann B. The role of leptin in anorexia nervosa: clinical implications. Mol Psychiatry. 2007;12(1): 23–35.
25. Monteleone P, Fabrazzo M, Tortorella A, Fuschino A, Maj M. Opposite modifications in circulating leptin and soluble leptin receptor across the eating disorder spectrum. Mol Psychiatry. 2002;7(6): 641–6.
26. Krizova J, Papezova H, Haluzikova D, Parizkova J, Jiskra J, Kotrlikova E, et al. Soluble leptin receptor levels in patients with anorexia nervosa. Endocr Res. 2002;28(3):199–205.
27. Misra M, Miller KK, Almazan C, Ramaswamy K, Aggarwal A, Herzog DB, et al. Hormonal and body composition predictors of soluble leptin receptor, leptin, and free leptin index in adolescent girls with anorexia nervosa and controls and relation to insulin sensitivity. J Clin Endocrinol Metab. 2004;89(7): 3486–95.
28. Kratzsch J, Lammert A, Bottner A, Seidel B, Mueller G, Thiery J, et al. Circulating soluble leptin receptor and free leptin index during childhood, puberty, and adolescence. J Clin Endocrinol Metab. 2002;87(10): 4587–94.
29. Laughlin GA, Yen SS. Hypoleptinemia in women athletes: absence of a diurnal rhythm with amenorrhea. J Clin Endocrinol Metab. 1997;82(1):318–21.
30. Ackerman KE, Slusarz K, Guereca G, Pierce L, Slattery M, Mendes N, et al. Higher ghrelin and lower leptin secretion are associated with lower LH secretion in young amenorrheic athletes compared with eumenorrheic athletes and controls. Am J Physiol Endocrinol Metab. 2012;302(7):E800–6.
31. Stoving RK, Vinten J, Handberg A, Ebbesen EN, Hangaard J, Hansen-Nord M, et al. Diurnal variation of the serum leptin concentration in patients with anorexia nervosa. Clin Endocrinol (Oxf). 1998;48(6): 761–8.
32. Puder JJ, Monaco SE, Sen Gupta S, Wang J, Ferin M, Warren MP. Estrogen and exercise may be related to body fat distribution and leptin in young women. Fertil Steril. 2006;86(3):694–9.
33. Chan JL, Heist K, DePaoli AM, Veldhuis JD, Mantzoros CS. The role of falling leptin levels in the neuroendocrine and metabolic adaptation to short-term starvation in healthy men. J Clin Invest. 2003;111(9):1409–21.
34. Boden G, Chen X, Mozzoli M, Ryan I. Effect of fasting on serum leptin in normal human subjects. J Clin Endocrinol Metab. 1996;81(9):3419–23.
35. Chan JL, Matarese G, Shetty GK, Raciti P, Kelesidis I, Aufiero D, et al. Differential regulation of metabolic, neuroendocrine, and immune function by

leptin in humans. Proc Natl Acad Sci U S A. 2006;103(22):8481–6.
36. Kolaczynski JW, Considine RV, Ohannesian J, Marco C, Opentanova I, Nyce MR, et al. Responses of leptin to short-term fasting and refeeding in humans: a link with ketogenesis but not ketones themselves. Diabetes. 1996;45(11):1511–5.
37. Kostrzewa E, van Elburg AA, Sanders N, Sternheim L, Adan RA, Kas MJ. Longitudinal changes in the physical activity of adolescents with anorexia nervosa and their influence on body composition and leptin serum levels after recovery. PLoS One. 2013;8(10):e78251.
38. Dei M, Seravalli V, Bruni V, Balzi D, Pasqua A. Predictors of recovery of ovarian function after weight gain in subjects with amenorrhea related to restrictive eating disorders. Gynecol Endocrinol. 2008;24(8):459–64.
39. Michopoulos V, Mancini F, Loucks TL, Berga SL. Neuroendocrine recovery initiated by cognitive behavioral therapy in women with functional hypothalamic amenorrhea: a randomized, controlled trial. Fertil Steril. 2013;99(7):2084–91.e1.
40. Genazzani AD, Ricchieri F, Lanzoni C, Strucchi C, Jasonni VM. Diagnostic and therapeutic approach to hypothalamic amenorrhea. Ann N Y Acad Sci. 2006;1092:103–13.
41. Genazzani AD, Bersi C, Luisi S, Fruzzetti F, Malavasi B, Luisi M, et al. Increased adrenal steroid secretion in response to CRF in women with hypothalamic amenorrhea. J Steroid Biochem Mol Biol. 2001;78(3):247–52.
42. Lindahl MS, Olovsson M, Nyberg S, Thorsen K, Olsson T, Sundstrom Poromaa I. Increased cortisol responsivity to adrenocorticotropic hormone and low plasma levels of interleukin-1 receptor antagonist in women with functional hypothalamic amenorrhea. Fertil Steril. 2007;87(1):136–42.
43. Gordon CM. Clinical practice. Functional hypothalamic amenorrhea. N Engl J Med. 2010;363(4):365–71.
44. Bomba M, Gambera A, Bonini L, Peroni M, Neri F, Scagliola P, et al. Endocrine profiles and neuropsychologic correlates of functional hypothalamic amenorrhea in adolescents. Fertil Steril. 2007;87(4):876–85.
45. Loucks AB, Mortola JF, Girton L, Yen SS. Alterations in the hypothalamic-pituitary-ovarian and the hypothalamic-pituitary-adrenal axes in athletic women. J Clin Endocrinol Metab. 1989;68(2):402–11.
46. Meczekalski B, Tonetti A, Monteleone P, Bernardi F, Luisi S, Stomati M, et al. Hypothalamic amenorrhea with normal body weight: ACTH, allopregnanolone and cortisol responses to corticotropin-releasing hormone test. Eur J Endocrinol. 2000;142(3):280–5.
47. Berga SL, Mortola JF, Girton L, Suh B, Laughlin G, Pham P, et al. Neuroendocrine aberrations in women with functional hypothalamic amenorrhea. J Clin Endocrinol Metab. 1989;68(2):301–8.
48. Couzinet B, Young J, Brailly S, Le Bouc Y, Chanson P, Schaison G. Functional hypothalamic amenorrhoea: a partial and reversible gonadotrophin deficiency of nutritional origin. Clin Endocrinol (Oxf). 1999;50(2):229–35.
49. De Souza MJ, Lee DK, VanHeest JL, Scheid JL, West SL, Williams NI. Severity of energy-related menstrual disturbances increases in proportion to indices of energy conservation in exercising women. Fertil Steril. 2007;88(4):971–5.
50. Laughlin GA, Yen SS. Nutritional and endocrine-metabolic aberrations in amenorrheic athletes. J Clin Endocrinol Metab. 1996;81(12):4301–9.
51. Misra M, Miller KK, Bjornson J, Hackman A, Aggarwal A, Chung J, et al. Alterations in growth hormone secretory dynamics in adolescent girls with anorexia nervosa and effects on bone metabolism. J Clin Endocrinol Metab. 2003;88(12):5615–23.
52. Chan JL, Williams CJ, Raciti P, Blakeman J, Kelesidis T, Kelesidis I, et al. Leptin does not mediate short-term fasting-induced changes in growth hormone pulsatility but increases IGF-I in leptin deficiency states. J Clin Endocrinol Metab. 2008;93(7):2819–27.
53. Genazzani AD, Petraglia F, Gastaldi M, Gamba O, Corazza F, D'Ambrogio G, et al. Growth hormone (GH)-releasing hormone-induced GH response in hypothalamic amenorrhea: evidence of altered central neuromodulation. Fertil Steril. 1996;65(5):935–8.
54. Baumann G. Growth hormone-binding proteins: state of the art. J Endocrinol. 1994;141(1):1–6.
55. Kojima M, Hosoda H, Date Y, Nakazato M, Matsuo H, Kangawa K. Ghrelin is a growth-hormone-releasing acylated peptide from stomach. Nature. 1999;402(6762):656–60.
56. Devesa J, Lima L, Tresguerres JA. Neuroendocrine control of growth hormone secretion in humans. Trends Endocrinol Metab. 1992;3(5):175–83.
57. Meczekalski B, Podfigurna-Stopa A, Warenik-Szymankiewicz A, Genazzani AR. Functional hypothalamic amenorrhea: current view on neuroendocrine aberrations. Gynecol Endocrinol. 2008;24(1):4–11.
58. Singhal V, Misra M, Klibanski A. Endocrinology of anorexia nervosa in young people: recent insights. Curr Opin Endocrinol Diabetes Obes. 2014;21(1):64–70.
59. Kelesidis T, Kelesidis I, Chou S, Mantzoros CS. Narrative review: the role of leptin in human physiology: emerging clinical applications. Ann Intern Med. 2010;152(2):93–100.
60. Khan SM, Hamnvik OP, Brinkoetter M, Mantzoros CS. Leptin as a modulator of neuroendocrine function in humans. Yonsei Med J. 2012;53(4):671–9.
61. Sanchez-Garrido MA, Tena-Sempere M. Metabolic control of puberty: roles of leptin and kisspeptins. Horm Behav. 2013;64(2):187–94.
62. Farooqi IS, Matarese G, Lord GM, Keogh JM, Lawrence E, Agwu C, et al. Beneficial effects of

leptin on obesity, T cell hyporesponsiveness, and neuroendocrine/metabolic dysfunction of human congenital leptin deficiency. J Clin Invest. 2002;110(8):1093–103.

63. Licinio J, Caglayan S, Ozata M, Yildiz BO, de Miranda PB, O'Kirwan F, et al. Phenotypic effects of leptin replacement on morbid obesity, diabetes mellitus, hypogonadism, and behavior in leptin-deficient adults. Proc Natl Acad Sci U S A. 2004;101(13):4531–6.
64. Garcia-Mayor RV, Andrade MA, Rios M, Lage M, Dieguez C, Casanueva FF. Serum leptin levels in normal children: relationship to age, gender, body mass index, pituitary-gonadal hormones, and pubertal stage. J Clin Endocrinol Metab. 1997;82(9):2849–55.
65. Mantzoros CS, Flier JS, Rogol AD. A longitudinal assessment of hormonal and physical alterations during normal puberty in boys. V. Rising leptin levels may signal the onset of puberty. J Clin Endocrinol Metab. 1997;82(4):1066–70.
66. Quennell JH, Mulligan AC, Tups A, Liu X, Phipps SJ, Kemp CJ, et al. Leptin indirectly regulates gonadotropin-releasing hormone neuronal function. Endocrinology. 2009;150(6):2805–12.
67. Pinilla L, Aguilar E, Dieguez C, Millar RP, Tena-Sempere M. Kisspeptins and reproduction: physiological roles and regulatory mechanisms. Physiol Rev. 2012;92(3):1235–316.
68. Kalra SP, Kalra PS. Nutritional infertility: the role of the interconnected hypothalamic neuropeptide Y-galanin-opioid network. Front Neuroendocrinol. 1996;17(4):371–401.
69. Sheffer-Babila S, Sun Y, Israel DD, Liu SM, Neal-Perry G, Chua Jr SC. Agouti-related peptide plays a critical role in leptin's effects on female puberty and reproduction. Am J Physiol Endocrinol Metab. 2013;305(12):E1512–20.
70. Tena-Sempere M. Roles of ghrelin and leptin in the control of reproductive function. Neuroendocrinology. 2007;86(3):229–41.
71. Bluher S, Mantzoros CS. Leptin in reproduction. Curr Opin Endocrinol Diabetes Obes. 2007;14(6):458–64.
72. Roubos EW, Dahmen M, Kozicz T, Xu L. Leptin and the hypothalamo-pituitary-adrenal stress axis. Gen Comp Endocrinol. 2012;177(1):28–36.
73. Glaum SR, Hara M, Bindokas VP, Lee CC, Polonsky KS, Bell GI, et al. Leptin, the obese gene product, rapidly modulates synaptic transmission in the hypothalamus. Mol Pharmacol. 1996;50(2):230–5.
74. Jethwa PH, Smith KL, Small CJ, Abbott CR, Darch SJ, Murphy KG, et al. Neuromedin U partially mediates leptin-induced hypothalamo-pituitary adrenal (HPA) stimulation and has a physiological role in the regulation of the HPA axis in the rat. Endocrinology. 2006;147(6):2886–92.
75. Heiman ML, Ahima RS, Craft LS, Schoner B, Stephens TW, Flier JS. Leptin inhibition of the hypothalamic-pituitary-adrenal axis in response to stress. Endocrinology. 1997;138(9):3859–63.
76. Wilson ME, Fisher J, Brown J. Chronic subcutaneous leptin infusion diminishes the responsiveness of the hypothalamic-pituitary-adrenal (HPA) axis in female rhesus monkeys. Physiol Behav. 2005;84(3):449–58.
77. Dardeno TA, Chou SH, Moon HS, Chamberland JP, Fiorenza CG, Mantzoros CS. Leptin in human physiology and therapeutics. Front Neuroendocrinol. 2010;31(3):377–93.
78. Rosenbaum M, Goldsmith R, Bloomfield D, Magnano A, Weimer L, Heymsfield S, et al. Low-dose leptin reverses skeletal muscle, autonomic, and neuroendocrine adaptations to maintenance of reduced weight. J Clin Invest. 2005;115(12):3579–86.
79. Saleri R, Giustina A, Tamanini C, Valle D, Burattin A, Wehrenberg WB, et al. Leptin stimulates growth hormone secretion via a direct pituitary effect combined with a decreased somatostatin tone in a median eminence-pituitary perifusion study. Neuroendocrinology. 2004;79(4):221–8.
80. Watanobe H, Habu S. Leptin regulates growth hormone-releasing factor, somatostatin, and alpha-melanocyte-stimulating hormone but not neuropeptide Y release in rat hypothalamus in vivo: relation with growth hormone secretion. J Neurosci. 2002;22(14):6265–71.
81. Argente J, Caballo N, Barrios V, Munoz MT, Pozo J, Chowen JA, et al. Multiple endocrine abnormalities of the growth hormone and insulin-like growth factor axis in patients with anorexia nervosa: effect of short- and long-term weight recuperation. J Clin Endocrinol Metab. 1997;82(7):2084–92.
82. Foo JP, Aronis KN, Chamberland JP, Paruthi J, Moon HS, Mantzoros CS. Fibroblast growth factor 21 levels in young healthy females display day and night variations and are increased in response to short-term energy deprivation through a leptin-independent pathway. Diabetes Care. 2013;36(4):935–42.
83. Confavreux CB, Levine RL, Karsenty G. A paradigm of integrative physiology, the crosstalk between bone and energy metabolisms. Mol Cell Endocrinol. 2009;310(1–2):21–9.
84. Christo K, Prabhakaran R, Lamparello B, Cord J, Miller KK, Goldstein MA, et al. Bone metabolism in adolescent athletes with amenorrhea, athletes with eumenorrhea, and control subjects. Pediatrics. 2008;121(6):1127–36.
85. Misra M. Bone density in the adolescent athlete. Rev Endocr Metab Disord. 2008;9(2):139–44.
86. Lee KC, Lanyon LE. Mechanical loading influences bone mass through estrogen receptor alpha. Exerc Sport Sci Rev. 2004;32(2):64–8.
87. Ducher G, Turner AI, Kukuljan S, Pantano KJ, Carlson JL, Williams NI, et al. Obstacles in the optimization of bone health outcomes in the female athlete triad. Sports Med. 2011;41(7):587–607.
88. Cobb KL, Bachrach LK, Sowers M, Nieves J, Greendale GA, Kent KK, et al. The effect of oral contraceptives on bone mass and stress fractures in female runners. Med Sci Sports Exerc. 2007;39(9):1464–73.

89. Grinspoon S, Thomas L, Miller K, Herzog D, Klibanski A. Effects of recombinant human IGF-I and oral contraceptive administration on bone density in anorexia nervosa. J Clin Endocrinol Metab. 2002;87(6):2883–91.
90. Gordon CM, Grace E, Emans SJ, Goodman E, Crawford MH, Leboff MS. Changes in bone turnover markers and menstrual function after short-term oral DHEA in young women with anorexia nervosa. J Bone Miner Res. 1999;14(1):136–45.
91. Dalamaga M, Chou SH, Shields K, Papageorgiou P, Polyzos SA, Mantzoros CS. Leptin at the intersection of neuroendocrinology and metabolism: current evidence and therapeutic perspectives. Cell Metab. 2013;18(1):29–42.
92. Hamrick MW, Ferrari SL. Leptin and the sympathetic connection of fat to bone. Osteoporos Int. 2008;19(7):905–12.
93. Bartell SM, Rayalam S, Ambati S, Gaddam DR, Hartzell DL, Hamrick M, et al. Central (ICV) leptin injection increases bone formation, bone mineral density, muscle mass, serum IGF-1, and the expression of osteogenic genes in leptin-deficient ob/ob mice. J Bone Miner Res. 2011;26(8):1710–20.
94. Fazeli PK, Bredella MA, Misra M, Meenaghan E, Rosen CJ, Clemmons DR, et al. Preadipocyte factor-1 is associated with marrow adiposity and bone mineral density in women with anorexia nervosa. J Clin Endocrinol Metab. 2010;95(1):407–13.
95. Aronis KN, Kilim H, Chamberland JP, Breggia A, Rosen C, Mantzoros CS. Preadipocyte factor-1 levels are higher in women with hypothalamic amenorrhea and are associated with bone mineral content and bone mineral density through a mechanism independent of leptin. J Clin Endocrinol Metab. 2011;96(10):E1634–9.
96. Roemmich JN, Clark PA, Mantzoros CS, Gurgol CM, Weltman A, Rogol AD. Relationship of leptin to bone mineralization in children and adolescents. J Clin Endocrinol Metab. 2003;88(2):599–604.
97. Goulding A, Taylor RW. Plasma leptin values in relation to bone mass and density and to dynamic biochemical markers of bone resorption and formation in postmenopausal women. Calcif Tissue Int. 1998;63(6):456–8.
98. Carbone F, La Rocca C, Matarese G. Immunological functions of leptin and adiponectin. Biochimie. 2012;94(10):2082–8.
99. Matarese G, Moschos S, Mantzoros CS. Leptin in immunology. J Immunol. 2005;174(6):3137–42.
100. Chan JL, Moschos SJ, Bullen J, Heist K, Li X, Kim YB, et al. Recombinant methionyl human leptin administration activates signal transducer and activator of transcription 3 signaling in peripheral blood mononuclear cells in vivo and regulates soluble tumor necrosis factor-alpha receptor levels in humans with relative leptin deficiency. J Clin Endocrinol Metab. 2005;90(3):1625–31.
101. Allende LM, Corell A, Manzanares J, Madruga D, Marcos A, Madrono A, et al. Immunodeficiency associated with anorexia nervosa is secondary and improves after refeeding. Immunology. 1998;94(4):543–51.
102. Mustafa A, Ward A, Treasure J, Peakman M. T lymphocyte subpopulations in anorexia nervosa and refeeding. Clin Immunol Immunopathol. 1997;82(3):282–9.
103. Marcos A, Varela P, Toro O, Lopez-Vidriero I, Nova E, Madruga D, et al. Interactions between nutrition and immunity in anorexia nervosa: a 1-y follow-up study. Am J Clin Nutr. 1997;66(2):485S–90.
104. Scheid JL, Williams NI, West SL, VanHeest JL, De Souza MJ. Elevated PYY is associated with energy deficiency and indices of subclinical disordered eating in exercising women with hypothalamic amenorrhea. Appetite. 2009;52(1):184–92.
105. Gale SM, Castracane VD, Mantzoros CS. Energy homeostasis, obesity and eating disorders: recent advances in endocrinology. J Nutr. 2004;134(2):295–8.
106. van Zessen R, van der Plasse G, Adan RA. Contribution of the mesolimbic dopamine system in mediating the effects of leptin and ghrelin on feeding. Proc Nutr Soc. 2012;71(4):435–45.
107. Russell M, Misra M. Influence of ghrelin and adipocytokines on bone mineral density in adolescent female athletes with amenorrhea and eumenorrheic athletes. Med Sport Sci. 2010;55:103–13.
108. Wren AM, Small CJ, Ward HL, Murphy KG, Dakin CL, Taheri S, et al. The novel hypothalamic peptide ghrelin stimulates food intake and growth hormone secretion. Endocrinology. 2000;141(11):4325–8.
109. Kluge M, Schussler P, Uhr M, Yassouridis A, Steiger A. Ghrelin suppresses secretion of luteinizing hormone in humans. J Clin Endocrinol Metab. 2007;92(8):3202–5.
110. Misra M, Miller KK, Kuo K, Griffin K, Stewart V, Hunter E, et al. Secretory dynamics of ghrelin in adolescent girls with anorexia nervosa and healthy adolescents. Am J Physiol Endocrinol Metab. 2005;289(2):E347–56.
111. Lawson EA, Eddy KT, Donoho D, Misra M, Miller KK, Meenaghan E, et al. Appetite-regulating hormones cortisol and peptide YY are associated with disordered eating psychopathology, independent of body mass index. Eur J Endocrinol. 2011;164(2):253–61.
112. Chan JL, Bullen J, Lee JH, Yiannakouris N, Mantzoros CS. Ghrelin levels are not regulated by recombinant leptin administration and/or three days of fasting in healthy subjects. J Clin Endocrinol Metab. 2004;89(1):335–43.
113. Hwang JJ, Chan JL, Ntali G, Malkova D, Mantzoros CS. Leptin does not directly regulate the pancreatic hormones amylin and pancreatic polypeptide: interventional studies in humans. Diabetes Care. 2008;31(5):945–51.
114. Russell M, Stark J, Nayak S, Miller KK, Herzog DB, Klibanski A, et al. Peptide YY in adolescent athletes with amenorrhea, eumenorrheic athletes and non-athletic controls. Bone. 2009;45(1):104–9.

115. Bruni V, Dei M, Morelli C, Schettino MT, Balzi D, Nuvolone D. Body composition variables and leptin levels in functional hypothalamic amenorrhea and amenorrhea related to eating disorders. J Pediatr Adolesc Gynecol. 2011;24(6):347–52.
116. Kolaczynski JW, Nyce MR, Considine RV, Boden G, Nolan JJ, Henry R, et al. Acute and chronic effects of insulin on leptin production in humans: studies in vivo and in vitro. Diabetes. 1996;45(5):699–701.
117. Lee JH, Chan JL, Sourlas E, Raptopoulos V, Mantzoros CS. Recombinant methionyl human leptin therapy in replacement doses improves insulin resistance and metabolic profile in patients with lipoatrophy and metabolic syndrome induced by the highly active antiretroviral therapy. J Clin Endocrinol Metab. 2006;91(7):2605–11.
118. Magkos F, Brennan A, Sweeney L, Kang ES, Doweiko J, Karchmer AW, et al. Leptin replacement improves postprandial glycemia and insulin sensitivity in human immunodeficiency virus-infected lipoatrophic men treated with pioglitazone: a pilot study. Metab Clin Exp. 2011;60(7):1045–9.
119. Petersen KF, Oral EA, Dufour S, Befroy D, Ariyan C, Yu C, et al. Leptin reverses insulin resistance and hepatic steatosis in patients with severe lipodystrophy. J Clin Invest. 2002;109(10):1345–50.
120. Paruthi J, Gill N, Mantzoros CS. Adipokines in the HIV/HAART-associated lipodystrophy syndrome. Metab Clin Exp. 2013;62(9):1199–205.
121. Moon HS, Dalamaga M, Kim SY, Polyzos SA, Hamnvik OP, Magkos F, et al. Leptin's role in lipodystrophic and nonlipodystrophic insulin-resistant and diabetic individuals. Endocr Rev. 2013;34(3):377–412.
122. Lee YH, Magkos F, Mantzoros CS, Kang ES. Effects of leptin and adiponectin on pancreatic beta-cell function. Metab Clin Exp. 2011;60(12):1664–72.
123. Misra M, Miller KK, Cord J, Prabhakaran R, Herzog DB, Goldstein M, et al. Relationships between serum adipokines, insulin levels, and bone density in girls with anorexia nervosa. J Clin Endocrinol Metab. 2007;92(6):2046–52.
124. Terra X, Auguet T, Aguera Z, Quesada IM, Orellana-Gavalda JM, Aguilar C, et al. Adipocytokine levels in women with anorexia nervosa. Relationship with weight restoration and disease duration. Int J Eat Disord. 2013;46(8):855–61.
125. Modan-Moses D, Stein D, Pariente C, Yaroslavsky A, Ram A, Faigin M, et al. Modulation of adiponectin and leptin during refeeding of female anorexia nervosa patients. J Clin Endocrinol Metab. 2007;92(5):1843–7.
126. Kang ES, Magkos F, Sienkiewicz E, Mantzoros CS. Circulating vaspin and visfatin are not affected by acute or chronic energy deficiency or leptin administration in humans. Eur J Endocrinol. 2011;164(6):911–7.
127. Lawson EA, Miller KK, Blum JI, Meenaghan E, Misra M, Eddy KT, et al. Leptin levels are associated with decreased depressive symptoms in women across the weight spectrum, independent of body fat. Clin Endocrinol (Oxf). 2012;76(4):520–5.
128. Brinkoetter M, Magkos F, Vamvini M, Mantzoros CS. Leptin treatment reduces body fat but does not affect lean body mass or the myostatin-follistatin-activin axis in lean hypoleptinemic women. Am J Physiol Endocrinol Metab. 2011;301(1):E99–104.
129. Heymsfield SB, Greenberg AS, Fujioka K, Dixon RM, Kushner R, Hunt T, et al. Recombinant leptin for weight loss in obese and lean adults: a randomized, controlled, dose-escalation trial. JAMA. 1999;282(16):1568–75.
130. Beltrand J, Lahlou N, Le Charpentier T, Sebag G, Leka S, Polak M, et al. Resistance to leptin-replacement therapy in Berardinelli-Seip congenital lipodystrophy: an immunological origin. Eur J Endocrinol. 2010;162(6):1083–91.
131. Steppan CM, Crawford DT, Chidsey-Frink KL, Ke H, Swick AG. Leptin is a potent stimulator of bone growth in ob/ob mice. Regulatory peptides. 2000;92(1–3):73–8.

20 Leptin Therapy as a Substitute for Insulin Replacement in Experimental Models of Diabetes: Clinical Implications in Humans

Satya Paul Kalra

Introduction

The minute to minute participation of the central nervous system (CNS) in imposing glucose homeostasis for lifetime was firmly established in the early twentieth century when ablation of selected sites in the hypothalamus or interruption of afferent signals to the periphery reliably affected ingestive behavior, adiposity, and metabolic balance, accompanied by accelerated secretion and excretion of glucose [1–5]. On the one hand, this revelation led to an upsurge in research focused on a deeper understanding of the ways the brain regulates appetite and adiposity accretion in response to ever-changing daily energy intake and disposal during lifetime, and on the other, it engendered an appreciation of the notion that hormones are indispensable for relaying regulatory signals between the CNS and peripheral organs for sustenance of metabolic homeostasis [2–6]. A major breakthrough emanating from these endeavors was the identification, isolation, chemical characterization, and soon, thereafter, availability of pancreatic insulin for treatment of diabetic patients in the 1920s [3, 4, 7]. Following the recognition of insulin as the indispensable signal in sustaining glucose homeostasis and as a miracle molecule of modern medicine, multidisciplinary research has been devoted to the better understanding of (1) the external and internal environmental factors at systemic, cellular, and molecular levels critical in regulation of insulin secretion, (2) delineation of pathways in the body that participate in integration of glucose disposal for glycemic control and (3) fine-tuning the insulin delivery technology to optimally simulate the normal pattern of glucose fluctuations on a 24-h basis in diabetics. Looking back on this history, one is stuck by the revelation that until the 1970s, there was a paucity of research aimed both at identifying the existence of additional signal molecules, as efficient as insulin, that regulate glucose homeostasis and at mapping metabolic and neural pathways that orchestrate and mediate the homeostatic cues for tight glycemic control. Fortunately, history is replete with instances when serendipitous observations herald a revolution in our understanding of the etiology of diseases that lead to the discovery of newer therapies. In this context, one can assign the serendipitous discovery of a few morbidly obese, diabetic mutants in a rodent colony and the diligent pursuit by elegant experimentation in vivo aimed to decipher the underlying pathogenesis of these metabolic aberrations, that culminated decades later, first in the discovery and isolation of leptin hormone from adipocytes [6, 8–12], and subsequently establishing the adipocyte leptin-hypothalamus axis as obligatory in maintenance

S.P. Kalra, Ph.D. (✉)
Department of Neuroscience, College of Medicine, University of Florida, 1149 Newell Drive, Room L1-100, Gainesville, FL 32611, USA
e-mail: skalra@ufl.edu

S. Dagogo-Jack (ed.), *Leptin: Regulation and Clinical Applications*,
DOI 10.1007/978-3-319-09915-6_20,

of glucose homeostasis [5, 11–14]. The outcome as summarized here is an ongoing mini revolution in the newer and deeper understanding of the etiology of diabetes mellitus type 1 (T1DM) and type 2 (T2DM), coupled with the findings from ingenious experimental paradigms that have compellingly endorsed the therapeutic potential of leptin.

New Conceptual Revelations

Pancreatic Insulin-Adipocyte Leptin-Hypothalamus Axis

Pancreatic insulin: Normally insulin is secreted in a pulsatile manner characterized by stable pulse frequency and wide amplitude fluctuations throughout the day. The strength of pulse discharge is quantitatively regulated by blood glucose concentrations, the higher range prevailing postprandially and return to basal range during the inter-meal interval. Hyperinsulinemia is invariably a consequence of increased episodes of insulin discharge in response to increments in quantity and quality of macronutrient intake [15–18]. Furthermore, substantial experimental evidence supports the emerging notion that sustenance of increased insulin pulse amplitude results in loss of target effectiveness engendered initially by down regulation of target receptor response followed sequentially by development of insulin insensitivity, resistance and extinction of intracellular signaling, breakdown in glucose homeostasis, thereby, progressively precipitating T2DM, fat accumulation, and obesity [7, 17, 18]. This new understanding of the chain of events in the pathophysiology of T2DM and obesity radically contrasts the widely prevailing conventional wisdom that it is the sustenance of increased fat depots over considerable periods that precipitates the development of insulin resistance leading to T2DM, instead of the antecedent increased energy intake-dependent hyperinsulinemia, insulin resistance, hyperglycemia, and T2DM [7, 19, 20] being the initial etiologic sequences that promote increased accretion of body fat and obesity.

Adipocyte Leptin

A critical reappraisal of recent experimental evidence has also affirmed that insulin is adipogenic and stimulates the secretion of a host of adipokines, including leptin [12, 13, 16, 21–24]. Quantitatively, rhythmic fluctuations in blood leptin levels are driven by pulsatile variations in insulin which, in turn, are dependent upon the strength of blood glucose signals generated in response to energy intake [25–28]. Further, just as observed in the case of hyperinsulinemia, hyperleptinemia readily engenders leptin receptor down regulation, leptin insensitivity and/or resistance at peripheral targets [17, 25, 29].

Hypothalamus and Leptin Insufficiency

As expected, soon after the identification of leptin as an anorexigenic peripheral signal, it became evident that the hypothalamus was the singular site of leptin action in inhibiting appetite, an essential component of brain control of body weight homeostasis [5, 6, 17, 26, 30–33] mediated by activation of leptin receptors located on the interconnected network of orexigenic and anorexigenic neurotransmitter producing neurons (Fig. 20.1) [5, 6, 17, 26, 30–33]. A major breakthrough that subsequently uncovered the etiology of hyperglycemia, diabetes, and augmented rate of fat accretion was the obligatory participation of the blood–brain barrier (BBB) in the control of leptin transport into the CNS [34–42]. It was observed that a sustained rise in circulating leptin levels readily down regulated leptin receptors on endothelial cells involved in the transport of leptin, leading thereby to decreased availability of leptin in various CNS sites, including the hypothalamus. Indeed , the resultant leptin insufficiency for extended periods in the hypothalamus was shown to be intimately associated with breakdown in glucose homeostasis as reflected by hyperglycemia, hyperinsulinemia, and rise in circulating adipokines titers, the major symptoms of T2DM

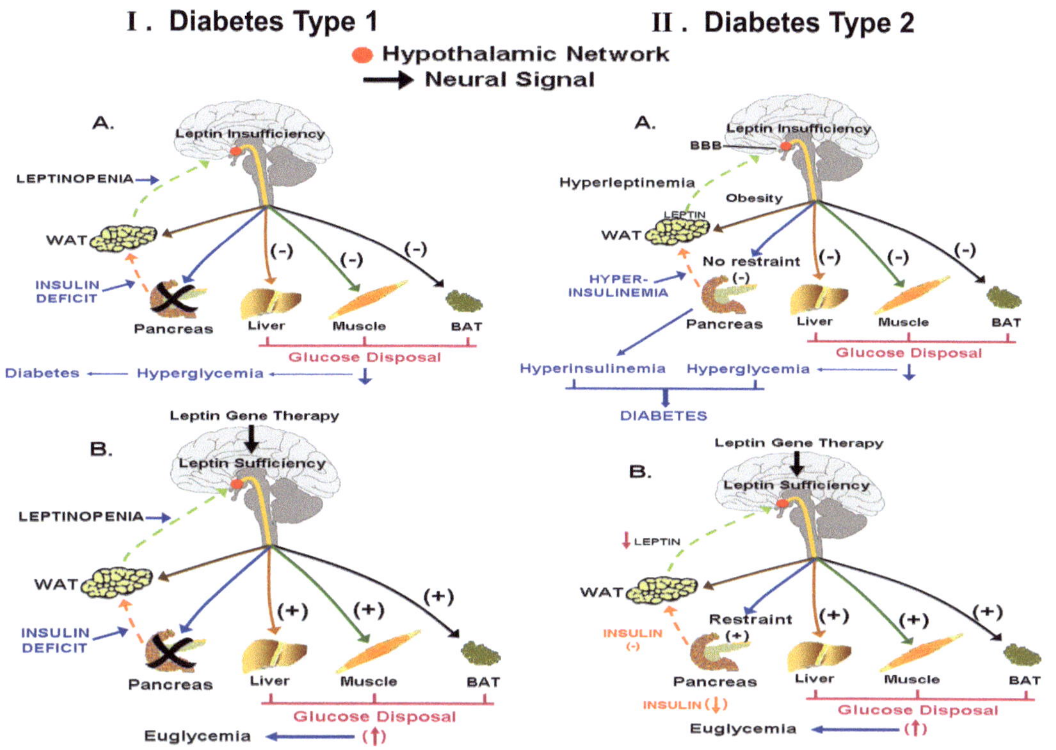

Fig. 20.1 Schematically depicts the role of hypothalamic leptin insufficiency and sufficiency reinstated with leptin gene therapy on glucose homeostasis. (I) Diabetes type 1 (*left*) (**a**) absence of insulin due to a loss of pancreatic b-cells secondarily results in leptinopenia, which, in turn, produces leptin insufficiency in the hypothalamus responsible for neurally reducing (–) glucose disposal in liver, skeletal muscle, and brown adipose tissue (BAT) in the periphery, and facilitating the development of chronic hyperglycemia (for details see text). (**b**) Leptin sufficiency in the hypothalamus transduced by leptin gene therapy optimally reinstates euglycemia by restoring enhanced rate (+) of glucose metabolism in peripheral sites, even in the absence of insulin (for details see text). (II) Diabetes type 2 (*right*) (**a**) through descending relays, leptin insufficiency in the hypothalamus produced by imperviousness of BBB transduced by environmentally acquired hyperleptinemia due to obesity, curtails (–) the central restraint on pancreatic insulin secretion and glucose disposal in peripheral targets leading to the development of chronic hyperinsulinemia and hyperglycemia, respectively. These two metabolic abnormalities in concert, sustain diabetes type 2. (**b**) Leptin sufficiency in the hypothalamus transduced by leptin gene therapy reinstates euglycemia by neurally suppressing hyperleptinemia, restoring the regulatory restrain on insulin secretion and upregulation of glucose metabolism in peripheral sites (+) (for details see text, reproduced from [43])

[19, 31, 41, 43], and increased rate of fat deposition . Remarkably, a similar hypothalamic insufficiency manifests in T1DM primarily due to the prevalence of extreme leptinopenia attributed to lack of insulin-induced leptin secretion from adipocytes [5, 12, 19]. That optimal leptin transport to the hypothalamus across BBB is mandatory was amply endorsed when leptin replenishment locally readily abrogated these metabolic disorders and reinstated glucose homeostasis in T1DM models [5, 42–44].

Leptin Targets in the Hypothalamus

A complex interconnected network of leptin receptor producing neurons spanning almost the entire basal hypothalamus was diligently mapped during the last decade (Fig. 20.1) [6, 17, 19, 45–48]. Rostrally from the medial preoptic area (MPOA), this circuit projects caudally and ventrally to the arcuate nucleus (ARC) and caudally and laterally to the paraventicular nucleus (PVN), ventromedial hypothalamus (VMH), and lateral hypothalamus (LH). The neurons within this circuitry coexpress diverse neuropeptides and amino acid neurotransmitters that communicate with each other and relay regulatory messages to multiple peripheral targets for energy balance under the direction of the ever-changing leptin milieu in the hypothalamus. More recently, the existence and dynamic operation of a discrete anatomical substrate within this circuitry concerned singularly with leptin-glucose homeostasis, has been detailed extensively [5, 6, 12–14, 17, 32, 48] and is presented in condensed form in the following sections.

Descending Neural Pathways

Extensive tracing studies aimed at delineating the paths of the leptin-induced descending relays from various nuclei in the hypothalamus revealed three distinct pathways namely, the appetite regulating network (ARN) to the gastrointestinal tract to control energy intake, the energy expending network (EEN) to brown adipose tissue to stimulate nonthermogenic energy expenditure, and the fat accrual network (FAN) to the pancreas to control insulin efflux and adipogenesis, and to skeletal muscles, liver, and white adipose tissue (WAT) to upregulate glucose disposal (Fig. 20.1) [48–55]. It is now well established that a coordinated operation of these afferent signals to the periphery is necessary for maintaining glucose homeostasis and a breakdown in any of the afferent relays rapidly precipitates hyperglycemia, diabetes, and fat accumulation [5, 12, 18, 19, 56].

Temporal Relationship Between Centrally Mediated Adipocyte-Leptin and Pancreatic-Insulin Feedback Underlying Glucose Homeostasis

Close evaluation of the temporal relationships among circulating concentrations of insulin and leptin and CNS leptin levels showed that either the complete absence or diminution of insulin secretion as seen in T1DM or that inflicted experimentally, is always concomitant with markedly low levels of leptin in the circulation as well as in the CNS [13, 15, 19, 21, 23, 34, 35, 38, 39, 57–59]. That this leptinopenia is the major etiologic cause of disruption in glucose homeostasis is reenforced by extensive experimental evidence showing that replenishment of leptin alone, either by systemic or by local central routes, reinstated glucose homeostasis, even in the complete absence of insulin in the circulation and unchanged fat depots [40, 43, 44, 57, 59–62]. On the other hand, insulin hypersecretion in response to increased energy intake is followed by augmented leptin secretion, but attenuated transport across BBB and disruption of glucose homeostasis in young and adult wild (WT) rodents [38, 41, 42, 60]. Under these conditions, whereas leptin administration by systemic routes was found to be completely ineffective, direct delivery into the CNS rapidly decreased insulin secretion and corrected glucose homeostasis along with a gradual decrease in body fat during the entire course of treatment [5, 12, 13, 26, 27, 29, 49, 55–57, 60]. Consequently, operation of the feedback loop between pancreatic insulin and adipocytic leptin was found to be essential in the regulation of glucose homeostasis via the hypothalamus [19, 32, 40, 43, 46, 56, 60]. This feedback loop is now known to normally operate as follows: rising blood glucose levels in response to food intake stimulate insulin secretion from pancreas, which in turn stimulates leptin secretion from adipocytes and transportation of leptin into the hypothalamus. Glucose homeostasis is then reinstated by activation by leptin of FAN and EEN afferent signaling in order to restrain insulin secretion and activate glucose disposal, as elaborated in the preceding sections.

Leptin, a New Therapy for Diabetes

The highlights of the new insight enumerated above are that optimal leptin signaling to the hypothalamus is mandatory for sustaining glucose homeostasis which is regulated by a tight centrally mediated feedback relationship between insulin and leptin. The follow-up discovery that leptin insufficiency in the hypothalamus is the common etiologic factor in causation of T1DM and T2DM [19], has triggered research towards comprehensively evaluating leptin as a new therapy to replace insulin for both types of diabetes in a variety of animal and clinical paradigms [5]. An account of these endeavors in the last decade is summarized in the following sections.

Type 1 Diabetes

Leptin mutant ob/ob mice are morbidly obese due to incessant hyperphagia in association with hyperglycemia and hyperinsulinemia [8–10]. Leptin replacement by systemic routes resulted in diminished energy intake, loss of fat depots, a slight diminution in insulin secretion accompanied by euglycemia, all of these metabolic changes were initially attributed solely to the disappearance of adiposity [3, 6, 7, 11, 22, 33]. In another leptinopenic rodent model exhibiting lipodystrophia but with severe hyperglycemia and hyperinsulinemia, daily leptin replacement systemically also corrected these pathologies [5, 60]. Most interestingly , these metabolic benefits were reproduced by central infusion of leptin alone with a slightly disparate temporal sequence, an antecedent decrease in circulating insulin levels and euglycemia followed by decrements in appetite and weight in various T1DM paradigms [5, 14, 18, 21, 23, 26, 28, 29, 31, 32, 41, 46, 56, 59]. These revelations clearly reinforced the notion that leptin action alone in the hypothalamus, while restraining insulin secretion from the pancreas, concurrently augmented glucose metabolism in order to impose a stable state of euglycemia (Fig. 20.1). To reaffirm the singularity of central site of leptin action in promoting stable euglycemia over extended intervals, a series of follow up investigations employed central leptin gene therapy to replenish leptin selectively within the hypothalmic sites for local actions, without diffusion either to adjoining brain sites or into the general circulation for actions on the peripheral targets (Fig. 20.1, Table 20.1).

This novel paradigm of selective and stable availability of biologically active leptin in minute amounts not only corroborated the earlier findings of metabolic benefits, but further showed that even in WT young and aging rodents leptin action selectively in the hypothalamus suppressed blood glucose and insulin levels (Table 20.1) [18, 19, 23, 26, 29, 32, 43, 57, 58]. Most surprisingly, similar central leptin gene therapy imposed euglycemia during the extended course of the experiment, lasting lifetime, in the T1DM rodent model, the insulin-deficient diabetic Akita mice and the leptin-deficient hyperinsulinemic diabetic ob/ob mice [44, 57–61]. Notably, whereas stable euglycemia manifested in both rodent models, it manifested independent of any appreciable change in energy consumption and body weight in Akita mice [58]. Recently, long-term normoglycemia was also established by hyperleptinemia induced in the progeny of these insulin deficient Akita mice crossbred with leptin-expressing transgenic (lepTG) mice [63], another experimental modality affirming that lack of leptin in insulin-deficient Akita mice underlies the diabetic state.

The robust ability of leptin delivered by systemic or central routes to ameliorate hyperglycemia and early mortality in the absence of insulin in Akita mice was replicated in WT adult mice pretreated with streptozotocin (STZ) to induce insulitis following destruction of pancreatic beta cells [59]. In another paradigm, skin transplants from transgenic mice overexpressing leptin, also induced glycemia when grafted into the leptin-deficient ob/ob mice, thereby reaffirming the ability of systemic leptin in insulin-deficient T1DM subjects [64]. As far as institution of stable glycemic control, leptin therapy was found to be superior when compared with insulin therapy in the commonly employed T1DM model, the nonobese diabetic (NOD) mouse (Table 20.1) [44].

Genetic defects in leptin signaling in target cells due to receptor gene mutation as in db/db mice, fa/fa Zucker rats and f/f Koletsky rats result in obesity, accompanied by hyperinsulinemia and hyperglycemia [19, 65]. Selective instillation of leptin receptor (OB-Rb) in discrete hypothalmic site(s) with the aid of leptin receptor gene therapy also markedly decreased body weight along with circulating insulin and normalization of glucose concentrations [65]. Consequently, all the adverse consequences on glucose homeostasis inflicted

Table 20.1 Effects of leptin on diabetes in animal paradigms

	Paradigm	Pathophysiology	Route of administration	Benefits
T1DM	ob/ob	Hyperglycemia, hyperinsulinemia, leptinonemia	Systemic, central	Euglycemia
	Akita	Hyperglycemia, insulinemia, leptinopenia	Systemic, central	Euglycemia
	NOD	Hyperglycemia, insulinopenia	Systemic	Euglycemia
	WT+STZ	Hyperglycemia, insulinemia	Central	Euglycemia
	Congenital lipodystrophy	Hyperglycemia, hyperinsulinemia	Systemic	Euglycemia
T2DM	WT aging, obese	Hyperglycemia, hyperinsulinemia, hyperleptinemia	Central	Euglycemia
	WT HFD, obese	Hyperglycemia, hyperinsulinemia, hyperleptinemia	Central	Euglycemia
	UCD-T2DM	Hyperinsulinemia, hyperinsulinemia, hyperleptinemia	Systemic	Euglycemia

by the loss of intracellular signal relay resulting from mutations in leptin receptor gene can be mitigated by reinstatement of leptin receptor, just in those hypothalmic sites previously found to be essential for glucose homeostasis [5, 32, 46].

Seemingly, in diabetics displaying either coexistent hyperinsulinemia and leptinopenia or insulinemia and leptinopenia, leptin therapy is highly effective in restoring normoglycemia. Further, it is now well established that insulin stimulates leptin secretion from adipocytes and it is this lack of insulin stimulus due to loss of pancreatic beta cells, the hallmark of T1DM, produces a state of leptinopenia leading sequentially to leptin deficiency in the hypothalamus and absence of neural afferents involved in sustenance of glucose homeostasis [5, 32, 46, 57–59, 61]. That leptinopenia is the singular etiologic factor of T1DM is further corroborated by the finding that leptinopenia due to experimentally induced lipodystrophia also results in breakdown in glucose homeostasis and it is readily corrected by leptin replacement [20, 57, 60, 66]. Consequently, optimal supply of leptin to hypothalmic targets either by systemic routes or directly into the hypothalamus is the treatment of choice for T1DM (Table 20.1) [67–73] and it can replace the currently in-vogue insulin monotherapy which is riddled with a host of shortcomings due to difficulties in simulating the normal minute-to-minute blood glucose fluctuations, ensuing frequent episodes of hypoglycemia and several related multiple metabolic inflictions emanating over the extended periods of energy imbalance [5, 12, 19, 32].

Type 2 Diabetes

The pathophysiology of T2DM characterized by high titers of circulating insulin and glucose, concomitant with insulin resistance and decrease in the rate of glucose disposal is commonly observed in association with obesity manifesting either gradually in an aged-related fashion or rapidly in response to consumption of calorie-rich high fat diet (HFD) [6, 17, 27, 46]. Furthermore, according to the conventional notion, the onset and sustenance of T2DM is engendered initially by a steady rise in the rate of visceral fat accumulation which impels the development of insulin resistance and decrements in glucose disposal to culminate in hyperglycemia [5, 7, 20, 24]. However, as described earlier, the age-related as well as HFD-induced obesity are also associated with the BBB-induced diminished leptin transport to the CNS in response to hyperleptinemia [19] and it is the ensuing insufficient leptin signaling within the hypothalmic targets that evokes diminished afferent relays to the periphery and breakdown in glucose homeostasis [5, 19]. That central leptin insufficiency in obese rodents may be the primary underlying cause of T2DM was amply affirmed by the findings that reinstatement of optimal leptin supply selectively in the hypothalmic targets ameliorated the age-related and HFD-induced T2DM, as reflected by the observation of stable glycemia, normalization of insulin sensitivity, and rate of glucose disposal (Fig. 20.1, Table 20.1) [2, 17, 18, 23, 26–29, 61].

In accord with these various lines of evidence gathered from WT animals, it was recently shown that UC Davis-type 2 diabetes mellitus (UCD-T2DM) rats that exhibit adult onset of obesity, diabetes, insulin resistance, and hyperglycemia when administered leptin subcutaneously for extended periods normalized blood glucose, by imparting increased insulin sensitivity in conjunction with diminution in insulin secretion in these rats [74]. Overall, it is clear that leptin insufficiency in the CNS engendered by imperviousness of the BBB due to increased adiposity-dependent hyperleptinemia underlies the development of T2DM (Fig. 20.1, Table 20.1) [5, 17].

Mode of Action of Leptin in the Hypothalamus in Regulation of Glucose Homeostasis

Detailed mapping of neuronal targets in the hypothalamus disclosed an interconnected network of two primary populations of neurons in the ARC, one that coexpresses neuropeptide Y, agouti-related peptide, and gamma-aminobutyric acid (GABA) and the other that coexpress proopiomelanocortin and GABA. These populations project into various sites within the hypothalamus to regulate leptin-induced afferent relays along the ARN, EEN, and FAN pathways associated with energy homeostasis (Fig. 20.1) [6, 13, 17, 46]. Evidently, inhibition of appetite by leptin is mediated by ARN that operates independently of its control on glucose homeostasis [18, 46]. Activation by leptin of EEN from the MPOA to brown adipose tissue controls nonthermogenic energy expenditure, while activation of FAN from ARC, VMH, and LH restrains pulsatile insulin secretion and insulin sensitivity, on the one hand, and stimulates glucose metabolism from skeletal muscles, liver, and WAT, on the other (Fig. 20.1) [18, 19, 32, 42, 60–62, 67–83]. Thus, diminution in leptin signaling in the hypothalamus, as it manifests in response to either leptinopenia or impaired entry of leptin across BBB, results in the breakdown in these hypothalamic regulatory relays on energy intake and glucose homeostasis, all of which can be rapidly reinstated with resupply of leptin [17–19, 30, 31, 42, 43, 46, 56, 57].

A Perspective: Future Clinical Testing

Early results of clinical studies to evaluate the benefits of leptin therapy delivered systemically on appetite and obesity were disappointing [7, 12, 84]. These failures are attributable now to multiple shortcomings, such as dose and frequency of administration in relation to preexisting levels of leptin, combined with a lack of appreciation of the pivotal role of BBB in transporting leptin to targets in the hypothalamus [12, 14, 19, 22, 38, 39, 46]. Soon after, however, it was reported that both in patients harboring congenital leptin-deficiency and a small population of obese patients displaying low circulating concentrations of leptin due to unknown causes, leptin replacement effectively imposed normoglycemia concomitant with reduced food intake and body weight [20, 22, 24, 33, 83]. Indeed, a small population of congenitally leptin-deficient pediatric and adult patients on leptin therapy has displayed improved glycemia for years without any discernible untoward metabolic disruptions. In response to these reports, leptin replacement therapy has also been tested worldwide in patients suffering from impaired glucose homeostasis in association with either leptinopenia due to congenital lipodystrophy or hypoleptinemia of acquired lipoatrophy. Leptin administration readily reinstated diverse centrally mediated metabolic responses, notably diabetes, for the entire course of treatments lasting several months to years [20, 22, 24, 33, 59, 66, 69, 70, 73, 75, 79–83]. Consequently, these clinical successes have boosted the discovery emanating from diverse experimental paradigms in rodents that the adipocytic leptin is an obligatory signal in maintenance of glucose homeostasis (Table 20.1).

Another significant outcome of these clinical investigations is that systemic administration of leptin only 2–3 times a day engendered stable glycemia. Because hypoleptinemia normally exists in newly diagnosed untreated T1DM patients and the fact that leptin under conditions of hypoleptinemia can restore euglycemia, leptin replacement therapy alone, or in adjunct with insulin therapy, is being clinically investigated.

In contrast, leptin administration systemically in obese, hyperleptinemic subjects suffering from T2DM has generally failed to exert any appreciable impact on blood glucose concentrations [7, 12, 84]. This outcome is not surprising in view of the clear evidence expounded earlier that BBB is rendered impervious by hyperleptinemia in humans and animals, alike. Therefore, one can easily surmise that raising blood leptin levels further in hyperleptinemic human subjects is unlikely to provide optimal leptin signals to the hypothalamus required to reinstate glucose homeostasis. On the other hand, the possibility that leptin delivery directly to the hypothalamus, as demonstrated by irrevocable findings from experiments in rodents (Table 20.1, Fig. 20.1), would ameliorate T2DM remains to be tested clinically.

Collectively on balance, to ameliorate both types of diabetes and to reduce or alleviate the accompanying well-documented adverse metabolic consequences, leptin therapy has immense potential to replace or be employed as a conjunct to insulin monotherapy [5, 12, 18, 32, 33]. As the incidence of diabetes has attained epidemic status worldwide [85], the societal burden of ever soaring treatment costs, in concert with the new expanding knowledge of the diabetes-associated multiple metabolic and neurological disorders, including cognition impairment [5, 12, 19], this discovery is highly significant . Consequently, there is a dire urgency to improve and identify new long-acting leptin mimetics that can bypass BBB enroute to CNS, and rigorously evaluate in humans the efficacy of leptin and /or mimetics delivery directly to CNS sites via well-tested gene therapy and intranasal routes [5, 18, 19, 86–88].

References

1. Haymaker W, Anderson E, Nauta WJH, editors. The hypothalamus. USA: Charles C Thomas; 1969.
2. Brobeck JR. Mechanisms of the development of obesity in animals with hypothalmic lesions. Physiol Rev. 1946;26:123–46.
3. Bray GA. Historical framework for the development of ideas about obesity. In Bray, Ga, Bouchard V, James WPT (eds) Handbook of obesity 1998:1–29, Marcel Dekker Inc., New York.
4. Banting FG, Best CH. Pancreatic extracts 1922. J Lab Clin Med. 1990;115:254–72.
5. Kalra SP. Should leptin replace insulin as a monotherapy for diabetes 1 and 2? Indian J Endocrinol Metab. 2013;17 Suppl 1:S23–4.
6. Kalra SP, Dube MG, Pu S, Xu B, Horvath TL, Kalra PS. Interacting appetite-regulating pathways in the hypothalamic regulation of body weight. Endocr Rev. 1999;20:68–100.
7. Kahn SE, Hull RL, Utzschneider KM. Mechanisms linking obesity to insulin resistance and type 2 diabetes. Nature. 2006;444:840–6.
8. Coleman DL. Effects of parabiosis of obese with diabetics and normal mice. Diabetologia. 1973;9:894–8.
9. Coleman DL. Obese and diabetics: two mutant genes causing diabetes-obesity syndromes. Diabetologia. 1978;14:141–8.
10. Zhang Y, Proenca R, Maffei M, Barone M, Leopold L, Friedman JM. Positional cloning of the mouse obese gene and its human homologue. Nature. 1994;372: 425–32.
11. Kamohara S, Burcelin R, Halaas JL, Friedman JM, Charron MJ. Acute stimulation of glucose metabolism in mice by leptin treatment. Nature. 1997;389: 374–7.
12. Kalra SP. A case for new therapy for diabetes, is it leptin? Indian J Endocrinol Metab. 2012;16 Suppl 3:S525–8.
13. Amitani M, Asakawa A, Amitani H, Inui A. The role of leptin in the control of insulin–glucose axis. Front Neurosci. 2013;7:1–12.
14. Marino JS, Xu Y, Hill W. Central insulin and leptin-mediated autonomic control of glucose homeostasis. Trends Endocrinol Metab. 2011;22:275–85.
15. Otukonyong EE, Dube MG, Torto R, Kalra PS, Kalra SP. Central leptin differentially modulates ultradian secretory patterns of insulin, leptin and ghrelin independent of effects on food intake and body weight. Peptides. 2005;26:2559–66.
16. Otukonyong EE, Dube MG, Torto R, Kalra PS, Kalra SP. High fat diet-induced ultradian leptin and insulin hypersecretion and ghrelin is absent in obesity-resistant rats. Obes Res. 2005;113:991–9.
17. Kalra SP, Kalra PS. NPY and cohorts in regulating appetite, obesity and metabolic syndrome: beneficial effects of gene therapy. Neuropeptides. 2004;38:201–11.

18. Kalra SP. Central leptin gene therapy ameliorates diabetes type 1 and 2 through two independent hypothalmic relays a benefit beyond weight and appetite regulation. Peptides. 2009;30:1957–63.
19. Kalra SP. Central leptin insufficiency syndrome: an interactive etiology for obesity, metabolic and neural diseases and for designing new therapeutic interventions. Peptides. 2008;29:127–38.
20. Moon H-S, Dalamaga M, Kim S, Polyzos SA, Hamnvik O-P, Magkos F, et al. Leptin's role in lipodystrophic and nonlipodystrophic insulin-resistant and diabetic individuals. Endocr Rev. 2013;34:377–412.
21. Kalra SP, Bagnasco M, Otukonyong EE, Dube MG, Kalra PS. Rhythmic, reciprocal ghrelin and leptin signaling: new insight in the development of obesity. Regul Pept. 2003;111:1–11.
22. Dalamaga M, Chou SH, Shields K, Papageorgious P, Polyzos SA, Mantzoros CH. Leptin at the intersection of neuroendocrinology and metabolism: Current evidence and therapeutic perspectives. Cell Metab. 2013; 8:29–43.
23. Boghossian S, Dube MG, Torto R, Kalra PS, Kalra SP. Hypothalmic clamp on insulin release by leptin-transgene expression. Peptides. 2006;27:3245–54.
24. Cummings BP. Leptin therapy in type 2 diabetes. Diabetes Obes Metab. 2013;15:1–6. Blackwell Publishing Ltd.
25. Bagnasco M, Kalra PS, Kalra SP. Plasma leptin levels are pulsatile in adult rats: effects of gonadectomy. Neuroendocrinology. 2002;75:257–63.
26. Dhillon H, Kalra SP, Prima V, et al. Central leptin gene therapy suppresses body weight gain, adiposity and serum insulin without affecting food consumption in normal rats: a long-term study. Regul Pept. 2001;99:69–77.
27. Dube MG, Beretta E, Dhillon H, Ueno N, Kalra PS, Kalra SP. Central leptin gene therapy blocks high fat diet-induced weight gain, hyperleptinemia and hyperinsulinemia: effects on serum ghrelin levels. Diabetes. 2002;51:1729–36.
28. Dube MG, Torto R, Kalra SP. Increased leptin expression selectively in the hypothalamus suppresses inflammatory markers CRP and IL-6 in leptin-deficient diabetic obese mice. Peptides. 2008;29:593–8.
29. Bagnasco M, Dube MG, Katz A, Kalra PS, Kalra SP. Leptin expression in hypothalamic PVN reverses dietary obesity and hyperinsulinemia but stimulates ghrelin. Obes Res. 2003;11:463–70.
30. Kalra SP, Kalra PS. Viral vectors as probes to decipher brain circuitry for weight control. Trends Endocrinol Metab. 2001;12:377–8.
31. Kalra SP. Circumventing leptin resistance for weight control. Proc Natl Acad Sci U S A. 2001;9:84279–81.
32. Kalra SP, Kalra PS. Gene transfer technology: a preventive neurotherapy to curb obesity, ameliorate metabolic syndrome and extend life-expectancy. Trends Pharmacol Sci. 2005;26:488–95.
33. Farooqi IS, O'Rahilly S. Leptin: a pivotal regulator of human energy homeostasis. Am J Clin Nutr. 2009;89:980S–4.
34. Kastin AJ, Pan W, Maness LM, Koletsky RJ, Ernsberger P. Decreased transport of leptin across the blood-brain barrier in rats lacking the short form of the leptin receptor. Peptides. 1999;20:1449–53.
35. Kastin AJ, Pan W. Dynamic regulation of leptin entry into brain by the blood-brain barrier. Regul Pept. 2000;92:37–43.
36. Banks WA, DiPalma CR, Farrell CL. Impaired transport of leptin across the blood-brain barrier in obesity. Peptides. 1999;20:1341–5.
37. Banks WA, Farr SA, Morley JE. The effects of high fat diets on the blood-brain barrier transport of leptin: failure or adaptation? Physiol Behav. 2006;88:244–8.
38. Kurrimbux D, Gaffen Z, Farrell CL, Martin D, Thomas SA. The involvement of the blood-brain and the blood-cerebrospinal fluid barriers in the distribution of leptin into and out of the rat brain. Neuroscience. 2004;123:527–36.
39. Ziylan YZ, Baltaci AK, Mogulkoc R. Leptin transport in the central nervous system. Cell Biochem Funct. 2009;27:63–70.
40. Miyanaga F, Ogawa Y, Ebihara K, Hidaka S, Tanaka T, Hayashi S, et al. Leptin as an adjunct of insulin therapy in insulin-deficient diabetes. Diabetologia. 2003;46:1329–37.
41. Burguera B, Couce ME, Curran GL, Jensen MD, Lloyd RV, Cleary MP, et al. Obesity is associated with a decreased leptin transport across the blood-brain barrier in rats. Diabetes. 2000;49:1219–23.
42. Caro JF, Kolaczynski JW, Nyce MR, Ohannesian JP, Opentanova I, Goldman WH, et al. Decreased cerebrospinal-fluid/serum leptin ratio in obesity: a possible mechanism for leptin resistance. Lancet. 1996;348:159–61.
43. Kalra SP. Pivotal role of leptin-hypothalamus signaling in the etiology of diabetes uncovered by gene therapy; a new therapeutic intervention? Gene Therapy. 2011;18:319–29.
44. Wang MY, Chen L, Clark GO, Lee Y, Stevens RD, Ilkayeva OR, et al. Leptin therapy in insulin-deficient type 1 diabetes. Proc Natl Acad Sci U S A. 2010; 107:4813–9.
45. Michael J, Krashes I, Bhavik P, Shah I, Joseph C, Madara I, et al. An excitatory paraventricular nucleus to AgRP neuron circuit that drives hunger. Nature. 2014;507:238–42.
46. Minokoshi Y, Haque MS, Shimazu T. Microinjection of leptin into the ventromedial hypothalamus increases glucose uptake in peripheral tissues in rats. Diabetes. 1999;48:287–91.
47. Cohen P, Zhao C, Cai X, Montez JM, Rohani SC, Feinstein P, et al. Selective deletion of leptin receptor in neurons leads to obesity. J Clin Invest. 2001; 108:1113–21.
48. Kalra SP, Kalra PS. Neuroendocrine update of energy homeostasis. Update and insight. Prog Brain Res. Martini L (Ed) 2010:181;17–33
49. Bartness TJ, Kay Song C, Shi H, Bowers RR, Foster MT. Brain-adipose tissue cross talk. Proc Nutr Soc. 2005;64:53–64.

50. Bamshad M, Song CK, Bartness TJ. CNS origins of the sympathetic nervous system outflow to brown adipose tissue. Am J Physiol. 1999;276(6 Pt 2): R1569–78.
51. Wang ZW, Zhou YT, Kakuma T, Lee Y, Higa M, Kalra SP, et al. Comparing the hypothalamic and extrahypothalamic actions of endogenous hyperleptinemia. Proc Natl Acad Sci U S A. 1999;96:10373–8.
52. Kreier F, Kap YS, Mettenleiter TC, van Heijningen C, van der Vliet J, Kalsbeek A, et al. Tracing from fat tissue, liver, and pancreas: a neuroanatomical framework for the role of the brain in type 2 diabetes. Endocrinology. 2006;147:1140–7.
53. Uyama N, Geerts A, Reynaert H. Neural connections between the hypothalamus and the liver. Anat Rec A Discov Mol Cell Evol Biol. 2004;280:808–20.
54. Buijs RM, Chun SJ, Niijima A, Romijn HJ, Nagai K. Parasympathetic and sympathetic control of the pancreas: a role for the suprachiasmatic nucleus and other hypothalamic centers that are involved in the regulation of food intake. J Comp Neurol. 2001;431: 405–23.
55. Fujikawa T, Berglund ED, Patel VR, Ramadori G, Vianna CR, Vonga L, et al. Leptin engages a hypothalmic neurocircuitry to permit survival in the absence of insulin. Cell Metab. 2013;18:431–44.
56. Koyama K, Shimabukuro M, Chen G, Wang MY, Lee Y, Kalra PS, et al. Resistance to adenovirally induced hyperleptinemia in rats: comparison of ventromedial hypothalamic lesions and mutated leptin receptors. J Clin Invest. 1998;102:728–33.
57. Fujikawa T, Coppari R. Hypothalamic-mediated control of glucose balance in the presence and absence of insulin. Aging. 2014;6:92–7.
58. Ueno N, Inui A, Kalra SP, Kalra PS. Leptin transgene expression in the hypothalamus enforces euglycemia in diabetic, insulin-deficient nonobese Akita mice and leptindeficient obese ob/ob mice. Peptides. 2006;27: 2332–42.
59. Kojima S, Asakawa A, Amitani H, Sakoguchi T, Ueno N, Inui A, et al. Central leptin gene therapy, a substitute for insulin therapy to ameliorate hyperglycemia and hyperphagia, and promote survival in insulin-deficient diabetic mice. Peptides. 2009; 30:962–6.
60. Shimomura I, Hammer RE, Ikemoto S, Brown MS, Goldstein JL. Leptin reverses insulin resistance and diabetes mellitus in mice with congenital lipodystrophy. Naure. 1999;401:73–6.
61. Chinookoswong N, Wang JL, Shi ZQ. Leptin restores euglycemia and normalizes glucose turnover in insulin- deficient diabetes in the rat. Diabetes. 1999;48: 1487–92.
62. Masuzaki H, Ogawa Y, Aizawa-Abe M, Hosoda K, Suga J, Ebihara K, et al. Glucose metabolism and leptin with lethal yellow agouti mutation: usefulness of leptin for the treatment of obesity-associated diabetes. Diabetes. 1999;48:1615–22.
63. Yoshioka M, Kayo T, Ikeda T, Koizumi A. A novel locus, Mody4, distal to D7Mit189 on chromosome 7 determines early-onset NIDDM in nonobese C57BL/6 (Akita) mutant mice. Diabetes. 1997;46:887–94.
64. Larcher F, Del Rio M, Serrano F, Segovia JC, Ramirez A, Meana A, et al. A cutaneous gene therapy approach to human leptin deficiencies, correction of the marine ob/phenotype using leptin-targeted keratinocytes grafts. FASEB. 2001;15:1529–38.
65. Keen-Rhinehart E, Kalra SP, Kalra PS. AAV mediated leptin receptor installation improves energy balance and the reproductive status of obese female Koletsky rats. Peptides. 2005;26:2567–78.
66. Park JY, Chong AY, Cochran EK, Haller MJ, Schatz DA, Gordon P. Type 1diabetes associated with acquired generalized lipodystrophy and insulin resistance: the effects of long-term leptin therapy. J Clin Endocrinol Metab. 2008;93:26–31.
67. Toyoshima Y, Gavrilova O, Yakar S, Jou W, Pack S, Asghar Z, et al. Leptin improves insulin resistance and hyperglycemia in a mouse model of type 2 diabetes. Endocrinology. 2005;146:4024–35.
68. Masuzaki H, Ogawa Y, Aizawa-Abe M, Hosoda K, Suga J, Ebihara K, et al. Glucose metabolism and leptin with lethal yellow agouti mutation: usefulness of leptin for the treatment of obesity-associated diabetes. Diabetes. 1999;48:1613–22.
69. Boghossian S, Ueno N, Dube MG, Kalra P, Kalra S. Leptin gene transfer in the hypothalamus enhances longevity in adult monogenic mutant mice in the absence of circulating leptin. Neurobiol Aging. 2007; 28:1594–604.
70. Murphy JE, Zhou S, Giese K, Williams LT, Escobedo JA, Dwarki VJ. Long-term correction of obesity and diabetes in genetically obese mice by a single intramuscular injection of recombinant adeno-associated virus encoding mouse leptin. Proc Natl Acad Sci U S A. 1997;94:13921–6.
71. Muzzin P, Eisensmith RC, Copeland KC, Woo SL. Correction of obesity and diabetes in genetically obese mice by leptin gene therapy. Proc Natl Acad Sci U S A. 1996;93:14804–8.
72. Ogawa Y, Masuzaki H, Hosoda K, Aizawa-Abe M, Suga J, Suda M, et al. Increased glucose metabolism and insulin sensitivity in transgenic skinny mice overexpressing leptin. Diabetes. 1999;48:1822–9.
73. Farooqi IS, O'Rahilly S. Monogenic obesity in humans. Ann Rev Med. 2005;56:443–58.
74. Cummings PB, Bettaleb A, Graham JL, Stanhope KL, Dill R, Morton JL, et al. Subcutaneous administration of leptin normalizes fasting plasma glucose in obese type 2 diabetics UCD-T2DM rats. PNAS. 2011;108: 14670–5.
75. Naito M, Fujikura J, Ebihara K, Miyanaga I, Yokoi H, Kusakabe T, et al. Therapeutic impact of leptin on diabetes, diabetic complications and longevity in insulin deficient diabetic mice. Diabetes. 2011;60(9):2265–73.
76. Bagnasco M, Dube MG, Kalra PS, Kalra SP. Evidence for the existence of distinct central appetite and energy expenditure pathways and stimulation of ghrelin as revealed by hypothalamic site-specific leptin gene therapy. Endocrinology. 2002;143:4409–21.

77. Hidaka S, Yoshimatsu H, Kondou S, Oka K, Tsuruta Y, Sakino H, et al. Hypoleptinemia, but not hypoinsulinemia, induces hyperphagia in streptozotocin-induced diabetic rats. J Neurochem. 2001;77: 993–1000.
78. Hidaka S, Yoshimatsu H, Kondou S, Tsuruta Y, Oka K, Noguchi H, et al. Chronic central leptin infusion restores hyperglycemia independent of food intake and insulin level in streptozotocin-induced diabetic rats. FASEB J. 2002;16:509–18.
79. Oral EA, Simha V, Ruiz E, Andewelt A, Premkumar A, Snell P, et al. Leptin-replacement therapy for lipodystrophy. N Engl J Med. 2002;346:570–8.
80. Lin CY, Higginbotham DA, Judd RL, White BD. Central leptin increases insulin sensitivity in streptozotocin-induced diabetic rats. Am J Physiol Endocrinol Metab. 2002;282:E1084–91.
81. Shi ZQ, Nelson A, Whitcomb L, Wang J, Cohen AM. Intracerebroventicular administration of leptin markedly enhances insulin sensitivity and systemic glucose utilization in conscious rats. Metabolism. 1998;47:1274–80.
82. Wang JL, Chinookoswong N, Scully S, Qi M, Shi ZQ. Differential effects of leptin in regulation of tissue glucose utilization in vivo. Endocrinology. 1999;140:2117–24.
83. Ebihara K, Kusakabe T, Hirata M, et al. Efficacy and safety of leptin-replacement therapy and posible mechanisms of leptin actions in patients with generalizad lipodystrophy. J Clin Endocrinol Metab. 2007;92:532–41.
84. Heymsfield SB, Greenberg AS, Fujioka K, et al. Recombinant leptin for weight loss in obese and lean adults: a randomized, controlled, dose-escalation trial. JAMA. 1999;282:1568–75.
85. Scully T. Diabetes in numbers. Nature. 2012;485: S2–376.
86. Kastin AJ, Pan W. Intranasal leptin: blood-brain barrier bypass (BBBB) for obesity? Endocrinology. 2006;147:2086–7.
87. Chapman CD, Frey II WH, Craft S, Danielyan L, Hallschmid M, Schoth H, et al. Intranasal treatment of central nervous system dysfunction in human. Pharm Res. 2013;30:2475–84.
88. Harmon BT, Aly AE, Padegimas L, Sesenogulu-Laird O, Cooper MJ, Waszczak BL. Intranasal administration of plasmid DNA nanoparticles yields successful transfection and expression of a reporter protein in the rat brain. Gene Therapy. 2014;21:514–21.

Novel Combinatorial Therapies Involving Leptin: Opportunities for Mechanistic Advances and Therapeutic Translation in Human Diseases

21

Timo D. Müller, Christoffer Clemmensen, Brian Finan, Richard D. DiMarchi, and Matthias H. Tschöp

Introduction

The prevalence of global obesity has reached epidemic proportions with excess weight being a causal factor associated with the accelerated development of various chronic diseases, such as diabetes, cardiovascular diseases, and certain types of cancer [1]. The World Health Organization (WHO) estimates that in 2035, approximately 300 million people will be obese [2] and in the United States alone, it is estimated that each year more than a quarter of a million adults die prematurely due to the consequences of obesity [3]. In light of the growing socioeconomic burden of obesity and diabetes, the development of new treatment options to safely and efficiently combat this epidemic of "diabesity" is a global priority. Apart from bariatric surgery, which is expensive, mostly irreversible and not without risk, clinical approaches to tackle obesity have been disappointing overall. To this end, selected groups of weight lowering drugs have been commercialized over the last few decades. Nearly all of them were withdrawn after a short time due to limited efficacy and/or unacceptable adverse effects [4]. However, whereas the history of anti-obesity drugs is filled with disappointments, hope remains for recent advances in the development of novel combination therapies. Such poly-pharmacotherapy can constitute adjunctive administration of several hormones, each possessing beneficial effects on body weight and/or glycemic control, or the administration of single molecules engineered to simultaneously target multiple receptors. The approach to combine pharmacology in a single molecule of sustained action and improved pharmacokinetics rests upon the idea that simultaneous targeting of multiple signaling mechanisms improves overall metabolism beyond what is achieved with single molecule treatment alone. The ultimate goal is to administer low drug concentrations that sustainably maximize the metabolic benefits while minimizing adverse effects [5]. In an ideal case, such poly-pharmacotherapy would enhance metabolism in a synergistic manner, providing efficacy and safety greater than the sum of the effects possible by the respective monotherapies. The aim of this chapter is to summarize recent advances in preclinical and clinical approaches to combat obesity and diabetes by either adjunctive

T.D. Müller, Ph.D. • C. Clemmensen, Ph.D.
B. Finan, Ph.D. • M.H. Tschöp, M.D. (✉)
Institute for Diabetes and Obesity, Helmholtz Zentrum München and Department of Medicine, Technische Universität München, Munich, Germany
e-mail: timo.mueller@helmholtz-muenchen.de

R.D. DiMarchi, Ph.D.
Department of Chemistry, Indiana University, Bloomington, IN, USA

S. Dagogo-Jack (ed.), *Leptin: Regulation and Clinical Applications*,
DOI 10.1007/978-3-319-09915-6_21, © Springer International Publishing Switzerland 2015

administration of several hormones, or by using unimolecular co-agonists, with a special emphasis on leptin.

Adjunctive Administration of Two Hormones

When used as monotherapy, most hormones have only limited efficacy to improve metabolism in common forms of obesity, which is mainly lifestyle/dietary-induced and does not result from rare single gene mutations. Increasing the dose of a single hormone therapy can improve the metabolic efficacy but is often hampered by enhanced incidence of adverse effects [6]. Therefore adjunctive administration of more than one drug is an intuitively promising alternative to more safely improve systems metabolism beyond what can be achieved with monotherapies.

The strategy to coadminister two hormones is not completely novel and was already popularly practiced by physicians in the 1980s with prescription of Fen-Phen, the combination of fenfluramine and phentermine [7]. However, in 1996 fenfluramine was withdrawn from clinical practice because of fatal pulmonary hypertension [8, 9] and an increased risk for valvular heart disease [10]. Phentermine, however, remains available as monotherapy in many countries, including the United States and in 2012, the U.S. Food and Drug Administration (FDA) approved the use of Qsymia® (Vivus Inc., California), a combination of phentermine and topiramate, as an addition to diet and exercise for weight management. Depending on the dose, weight-loss attributed to treatment with Qsymia® is between 8.1 and 10.9 % relative to 1.4–1.8 % in placebo-treated controls. The weight loss is accompanied by improvements in lipid, cholesterol, and glucose metabolism [11].

The Use of Leptin as a Stand-Alone Therapy for Obesity

The discovery of leptin in 1994 [12] has pioneered our understanding of how peripheral signals, that rise or fall in response to fuel availability, integrate in a complex central network that controls systemic metabolism [13]. To this end, 20 years of leptin research has revealed that leptin modulates energy metabolism via central regulation of food intake and energy expenditure [13]. We have also witnessed how leptin is involved in regulating diverse biological functions including the immune system, endocrine systems, reproduction (see Chap. 13), glucose homeostasis (see Chap. 7), hematopoiesis, angiogenesis, and inflammation (see Chap. 11). The discovery of leptin has furthermore not only revolutionized our view about the adipose tissue as an endocrine organ, it has also paved the way for a better understanding and targeting of lipid metabolism in general [14].

Shortly, after leptin was discovered by positional cloning of the mouse *ob* gene [12] several studies reported that leptin replacement corrects the obesity of leptin-deficient ob/ob mice [15–17]. Beyond the early notion that leptin promotes it's biological action through central neuronal networks [16], these early studies also noted that leptin supplementation potently improves insulin sensitivity in leptin deficient mice, remarkably even prior to leptin induced weight loss [15, 18]. Together, these findings created much excitement for leptin as the pharmacological "silver bullet" to correct imbalances associated with the metabolic syndrome. Indeed, it is nowadays solidly confirmed that leptin replacement therapy corrects obesity and insulin resistance in individuals with endogenous deficiency of leptin, as occurs in ob/ob mice [15–17], in congenitally leptin-deficient humans [19–22] and in individuals with lipodystrophy [23–27]. Unfortunately, however leptin has little to no anorectic or glycemic effect under conditions where endogenous leptin levels are elevated, which represents the vast majority of diet-induced human obesity [28, 29].

The inability of leptin to promote weight loss in conditions of common obesity has eliminated its pharmacological use as a stand-alone therapy. Accordingly, administration of further enhanced doses of leptin or analogs of sustained pharmacokinetics failed to promote weight loss in common forms of human obesity [29–31]. Failure to respond to the anorectic action of the hormone is generally referred to as leptin-resistance (as reviewed in [32]). The mechanisms leading to leptin-resistance are complex and might include impaired transport of leptin across the blood-brain barrier (BBB) [33, 34], impaired leptin signaling in first-order CNS neurons [35–37], or impaired leptin signaling in downstream second-order neurocircuits (as reviewed in [38]). The hypothalamic arcuate nucleus (ARC) seems to serve a major role in the development of leptin resistance, as exposure of mice to a high-fat diet (HFD) rapidly decreases phosphorylation of signal transducer and activator of transcription 3 (P-STAT3) in the ARC, while leptin-sensitivity is simultaneously maintained in other hypothalamic and extrahypothalamic nuclei [35]. Whereas the cellular mechanisms leading to leptin-resistance are still an area of intense scientific investigation (see also Chap. 6) there is growing evidence indicating that dietary macronutrients, especially fat and sugar are detrimental to leptin-sensitivity and impose leptin-resistance before the onset of obesity and hyperleptinemia [39–42]. Impaired levels of P-STAT3 in the ARC are accordingly observed as early as after 6 days of HFD exposure [35] and even short-term overfeeding of otherwise normal weight rats rapidly induces leptin-resistance and imbalances in glycemic control [42]. Consistent with these observations, leptin therapy does not prevent the development of obesity when lean mice are switched to a high-fat, high-sugar diet at the beginning of leptin therapy (Fig. 21.1), and long-term exposure of mice to HFD decreases POMC immunoreactivity in the hypothalamus [43]. In summary, these data indicate that leptin has only limited potential as a stand-alone therapy under conditions where endogenous leptin levels are elevated. Furthermore, dietary fat and sugar contribute to the development of leptin-resistance and thus constitute a major impediment for the development of leptin-based pharmacotherapies.

The Use of Leptin in Combination Therapies

Adjunctive administration of leptin with therapy that might unlock the beneficial pharmacology that endogenously resides in leptin, but remains suppressed in common obesity constitutes a promising approach to successfully address the "diabesity" epidemic. In an ideal case, such pharmacotherapy would safely and sustainably unleash leptin pharmacology as a supplement to lifestyle change and diet modification.

The Combination of Leptin and Metformin

Metformin is a drug reported to modestly improve leptin-sensitivity under conditions of common obesity [44]. Metformin promotes body weight loss

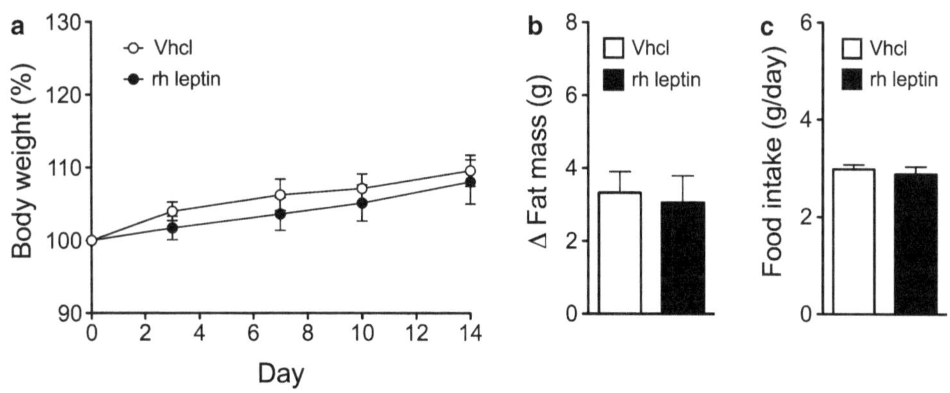

Fig. 21.1 Leptin therapy does not prevent the development of diet-induced obesity in mice. Effect of daily administration of vehicle (PBS) or human recombinant (rh) leptin (1 mg/kg/day) on body weight (**a**), fat mass (**b**) and food intake (**c**) of lean 15 weeks old chow-fed C57BL/6J mice that were switched to HFD (56 % kcal fat, Research Diets, New Brunswick, USA) at study day 0. $N=8$ mice each group. Data represent means ± SEM

while improving glycemic control via enhanced insulin-stimulated glucose uptake in skeletal muscle and adipose tissue with inhibition of hepatic gluconeogenesis [45, 46]. The mechanism of how metformin promotes weight loss is not exactly clear, yet it's ability to improve body weight and glucose metabolism under conditions of common obesity has been shown in a series of clinical studies [47–53]. Several studies suggest that metformin's effects on systems metabolism are, at least in part, mediated via leptin signaling. Accordingly, metformin decreases hyperleptinemia in morbidly obese individuals [47, 48], an effect seemingly independent of metformin's effect on body weight [54]. Furthermore, metformin stimulates leptin receptor expression in the ARC [55] and treatment of obese rats with metformin increases levels of P-STAT3 in the hypothalamus while decreasing expression of neuropeptide Y (NPY) and agouti-related protein (AgRP) [56]. Interestingly, 4-weeks pretreatment of leptin-resistant DIO rats with metformin restored the anorectic effect of intracerebroventricular (icv) leptin infusion and 2-day treatment of rats with metformin enhanced the acute central effect of leptin on 24 h food intake and phosphorylation of STAT3 in the hypothalamus [44]. In summary, these data indicate that leptin-sensitivity can be enhanced using pharmacology and constitute a valuable adjunct to other weight lowering agents.

The Combination of Leptin and Amylin

Amylin (a.k.a. islet amyloid polypeptide; IAPP) is co-secreted with insulin from the pancreatic β-cells. Like insulin, plasma levels of amylin increase in response to ingested nutrients (especially glucose) and subsequently decrease upon fasting [57, 58]. In line with the β-cells being the primary source of amylin secretion, the increase of amylin in response to a meal is impaired in individuals with type 2 diabetes and is absent in individuals with type 1 diabetes (reviewed in [59]). Plasma concentrations of amylin are higher in obese compared to lean individuals [60, 61] and subsequently decrease upon weight loss [61, 62]. In the gastrointestinal tract amylin delays gastric emptying, decreases gastric acid secretion, and inhibits glucagon secretion from the pancreatic α-cells (as reviewed in [63]). When injected in either the brain or the periphery, amylin dose-dependently decreases food intake due to a reduction in meal size [64, 65]. Amylin seems to promote its anorectic action via the area postrema (AP), as administration of amylin into the AP decreases food intake whereas selective blockade of amylin in the AP has the opposite effect. Peripheral administration of amylin further increases c-fos immunoreactivity in the AP whereas lesions of the AP abolish amylin's effect on food intake and adiposity [66–69]. Due to its beneficial effects on energy and glucose metabolism, amylin has gained much attention for its pharmacological use to treat obesity and diabetes. Accordingly, in 2005, the FDA approved pramlintide (trade name Symlin®; Amylin Pharmaceuticals Inc., San Diego, USA), a synthetic amylin receptor agonist, for the treatment of type 1 and type 2 diabetes. The mechanisms of how amylin affects systems metabolism are complex and remain an area of intense scientific investigation. However, amylin was shown to restore leptin-sensitivity in DIO rats and when combined with leptin synergistically lowered body weight relative to treatment with the respective monotherapies alone [70–72]. Directionally similar results were observed in calorie-restricted overweight/-obese humans that were treated with the combination of pramlintide and recombinant methionyl human leptin (a.k.a. metreleptin) [70, 72, 73]. In a 24-week, randomized, double blind trial, treatment of overweight/obese individuals with a combination of pramlintide/metreleptin and a 40 % calorie-reduced diet led to greater body weight loss (−12.7 ± 0.9 %) relative to treatment with pramlintide (−8.4 ± 0.9 %) or metreleptin (−8.2 ± 1.3 %;) alone [73]. Notably, in DIO rats, leptin had no effect on body weight when administered to animals that were pair-fed to the amylin-treated group [70], thus indicating that the pharmacology of amylin rather than the weight loss in general accounts for the observed restoration of leptin sensitivity. The weight loss induced by the amylin/leptin combination seems to be fat-specific [71, 72, 74] and attributable to a direct effect of amylin on leptin signaling. Accordingly, mice that lack amylin show decreased expression of the leptin receptor in the hypothalamus and impaired leptin stimulated levels of P-STAT3 in the ARC and in the ventromedial hypothalamus (VMH) [75]. In line with this finding, amylin potentiates leptin-stimulated phosphorylation of STAT3 in the ARC of lean rats [75] and in the VMH of DIO rats [72]. Pramlintide/metreleptin was generally well tolerated and no major adverse effects were reported in the clinical studies [59, 70, 72, 73]. Surprisingly, however, Amylin Inc. recently announced in a press release that the development of a pramlintide/metreleptin combination therapy has been stopped due to potential safety concerns. Whether this relates to the reported instances of anti-leptin antibodies in a subset of the patients remains speculative. The potential of amylin/leptin to improve leptin-sensitivity spurred scientific interest in combining leptin with other weight lowering agents. Positive results, albeit with additive rather than synergistic effects, were already reported by Amylin Inc. with the combination of leptin with peptide YY (PYY_{3-36}) and the GLP-1 analog AC3174 [70]. Whereas the data provided by Amylin Inc. are encouraging, it is noteworthy that only a moderate HFD (32 % kcal from fat) was used in the rodent studies [70, 71]. Likewise, the clinical studies used the combination of pramlintide/metreleptin along with a 40 % calorie-reduced diet [70, 73]. As dietary macronutrients play an important role in the development of leptin-resistance [39–42] it would be interesting to determine how this polypharmacy affects metabolism under exposure to a more pathological HFD.

The Combination of Leptin with Exendin4 or FGF21

Encouraged by the observation that leptin resistance can be reversed by pharmacology, several subsequent studies assessed whether leptin responsiveness can also be restored by weight lowering agents independent of amylin signaling. Treatment of DIO mice with the GLP-1 analog exendin-4, which were switched from HFD to a chow diet at treatment initiation, restores leptin sensitivity after an initial weight loss of approximately 25 % [76]. Accordingly, the combination of exendin-4 with an optimized pegylated (PEG) leptin analog of sustained action and improved pharmacokinetics synergistically enhances weight loss, decreases food intake, and improves glucose tolerance beyond what can be achieved with the respective monotherapies alone. PEG-leptin monotherapy following the combination therapy was sufficient to maintain a lower body weight, in line with restored leptin responsiveness [76]. Notably, treatment of DIO mice with fibroblast growth factor 21 (FGF21) likewise restores leptin sensitivity after an initial weight loss identical to what has been observed for exendin-4. Using either combination, weight loss was enhanced compared with either exendin-4 or FGF21 monotherapy, and leptin monotherapy without prior combination therapy had no effect on body weight and glycemic control relative to saline-treated controls [76]. Notably, and in line with the amylin/leptin combination, leptin monotherapy proved ineffective when identical weight loss was induced over a comparable time by caloric restriction alone, thus indicating that restoration of leptin-sensitivity requires pharmacotherapy, but is not directly attributable to weight loss or a unique signaling mechanism. Supportive of this finding, treatment of DIO mice with exendin-4 decreased immunoreactivity of agouti-related protein (AgRP) in the ARC, an effect that was not seen in DIO mice that were calorie-restricted to match the body weight of the exendin-4-treated group [76]. In summary, these data indicate that leptin-resistance can be reversed by pharmacology but also indicate that restoration of leptin responsiveness does not appear to be restricted to a unique signaling pathway. Of appreciable note, restoration of leptin-sensitivity using either amylin, PYY_{3-36}, exendin4, or FGF21 were only shown in the presence of a moderately low content of dietary lipids [70, 76]. In fact, the combination of leptin with exendin-4 or FGF21 had no greater effect than the respective monotherapies when DIO mice were continued on a high-fat, high-sugar diet comprising 58 % kcal fat [76], emphasizing once again that dietary fat and sugar are detrimental to leptin-sensitivity.

Unimolecular Co-agonists for the Treatment of the Metabolic Syndrome

GLP-1/Glucagon Co-agonism Reverses the Metabolic Syndrome in DIO Mice

The gastrointestinal peptide hormone GLP-1 acts directly on the pancreas to enhance glucose-stimulated insulin secretion [77–79] and to inhibit the release of glucagon [80]. Beyond this insulinotropic effect, GLP-1 increases β-cell proliferation, and β-cell mass in rodents [81–87], enhances insulin sensitivity in skeletal muscle [88–90], inhibits hepatic gluconeogenesis [91–95] and promotes body weight loss through inhibition of food intake and by slowing down gastric emptying [96]. Collectively, this renders GLP-1 a uniquely attractive option for treatment of the metabolic syndrome. As of today, several dipeptidyl peptidase-IV (DPP-IV) resistant GLP-1 analogs, such as exenatide (Byetta®; Eli Lilly & Co, USA) and liraglutide (Victoza®; Novo Nordisk, Denmark) are approved by the FDA for the treatment of diabetes. The efficacy of these GLP-1 analogs to improve systems metabolism has been shown in numerous preclinical and clinical studies (as reviewed in [97]). However, GLP-1 action confers dose-dependent adverse effects, most prominently nausea and vomiting [6], which limits the maximal pharmacological potential of such drugs.

A major breakthrough in the development of novel anti-obesity, anti-diabetic polypharmacotherapies was the development of single peptides with balanced co-agonism at the glucagon and GLP-1 receptors [98, 99]. The counterintuitive recruitment of glucagon agonism in combination with GLP-1 agonism has transformed the perspective use of a hormone where its antagonism was broadly pursued. These GLP-1/glucagon co-agonists combined the glycemic and anorectic effects of GLP-1 with the lipolytic and thermogenic properties of glucagon in single molecules of sustained action, with improved pharmacokinetics as compared to the native peptides. Accordingly, single subcutaneous treatment of persistently HFD-exposed DIO mice with 70 nmol/kg of a 40k pegylated GLP-1/glucagon co-agonist (Aib2 C24 lactam 40k) decreased body weight within 7 days by 25.8 %, while body weight was notably unaffected in saline-treated controls [98]. The name "Aib2 C24 lactam 40k" indicates that an aminoisobutyric acid (Aib) at position two protects from DPP-IV cleavage, and a lactam bridge is used to stabilize the secondary structure, with the cysteine residue 24 (C24) conjugated to a linear 40k polyethylene glycol (PEG) to prolonged in vivo action. The weight loss induced by this nearly-balanced GLP-1/glucagon co-agonist was primarily the result of decreased body fat mass and was accompanied by decreased food intake. In a subsequent study, once-weekly treatment of DIO mice with 70 nmol/kg of this co-agonist reversed diet-induced obesity and hepatosteatosis, and normalized glycemic control within only 4 weeks of treatment [98]. In line with glucagon's lipolytic and thermogenic effects, weight loss induced by the co-agonist was reflected by enhanced energy expenditure and increased lipolysis, as indicated by increased phosphorylation of hormone sensitive lipase (P-HSL) in the white adipose tissue. Albeit with lower potency, the co-agonist further lowered body weight and body fat mass in GLP-1R-deficient DIO mice, thus emphasizing the role of glucagon in the metabolic benefits achieved by this co-agonist [98]. Subsequent preclinical and clinical studies are currently evaluating the mechanistic underpinnings as well as the translational value and safety of these molecules. More mechanistic data on e.g. post-receptor signaling and clearance will further help to fully appreciate the therapeutic potential of these molecules.

Restoration of Leptin Responsiveness by GLP-1/Glucagon Co-agonism

The mechanistic underpinnings underlying the synergistic efficacy derived from the GLP-1/glucagon co-agonist remain an object of intense scientific investigation. However, a recent study that used the exact same GLP-1/glucagon co-agonist showed that this peptide restores leptin-sensitivity in otherwise leptin-resistant DIO mice [100]. Accordingly, treatment of DIO mice with a combination of PEG-leptin and the GLP-1/glucagon co-agonist resulted in greater weight loss, decreased food intake, improved glucose and lipid metabolism as compared to treatment with PEG-leptin or the GLP-1/glucagon co-agonist alone [100]. It is noteworthy that the GLP-1/glucagon co-agonist restored leptin action in DIO mice after an initial body weight loss similar to what has been reported for exendin-4 or FGF21 [76, 100]. However, in contrast to exendin-4 and FGF21, the GLP-1/glucagon co-agonist restored leptin-sensitivity under chronic exposure to an extremely high-fat, high-sugar diet (58 % kcal from fat). Under similar dietary management exendin-4 and fibroblast growth factor 21 (FGF21) failed to improve leptin-sensitivity and combinations such as amylin/leptin have yet to be tested [76].

Unimolecular Co-agonists at the Receptors for GLP-1 and GIP

The strategy to combine the pharmacology of several hormones into a single molecule of optimized pharmacokinetics was recently extended to lead to the discovery of an unimolecular dual incretin co-agonist with balanced agonism at the receptors for GLP-1 and the glucose-dependent insulinotropic polypeptide (GIP) [101]. This "twincretin" potently reversed several hallmarks of the metabolic syndrome, such as obesity, hyperglycemia, and dyslipidemia, through synergistic pharmacology in rodent models of common obesity, insulin resistance, and type 2 diabetes, such as DIO mice, db/db mice, and ZDF rats. The balanced GLP-1/GIP co-agonist improved glycemic control through a potent effect on glucose-stimulated insulin secretion and this enhanced insulinotropic efficacy translated from rodent models of obesity and diabetes to both nonhuman primates and humans [101]. The observations put to rest a long-standing controversy regarding the wisdom of GIP agonism relative to antagonism. Accordingly, treatment of healthy nondiabetic human subjects with this balanced GLP-1/GIP co-agonist reduced blood glucose excursion through potentiation of glucose-stimulated insulin secretion. Of particular note, and in contrast to exendin-4 was the absence of any effect on gut motility leading to gastric discomfort, as assessed my acetaminophen absorption [101]. Improved glycemic control was also observed in a subsequent clinical study, in which type 2 diabetic individuals were treated for 6 weeks with escalating doses of the GLP-1/GIP co-agonist. In this study, the GLP-1/GIP co-agonist dose-dependently decreased plasma levels of glycosylated hemoglobin A_{1c} (HbA_{1c}) in the range of −0.53 to −1.11 % relative to −0.16 % in placebo-treated controls [101]. Notably, no major adverse effects were reported from the clinical studies.

Targeted Delivery of Nuclear Hormones

Hormones acting via nuclear receptors, such as glucocorticoids, thyroid hormone, and testosterone are implicated in a myriad of key metabolic functions, such as the regulation of the hypothalamic-pituitary-gonadal (HPG) and adrenal (HPA) axis, thermogenesis, and inflammation [102, 103]. Several of these nuclear hormones have beneficial effects on glucose and lipid metabolism [102], such as e.g. estrogen, which acts on hypothalamic neurocircuits to inhibit food intake and to increase energy expenditure [104–107]. In mice, estrogen further protects from HFD-induced glucose intolerance and insulin resistance [108] and several previous studies have highlighted the potential of estrogen receptor agonists to treat obesity and diabetes [109, 110]. However, the oncogenic potential and gynecological action of estrogen limits its pharmacological use in weight management. Aiming to make estrogen therapeutically more viable, unimolecular biomolecules were generated, which covalently linked estrogen to the peptide carrier GLP-1 using either an ether bond or an aromatic ester [111]. The resulting conjugates varied in linkage biostability, which renders the more stable ether-linked estrogen to be targeted only to cells in which there is GLP-1R-mediated uptake. The unstable ester-linked conjugate readily decomposes to active peptide and free estrogen in circulating blood leading to nontargeted estrogen therapy [111]. Treatment of DIO mice for 14 days with escalating doses of these conjugates showed a more profound effect of the stable conjugate to reverse several acute hallmarks of the metabolic syndrome, such as obesity, insulin resistance, and abnormalities in cholesterol and lipid metabolism [111]. In contrast to the labile conjugate, the stable conjugate also showed no off-target effects in GLP-1R negative tissues. The off-target effects were assessed by uterine weight, as well as estrogen-dependent tumor growth in MCF-7 xenograft mice. Whereas subcutaneous treatment of ovarectomized lean mice for 7 days revealed a strong uterotrophic effect of the labile conjugate but even at doses tenfold greater than the maximally effective dose for weight lowering. There was no apparent difference in uterus weight between the GLP-1-treated negative controls and mice treated with the stable estrogen conjugate. Notably, neither GLP-1 nor the stable conjugate were able to induce weight loss in mice with CNS-specific GLP-1R deletion, demonstrating that the metabolic benefits of the stable conjugate are mediated by GLP-1R signaling in the CNS. Consistent with a primarily CNS-mediated mode of action, the stable conjugate increased expression of proopiomelanocortin (POMC) and the leptin receptor in the ARC to a greater extent as compared to treatment with GLP-1 or estrogen alone. Together these findings suggest that GLP-1-mediated estrogen delivery promotes its beneficial effects on systemic metabolism through the hypothalamic melanocortinergic system [111]. Whereas the preclinical data overall show no gynecological or mitogenic effect of the stabile conjugate in GLP-1R negative tissues, long-term toxicology studies are clearly warranted to assess the oncogenic potential of this conjugate in tissues that express the GLP-1 receptor. More importantly, this strategy of using macromolecules to target conventional small molecule drugs for purposes of enhanced therapeutic outcome with greater safety should extend to other peptides and nuclear hormones. It clearly warrants further clarification whether and to what extent these studies translate to humans, and whether they can safely induce sustained efficacy in large study cohorts and over a sustained time period.

Conclusion

The global epidemic of diabetes and obesity challenges us to rapidly identify an effective approach to address primary disease and the subsequent chronic outcomes associated with elevated body weight and blood glucose. The emergence of individual hormones such as GLP-1, leptin, and FGF-21 to name just a few hold appreciable promise, but have proven limited in their individual ability to correct excess body weight. A new class of tailored biomolecules has emerged that offer unique efficacy and safety relative to traditional monoagonists. In certain instances such as GLP-1/GIP co-agonist the combination appears physiologically logically given the combined action of these two independent incretins to improve systems metabolism. In other examples the combination is counterintuitive such as the recruitment of glucagon as a therapeutic agonist in combination with GLP-1 agonism, where for decades the focus for this same therapeutic application has been on glucagon antagonism. Finally, the combination of a targeting peptide with a hormone such as estrogen might provide access to selective nuclear hormones that have proven so elusive for conventional small molecule medicinal chemistry. These molecules emphasize the principle that new highly active peptides that simultaneously target multiple signaling pathways can be designed to safely and efficiently improve systemic metabolism, paving the way for a new era in obesity and diabetes research. Without doubt, extension of these principles to include additional endocrine factors implicated in systems metabolism as well as transfer of these strategies to other diseases, such as cancer, cachexia, or cardiovascular diseases, might lead to an enormous boom in the development of novel future pharmacotherapies.

References

1. Ebbeling CB, Pawlak DB, Ludwig DS. Childhood obesity: public-health crisis, common sense cure. Lancet. 2002;360(9331):473–82. PubMed PMID: 12241736. Epub 2002/09/21. eng.
2. Organization WH. Obesity: preventing and managing the global epidemic. Report of a WHO consultation on obesity 1997 June 3–5;Geneva, Switzerland. Publication WHO/NUT/NCD/98.1.
3. Allison DB, Fontaine KR, Manson JE, Stevens J, VanItallie TB. Annual deaths attributable to obesity in the United States. JAMA. 1999;282(16):1530–8. PubMed PMID: 10546692. Epub 1999/11/05. eng.
4. Rodgers RJ, Tschop MH, Wilding JP. Anti-obesity drugs: past, present and future. Dis Model Mech. 2012;5(5):621–6. PubMed PMID: 22915024. Pubmed Central PMCID: 3424459. Epub 2012/08/24. eng.
5. Tschop MH, DiMarchi RD. Outstanding Scientific Achievement Award Lecture 2011: defeating diabesity: the case for personalized combinatorial therapies. Diabetes. 2012;61(6):1309–14. PubMed PMID: 22618765. Pubmed Central PMCID: 3357302. Epub 2012/05/24. eng.
6. Marino AB, Cole SW, Nuzum DS. Alternative dosing strategies for liraglutide in patients with type 2 diabetes mellitus. Am J Health-Syst Pharm AJHP. 2014;71(3):223–6. PubMed PMID: 24429016. Epub 2014/01/17. eng.
7. Weintraub M, Hasday JD, Mushlin AI, Lockwood DH. A double-blind clinical trial in weight control. Use of fenfluramine and phentermine alone and in combination. Arch Intern Med. 1984;144(6):1143–8. PubMed PMID: 6375610. Epub 1984/06/01. eng.
8. Voelkel NF, Clarke WR, Higenbottam T. Obesity, dexfenfluramine, and pulmonary hypertension. A lesson not learned? Am J Resp Crit Care Med. 1997; 155(3):786–8.
9. Fishman AP. Appetite-suppressant drugs and primary pulmonary hypertension. N Engl J Med. 1997;336(7):511. PubMed PMID: 9019650. Author reply 2–3. Epub 1997/02/13. eng.
10. Connolly HM, Crary JL, McGoon MD, Hensrud DD, Edwards BS, Edwards WD, et al. Valvular heart disease associated with fenfluramine-phentermine. N Engl J Med. 1997;337(9):581–8. PubMed PMID: 9271479. Epub 1997/08/28. eng.
11. Kiortsis DN. A review of the metabolic effects of controlled-release Phentermine/Topiramate. Hormones (Athens). 2013;12(4):507–16. PubMed PMID: 24457398. Epub 2014/01/25. eng.
12. Zhang Y, Proenca R, Maffei M, Barone M, Leopold L, Friedman JM. Positional cloning of the mouse obese gene and its human homologue. Nature. 1994;372(6505):425–32. PubMed PMID: 7984236. Epub 1994/12/01. eng.
13. Schwartz MW, Woods SC, Porte Jr D, Seeley RJ, Baskin DG. Central nervous system control of food intake. Nature. 2000;404(6778):661–71. PubMed PMID: 10766253. Epub 2000/04/15. eng.
14. Rosen ED, Spiegelman BM. What we talk about when we talk about fat. Cell. 2014;156(1–2):20–44. PubMed PMID: 24439368. Pubmed Central PMCID: 3934003. Epub 2014/01/21. eng.
15. Pelleymounter MA, Cullen MJ, Baker MB, Hecht R, Winters D, Boone T, et al. Effects of the obese gene product on body weight regulation in ob/ob mice. Science. 1995;269(5223):540–3. PubMed PMID: 7624776. Epub 1995/07/28. eng.
16. Campfield LA, Smith FJ, Guisez Y, Devos R, Burn P. Recombinant mouse OB protein: evidence for a peripheral signal linking adiposity and central neural networks. Science. 1995;269(5223):546–9. PubMed PMID: 7624778. Epub 1995/07/28. eng.
17. Halaas JL, Gajiwala KS, Maffei M, Cohen SL, Chait BT, Rabinowitz D, et al. Weight-reducing effects of the plasma protein encoded by the obese gene. Science. 1995;269(5223):543–6. PubMed PMID: 7624777. Epub 1995/07/28. eng.
18. Hedbacker K, Birsoy K, Wysocki RW, Asilmaz E, Ahima RS, Farooqi IS, et al. Antidiabetic effects of IGFBP2, a leptin-regulated gene. Cell Metab. 2010;11(1):11–22. PubMed PMID: 20074524. Epub 2010/01/16. eng.
19. Licinio J, Caglayan S, Ozata M, Yildiz BO, de Miranda PB, O'Kirwan F, et al. Phenotypic effects of leptin replacement on morbid obesity, diabetes mellitus, hypogonadism, and behavior in leptin-deficient adults. Proc Natl Acad Sci U S A. 2004;101(13):4531–6. PubMed PMID: 15070752. Pubmed Central PMCID: 384781. Epub 2004/04/09. eng.
20. Farooqi IS, Matarese G, Lord GM, Keogh JM, Lawrence E, Agwu C, et al. Beneficial effects of leptin on obesity, T cell hyporesponsiveness, and neuroendocrine/metabolic dysfunction of human congenital leptin deficiency. J Clin Invest. 2002;110(8):1093–103. PubMed PMID: 12393845. Pubmed Central PMCID: 150795. Epub 2002/10/24. eng.
21. Farooqi IS, Jebb SA, Langmack G, Lawrence E, Cheetham CH, Prentice AM, et al. Effects of recombinant leptin therapy in a child with congenital leptin deficiency. N Engl J Med. 1999;341(12):879–84. PubMed PMID: 10486419. Epub 1999/09/16. eng.
22. Montague CT, Farooqi IS, Whitehead JP, Soos MA, Rau H, Wareham NJ, et al. Congenital leptin deficiency is associated with severe early-onset obesity in humans. Nature. 1997;387(6636):903–8. PubMed PMID: 9202122. Epub 1997/06/26. eng.
23. Chong AY, Lupsa BC, Cochran EK, Gorden P. Efficacy of leptin therapy in the different forms of human lipodystrophy. Diabetologia. 2010;53(1):

27–35. PubMed PMID: 19727665. Epub 2009/09/04. eng.

24. Ebihara K, Kusakabe T, Hirata M, Masuzaki H, Miyanaga F, Kobayashi N, et al. Efficacy and safety of leptin-replacement therapy and possible mechanisms of leptin actions in patients with generalized lipodystrophy. J Clin Endocrinol Metab. 2007; 92(2):532–41. PubMed PMID: 17118991. Epub 2006/11/23. eng.
25. Oral EA, Simha V, Ruiz E, Andewelt A, Premkumar A, Snell P, et al. Leptin-replacement therapy for lipodystrophy. N Engl J Med. 2002;346(8):570–8. PubMed PMID: 11856796. Epub 2002/02/22. eng.
26. Petersen KF, Oral EA, Dufour S, Befroy D, Ariyan C, Yu C, et al. Leptin reverses insulin resistance and hepatic steatosis in patients with severe lipodystrophy. J Clin Invest. 2002;109(10):1345–50. PubMed PMID: 12021250. Pubmed Central PMCID: 150981. Epub 2002/05/22. eng.
27. Shimomura I, Hammer RE, Ikemoto S, Brown MS, Goldstein JL. Leptin reverses insulin resistance and diabetes mellitus in mice with congenital lipodystrophy. Nature. 1999;401(6748):73–6. PubMed PMID: 10485707. Epub 1999/09/15. eng.
28. Heymsfield SB, Greenberg AS, Fujioka K, Dixon RM, Kushner R, Hunt T, et al. Recombinant leptin for weight loss in obese and lean adults: a randomized, controlled, dose-escalation trial. JAMA. 1999;282(16):1568–75. PubMed PMID: 10546697. Epub 1999/11/05. eng.
29. Hukshorn CJ, Saris WH, Westerterp-Plantenga MS, Farid AR, Smith FJ, Campfield LA. Weekly subcutaneous pegylated recombinant native human leptin (PEG-OB) administration in obese men. J Clin Endocrinol Metab. 2000;85(11):4003–9. PubMed PMID: 11095423. Epub 2000/11/30. eng.
30. Westerterp-Plantenga MS, Saris WH, Hukshorn CJ, Campfield LA. Effects of weekly administration of pegylated recombinant human OB protein on appetite profile and energy metabolism in obese men. Am J Clin Nutr. 2001;74(4):426–34. PubMed PMID: 11566639. Epub 2001/09/22. eng.
31. Hukshorn CJ, van Dielen FM, Buurman WA, Westerterp-Plantenga MS, Campfield LA, Saris WH. The effect of pegylated recombinant human leptin (PEG-OB) on weight loss and inflammatory status in obese subjects. Int J Obes Relat Metab Disord. 2002;26(4):504–9. PubMed PMID: 12075577. Epub 2002/06/22. eng.
32. Myers Jr MG, Heymsfield SB, Haft C, Kahn BB, Laughlin M, Leibel RL, et al. Challenges and opportunities of defining clinical leptin resistance. Cell Metab. 2012;15(2):150–6. PubMed PMID: 22326217. Pubmed Central PMCID: 3281561. Epub 2012/02/14. eng.
33. Caro JF, Kolaczynski JW, Nyce MR, Ohannesian JP, Opentanova I, Goldman WH, et al. Decreased cerebrospinal-fluid/serum leptin ratio in obesity: a possible mechanism for leptin resistance. Lancet. 1996;348(9021):159–61. PubMed PMID: 8684156. Epub 1996/07/20. eng.
34. Banks WA, DiPalma CR, Farrell CL. Impaired transport of leptin across the blood-brain barrier in obesity. Peptides. 1999;20(11):1341–5. PubMed PMID: 10612449. Epub 1999/12/28. eng.
35. Munzberg H, Flier JS, Bjorbaek C. Region-specific leptin resistance within the hypothalamus of diet-induced obese mice. Endocrinology. 2004; 145(11):4880–9. PubMed PMID: 15271881. Epub 2004/07/24. eng.
36. Wilsey J, Zolotukhin S, Prima V, Scarpace PJ. Central leptin gene therapy fails to overcome leptin resistance associated with diet-induced obesity. Am J Physiol Regul Integr Comp Physiol. 2003;285(5):R1011–20. PubMed PMID: 14557234. Epub 2003/10/15. eng.
37. El-Haschimi K, Pierroz DD, Hileman SM, Bjorbaek C, Flier JS. Two defects contribute to hypothalamic leptin resistance in mice with diet-induced obesity. J Clin Invest. 2000;105(12):1827–32. PubMed PMID: 10862798. Pubmed Central PMCID: 378516. Epub 2000/06/23. eng.
38. Coppari R, Bjorbaek C. Leptin revisited: its mechanism of action and potential for treating diabetes. Nat Rev Drug Discov. 2012;11(9):692–708. PubMed PMID: 22935803. Epub 2012/09/01. eng.
39. Vasselli JR, Scarpace PJ, Harris RB, Banks WA. Dietary components in the development of leptin resistance. Adv Nutr. 2013;4(2):164–75. PubMed PMID: 23493533. Pubmed Central PMCID: 3649097. Epub 2013/03/16. eng.
40. Vasselli JR. The role of dietary components in leptin resistance. Adv Nutr. 2012;3(5):736–8. PubMed PMID: 22983859. Pubmed Central PMCID: 3648762. Epub 2012/09/18. eng.
41. Vasselli JR. Fructose-induced leptin resistance: discovery of an unsuspected form of the phenomenon and its significance. Focus on "Fructose-induced leptin resistance exacerbates weight gain in response to subsequent high-fat feeding," by Shapiro et al. Am J Physiol Regul Integr Comp Physiol. 2008;295(5):R1365–9. PubMed PMID: 18784330. Epub 2008/09/12. eng.
42. Wang J, Obici S, Morgan K, Barzilai N, Feng Z, Rossetti L. Overfeeding rapidly induces leptin and insulin resistance. Diabetes. 2001;50(12): 2786–91. PubMed PMID: 11723062. Epub 2001/11/28. eng.
43. Thaler JP, Yi CX, Schur EA, Guyenet SJ, Hwang BH, Dietrich MO, et al. Obesity is associated with hypothalamic injury in rodents and humans. J Clin Invest. 2012;122(1):153–62. PubMed PMID: 22201683. Pubmed Central PMCID: 3248304. Epub 2011/12/29. eng.
44. Kim YW, Kim JY, Park YH, Park SY, Won KC, Choi KH, et al. Metformin restores leptin sensitivity in high-fat-fed obese rats with leptin resistance. Diabetes. 2006;55(3):716–24. PubMed PMID: 16505235. Epub 2006/03/01. eng.
45. Hundal HS, Ramlal T, Reyes R, Leiter LA, Klip A. Cellular mechanism of metformin action involves glucose transporter translocation from an intracellu-

lar pool to the plasma membrane in L6 muscle cells. Endocrinology. 1992;131(3):1165–73. PubMed PMID: 1505458. Epub 1992/09/01. eng.

46. Wiernsperger NF, Bailey CJ. The antihyperglycaemic effect of metformin: therapeutic and cellular mechanisms. Drugs. 1999;58 Suppl 1:31–9. PubMed PMID: 10576523. Discussion 75–82. Epub 1999/11/27. eng.
47. Glueck CJ, Fontaine RN, Wang P, Subbiah MT, Weber K, Illig E, et al. Metformin reduces weight, centripetal obesity, insulin, leptin, and low-density lipoprotein cholesterol in nondiabetic, morbidly obese subjects with body mass index greater than 30. Metab Clin Exp. 2001;50(7):856–61. PubMed PMID: 11436194. Epub 2001/07/04. eng.
48. Kay JP, Alemzadeh R, Langley G, D'Angelo L, Smith P, Holshouser S. Beneficial effects of metformin in normoglycemic morbidly obese adolescents. Metab Clin Exp. 2001;50(12):1457–61. PubMed PMID: 11735093. Epub 2001/12/06. eng.
49. Paolisso G, Amato L, Eccellente R, Gambardella A, Tagliamonte MR, Varricchio G, et al. Effect of metformin on food intake in obese subjects. Eur J Clin Invest. 1998;28(6):441–6. PubMed PMID: 9693934. Epub 1998/08/07. eng.
50. Kendall D, Vail A, Amin R, Barrett T, Dimitri P, Ivison F, et al. Metformin in obese children and adolescents: the MOCA trial. J Clin Endocrinol Metab. 2013;98(1):322–9. PubMed PMID: 23175691. Epub 2012/11/24. eng.
51. Mauras N, DelGiorno C, Hossain J, Bird K, Killen K, Merinbaum D, et al. Metformin use in children with obesity and normal glucose tolerance–effects on cardiovascular markers and intrahepatic fat. J Pediatr Endocrinol Metab JPEM. 2012;25(1–2):33–40. PubMed PMID: 22570948. Epub 2012/05/11. eng.
52. He H, Zhao Z, Chen J, Ni Y, Zhong J, Yan Z, et al. Metformin-based treatment for obesity-related hypertension: a randomized, double-blind, placebo-controlled trial. J Hypertens. 2012;30(7):1430–9. PubMed PMID: 22525206. Epub 2012/04/25. eng.
53. Ghandi S, Aflatoonian A, Tabibnejad N, Moghaddam MH. The effects of metformin or orlistat on obese women with polycystic ovary syndrome: a prospective randomized open-label study. J Assist Reprod Genet. 2011;28(7):591–6. PubMed PMID: 21484319. Pubmed Central PMCID: 3162050. Epub 2011/04/13. eng.
54. Fruehwald-Schultes B, Oltmanns KM, Toschek B, Sopke S, Kern W, Born J, et al. Short-term treatment with metformin decreases serum leptin concentration without affecting body weight and body fat content in normal-weight healthy men. Metab Clin Exp. 2002;51(4):531–6. PubMed PMID: 11912566. Epub 2002/03/26. eng.
55. Aubert G, Mansuy V, Voirol MJ, Pellerin L, Pralong FP. The anorexigenic effects of metformin involve increases in hypothalamic leptin receptor expression. Metab Clin Exp. 2011;60(3):327–34. PubMed PMID: 20303124. Epub 2010/03/23. eng.
56. Lv WS, Wen JP, Li L, Sun RX, Wang J, Xian YX, et al. The effect of metformin on food intake and its potential role in hypothalamic regulation in obese diabetic rats. Brain Res. 2012;1444:11–9. PubMed PMID: 22325091. Epub 2012/02/14. eng.
57. Ludvik B, Kautzky-Willer A, Prager R, Thomaseth K, Pacini G. Amylin: history and overview. Diabet Med. 1997;14 Suppl 2:S9–13. PubMed PMID: 9212323. Epub 1997/06/01. eng.
58. Thomaseth K, Pacini G, Clodi M, Kautzky-Willer A, Nolan JJ, Prager R, et al. Amylin release during oral glucose tolerance test. Diabet Med. 1997;14 Suppl 2:S29–34. PubMed PMID: 9212327. Epub 1997/06/01. eng.
59. Tam CS, Lecoultre V, Ravussin E. Novel strategy for the use of leptin for obesity therapy. Expert Opin Biol Ther. 2011;11(12):1677–85. PubMed PMID: 21910668. Epub 2011/09/14. eng.
60. Reda TK, Geliebter A, Pi-Sunyer FX. Amylin, food intake, and obesity. Obes Res. 2002;10(10):1087–91. PubMed PMID: 12376591. Epub 2002/10/12. eng.
61. Reinehr T, de Sousa G, Niklowitz P, Roth CL. Amylin and its relation to insulin and lipids in obese children before and after weight loss. Obesity (Silver Spring). 2007;15(8):2006–11. PubMed PMID: 17712118. Epub 2007/08/23. eng.
62. Sumithran P, Prendergast LA, Delbridge E, Purcell K, Shulkes A, Kriketos A, et al. Long-term persistence of hormonal adaptations to weight loss. N Engl J Med. 2011;365(17):1597–604. PubMed PMID: 22029981. Epub 2011/10/28. eng.
63. Lutz TA. The role of amylin in the control of energy homeostasis. Am J Physiol Regul Integr Comp Physiol. 2010;298(6):R1475–84. PubMed PMID: 20357016. Epub 2010/04/02. eng.
64. Chance WT, Balasubramaniam A, Zhang FS, Wimalawansa SJ, Fischer JE. Anorexia following the intrahypothalamic administration of amylin. Brain Res. 1991;539(2):352–4. PubMed PMID: 1675913. Epub 1991/01/25. eng.
65. Lutz TA, Del Prete E, Scharrer E. Reduction of food intake in rats by intraperitoneal injection of low doses of amylin. Physiol Behav. 1994;55(5):891–5. PubMed PMID: 8022910. Epub 1994/05/01. eng.
66. Becskei C, Grabler V, Edwards GL, Riediger T, Lutz TA. Lesion of the lateral parabrachial nucleus attenuates the anorectic effect of peripheral amylin and CCK. Brain Res. 2007;1162:76–84. PubMed PMID: 17617389. Epub 2007/07/10. eng.
67. Lutz TA, Senn M, Althaus J, Del Prete E, Ehrensperger F, Scharrer E. Lesion of the area postrema/nucleus of the solitary tract (AP/NTS) attenuates the anorectic effects of amylin and calcitonin gene-related peptide (CGRP) in rats. Peptides. 1998;19(2):309–17. PubMed PMID: 9493863. Epub 1998/03/11. eng.
68. Riediger T, Schmid HA, Lutz T, Simon E. Amylin potently activates AP neurons possibly via formation of the excitatory second messenger cGMP. Am J

Physiol Regul Integr Comp Physiol. 2001;281(6): R1833–43. PubMed PMID: 11705768. Epub 2001/11/14. eng.

69. Riediger T, Zuend D, Becskei C, Lutz TA. The anorectic hormone amylin contributes to feeding-related changes of neuronal activity in key structures of the gut-brain axis. Am J Physiol Regul Integr Comp Physiol. 2004;286(1):R114–22. PubMed PMID: 12958059. Epub 2003/09/06. eng.
70. Roth JD, Roland BL, Cole RL, Trevaskis JL, Weyer C, Koda JE, et al. Leptin responsiveness restored by amylin agonism in diet-induced obesity: evidence from nonclinical and clinical studies. Proc Natl Acad Sci U S A. 2008;105(20):7257–62. PubMed PMID: 18458326. Pubmed Central PMCID: 2438237. Epub 2008/05/07. eng.
71. Trevaskis JL, Coffey T, Cole R, Lei C, Wittmer C, Walsh B, et al. Amylin-mediated restoration of leptin responsiveness in diet-induced obesity: magnitude and mechanisms. Endocrinology. 2008;149(11): 5679–87. PubMed PMID: 18669592. Epub 2008/08/02. eng.
72. Roth JD, Trevaskis JL, Turek VF, Parkes DG. "Weighing in" on synergy: preclinical research on neurohormonal anti-obesity combinations. Brain Res. 2010;1350:86–94. PubMed PMID: 20096672. Epub 2010/01/26. eng.
73. Ravussin E, Smith SR, Mitchell JA, Shringarpure R, Shan K, Maier H, et al. Enhanced weight loss with pramlintide/metreleptin: an integrated neurohormonal approach to obesity pharmacotherapy. Obesity (Silver Spring). 2009;17(9):1736–43. PubMed PMID: 19521351. Pubmed Central PMCID: 2754219. Epub 2009/06/13. eng.
74. Seth R, Knight WD, Overton JM. Combined amylin-leptin treatment lowers blood pressure and adiposity in lean and obese rats. Int J Obes (Lond). 2011;35(9):1183–92. PubMed PMID: 21179001. Epub 2010/12/24. eng.
75. Turek VF, Trevaskis JL, Levin BE, Dunn-Meynell AA, Irani B, Gu G, et al. Mechanisms of amylin/leptin synergy in rodent models. Endocrinology. 2010;151(1):143–52. PubMed PMID: 19875640. Epub 2009/10/31. eng.
76. Muller TD, Sullivan LM, Habegger K, Yi CX, Kabra D, Grant E, et al. Restoration of leptin responsiveness in diet-induced obese mice using an optimized leptin analog in combination with exendin-4 or FGF21. J Pept Sci. 2012;18(6):383–93. PubMed PMID: 22565812. Epub 2012/05/09. eng.
77. Kreymann B, Williams G, Ghatei MA, Bloom SR. Glucagon-like peptide-1 7-36: a physiological incretin in man. Lancet. 1987;2(8571):1300–4. PubMed PMID: 2890903. Epub 1987/12/05. eng.
78. Mojsov S, Weir GC, Habener JF. Insulinotropin: glucagon-like peptide I (7-37) co-encoded in the glucagon gene is a potent stimulator of insulin release in the perfused rat pancreas. J Clin Invest. 1987; 79(2):616–9. PubMed PMID: 3543057. Pubmed Central PMCID: 424143. Epub 1987/02/01. eng.
79. Drucker DJ, Philippe J, Mojsov S, Chick WL, Habener JF. Glucagon-like peptide I stimulates insulin gene expression and increases cyclic AMP levels in a rat islet cell line. Proc Natl Acad Sci U S A. 1987;84(10):3434–8. PubMed PMID: 3033647. Pubmed Central PMCID: 304885. Epub 1987/05/01. eng.
80. Schirra J, Nicolaus M, Roggel R, Katschinski M, Storr M, Woerle HJ, et al. Endogenous glucagon-like peptide 1 controls endocrine pancreatic secretion and antro-pyloro-duodenal motility in humans. Gut. 2006;55(2):243–51. PubMed PMID: 15985560. Pubmed Central PMCID: 1856508. Epub 2005/06/30. eng.
81. Stoffers DA, Kieffer TJ, Hussain MA, Drucker DJ, Bonner-Weir S, Habener JF, et al. Insulinotropic glucagon-like peptide 1 agonists stimulate expression of homeodomain protein IDX-1 and increase islet size in mouse pancreas. Diabetes. 2000;49(5):741–8. PubMed PMID: 10905482. Epub 2000/07/25. eng.
82. Rolin B, Larsen MO, Gotfredsen CF, Deacon CF, Carr RD, Wilken M, et al. The long-acting GLP-1 derivative NN2211 ameliorates glycemia and increases beta-cell mass in diabetic mice. Am J Physiol Endocrinol Metab. 2002;283(4):E745–52. PubMed PMID: 12217892. Epub 2002/09/10. eng.
83. Kim JG, Baggio LL, Bridon DP, Castaigne JP, Robitaille MF, Jette L, et al. Development and characterization of a glucagon-like peptide 1-albumin conjugate: the ability to activate the glucagon-like peptide 1 receptor in vivo. Diabetes. 2003;52(3):751–9. PubMed PMID: 12606517. Epub 2003/02/28. eng.
84. Hui H, Nourparvar A, Zhao X, Perfetti R. Glucagon-like peptide-1 inhibits apoptosis of insulin-secreting cells via a cyclic 5′-adenosine monophosphate-dependent protein kinase A- and a phosphatidylinositol 3-kinase-dependent pathway. Endocrinology. 2003;144(4):1444–55. PubMed PMID: 12639928. Epub 2003/03/18. eng.
85. Edvell A, Lindstrom P. Initiation of increased pancreatic islet growth in young normoglycemic mice (Umea +/?). Endocrinology. 1999;140(2):778–83. PubMed PMID: 9927305. Epub 1999/02/02. eng.
86. Wang X, Cahill CM, Pineyro MA, Zhou J, Doyle ME, Egan JM. Glucagon-like peptide-1 regulates the beta cell transcription factor, PDX-1, in insulinoma cells. Endocrinology. 1999;140(10):4904–7. PubMed PMID: 10499550. Epub 1999/09/28. eng.
87. Farilla L, Hui H, Bertolotto C, Kang E, Bulotta A, Di Mario U, et al. Glucagon-like peptide-1 promotes islet cell growth and inhibits apoptosis in Zucker diabetic rats. Endocrinology. 2002;143(11):4397–408. PubMed PMID: 12399437. Epub 2002/10/26. eng.
88. Idris I, Patiag D, Gray S, Donnelly R. Exendin-4 increases insulin sensitivity via a PI-3-kinase-dependent mechanism: contrasting effects of GLP-1. Biochem Pharmacol. 2002;63(5):993–6. PubMed PMID: 11911852. Epub 2002/03/26. eng.
89. Scalzetti EM, Heitzman ER, Groskin SA, Randall PA, Katzenstein AL. Developmental lymphatic

disorders of the thorax. Radiographics. 1991;11(6): 1069–85. PubMed PMID: 1749850. Epub 1991/11/01. eng.

90. Gonzalez N, Acitores A, Sancho V, Valverde I, Villanueva-Penacarrillo ML. Effect of GLP-1 on glucose transport and its cell signalling in human myocytes. Regul Pept. 2005;126(3):203–11. PubMed PMID: 15664668. Epub 2005/01/25. eng.
91. Prigeon RL, Quddusi S, Paty B, D'Alessio DA. Suppression of glucose production by GLP-1 independent of islet hormones: a novel extrapancreatic effect. Am J Physiol Endocrinol Metab. 2003; 285(4):E701–7. PubMed PMID: 12773303. Epub 2003/05/30. eng.
92. Valverde I, Morales M, Clemente F, Lopez-Delgado MI, Delgado E, Perea A, et al. Glucagon-like peptide 1: a potent glycogenic hormone. FEBS Lett. 1994;349(2):313–6. PubMed PMID: 8050588. Epub 1994/08/01. eng.
93. Alcantara AI, Morales M, Delgado E, Lopez-Delgado MI, Clemente F, Luque MA, et al. Exendin-4 agonist and exendin(9-39)amide antagonist of the GLP-1(7-36)amide effects in liver and muscle. Arch Biochem Biophys. 1997;341(1):1–7. PubMed PMID: 9143346. Epub 1997/05/01. eng.
94. Redondo A, Trigo MV, Acitores A, Valverde I, Villanueva-Penacarrillo ML. Cell signalling of the GLP-1 action in rat liver. Mol Cell Endocrinol. 2003;204(1–2):43–50. PubMed PMID: 12850280. Epub 2003/07/10. eng.
95. Lee YS, Shin S, Shigihara T, Hahm E, Liu MJ, Han J, et al. Glucagon-like peptide-1 gene therapy in obese diabetic mice results in long-term cure of diabetes by improving insulin sensitivity and reducing hepatic gluconeogenesis. Diabetes. 2007;56(6):1671–9. PubMed PMID: 17369525. Epub 2007/03/21. eng.
96. Willms B, Werner J, Holst JJ, Orskov C, Creutzfeldt W, Nauck MA. Gastric emptying, glucose responses, and insulin secretion after a liquid test meal: effects of exogenous glucagon-like peptide-1 (GLP-1)-(7-36) amide in type 2 (noninsulin-dependent) diabetic patients. J Clin Endocrinol Metab. 1996;81(1): 327–32. PubMed PMID: 8550773. Epub 1996/01/01. eng.
97. Drucker DJ. The biology of incretin hormones. Cell Metab. 2006;3(3):153–65. PubMed PMID: 16517403. Epub 2006/03/07. eng.
98. Day JW, Ottaway N, Patterson JT, Gelfanov V, Smiley D, Gidda J, et al. A new glucagon and GLP-1 co-agonist eliminates obesity in rodents. Nat Chem Biol. 2009;5(10):749–57. PubMed PMID: 19597507. Epub 2009/07/15. eng.
99. Day JW, Gelfanov V, Smiley D, Carrington PE, Eiermann G, Chicchi G, et al. Optimization of co-agonism at GLP-1 and glucagon receptors to safely maximize weight reduction in DIO-rodents. Biopolymers. 2012;98(5):443–50. PubMed PMID: 23203689. Epub 2012/12/04. eng.
100. Clemmensen C, Chabenne J, Finan B, Sullivan L, Fischer K, Kuchler D, et al. GLP-1/glucagon coagonism restores leptin responsiveness in obese mice chronically maintained on an obesogenic diet. Diabetes. 2014;63(4):1422–7. PubMed PMID: 24379349. Epub 2014/01/01. eng.
101. Finan B, Ma T, Ottaway N, Muller TD, Habegger KM, Heppner KM, et al. Unimolecular dual incretins maximize metabolic benefits in rodents, monkeys, and humans. Science translational medicine. 2013;5(209):209ra151. PubMed PMID: 24174327. Epub 2013/11/01. eng.
102. Hong SH, Ahmadian M, Yu RT, Atkins AR, Downes M, Evans RM. Nuclear receptors and metabolism: from feast to famine. Diabetologia. 2014;12. PubMed PMID: 24619218. Epub 2014/03/13. Eng.
103. Kadmiel M, Cidlowski JA. Glucocorticoid receptor signaling in health and disease. Trends Pharmacol Sci. 2013;34(9):518–30. PubMed PMID: 23953592. Pubmed Central PMCID: 3951203. Epub 2013/08/21. eng.
104. Musatov S, Chen W, Pfaff DW, Mobbs CV, Yang XJ, Clegg DJ, et al. Silencing of estrogen receptor alpha in the ventromedial nucleus of hypothalamus leads to metabolic syndrome. Proc Natl Acad Sci U S A. 2007;104(7):2501–6. PubMed PMID: 17284595. Pubmed Central PMCID: 1892990. Epub 2007/02/08. eng.
105. Gao Q, Mezei G, Nie Y, Rao Y, Choi CS, Bechmann I, et al. Anorectic estrogen mimics leptin's effect on the rewiring of melanocortin cells and Stat3 signaling in obese animals. Nat Med. 2007;13(1):89–94. PubMed PMID: 17195839. Epub 2007/01/02. eng.
106. Gao Q, Horvath TL. Cross-talk between estrogen and leptin signaling in the hypothalamus. Am J Physiol Endocrinol Metab. 2008;294(5):E817–26. PubMed PMID: 18334610. Epub 2008/03/13. eng.
107. Xu Y, Nedungadi TP, Zhu L, Sobhani N, Irani BG, Davis KE, et al. Distinct hypothalamic neurons mediate estrogenic effects on energy homeostasis and reproduction. Cell Metab. 2011;14(4):453–65. PubMed PMID: 21982706. Pubmed Central PMCID: 3235745. Epub 2011/10/11. eng.
108. Riant E, Waget A, Cogo H, Arnal JF, Burcelin R, Gourdy P. Estrogens protect against high-fat diet-induced insulin resistance and glucose intolerance in mice. Endocrinology. 2009;150(5):2109–17. PubMed PMID: 19164473. Epub 2009/01/24. eng.
109. Mauvais-Jarvis F. Estrogen and androgen receptors: regulators of fuel homeostasis and emerging targets for diabetes and obesity. Trends Endocrinol Metab TEM. 2011;22(1):24–33. PubMed PMID: 21109497. Pubmed Central PMCID: 3011051. Epub 2010/11/27. eng.
110. Nilsson S, Koehler KF, Gustafsson JA. Development of subtype-selective oestrogen receptor-based therapeutics. Nat Rev Drug Discov. 2011;10(10):778–92. PubMed PMID: 21921919. Epub 2011/09/17. eng.
111. Finan B, Yang B, Ottaway N, Stemmer K, Muller TD, Yi CX, et al. Targeted estrogen delivery reverses the metabolic syndrome. Nat Med. 2012;18(12):1847–56. PubMed PMID: 23142820. Pubmed Central PMCID: 3757949. Epub 2012/11/13. eng.

Index

S. Dagogo-Jack (ed.), *Leptin: Regulation and Clinical Applications*,
DOI 10.1007/978-3-319-09915-6, © Springer International Publishing Switzerland 2015

N

O

P

R

MIX
Papier aus verantwortungsvollen Quellen
Paper from responsible sources
FSC® C105338

If you have any concerns about our products,
you can contact us on
ProductSafety@springernature.com

In case Publisher is established outside the EU,
the EU authorized representative is:
Springer Nature Customer Service Center GmbH
Europaplatz 3, 69115 Heidelberg, Germany

Printed by Libri Plureos GmbH
in Hamburg, Germany